AF248704

Proceedings of the International Symposium on

Diversity in Auditory Mechanics

University of California, Berkeley   *24 – 28 June 1996*

editors

E R Lewis *(University of California, Berkeley)*

G R Long *(Purdue University)*

R F Lyon *(Apple Computer Inc.)*

P M Narins *(University of California, Los Angeles)*

C R Steele *(Stanford University)*

E Hecht-Poinar *(University of California, Berkeley)*

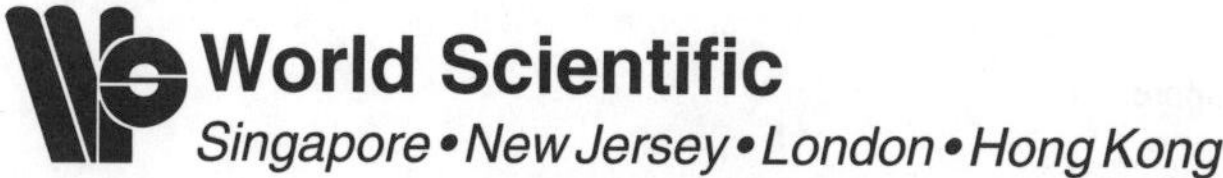

World Scientific
Singapore • New Jersey • London • Hong Kong

Published by

World Scientific Publishing Co. Pte. Ltd.

P O Box 128, Farrer Road, Singapore 912805

USA office: Suite 1B, 1060 Main Street, River Edge, NJ 07661

UK office: 57 Shelton Street, Covent Garden, London WC2H 9HE

British Library Cataloguing-in-Publication Data
A catalogue record for this book is available from the British Library.

DIVERSITY IN AUDITORY MECHANICS

Copyright © 1997 by World Scientific Publishing Co. Pte. Ltd.

All rights reserved. This book, or parts thereof, may not be reproduced in any form or by any means, electronic or mechanical, including photocopying, recording or any information storage and retrieval system now known or to be invented, without written permission from the Publisher.

For photocopying of material in this volume, please pay a copying fee through the Copyright Clearance Center, Inc., 222 Rosewood Drive, Danvers, MA 01923, USA. In this case permission to photocopy is not required from the publisher.

ISBN 981-02-2712-4

Printed in Singapore.

Diversity in
Auditory Mechanics

The sixth international symposium on the mechanics of hearing and this volume, which was based on that symposium, were sponsored by the National Institute on Deafness and other Communicative Disorders (National Institutes of Health), under grant 1 R13 DC03060. The meeting was held at the Bechtel Engineering Center on the campus of the University of California, Berkeley, California. Local support for the meeting was provided by the Meakin Interdisciplinary Studies Center of the University of California College of Engineering and by Tucker-Davis Technologies.

Organizing committee:
E.R. Lewis, G.R. Long, R.F. Lyon, P.M. Narins and C.R. Steele

Previous publications from this series of symposia:

Mechanics of Hearing. Edited by E. de Boer and M.A. Viergever. Nijhoff, The Hague/Delft University Press, 1983.

Peripheral Auditory Mechanisms. Edited by J.B. Allen, J.L. Hall, A. Hubbard, S.T. Neely and A. Tubis. Springer, Berlin, 1986

Cochlear Mechanisms: Structure, Function and Models. Edited by J.P. Wilson and D.T. Kemp. Plenum, New York, 1989.

The Mechanics and Biophysics of Hearing. Edited by P. Dallos, C.D. Geisler, J.W. Matthews, M.A. Ruggero and C.R. Steele. Springer, Berlin, 1990.

Biophysics of Hair Cell Sensory Systems. Edited by H. Duifhuis, J.W. Horst, P. van Dijk and S.M. van Netten. World Scientific, Singapore, 1993.

Preface: toward rational reductionism

This conference, and each of those that preceded it in this series, was devoted to quantitative modeling of the auditory periphery. Since the time of Newton, at least, quantitative modeling has played a crucial role in the advancement of science; but that role itself is not often analyzed or discussed explicitly. To facilitate such analysis and discussion, it is useful to construct a *model* of this quantitative modeling process as it was used by Newton and is used widely today in biophysics and other natural sciences. One can consider the physical laws (e.g., the Galileo-Newton laws of motion, Fourier's law, Stokes's law, Ohm's law, Fick's laws, Coulomb's law) upon which we base much of our fundamental biophysical modeling to be descriptions (*descriptive models*) of natural phenomena, derived from repeated observation and induction. A quantitative modeler, in the tradition of Newton, would combine such descriptive models with a set of structural constraints (a *structural model*) to form a *synthetic model*. Thus one might combine the microscopic version of Ohm's law (a descriptive model) with the putative dimensions (a structural model) of a resistive electric current path to form a (synthetic) model of a resistor. One also could measure voltage-current characteristics of the resistor directly, and translate them directly into a descriptive model of the device. I believe that one can describe the modeling enterprise that has been applied so profitably since the time of Newton as interplay between descriptive models and synthetic models of these kinds. The first evidence for the inverse-square law of gravitational force is an instructive example. Kepler's laws form a descriptive model of planetary orbits. Newton combined a structural model (comprising two point mass elements along with their initial positions and motions) with descriptive models (the laws of motion) and a conjectural model (concerning the force of gravity) to form a synthetic model (*Newton's synthesis*) of an orbiting object. He tested the synthetic model by comparing the orbital properties that emerged from it with Kepler's descriptive model, and he sculpted the conjectural model to make the synthetic model fit Kepler's model (only the inverse square law would work).

Another example is provided by the Hodgkin-Huxley model of spike generation. An extremely good descriptive model of spike generation had been published independently by Rashevsky, Monnier and Hill.[1] Hodgkin and Huxley hypothesized that the elements underlying spike production were charge flows carried by sodium ions and potassium ions, interacting through accumulation of charge dipoles across a dielectric medium (cell membrane). Through observation and induction, they constructed descriptive models of the ion currents and the dipole accumulation process. Then they combined these descriptive models with a structural model (a circuit graph, placing the ion-flow paths in parallel with each other and with a capacitive branch representing the locale of dipole accumulation) to form a synthetic model of a patch of axonal membrane. In testing this synthetic model, among other things, Hodgkin and

Huxley compared its emergent behavior with that of the descriptive model of Rashevsky, Monnier and Hill. The emergent properties of the Hodgkin-Huxley model are sufficiently close to those of the real axon to convince us of the validity of their hypothesis; but with respect to the behavior (accommodation of threshold) that the Rashevsky-Monnier-Hill model was intended to describe, that model remains a more faithful descriptor of real spike generation. Therein, I believe, lies an important message for reductionists, especially in this emerging era of accessible, powerful computers that make synthetic modeling so easy. A synthetic model of a system may be an excellent tool for hypothesis testing and advancing science, but its approximations and imperfections will make its representation of the *system or subsystem as a whole* less faithful than that of the best achievable descriptive model of that system or subsystem.

In the mid-1960's, as biological modeling was growing very rapidly, Louis Fein challenged modelers to show an example of a modeling endeavor that actually provided some understanding of a biological system.[2] He used engineering as a model to define *understanding*. Understanding, to an engineer, is reflected in ability to *design, construct, use, maintain and repair* a system. Although biophysicists might seek other definitions, it is instructive to reflect on how engineers achieve their kind of understanding. Extensive history with synthetic modeling in engineering reveals that synthetic models always are approximate and imperfect (sometimes crudely so)-- even when they are based on elements that are manufactured with considerable precision. For that reason, and for one other, engineers use hierarchical modeling. They use a synthetic model to understand (design, construct, repair, redesign) an object at a given hierarchical level; but they use a descriptive model of that object when combining it with other objects at the same level to synthesize an object at the next higher hierarchical level. Thus an engineer may consider basic physics (quantum statistics, charge diffusion processes, and the like) when trying to understand the operation of a transistor; but he or she will use a descriptive model of the transistor, with its parameters (junction capacitances, common-emitter current gain, etc.) determined by observation, when trying to understand the role of that transistor in the operation of a switching circuit; and he or she will use a descriptive model of the switching circuit, again with its parameters (threshold, switching times, etc.) determined by observation, when trying to understand the role of that switching circuit in the operation of a logical element (such as a register) in the central processing unit (CPU) of a computer; and he or she will use a descriptive model of the register (in terms of bit capacity and the like) when trying to understand its role in the operation of the CPU. Experience, so far, tells us that attempting to understand the operation of the CPU directly in terms of the language of basic physics (quantum statistics, etc.) will not be instructive-- at the CPU level of the hierarchy, insightful modeling is carried out with a different language, one that concisely expresses concepts appropriate to that level. That is the second reason for the hierarchical approach. The first reason is the inherent lack of fidelity in synthetic models. For the first reason alone, the use of synthetic models (in place of descriptive models with observed parameter values) as elements of a synthetic model at a higher hierarchical level (especially at a level more than one step higher) is not good practice. It should be done as a last resort, when the properties of the element at the higher level cannot be observed directly or described more simply.

Those of us who are students of the nervous system attempt to identify its components and to observe the properties of those components and develop descriptive models of them, hoping that those models will be useful in helping us understand the system as a whole. Because we do not manufacture and assemble the components ourselves, our synthetic models are likely to be especially crude. Furthermore, without a faithful descriptive model of the operation of a neural system or subsystem as a whole, we will lack the ability to test, in the tradition of Newton, our synthetic models of that system or subsystem. This makes the use of the hierarchical approach to quantitative modeling especially imperative. In that context, a good descriptive model of a putatively-identified component at one hierarchical level is inherently neither less nor more valuable, scientifically, than a good descriptive model of a putatively-identified component at the next lower level, or the level below that. This, I believe, is compelling justification for a multilevel integrative approach to neurobiology.

A challenge for the neurobiologist, of course, is to invent the concepts and language appropriate at each level. This is closely related to an argument, often cited, in favor of integrative approaches—namely the value of top-down perspective. Is it possible to achieve strong inferences about what it is that a particular biological system or subsystem does (i.e., what is its function or what selective advantage does it provide the individual organism or the species, and what concepts and language are appropriate for describing that function) by looking only at the elements of the system? I believe not. I believe that such strong inferences can be derived only from thorough top-down (integrative) perspective-- thorough knowledge of the evolutionary, ecological, and behavioral contexts of the species and the developmental and physiological contexts of the system. If one does not possess strong inferences about what it is that a system does, how can he or she ever expect to explain how the system does it?

Edwin R. Lewis
Berkeley, California
November 8, 1996

[1] MacGregor, R.J. and Lewis, E.R. (1977). *Neural Modeling* (Plenum Press, New York) pp. 159-169.
[2] Fein, L. (1966). Biological investigations by information-processing simulations. In: *Natural Automata and Useful Simulations,* eds. H.H. Pattee, E.A. Edelsack, L. Fein and A.B. Callahan (Spartan Books, Washington) pp. 181-202.

Introduction

This conference was held in the Bechtel Engineering Center at the University of California at Berkeley, between June 24 and June 28, 1996. It was the sixth in a series that started in 1983 at Delft. The next will be held in 1999 in Sendai, Japan. Previous meetings:

1983, Delft, The Netherlands (organized by E. de Boer and M.A. Viergever)
1985, Boston, Massachusetts, USA (organized by J. Allen, J.L. Hall, A.E. Hubbard, S.T. Neely and A.Tubis)
1988, Keele, UK (organized by J.P. Wilson and D.T. Kemp)
1990, Madison, Wisconsin, USA (organized by P. Dallos, C.D. Geisler, J.W. Matthews, M.A. Ruggero, and C.R. Steele)
1993, Paterswolde, The Netherlands(organized by H.Duifhuis, J.W. Horst, P. van Dijk and S.M. van Netten)

This volume and the conference on which it is based was supported by grant 1 R13 DC03060 from the National Institutes of Health, National Institute on Deafness and other Communicative Disorders. We thank Tucker-Davis Technologies for sponsoring the conference reception and the Meakin Interdisciplinary Studies Center for providing facilities as well as administrative and logistic support for the conference. We are especially grateful to Eva Hecht Poinar and Angela Corral for their tireless assistance in the organization and running of the conference, to Ms. Poinar for extensive assistance in editing this volume.

We believe that the papers presented at the conference and in this volume reflect the hearing research community at its best, with a very healthy balance of excellent biology at many levels, including evolutionary, ecological, behavioral, developmental, physiological and molecular. The organizers of this conference are happy to be members of a community that openly values such an integrative approach to neurobiology. We thank the National Institute on Deafness and other Communicative Disorders for its recognition of the value of the integrative approach and its generous support of this conference.

E.R. Lewis
G.R. Long
R.F. Lyon
P.M. Narins
C.R. Steele

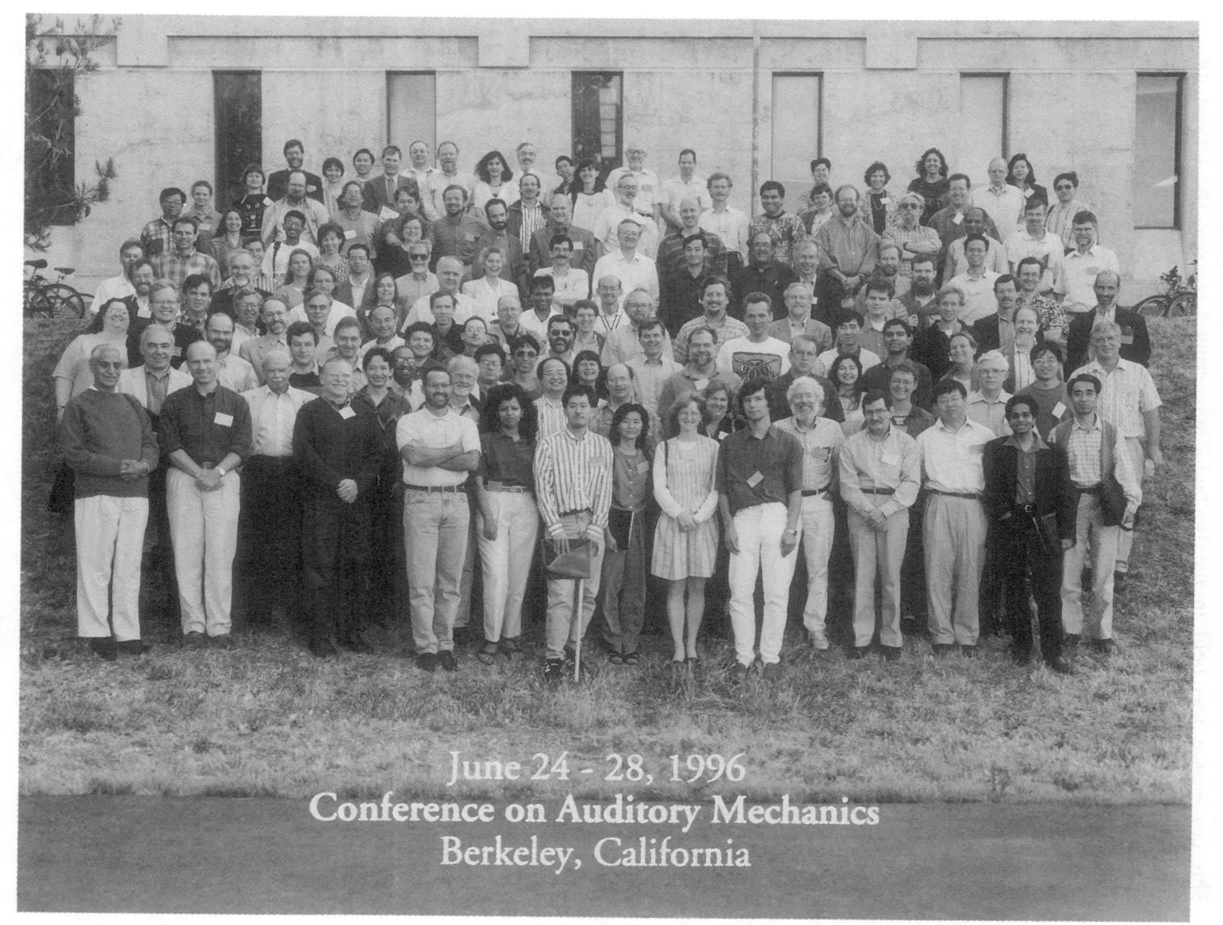

June 24 - 28, 1996
Conference on Auditory Mechanics
Berkeley, California

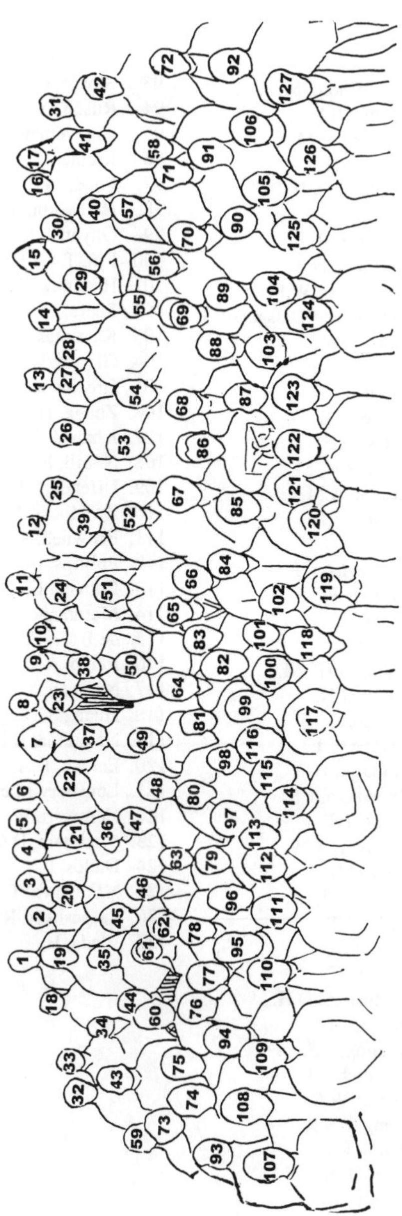

xii

PHOTOLEGEND

1. Walsh, E.J.
2. Köppl, C.
3. Lai, T.
4. Lewis, E.R.
5. Spector, A.A.
6. Simmons, J.A.
7. Simmons, A
8. Manley, G.A.
9. Yamada, W.M.
10. Voss, S.E.
11. Peake, W.T.
12. Cohen, A.
13. Escabi, M. A.
14. Hecht-Poinar, E.I.
15. Cortopassi, K.A.
16. Tubis, A.
17. Chan, E.
18. Prijs, V.F.
19. Rosowski, J.J.
20. Chadwick, R.S.
21. Iwasa, K.H.
22. Dimitriades, E.K.
23. Ravicz, M.E.
24. Geisler, C.D.
25. Lukashkin, A.N.
26. Murugasu, E.
27. ?
28. Slaney, M.
29. Ruggero, M.A.
30. Talmadge, C.L.
31. Ren, T.
32. Li, Cheuk
33. Novoselova, S.M.
34. McGee, J.
35. Dhar, S.
36. Long, G.
37. Purgue, A.
38. Narins, P.M.
39. Kolston, P.J.
40. Kumaresan, R.
41. Dolan, D.F.
42. Nuttall, A.L.
43. Kachar, B.
44. Fay, J.
45. Shaffer, L.
46. Tolomeo, J.A.
47. Wiederhold, M.
48. Young, E.D.
49. Cheatham, M.A.
50. Neely, S.T.
51. Hubbard, A.E.
52. Xue, S.
53. Hafter, E.R.
54. Duifhuis, H.
55. Decraemer, W.F.
56. Christensen-Dalsgaard, J.
57. Teoh, S.W.
58. Cooper, N.P.
59. Sattel, T.
60. Steele, C.R.
61. Zetes, D.E.
62. Sanderson, M.
63. Brown, A.M.
64. Puria, S.
65. Avan, P.
66. Smurzynski, J.
67. Lyon, R.F.
68. Fay, R.R.
69. Meyer, J.
70. Kanneworff, M.
71. Miles, R.N.
72. Ashmore, J.F.
73. LePage, E.L.
74. van Dijk, P.
75. Uppenkamp, S.
76. Fahey, P.F.
77. Gummer, A.W.
78. Allen, J.B.
79. Russell, I.J.
80. Cody, A.R.
81. Dancer, A.
82. Kalinec, F.
83. Ehrenstein, D.H.
84. Holley, M.C
85. Dooling, R.J.
86. Faulstich, M.
87. Rhode, W.S.
88. Tsang, P.S.K.
89. Naidu, R.C.
90. Olson, E.S.
91. Guinan, J.J.
92. Mills, D.M.
93. Stover, L.
94. Rüsch, A.
95. van Netten, S.M.
96. Richter, C.-P.
97. Popel, A.S.
98. Hallworth, R.
99. Ohyama, K.
100. Lin, T.
101. Hackney, C.M.
102. Shera, C.
103. Karavitaki, K.D.
104. Glowatzki, E.
105. Greenwood, D.D.
106. Zhang, L.
107. Khanna, S.M.
108. Nobili, R.
109. Ulfendahl, M.
110. Zwislocki, J.J.
111. Brownell, W.E.
112. Phillips, B.
113. Ratnanather, J.T.
114. Mammano, F.
115. de Boer, E.
116. Recio, A.
117. Narayan, S.
118. Huang, G.T.
119. Nakajima, H.H.
120. Eatock, R.A.
121. Lonsbury-Martin, B.L.
122. Hemmert, W.
123. Mountain, D.C.
124. Dallos, P.
125. Nakagawa, T.
126. Sarpeshkar; R.
127. Wada, H.

PARTICIPANTS in the CONFERENCE on
DIVERSITY IN AUDITORY MECHANICS
{(numbers) refer to number on photo}

Allen, J.B. (78)
AT&T Research Laboratory, Murray Hill, NJ 07974   USA
jba@research.att.com

Avan, P. (65)
Biophysics and Neurosurgery Departments, University Medical School PO Box 38
Clermont-Ferrand, France
paul.avan@u-clermont1.fr

Ashmore, J.F. (72)
Dept. of Physiology, School of Medical Sciences, University of Bristol BS8 1TD, UK
j.ashmore@ucl.ac.uk

de Boer, E. (115)
Academic Medical Center, Meibergdreef 9, AZ, Amsterdam, Netherlands
e.deboer@amc.uva.nl

Brown, A.M. (63)
Laboratory of Experimental Psychology, University of Sussex, Brighton BN1 9QG   UK
annb@epunix.susx.ac.uk

Brownell; W.E. (111)
Dept of Otorhinolaryngology and Communicative Sciences
Baylor College of Medicine, One Baylor Plaza, Houston, TX 77030, USA
brownell@bcm.tmc.edu

Chadwick, R.S. (20)
Biomedical Engineering and Instrumentation Program, NCRR, National Institutes of Health, Bldg.
13/3N17, Bethesda, MD 20892
chadwick@helix.nih.gov

Chan, E. (17)
Dept of Physiology & Pharmacology, Div.Physiology II, Karolinska Institute,
Stockholm, Sweden
eliza.chan@fyfa.ki.se

Chatterjee, M.
Dept of Auditory Implants and Perception Research
House Ear Institute, 2100 W Third Strret, Los Angeles, CA 90057
mchatterje@hei.org

Cheatham, M.A. (49)
Auditory Physiology Laboratory (The Hugh Knowles Center),
Dept of Communication Sciences and Disorders,
Northwestern University, Evanston, IL 60208-3550 USA
m-cheatham@nwu.edu

Christensen-Dalsgaard, J. (56)
Center for Sound Communication, Institute of Biology, Odense University,
Campusvej 55. DK-5230 Odense M, Denmark
jcd@dou.dk

Cody, A.R. (80)
Dept. of Physiology and Pharmacology, The University of Queensland,
Queensland, 4072, Australia
a.cody@mailbox.uq.oz.au

Cohen, A. (12)
Dept of Electrical Engineering - Systems Faculty of Engineering, Tel Aviv University,
Tel Aviv 69978, Israel
azi@eng.tau.ac.il

xiii

Cooper, N.P. (58)
Dept of Neurophysiology, Medical Sciences Building, 1300 University Avenue
Madison, WI 53706   USA
cooper@mvg.neurophys.wisc.edu   USA

Cortopassi, K.A. (15)
Dept. of EECS, University of California, Berkeley,   Berkeley.CA 94720-1770
calamari@bandit.eecs.berkeley.edu

Dallos, P. (124)
Auditory Physiology Laboratory (The Hugh Knowles Center)
Depts of Neurobiology and Physiology and Communication Sciences and Disorders
Northwestern University, Evanston, IL 60208   USA
p-dallos@nwu.edu

Dancer, A. (81)
French-German Research Institute of Saint-Louis, Saint-Louis,   France
dancer@nucleus.fr

Decraemer, W.F. (55)
University of Antwerp, Ruca, 171 Groenenborgerlaan, Antwerpen, B-2020, Belgium
wimdec@ruca.ua.ac.be

Dhar, S. (35)
Dept of Audiology and Speech Sciences, Heavilon Hall, Purdue University,
West Lafayette, IN 47907
sumit@zwicker.aus.purdue.edu

van Dijk, P. (74)
ENT Department, Audiology, P.O.Box 30.001, RB Groningen, Netherlands
p.van.dijk@med.rug.nl

Dimitriades, E.K. (22)
Biomedical Engineering and Instrumentation Program, NCRR
National Institutes of Health, Bldg. 13/3N17, Bethesda, MD 20892
dimitria@helix.nih.gov

Dolan, D.F. (41)
Kresge Hearing Research Institute,, University of Michigan Medical School,
1301 East Ann Street, Ann Arbor, Michigan 48109, USA
ddolan@umich.edu

Dooling, R.J. (85)
Dept. of Psychology, University of Maryland, College Park, MD 20742   USA
dooling@bss3.umd.edu

Duifhuis, H. (54)
Dept. of Biophysics, Graduate School of Behavioral and Cognitive Neurosciences
University of Groningen, Nijenborgh 4, 9747 AG Groningen, Netherlands
duifhuis@bcn.rug.nl

Eatock; R.A. (120)
Dept. of Otorhinolaryngology and Communicative Sciences, Baylor College of Medicine,
One Baylor Plaza, Houston, TX 77030   USA
eatock@bcm.tmc.edu

Ehrenstein, D.H. (83)
Biophysics Section, NIDCD - NIH, Bethesda, MD 20892-0922   USA
david-e@nih.gov

Escabi, M.A. (13)
UCSF/UCB Joint Bioengineering Graduate Group, U. of California,San Francisco, CA 94143
escabim@garnet.berkeley.edu

Fahey, P (76)
Dept . of Physics, University of Scranton, Scranton, PA 18510-4672   USA
faheyp1@jaguar.uofs.edu

Faulstich, M. (86)
Zoologisches Institut, Universität München, Luisenstrasse 14, 80333 , München, Germany
brueck@zi.biologie.uni-muenchen.de

Fay, J. (44)
Dept of Mechanical Engineering, , Div of Applied Mechanics Durand Building,
Stanford University, Stanford, CA 94305 USA
jfay@leland.stanford.edu

Fay, R.R. (68)
Parmly Hearing Institute and Dept. of Psychology, Loyola University Chicago
North Sheridan Road, Chicago, IL 60626 USA
rfay@luc.edu

Geisler, C.D. (24)
Depts of.*wisc.edu*
Neurophysiology and of Electrical and Computer Engineering
University of Wisconsin-Madison, Madison, WI 53706, USA
geisler@mvg.neurophys

Glowatzki, E. (104)
Dept. of Sensory Biophysics, University of Tübingen, Röntgenweg 11
72076 Tübingen, Germany
elisabeth.glowatzki@uni-tuebingen.de

Greenwood, D.D. (105)
School of Audiology and Speech Sciences, Faculty of Medicine, Univ.of British Columbia
Fairview Ave, Vancouver, BC V6T 1V3   Canada
ddg@audiospeech.ubc.ca

Guinan, J.J. (91)
Eaton-Peabody Laboratory, Massachusetts Eye and Ear Infirmary,, Charles Street,
Boston, MA 02114, USA]
jjg@epl.meei.harvard.edu

Gummer, A.W. (77)
Section of Physiological Acoustics and Communication, Dept. of Otolaryngology,
University of Tübingen, Silcherstrasse 5, 72076 Tübingen,   Germany
anthony.gummer@uni-tuebingen.de

Hackney, C.M. (101)
Dept. of Communication and Neuroscience, Keele University, Keele, Staffs. ST5 5BG   UK
c.m.hackney@keele.ac.uk

Hafter, E.R. (53)
Dept of Psychology,University of California, Berkeley, Berkeley, CA 94720-1650
hafter@violet.berkeley.edu

Hallworth, R. (98)
Dept. of Otolaryngology, UTHSCSA., 7703, Floyd Curl Drive, San Antonio, TX 78284   USA
hallworth@uthscsa.edu

Hecht-Poinar, E.I. (14)
Dept. of EECS, University of California, Berkeley, Berkeley, CA 94720-1770
eva@bandit.eecs.berkeley.edu

Hemmert, W. (122)
Section of Physiological Acoustics and Communication, Dept. of Otolaryngology,
University of Tübingen, Silcherstrasse 5, 72076 Tübingen,   Germany
werner.hemmert@uni-tuebingen.de

Holley, M.C. (84)
Dept of Physiology, University of Bristol, Bristol, BS8 1TD, UK
m.c.holley@bris.ac.uk

Huang; G.T. (118)
McClean Place, Apt 10, Cambridge, MA 02140
gthuang@mit.edu

Hubbard, A.E. (51)
Boston University College of Engineering and Hearing Research Center
44 Cummington St, Boston, MA 02215 USA
aeh@enga.bu.edu

Iwasa, K.H. (21)
Biophysics Section, NIDCD, NIH, Bethesda, MD 20892-0922
kiwasa@helix.nih.gov

Kachar, B. (43)
Laboratory of Cellular Biology, NIDCD, Research Court/2A-03, Rockville, MD 20850
bkachar@pop.nidcd.nih.gov

Kalinec, F. (82)
Laboratory of Cellular Biology, NIDCD - NIH
Research Court, Room 2A03, Rockville, MD 20850-3320
fkalinec@pop.nidcd.nih.gov

Kanneworff, M. (70)
Center for Sound Communication, Institute of Biology, Odense University,
Campusvej 55, DK-5230 Odense M, Denmark
mka@dou.dk

Karavitaki, K.D. (103)
Boston University Hearing Research Center
44 Cummington Street, Boston, MA 02215   USA
dkk@enga.bu.edu

Khanna, S.M. (107)
Columbia University, 630 West 168th Street, New York, NY 10032   USA
smk3@columbia.edu

Kolston, P.J. (39)
Dept of Physiology, University of Bristol, Bristol *BS8 1TD, UK*
paul.j.kolston@bristol.ac.uk

Köppl, C. (2)
Institut für Zoologie der Technischen Universität München
Lichtenbergstrasse 4, 85747 Garching, Germany
CK@cip1.zoo.chemie.tu-muenchen.de

Kössl, M.
Zoologisches Institut, Universität München, Luisenstrasse 14, 80333 ,
München,   Germany
koessl@zi.biologie.uni-muenchen.de

Kumaresan, R. (40)
Dept of Electrical Engineering
University of Rhode Island, Kingston, RI 02881
kumar@ele.uri.edu

Lai, T. (3)
Tlai@WWPWP.MHS.Compuserve.com

LePage, E.L. (73)
Hearing Loss Prevention Research, National Acoustic Laboratories,
Chatswood, N.S.W. 2067 Australia
eric.lePage@nal.gov.au

Lewis,E.R. (4)
Dept of EECS, University of California, Berkeley,Berkeley, CA 94720-1770
lewis@eecs.berkeley.edu

Li, Cheuk (32)
Dept. of EECS, University of California, Berkeley, Berkeley, CA 94720-1770
cheukli@bandit.eecs.berkeley.edu

Lin, T. (100)
Eaton-Peabody Laboratory, Massachusetts Eye and Ear Infirmary, Charles Street,
Boston, MA 02114, USA]
tai@epl.meei.harvard.edu

Long, G. (36)
Dept of Audiology and Speech Sciences,, Purdue University, West Lafayette, IN 47907
long@physics.purdue.edu

Lonsbury-Martin, B.L. (121)
University of Miami Ear Institute (M805), Box 016960, Miami, FL 33101   USA
bmartin@mednet.med.miami.edu

Lukashkin, A.N. (25)
School of Biological Sciences, University of Sussex,, Falmer, Brighton, BN1 9QG, UK
a.lukashkin@sussex.ac.uk

Lyon, R.F. (67)
Apple Computer, Inc., One Infinite Loop, Cupertino, CA 94022   USA
lyon@apple.com

Mammano; F. (114)
International School for Advanced Studies, Laboratory of Biophysics, via Beirut 9
Trieste,   Italy
mammano@neumann.sissa.it

Manley, G.A. (8)
Institut für Zoologie der Technischen Universität München
Lichtenbergstrasse 4, 85747 Garching, Germany
GAM@cip1.zoo.chemie.tu-muenchen.de

Martin, G.K.
University of Miami Ear Institute (M805), Box 016960, Miami, FL 33101   USA
bmartin@mednet.med.miami.edu

McGee,J. (34)
Boys Town National Research Hospital, North 30th Street, Omaha, NE 68131 USA
walsh@boystown.org

Meyer, J. (69)
Section of Physiological Acoustics and Communication, Dept. of Otolaryngology,
University of Tübingen, Silcherstrasse 5, 72076 Tübingen,   Germany
jens.meyer@uni-tuebingen.de

Miles, R.N. (71)
Dept. of Mechanical Engineering, State University of New York at Binghamton
Binghamton, NY 13902-6000   USA
miles@binghamton.edu

Mills, D.M. (92)
Virginia Merrill Bloedel Hearing Research Center
University of Washington, Seattle, WA 98195-7923   USA
dmmills@u.washington.edu

Mountain, D.C. (123)
Boston University College of Engineering and Hearing Research Center
44 Cummington St, Boston, MA 02215 USA
dcm@enga.bu.edu

Murugasu,E. (26)
Dept of Otolaryngology, National University Hospital, Lower kent Ridge Road
Singapore, 119074
entem@leonis.nus.sg

Popel; A.S. (97)
Dept. of Biomedical Engineering, The Johns Hopkins University School of Medicine
Rutland Ave, Baltimore, MD 21205, USA
aspopel@bme.jhu.edu

Prijs, V.F. .(18)
ENT Department, University Hospital Leiden, PO Box 9600, 2300 RC Leiden,, Netherlands
prys@rullf2.LeidenUniv.nl

Purgue, A.P. (37)
Dept of Physiological Sciences , University of California, Los Angeles, CA 90095-1527
apurgue@UCLA.edu

Puria, S. (64)
Eaton-Peabody Laboratory, Massachusetts Eye and Ear Infirmary,, Charles Street,
Boston, MA 02114, USA]
sunil@epl.meei.harvard.edu

Ratnanather, J.T. (113)
Dept. of Biomedical Engineering, The Johns Hopkins University School of Medicine.
Rutland Ave, Baltimore, MD 21205, USA
tratnana@bme.jhu.edu

Ravicz, M.E. (23)
Eaton-Peabody Laboratory, Massachusetts Eye and Ear Infirmary, Charles Street,
Boston, MA 02114 USA
mer@epl.meei.harvard.edu

Recio, A. (116)
The Hugh Knowles Center and Institute for Neuroscience, Northwestern University,
Evanston, IL 60208, USA
ars@merle.acns.nwu.edu

Ren, T. (31)
Kresge Hearing Institute, University of Michigan Medical School
East Ann Street, Ann Arbor, MI 48109-0506 USA and
Dept. of Otolaryngology, Xian Medical University, The People's Republic of China
renty@umich.edu

Rhode, W.S. (87)
Dept. of Neurophysiology, 275 Medical Sciences Building, University Avenue,
Madison, WI 53706 USA
rhode@mvg.neurophys.wisc.edu

Richter, C.-P. (96)
Zentrum der Physiologie, J.W.Goethe - Universität, Theodor-Stern-Kai 7, 60590 Frankfurt/Main
Germany
Northwestern University, Frances Searle Bldg, 2299 North Campus Dr., Evanston, IL 60208
cri529@nwu.edu

Rosowski, J.J. (19)
Eaton-Peabody Laboratory, Massachusetts Eye and Ear Infirmary, Charles Street,
Boston, MA 02114, USA]
jjr@epl.meei.harvard.edu

Ruggero, M.A. (29)
The Hugh Knowles Center and Institute for Neuroscience Northwestern University,
Evanston, IL 60208, USA
mruggero@merle.acns.nwu.edu

Rüsch, A. (94)
Dept. of Otorhinolaryngology and Communicative Sciences, Baylor College of Medicine,
One Baylor Plaza, Houston, TX 77030 USA
alfons.rusch@uni-tuebingen.de

Russell, I.J. (79)
School of Biological Sciences, University of Sussex,, Falmer, Brighton, BN1 9QG, UK
i.j.russell@sussex.ac.uk

Sanderson, M. (62)
Dept of Neuroscience, Brown University, Providence, RI 02912
sander@brownvm.brown.edu

Sarpeshkar, R. (126)
Moore Building MS 136-93, California Institute I of Technology, Pasadena, CA 91125   USA
rahul@pcmp.caltech.edu

Sattel, T. (59)
Institut für Mechanik, Arbeitsgruppe Dynamik, Technische Hochschule Darmstadt
Hochschulstrasse 1, 64289 Darmstadt, Germany
sattel@kepler.mechanik.th-darmstadt.de

Shaffer, L. (45)
Dept of Audiology and Speech Sciences, Heavilon Hall, Purdue University,
West Lafayette, IN 47907
lauren@zwicker.aus.purdue.edu

Shera, C. (102)
Eaton-Peabody Laboratory, Massachusetts Eye and Ear Infirmary,, Charles Street,
Boston, MA 02114, USA]
shera@epl.meei.harvard.edu

Simmons, A. (7)
Dept of Neuroscience, Brown University, Providence, RI 02912
andrea_simmons@brown.edu

Simmons, J.A. (6)
Dept of Neuroscience, Box 1953, Brown University, Providence, RI 02912
james_simmons@brown.edu

Slaney,M (28)
Interval Research Corporation, 1801 Page Mill Rd. Palo Alto, CA 94304   USA
malcolm@interval.com

Smurzynski, J. (66)
Dept of Otorhinolaryngology, University of Basel, Kantonsspital Basel
Petersgraben 4, CH-4031 Basel,   Switzerland
smurzynski@ubaclu.unibas.ch

Spector, A.A. (5)
Dept. of Biomedical Engineering, The Johns Hopkins University School of Medicine
Rutland Ave, Baltimore, MD 21205, USA
aspector@bme.jhu.edu

Steele, C.R. (60)
Dept of Mechanical Engineering, , Div of Applied Mechanics Durand Building,
Stanford University, Stanford, CA 94305   USA
chas@am-sparc7.stanford.edu

Stover, L. (93)
Boys Town National Research Hospital, North 30th Street, Omaha, NE 68131 USA
stover@boystown.org

Talmadge, C.L. (30)
Dept of Physics, Purdue University, West Lafayette, IN 47907   USA
clt@physics.purdue.edu

Teoh, S.W. (57)
New Orleans #120, Dallas, TX 75235
teoh01@utsw.swmed.edu

Thurm, U.
Insitut für Neuro- und Verhaltensbiologie, University of Münster, Badestr.9,
D48149, Germany
thurm@uni-muenster.de

Tolomeo, J.A. (46)
Dept of Physiology, University of Bristol, Bristol, BS8 1TD, UK
j.tolomeo@bris.ac.uk
tolomeo@am-sun2.stanford.edu

Tsang, P.S.K. (88)
Dept. of Biophysics, Nijenborgh 4, University of Groningen,
9747 AG Groningen, Netherlands
tsang@bcn.rug.nl

Tubis, A. (16)
Dept of Physics, Purdue University,, West Lafayette, IN 47907
atu@physics.purdue.edu

Ulfendahl; M. (109)
Dept of Physiology & Pharmacology, Div.Physiology II, Karolinska Institute
Stockholm, Sweden
mats.ulfendahl@fyfa.ki.se

Uppenkamp, S. (75)
Fachbereich Physik, AG Medizinische Physik, , University of Oldenburg,
D-26111 Oldenburg, Germany
stefan@medi.physik.uni-oldenburg.de

Vater, M.
Institut für Zoologie, Universität Regensburg, Universitäts Str. 31,
93040 Regensburg, Germany
marianne.vater@biologie.uni-regensburg.de

Voss, S.E. (10)
Dept of Speech and Hearing Sciences, Massachusetts Institute of Technology,
Cambridge, MA 02139 USA
selawser@athena.mit.edu

Wada, H. (127)
Dept. of Mechanical Engineering, Tohoku University, Sendai 980-77 Japan
wada@cc.mech.tohoku.ac.jp

Walsh, E.J. (1)
Boys Town National Research Hospital, North 30th Street, Omaha, NE 68131 USA
walsh@boystown.org

Wiederhold, M. (47)
Health Science Center, Floyd Curl Dr, University of Texas, San Antonio, TX 78284-7966
wiederhold@uthscsa.edu

Wolodkin, G.J.
Dept of EECS, University of California, Berkeley, Berkeley, CA 94720-1770
greg@EECS.berkeley.edu
Dept of Aerospace Engineering and Mechanics, 107 Akerman Hall, 110 Union St. SE
Minneapolis, MN 55455 USA
wolodkin@aem.umn.edu

Xue, S. (52)
Div. of Otolaryngology-HNS, Box 3550, Duke University Medical Center.,
Durham, NC 27710 USA
sx@dukehrl.mc.duke.edu

Yamada, W.M. (9)
Dept of EECS, University of California, Berkeley. Berkeley, CA 94720-1770 USA
yamada@bandit.eecs.berkeley.edu

Young, E.D. (48)
Dept of Biomedical Engineering and Center for Hearing Sciences,
The Johns Hopkins University, Baltimore, MD 21205, USA
eyoung@bme.jhu.edu
Zetes, D.E. (61)
Div.of Applied Mechanics, Stanford University, Stanford, CA 94305   USA
dzetes@am-sun2.stanford.edu
Zhang, L. (106)
Hearing Research Center, Boston Univ., 44 Cummington Street,, Boston MA 02215   USA
lgzhang@engpub1.bu.edu
Zwislocki, J.J. (110)
Institute for Sensory Research, Syracuse University, Syracuse, NY 13244   USA
joe_zwislocki@isr.syr.edu

Contents

Part one **Diversity in auditory mechanics**

Part two   Descriptive models of middle and outer ear

Part three   Descriptive models of cochlear function

From ear canal to VIIIth nerve or higher

In terms of spontaneous and evoked cochlear emissions

In terms of basilar membrane motion

Part five   Descriptive models of cellular elements

Part six   Synthetic models of cellular elements

Part One

Diversity in auditory mechanics

Hoping to make the sixth symposium reflect the breadth of the hearing research community, the organizing committee selected "Diversity in Auditory Mechanics" as its central theme. The reader will see this theme reflected throughout this volume, but it is especially conspicuous in Part One, where we have collected 19 papers that focus on comparative and evolutionary issues in hearing.

MIDDLE-EAR STRUCTURAL AND FUNCTIONAL DEPENDENCE ON ANIMAL SIZE

W.T. PEAKE and J.J. ROSOWSKI

Eaton-Peabody Laboratory, Massachusetts Eye and Ear Infirmary,
243 Charles Street, Boston, MA 02114, USA
and
Research Laboratory of Electronics, M.I.T.
77 Massachusetts Avenue, Cambridge, MA 02139, USA
E-mail wmtpeake@mit.edu

To investigate how middle-ear performance depends on animal size we focus on the family Felidae. Measurements on 400 skulls from 34 species are fit with equations that express bullar and ear-canal dimensions as power functions of skull length L_{CB} (in mm). For low frequencies the cavity gain, G_{CAV} = (pressure acting on the ossicular chain)/ (pressure in the ear canal), can be related to structure, and the combination of structural data and structure-function relations leads to $G_{CAV} = (1 + 7.38 \; 10^3 \; L_{CB}^{-1.98})^{-1}$. This relation indicates that the smallest cats (L_{CB} = 65 mm) expend 2/3 of the sound pressure applied in the ear canal compressing the air in the middle-ear cavity. However, in the largest felids (L_{CB} = 400 mm) the effect of the cavities is very small and G_{CAV} is approximately 1. Measurements of G_{CAV} in four species (cat, bobcat, tiger and lion) are roughly consistent with this structure-based rule.

1. Introduction: Diversity in middle-ear structure and function

The same middle-ear components occur in most mammalian species, but some dramatic variations occur [1]. We will focus here on the middle-ear air space, which is usually enclosed in a bony wall. In many species part of this wall forms a distinct feature on the posterior skull, called the auditory bulla [2]. The prominence of the bulla varies: in some species it is undetectable (e.g. humans and elephants); in others it dominates the caudal end of the skull (e.g. kangaroo rat, chinchilla and gerbil)[3].

The consequences of these structural variations in middle-ear air space have attracted some attention. Hypertrophied bullae have been associated with arid habitat[4,5] and with relatively sensitive low-frequency hearing that is helpful in evading predators[6-9]. A physical basis for the air space's effect on hearing is apparent; the acoustic impedance introduced by the air spaces reduces the response of the middle ear. A measure of this effect, called the cavity gain G_{CAV}, varies from 0.1 to near 1 (at low frequencies) among 10 diverse species[10]. Interspecies comparisons in this group do not reveal a pattern relating G_{CAV} to structure or taxonomy; the species with the smallest and the largest values of G_{CAV} (hamster and mouse, respectively) are both rather small rodents with unprominent bullae; two species with prominent bullae, chinchilla and kangaroo rat, are also far apart in this measure. We propose here to develop a rule that relates this physiological measure (G_{CAV}) to animal size. Such a rule seems most likely to provide an accurate prediction of performance, if it is restricted to a taxonomic group that has many common structural features. We have chosen the cat family as a desirable taxon because it has qualitative structural uniformity among species, a large size range, a moderate number of species (37) and one member, domestic cat, that has been well studied physiologically. We describe here some features of the dependence of ear structure on animal size. We determine a rule that relates G_{CAV} (for low frequencies) to skull size. The rule is then tested with acoustic measurements from live domestic cats and a few post-mortem exotic cat species.

2. Methods

We used museum collections to measure dimensions of skulls and ears on about 400 specimens covering 34 of the 37 recognized felid species. For most species we have approximately 10 specimens in our data base, however, in 3 species we have 4 or fewer and in one case (mountain lion, *Puma concolor*) we have 65. In our treatment here we ignore the species of each specimen and regard all as members of the same group (Felidae).

We measured 13 skull dimensions and 5 ear dimensions on each skull. We describe the dependence of one dimension on another by allometric functions of the form $y = ax^b$, where x is the measure of size[11,12]. For the special case in which the exponent b equals 1, the equation indicates "isometry" or direct proportionality. In post-mortem material obtained from Boston's Franklin Park Zoo and from the Massachusetts Department of Fish and Wildlife we have measured the acoustic impedance of ears at the tympanic membrane and sound pressures within the middle ear. Results have been obtained on 1 lion, 1 tiger, and 1 bobcat. From CT scans of these specimens we traced boundaries of the middle-ear air space to determine the total volume V_{CAV} .

3. Structural rules

We use the midline "condylobasal length" L_{CB} (from the premaxilla just above the incisors to the posterior surfaces of the occipital condyles) as a convenient (and conventional) measure of skull size; it ranges in our sample from 65 to 375 mm. (Animal weight in felid species ranges from 1.5 to 300 kg.) Exponential relations provide a good description of each skull dimension's dependence on L_{CB}; for more than half of the relations the least-squares linear regression fit (to log-log plots of the measurements) explains over 96 percent of the variance. None of the dimensions varies isometrically with L_{CB}; the exponents vary from 0.70 to 1.16. The dimensions with exponents larger than 1 are from the facial skull; for the cerebral skull the values are less than 1. This dichotomy represents a well-known increase in size of the facial skull relative to the cerebral skull as size increases in carnivores[14-16].

Three dimensions of the auditory bulla (length L_B, width W_B and depth D_B) were measured. For each of these measures the exponent that describes growth with L_{CB} is 0.7. The product of these three dimensions is fit with an exponent of about 2 (Fig. 1) . This exponential relationship between the product of the bullar dimensions and the size measure L_{CB} is our first structural rule.

Figure 1. The product of bullar dimensions plotted versus skull length for 362 felid skulls. The linear regression fit is shown; the estimated SLOPE of log y vs. log x is shown with its (±) standard error. R^2, the square of the coefficient of determination, is the fraction of the variance in log y that is explained by the linear regression fit. The exponential relation for the plotted line is shown.

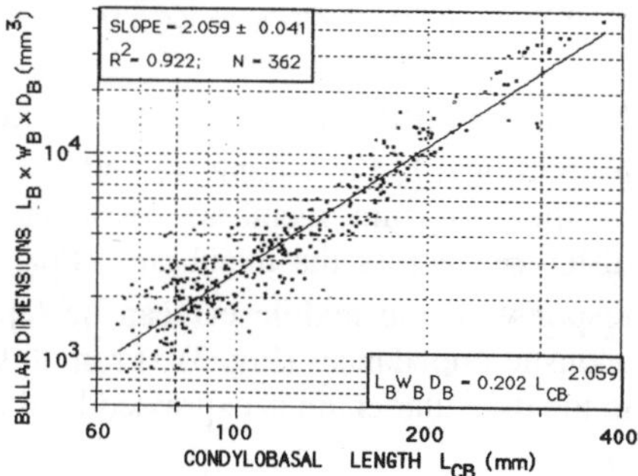

Two diameters of the bony external ear canal were measured: the longest diameter, which we call the width W_{EC} and the diameter perpendicular to this, the ear-canal height H_{EC}. The exponents for these dimensions are 0.298 (for W_{EC}) and 0.256 (for H_{EC}), both of which are substantially smaller than those for the bullar dimensions. Figure 2 shows that the regression fit to the product of these two diameters explains about half of the variance (R^2 =0.454). This exponential relation for the dependence of the product ($W_{EC} H_{EC}$) on L_{CB} is a second structural rule.

Figure 2. The product of ear-canal diameters versus skull length with an exponential fit to the measurements as in Fig. 1.

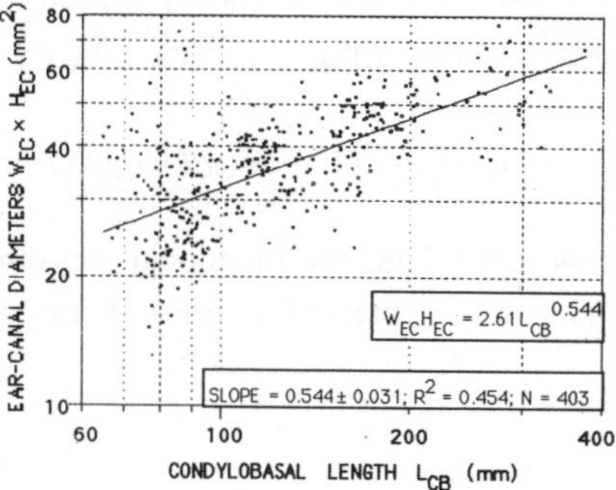

6

4. Functional model for cavity gain G_{CAV}

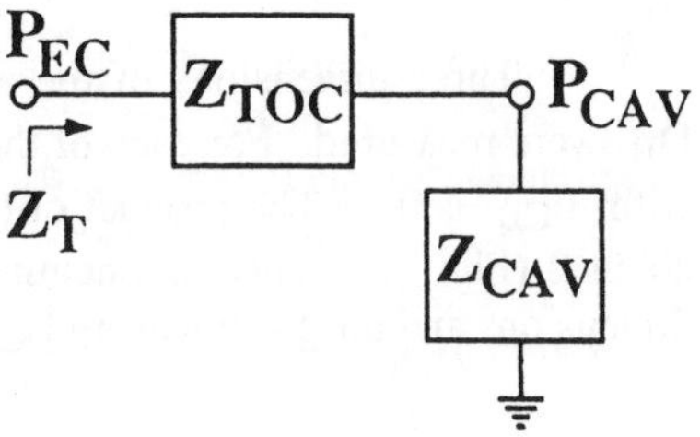

Figure 3. An analog circuit model for the relationship between sound pressures in the ear canal P_{EC} and in the middle-ear air space P_{CAV}. Z_{TOC} is the acoustic impedance of the TM and ossicular chain; Z_{CAV} is the acoustic impedance of the middle-ear air space. The impedance at the tympanic membrane is $Z_T = Z_{TOC} + Z_{CAV}$.

If it is assumed that the sound pressure generated in the tympanic cavity P_{CAV} is proportional to the volume velocity of the tympanic membrane and that the motion of the tympanic membrane-ossicular chain system is driven by the pressure difference across the membrane ($P_{EC} - P_{CAV}$), the effect of the cavities on the response of the middle ear can be represented by a series-circuit analog of two acoustic impedances (Fig. 3). From this model the effect of the cavities on the input to the ossicular chain is expressed by the cavity gain

$$G_{CAV} = (P_{EC} - P_{CAV})/P_{EC} = Z_{TOC}/(Z_{TOC} + Z_{CAV}) = (1 + Y_{TOC}/Y_{CAV})^{-1}. \tag{1}$$

This expression shows that, if the magnitude of the acoustic admittance of the cavities $|Y_{CAV}|$ is much larger than that of the admittance of the tympanic-membrane ossicular-chain linkage $|Y_{TOC}|$, the cavities have very little effect and $G_{CAV} = 1$.

To keep the functional dependence on structure simple, we will consider here only the low-frequency region, in which both admittances are compliance-like[10], so that $Y_{TOC} = j\, C_{TOC}$, $Y_{CAV} = j\, C_{CAV}$ and therefore

$$G_{CAV} = (1 + C_{TOC}/C_{CAV})^{-1} = (1 + V_{TOC}/V_{CAV})^{-1}. \tag{2}$$

This rule relates the functional measure G_{CAV} to the acoustic compliances, which can also be expressed in terms of equivalent air volumes V_{TOC} and V_{CAV}.

5. From structural rules to a functional rule

The acoustic compliance of a closed cavity with rigid walls is equal to the compressibility of air times the cavity volume. Therefore, the low-frequency cavity compliance can be found directly from the volume V_{CAV} of the middle-ear air space. The quantity given by the product of the three bullar dimensions (Fig. 1) should be closely related to V_{CAV}. To determine this relationship we used all the measured volumes that were available: the relation given by the regression fit (Fig. 4) is

$$V_{CAV} = 0.632 \ (L_B \ W_B \ D_B)^{0.963}. \qquad (4)$$

Inserting the exponential relation from Fig. 1 into this equation yields

$$V_{CAV} = 0.135 \ L_{CB}^{1.98}, \qquad (5)$$

which determines $Y_{CAV}(L_{CB})$, a functional measure expressed in terms of size.

Figure 4 .   Measured volume of the middle-ear air space versus the product of bullar dimensions for 16 specimens (1 lion, 1 tiger, 1 clouded leopard, 2 bobcats and 11 domestic cats). For the domestic cats these volumes were measured by water filling when the cats were alive[13]; the others were determined from CT scans of the frozen heads.

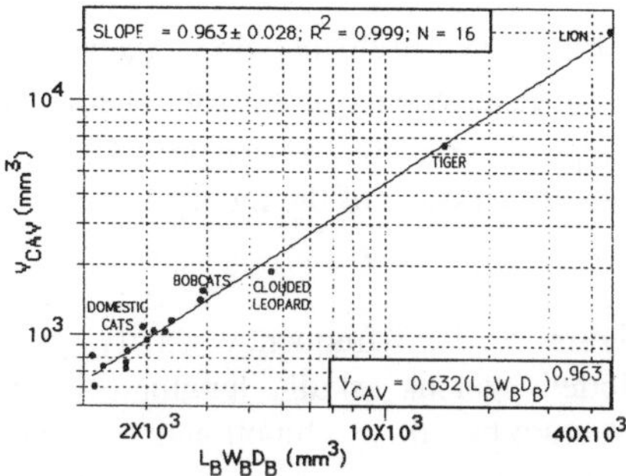

The structual dependence of the other relevant compliance C_{TOC} is not so easily related to size, because several structures are involved (TM, ossicular ligaments) and none of their compliances has been related to dimensions. As the tympanic membrane (TM) might be a major contributor to C_{TOC} we have looked for an empirical dependence on the area of the tympanic ring A_{TR} using measurements from 8 felid specimens, including 5 live cats and 3 dead specimens (1 bobcat, 1 tiger and 1 lion). The resulting plot does not show a tight dependence of C_{TOC} on A_{TR}. Only 35% of the variance is explained by the regression line, and the slope of the line (0.5 ± 0.3) is marginally different from zero. Two of the domestic cats have C_{TOC} within 20% of the lion's and the bobcat's C_{TOC} is 20% larger than the lion's. This weak dependence on tympanic ring size suggests the simplifying assumption that C_{TOC} is _independent_ of size and can be represented by

8

an average of the measurements. We chose $V_{TOC} = 10^3$ mm^3, where we have expressed the compliance in terms of its equivalent volume of air. The key conclusion here is that the increase of C_{TOC} with skull size L_{CB} is much less than the increase in V_{CAV}.

Substitution of this value for V_{TOC} and the V_{CAV} expression from equation (5) into equation (2) yields

$$G_{CAV} = (1 + 7.38 \ 10^3 \ L_{CB}^{-1.98})^{-1} , \qquad (6)$$

which predicts (Fig. 5) that as size increases (from the smallest to the largest felid) the cavity gain increases from about 0.3 to near 1. That is, for the smallest cats 70% of the input pressure is required to compress the air in the middle ear, but for the largest cats the middle-ear volume is so large that the cavities have an inconsequential effect.

6. Test of the function-size rule

In Fig. 5 measurements of G_{CAV} are plotted with the structurally based rule (Eq. 6). The measurements support the theory in that the two large felids have larger G_{CAV} values than the smaller species. Clearly more measurements are required to test the predictive power of the theory.

Figure 5. Low-frequency cavity gain plotted versus skull length. The structure-based functional rule expressed by the displayed equation is plotted as a dotted line. Measurements in 8 specimens (of 4 species) provided the measured G_{CAV} values. The cat values were taken from impedance measurements in Fig. 13 of reference 18; vertical and horizontal lines indicate one standard deviation. The lion measurement is from 17. The tiger and bobcat data are unpublished .

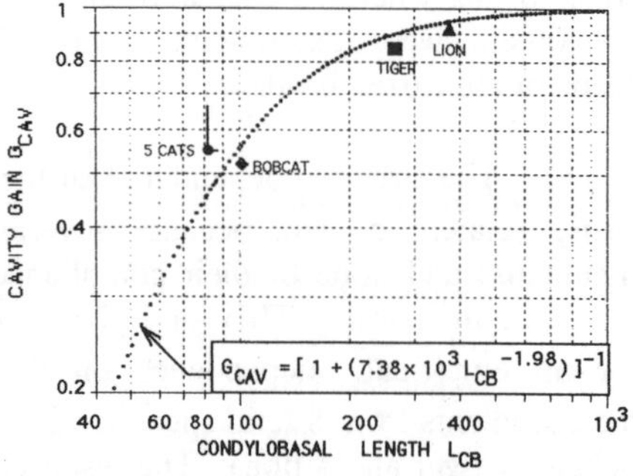

7. Future possibilities for this approach

These results show that quantitative rules relating function to size can be developed and tested. Other rules to describe trends within this taxon might include: (1) Other features of G_{CAV} such as the frequency of the dip in sensitivity introduced by an antiresonance in the two coupled middle-ear cavities[17]; (2) Measures of hearing function such as the dependence of frequency range on size.

Analyses of this kind can also demonstrate whether species deviate substantially from the family trends. For instance, if species that live in arid habitats prove to have unusually large bullae for their size, quantitative support will be provided for the proposed correlation of bullar inflation with habitat[4-9].

Acknowledgments

We enjoyed use of the collections of the Harvard U. Museum of Comparative Zoology in Cambridge, the Field Museum of Natural History in Chicago, the National Museum of Natural History in Washington DC, and the American Museum of Natural History in New York. Judy Chupasko and Maria Rutzmoser of the Harvard M.C.Z. have contributed in numerous ways. We have had essential cooperation from the Franklin Park Zoo of Boston, the National Zoo in Washington DC, and the Mass. Fish and Wildlife Department. Michael Ravicz, Deborah Flandermeyer and Barbara Kiang of the Eaton-Peabody Laboratory have made important contributions. Helen C. Peake has been a major contributor in the museum measurements, data processing, figure production and translation of papers. Supported in part by a grant from the National Institute of Deafness and Communicative Disorders (NIH).

References

1. Henson , O.W. (1974) Comparative anatomy of the middle ear. In: *Handbook of Sensory Physiology: The Auditory System V/1*, ed.W.D. Keidel and W.D. Neff (Springer-Verlag, New York) 39-110.
2. Novacek, M.J.(1977 Aspects of the problem of variation, origin and evolution of the eutherian auditory bulla. *Mammal Rev.* **7** 131-150.
3. Keen, J.A. and Grobbelaar ,C.S. (1941) The comparative anatomy of the tympanic bulla and auditory ossicles with a note suggesting their function. *Trans. R. Soc. S. Africa* **28** 307-329.
4. Heim de Balsac, H.(1936) Biogeographie de mammiferes et des oiseaux de l'Afrique de Nord. *Suppl. Bull. Fisiologique de France et Belgique.* **21** 371-445.

5. Lay, D.L. (1972). The anatomy, physiology, functional significance and evolution of specialized hearing organs of gerbilline rodents. *J. Morph.* **138** 41-120.

6. Legouix, J.P. and Wisner, A. (1955) Role functionnel des bulles tympaniques geantes de certains rongeurs. *Acustica* **5** 208-216.

7. Webster, D.B. (1965) Ears of <u>Dipodomys</u>. *Nat. Hist.* **74** 26-33.

8. Webster, D.B. (1982) A function of the enlarged middle ear cavities of the kangaroo rat <u>Dipodomys</u>. *Physiol. Zool.* **35** 248-255.

9. Webster , D.B. and Webster, M. (1984) The specialized auditory system of kangaroo rats. *Contrib. Sensory Physiol.* **8**, 161-196. Acad Press.

10. Rosowski, J.J. (1994) Outer and middle ear. In: *Comparative Hearing: Mammals* eds. R.R. Fay and A.N. Popper (Springer-Verlag). **6** 172-247.

11. Gould, S.J. (1966) Allometry and size in ontogeny and phylogeny. *Biol. Rev. Cambridge Phil. Soc.* **41**, 587-640.

12. Schmidt-Nielsen, K. (1984) Scaling: Why is Animal Size so Important? Cambridge.

13. Lynch, T.J.,III (1981) Signal processing by the cat middle ear: Admittance and transmission, measurements and models. *Ph.D. Thesis, M.I.T.*

14. Ewer, R.F. (1973) The Carnivores , Cornell/ Comstock.

15. Radinsky, L.B. (1985) Approaches in evolutionary morphology: A search for patterns. *Ann. Rev. Ecol. Syst.* **16**, 1-14.

16. Emerson, S.B. and Bramble, D.M.(1993) Scaling, allometry and skull design. In: *The Skull, Vol. 3; Functional and Evolutionary Mechanisms*, ed. J. Hanken and B.K.Hall (U. Chicago).

17. Huang, G., Rosowski, J.J., Flandermeyer, D., Lynch, T.J.,III and Peake, W.T. (1996) The middle ear of a lion: comparison of structure and function to domestic cat. *J.Acoust. Soc. Amer.* (in press)

18. Lynch, T.J.,III, Peake, W.T. and Rosowski, J.J.(1994) Measurements of acoustic input-impedance of cat ears: 10 Hz to 20 kHz. *J. Acoust. Soc. Am.* **96** 2184-2209.

ROLES OF INTRACRANIAL AIR PRESSURE IN BIRD AUDITION

O.N. LARSEN,
Centre for Sound Communication; Odense University
Campusvej 55, DK-5230 Odense M, Denmark

R.J. DOOLING
Department of Psychology; University of Maryland
College Park, MD 20742 USA

B.M. RYALS
Hearing and Speech Sciences; James Madison University
Harrisburg, VA. 22807 USA

The existence of an interaural pathway in birds has motivated a considerable amount of research on the mechanisms of avian hearing particularly those related to sound localization. Here we show that the tympanal frequency response changes with intracranial air pressure in several species of small birds providing a potential mechanism for directional hearing especially at low frequencies. Moreover, intracranial air pressure changes in some birds during vocal production, during intense noise exposure, under anesthesia, and when the bird is stimulated by intense pure tone bursts. These results confirm the existence of a functional interaural pathway and suggest an important role for intracranial air pressure in several aspects of avian hearing.

1 Introduction

1.1 The Avian Interaural Pathway

It has long been known that the middle ears of birds are connected through a pathway referred to as the interaural canal[1]. In some species it is tubelike, while in others it is criss-crossed with trabeculate bone which surrounds the brain ventrocaudally. The morphology suggests the air pressure is always the same on the interior surface of the two eardrums (tympana). Poor high frequency hearing in birds and small interaural distances have implicated the interaural canal as a mechanism by which sound may propagate from one ear to the other making the ears inherently directional pressure difference receivers.

The present series of studies involving five species of small birds (budgerigars, canaries, chicks, quail, and zebra finches) was conducted to extend earlier observations on the starling[2] to other species and explore the potential role of intracranial air (ICA) pressure changes on other aspects of hearing. These studies were also motivated in part by observations that a negative middle ear pressure in mammals develops during inflammation due to gas exchange over the middle ear mucosa[3] and more recent findings that the tympana slowly pull inwards during anesthesia in the quail[4]. Changes in the tympana could potentially influence the frequency response of the eardrums, the directionality of the ears, the efficacy of masking noise, and the susceptibility to damage from acoustic overexposure.

1.2 Hypotheses

The present studies test several hypotheses. The first is that changes of intracranial air (ICA) pressure are responsible for an inward movement of the tympanum. The second is that there is a relation between ICA pressure and the frequency response of tympanal vibration. The third is that in some species, biologically significant changes in ICA pressure occur in other situations such as anesthesia, continuous acoustic overexposure, self-produced vocalizations, and pure tone stimulation.

2 Methods

2.1 Measurement of Intracranial Air (ICA) Pressure.

Under Ketamine-Xylazine anesthesia, an 8 mm cut-and-polished 0.8 mm diameter injection needle was cemented into the bird skull in the trabeculated bone underneath the hind brain about 5 mm off the midline. For pressure measurements a FUJIKURA (type FPM-05PG) pressure transducer was connected to the cemented needle through a 40 mm flexible tube from a winged needle infusion set. The output from the pressure transducer electronics was low-pass filtered and A/D sampled with Labtech Notebook v. 8.1 software or Tucker-Davis Technologies hardware and software (sampling rate 1-1000 Hz depending on the experiment) and monitored on an oscilloscope. The pressure transducer was calibrated against a water column. For measurements on awake birds, the pressure transducer was suspended on a balanced arm such that the bird was free to move, introducing only minor movement artifacts in the recordings. Measurements were also made on anesthetized birds with vented and unvented skulls, birds exposed to continuous broadband noise or tone bursts and birds that were vocalizing. For assessing the relation between ICA pressure and tympanal vibration a second needle was cemented into the skull and connected to a 1 ml syringe to provide a means of artificially changing the pressure.

2.2 Measurement of Tympanal Frequency Response.

A 3.5 ms burst chirp sweep from a 2-channel spectrum analyzer (HP35665A) served as sound stimulus, delivered by either a normal free field speaker, mounted on a roundabout for the directional measurements, or by a 'local source', consisting of a speaker connected to a glass pipette via a plastic tube and placed next to the ear opening. The burst chirp output was also fed to channel A of the spectrum analyzer for calculation of transfer functions. The sound stimulus was recorded at the upper rim of the ear opening with a Bruel & Kjaer probe microphone (type 4182), the amplified output of which was fed to channel B of the spectrum analyzer and displayed as a transfer function (B/A) consisting of amplitude and phase versus frequency.

Tympanal vibrations were recorded as the velocity of a point on the extra columella indicated by a very small glass bead (about 0.5 µg). The vibrations were detected with a Dantec fiber optic Laser Doppler Vibrometer (type 55N21), placed 70 cm from the bird, and fed into channel B on the spectrum analyzer to produce transfer functions. The tympanal frequency response was then found by dividing the vibration transfer function with that of the sound stimulus.

Interaural transmission gain was estimated in a three step process: (1) the ear was stimulated with the local source from the ipsilateral side and the transfer function was determined,   (2) the ear was stimulated with the local source from the contralateral side and the transfer function determined, (3) the 'contralateral transfer function' was divided by the 'ipsilateral transfer function' to obtain the change (both attenuation and delay) of sound reaching the inner side of the tympanum after passing across the contralateral tympanum and through the interaural canal.

In computing the directional response, an anesthetized bird was suspended with its right ear in the center of the circular path described by the free field speaker mounted on the roundabout. The speaker position was changed in 30° steps through 360° and the frequency response of stimulus sound to the ear and of the tympanal response was measured and stored on disk. Amplitude and phase values at 4 frequencies were normalized relative to 0° (frontal direction) for calculation of directional effects off line.

3   Results

3.1 ICA Pressure and the Tympanal Frequency Response

In all awake birds tested the ICA pressure grows steadily negative over a period of seconds to minutes, but is reset once it reaches -2 to -4 mm H_2O probably by the bird opening its Eustachian tube. Depending on species this happens every 30-90 seconds. In anesthetized birds, the ICA pressure is not reset but continues to grow and may reach large negative values. For instance, in one anesthetized budgerigar, the ICA pressure moved negative by 120mm H_2O in just over 10 minutes. A qualitative aspect of the falling ICA pressure during anesthesia is an inward movement of the tympana. It is likely that control over the Eustachian tube is abolished under anesthesia allowing middle ear gases diffusing into the blood stream to cause a chronic, negative ICA pressure. This phenomenon has been extensively explored in mammals where the development of negative pressure is also thought to be caused by gas exchange across the middle ear mucosa, partially regulated by the blood flow rate[3].

In birds, the inward movement of the tympana has a dramatic effect on the tympanal transfer function as well as on any interaural transmission gain afforded by an interaural canal. Figure 1 shows the interaural transmission gain in an anesthetized budgerigar with a vented and an non-vented skull. The attenuation is about 5 dB below 1 kHz increasing to about 15 dB at 4-5 kHz in an anesthetized bird with a vented skull. If the vent is occluded and negative pressure is allowed to build up, the interaural transmission at low frequencies changes accordingly.

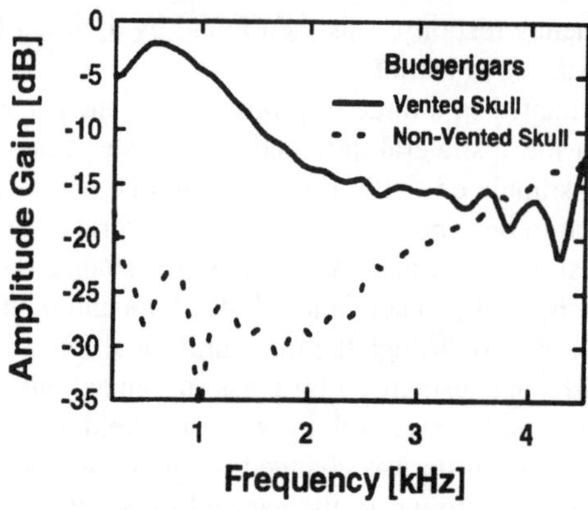

Figure 1 Interaural transmission gainin a budgerigar with a vented and non-vented skull. The upper cutoff frequency of the local sound source was 4.6 kHz. There are dramatic differences between the vented and non-vented skull conditions at low frequencies. Similar results were observed for other species.

We also observed similar effects on the ICA in some birds during continuous exposure to loud noise. This may explain the well known effects of both variability and relative insensitivity of birds to damage by continuous acoustic overexposure and the observation that birds with vented intracranial airspace suffer more damage from acoustic overexposure than those with intact intracranial airspaces[5].

3.2 Directional Effects of ICA Pressure Changes

Frequency specific changes in the tympanal transfer function and transmission gain through the interaural canal cause frequency specific directional effects. Figure 2 compares tympanal vibration amplitude and sound amplitude as a function of azimuth at 1.0 kHz for an anesthetized budgerigar with a vented and non-vented skull. When the skull is vented, there are large directional effects at 1.0 kHz and at other frequencies.

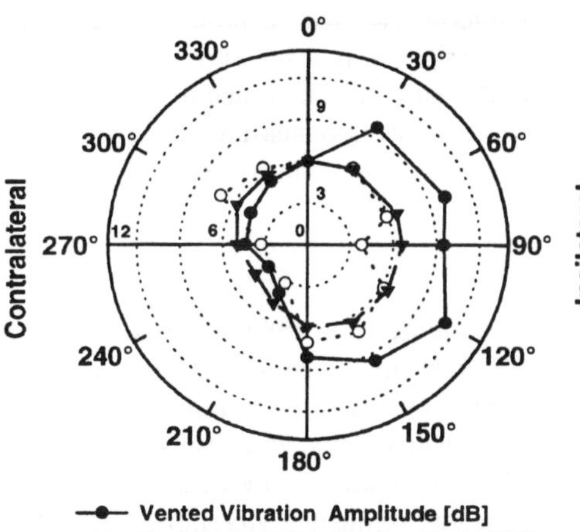

Figure 2: The directional effects of ICA pressure at 1 kHz for a budgerigar with a vented and a non-vented skull. ICA pressure in the non-vented skull reached -60 to -80 mm H_2O. When non-vented, variation in amplitude with azimuth is close to that of ipsilateral sound pressure. When the skull is vented, large directional effects can occur. Similar effects were also seen at 2, 4, and 8 kHz. Thus, the interaural pathway in small birds may play a role in a number of binaural phenomenal including spatial discrimination of sound sources, sound localization and binaural release from masking.

3.3 Middle Ear Muscle Reflex

A protective middle ear reflex associated with self-produced vocalizations in chicks has been reported earlier[6] and was confirmed in chicks using the present technique. There was a clear negative going ICA with each peep produced by a chick. It is not yet clear whether this response is observed in other species. ICA recordings in budgerigars producing contact calls tend to show a positive going ICA pressure change with vocal production and the significance of this is not yet clear.

Earlier work on chicks and starlings show that a middle ear reflex to external sounds is positively absent though it does exist in the Tawny Owl[6,7]. In the present experiments, we measured ICA pressure changes in chicks, quail, zebra finches, canaries, and budgerigars during stimulation by intense tone bursts.

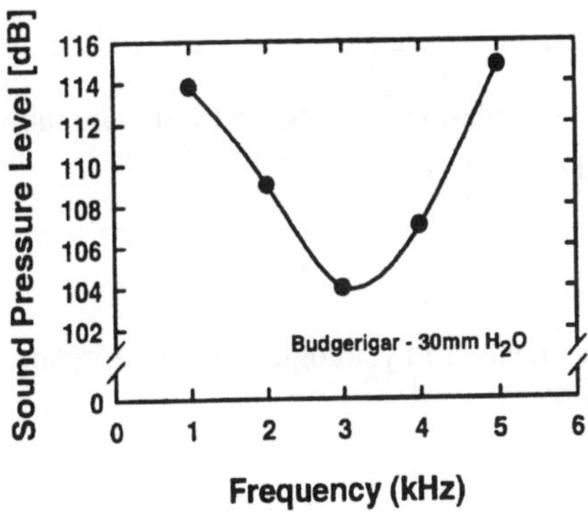

Figure 3: The SPL at each test frequency required to evoke a constant pressure response of 30 mm of H_2O in an awake budgerigar. The shape of this function parallels that of the audibility curve of this species. An evoked pressure response was consistently observed in budgerigars at SPLs greater than 95-100 dB but not in any other species.

Only budgerigars showed evidence of a middle ear muscle reflex to externally presented sounds. The SPL needed to evoke a criterion ICA pressure response of 30 mm H_2O at different frequencies is shown in Figure 3. The shape of this function is remarkably similar to the shape of the audibility function measured behaviorally in this species.

4 Conclusions

In awake birds intracranial air pressure deviates little from ambient pressure due to frequent resetting, probably by opening of the Eustachian tube. In anesthetized birds, and occasionally in birds being exposed to continuous noise, intracranial air pressure goes negative and may remain at a fairly large negative value with respect to ambient pressure. These pressures force the tympanal membranes inwards, change their frequency responses mainly by a reduction in low frequency vibration amplitudes, and may influence physiologically-based estimates of avian auditory system directionality. Venting the intracranial air space during physiological experiments should eliminate this problem.

It remains unclear to what extent there is active modulation of ICA pressure in different species of birds through control of the Eustachian tube. The present data suggest that such control may serve to protect the avian ear against damage from acoustic overexposure in a number of species. In chicks, short term protection during vocal production is accomplished by a middle ear muscle reflex. Of the five species tested, only budgerigars show clear evidence of a middle ear muscle reflex in response to external sound stimulation. The significance of species differences in the presence of a middle ear muscle reflex and the relation to other aspects of hearing and acoustic communication these species require further exploration. It seems clear, however, that ICA pressure may play a more significant role in avian hearing than heretofore realized.

Acknowledgments

Supported by Danish National Research Foundation to ONL and NIH Grants MH-00982, DC-00198 and DC-001372 to RJD

References

1. Wada, Y. (1924) Beiträge zur vergleichenden Physiologie des Gehörorgans, *Pflugers. Arch. Ges. Physiol.* **202** 46-49.

2. Klump, G.K. and Larsen, O.N. (1992). Azimuthal sound localization in the European starling (*Sturnus vulgaris*): I. Physical binaural cues, *J. Comp. Physiol(A)*. **170** 243-251.

3. Doyle, W.J, Seroky, J.T. and Alper, C.M. (1995). Gas exchange across the middle ear mucosa in monkeys, *Arch. Otolaryngol. Head Neck Surg.* **121** 887-892

4. Larsen, O.N. and Popov, A.V. (1995). The interaural canal does enhance directional hearing in quail, *Proc. 4th Internat. Conf. Neuroethol.*

5. Ryals, B.M, Dooling, R.J. and Larsen, O.N. (1995). Variability in acoustic trauma results from changes in middle ear pressure in birds. *Association for Research in Otolaryngology Abstracts.*

6. Counter, S.A. and Borg, E. (1982). The avian stapedius muscle, *Acta Otolaryngol.* **94** 267-274.

7. Oeckinghaus, H. and Schwartzkopff, J. (1983). Electrical and acoustical activation of the middle ear muscle in a songbird, *J. Comp. Physiol.* **150** 61-67.

A MECHANICAL ANALYSIS OF THE NOVEL EAR OF THE PARASITOID FLY *Ormia ochracea*

R. N. MILES and T. D. TIEU

Department of Mechanical Engineering,
State University of New York at Binghamton,
Binghamton, NY 13902-6000, USA
miles@binghamton.edu, tai.tieu@ped.gmeds.com

D. ROBERT and R. R. HOY

Section of Neurobiology and Behavior
Cornell University, Ithaca, NY 14853-2702, USA
drobert@zool.unizh.ch, rrh3@cornell.edu

An analysis is presented of the mechanical response to a sound field of the ears of the parasitoid fly *Ormia ochracea*. This animal shows a remarkable ability to detect the direction of an incident sound stimulus even though its acoustic sensory organs are in very close proximity to each other. A mathematical model of the mechanical response of the ear to a sound stimulus is presented. It is shown that the directional sensitivity of the system is achieved by processing the sum and the difference of the acoustic pressures acting on the tympana. In order to illustrate the mechanics of the system, an electronic circuit is developed which processes the output signals from two closely spaced omnidirectional microphones (which represent the eardrums) to construct two output signals (which represent the inputs to the sensory cells). Experimental results are shown which demonstrate that this electronic analogue possesses similar directional sensitivity to that of the fly's ears.

1　Introduction

We have shown recently that the mechanical structure of the ear of the parasitoid fly *Ormia ochracea* (Order: Diptera; Family: Tachinidae) [1,2] endows the fly with a remarkable ability to sense the direction of an incident sound wave [3]. Measurements of the mechanical response of the ears of this fly indicate that when sound arrives from one side, the ear that is closer to the sound source responds with significantly greater amplitude than the ear which is further from the source. This significant difference in tympanal response is surprising considering that the ears are so close together that the incident sound arrives at the two ears with a difference in arrival time of only 1 to 2 μsec. The close proximity of the ears causes any differences in the incident pressure due to diffraction to be unmeasurable. The interaural difference in mechanical response is due to the coupling of the ears' motion by a cuticular structure which joins the two tympana, known as the intertympanal bridge.

A simple mechanical model of the ears of *Ormia ochracea* has been shown to accurately represent the response due to sound from any incident direction[3]. An examination of this model shows that the system can be represented in terms of two, uncoupled resonant modes of vibration. One mode consists of the two tympana vibrating out of phase, or rocking about the fulcrum of the intertympanal bridge. The other mode, which has a higher natural frequency than the rocking mode, consists of the two tympana moving in-phase. With the right set of system parameters, these modes combine to give a response over a fairly broad range of frequencies in which one tympanum moves with substantially greater response than the other when sound arrives from one side. Other insects such as some cicadas [4,5] have coupled ears which respond in a similar way but *Ormia* appears to be the only animal to rely on a direct mechanical link between the ears to accomplish this. A goal of the present investigation is to mimic this system to construct a simple directionally sensitive receiver. This will help to illustrate the principles used in this animal for achieving directional hearing. It is found that the ears of *Ormia ochracea* employ a mechanical realization of a concept devised by Blumlein[6] in 1931 to electronically process signals from two closely spaced microphones in order to record a stereophonic signal.

In the following, we will briefly describe the analytical model of the fly's coupled ears. The governing equations will then be manipulated to motivate the design of a simple analog electronic circuit which accomplishes nearly the same task as the mechanical structure in the ears of *Ormia ochracea*. The inputs to the circuit are signals from two closely spaced omnidirectional microphones. The two outputs are shown to have Cardioid directivities which are oriented in opposite directions. With the proper orientation of the pair of microphones relative to a sound source, one output from the circuit will give the sound traveling away from the source and the other output will give the sound traveling in the opposite direction, toward the source. The circuit provides a means of constructing a small stereo microphone with excellent channel separation.

2 Analytical Model of the Response of the Ears of *Ormia ochracea*

Figure 1 shows the ears along with a mechanical system which is used to illustrate the mechanism employed to achieve directional sensitivity. The anatomy of the ears is discussed in detail by Robert, Read, Hoy[2] and Miles, Robert, and Hoy [3] . The tympanal membranes consist of the pair of corrugated regions. The model system consists of two rigid bars joined by a spring k_3 and dash-pot c_3. The remaining springs and dash-pots connect to the extreme ends of the bars. The responses $x_1(t)$ and $x_2(t)$ of the two ends of the bars represent the responses of the inputs to the acoustic sensory organs [3]. $x_1(t)$ and $x_2(t)$ may be determined by solving

$$\begin{bmatrix} k_1 + k_2 & k_3 \\ k_3 & k_2 + k_3 \end{bmatrix} \begin{pmatrix} x_1(t) \\ x_2(t) \end{pmatrix} + \begin{bmatrix} c_1 + c_2 & c_3 \\ c_3 & c_2 + c_3 \end{bmatrix} \begin{pmatrix} \dot{x}_1(t) \\ \dot{x}_2(t) \end{pmatrix}$$

$$+ \begin{bmatrix} m & 0 \\ 0 & m \end{bmatrix} \begin{pmatrix} \ddot{x}_1(t) \\ \ddot{x}_2(t) \end{pmatrix} = \begin{pmatrix} f_1(t) \\ f_2(t) \end{pmatrix} \tag{1}$$

where m is the effective mass at each end and $f_1(t)$ and $f_2(t)$ represent the forces applied at the two tympanal membranes. These two forces will have essentially identical amplitudes and very small phase differences due to the small amount of time it takes for sound to travel across the ears.

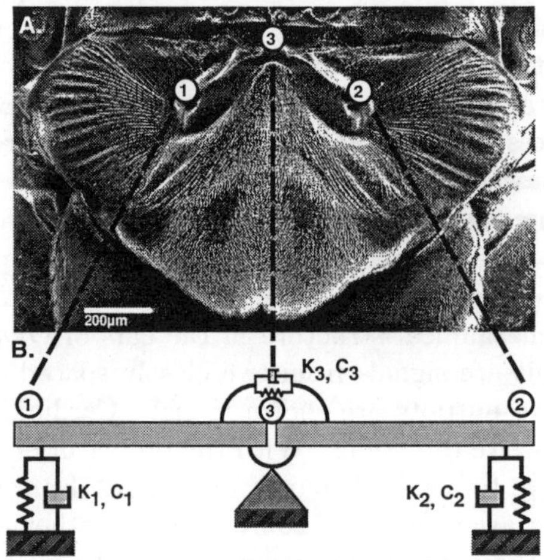

Figure 1. Ear of *Ormia ochracea* and mechanical model.

If the system is symmetric about the fulcrum then we can let $k_1 = k_2 = k$. The eigenvalues of the unforced, undamped system are found to be $\omega_1^2 = k/m$ and $\omega_2^2 = (k + 2k_3)/m$. The natural motion, or mode shape corresponding to the first eigenvalue, ω_1^2 is found to be $X_1 = -X_2$, so that the two coordinates move in opposite directions with equal magnitudes. The second mode shape, corresponding to ω_2^2 is $X_1 = X_2$ so that both tympana translate in the same manner. The directional sensitivity of the ears results from the combined responses of these two resonant modes. The parameters of the system are such that when sound arrives from one side, the responses of these two modes add on the ear closest to the source and they cancel on the ear furthest from the source. This will be shown in the following by manipulating equation (1).

If we consider the special case of excitation resulting from a plane, harmonic sound wave, the pressure at the pivot point may be written as $Pe^{\hat{i}\omega t}$, where $\hat{i} = \sqrt{-1}$. If $x_1(t)$ is the response of the ear closest to the sound source then

$$
\begin{aligned}
f_1(t) &= F_1 e^{\hat{i}\omega t} = Pse^{\hat{i}\omega(t+\frac{\tau}{2})} \\
f_2(t) &= F_2 e^{\hat{i}\omega t} = Pse^{\hat{i}\omega(t-\frac{\tau}{2})}
\end{aligned}
\tag{2}
$$

where s is the surface area of each tympanal membrane and τ is the transit time for the wave to travel between the two points of application of the force on the tympanal membranes. If the direction of propagation of the incident wave is at an angle ϕ relative to the fly's longitudinal axis, then the time delay between the ipsilateral and contralateral forces is $\tau = dsin(\phi)/c$, where d is the distance between the effective points of application of the force and c is the sound speed which is roughly 344 m/s. F_1 and F_2 are the complex amplitudes of the effective forces, $F_1 = Pse^{\hat{i}\omega\frac{\tau}{2}}$ and $F_2 = Pse^{-\hat{i}\omega\frac{\tau}{2}}$.

By manipulating equation (1), the response of each end of the tympanal bridge may be expressed as

$$
\begin{aligned}
x_1(t) &= \frac{e^{\hat{i}\omega t}}{2m}\left(\frac{F_1+F_2}{\omega_2^2-\omega^2+2\omega_2\xi_2\hat{i}\omega} - \frac{F_2-F_1}{\omega_1^2-\omega^2+2\omega_1\xi_1\hat{i}\omega}\right) \\
x_2(t) &= \frac{e^{\hat{i}\omega t}}{2m}\left(\frac{F_1+F_2}{\omega_2^2-\omega^2+2\omega_2\xi_2\hat{i}\omega} + \frac{F_2-F_1}{\omega_1^2-\omega^2+2\omega_1\xi_1\hat{i}\omega}\right),
\end{aligned}
\tag{3}
$$

where ξ_1 and ξ_1 are the damping ratios of the two modes. Examination of the numerator of each term in equation (3) shows that the responses $x_1(t)$ and $x_2(t)$ depend on combinations of the sum and difference of the forces on each side of the ear. The first mode (rocking mode) depends on the difference in the two forces while the second mode (translating mode) depends on the sum of the forces. The denominators in equation (3) determine the relative contribution of each mode and depend on the driving frequency ω. These terms represent the frequency response functions of the two modes. The mechanical system essentially combines the sums and differences of the pressures on the two ears in order to achieve a cancellation of the response on one side and an addition on the other. In the following, we will show that with the right set of parameters, a system having a response described by equation (3) will have a bi-cardioid directional response. An extensive comparison of measured results and predictions based on equation (3) has been presented by Miles, Robert

22

and Hoy[3]. It has been shown that the model gives excellent agreement with measurements.

In order to examine the sensitivity of the response to sound arriving from different directions we will replace F_1 and F_2 in equation (3) by the expressions in the discussion preceding equation (3). We will also assume that the system is operated in the frequency range near the rocking mode $\omega \approx \omega_1 \ll \omega_2$. Since $\omega \ll \omega_2$ the denominators of the first terms in equation (3) become approximately ω_2^2. Equation (3) may then be approximated by

$$
\begin{aligned}
x_1(t) &\approx \frac{sPe^{i\omega t}}{2m}\left(\frac{2\cos(\omega\tau/2)}{\omega_2^2} + \frac{\hat{i}\sin(\omega\tau/2)}{\omega_1\xi_1\hat{i}\omega}\right) \approx \frac{sPe^{i\omega t}}{m}\left(\frac{1}{\omega_2^2} + \frac{\tau}{4\omega_1\xi_1}\right) \\
x_2(t) &\approx \frac{sPe^{i\omega t}}{2m}\left(\frac{2\cos(\omega\tau/2)}{\omega_2^2} - \frac{\hat{i}\sin(\omega\tau/2)}{\omega_1\xi_1\hat{i}\omega}\right) \approx \frac{sPe^{i\omega t}}{m}\left(\frac{1}{\omega_2^2} - \frac{\tau}{4\omega_1\xi_1}\right)
\end{aligned}
\tag{4}
$$

where we have assumed that $\omega\tau/2 \ll 1$. From equation (4) we can see that if $\omega_2^2 \approx \frac{4\omega_1\xi_1}{d/c}$ then the responses of the two tympana as a function of the angle of incidence of the sound are

$$
\begin{aligned}
x_1(t) &\approx sP\frac{e^{i\omega t}}{m\omega_2^2}\left(1 + \sin(\phi)\right) \\
x_2(t) &\approx sP\frac{e^{i\omega t}}{m\omega_2^2}\left(1 - \sin(\phi)\right)
\end{aligned}
\tag{5}
$$

where we have again used the fact that $\tau = d\sin(\phi)/c$. Equations (5) show that the responses of the tympana $x_1(t)$ and $x_2(t)$ will have Cardioid directivity patterns which are oriented in opposite directions.

3   Biomimicry of the Ormiine Ear

Our analysis presented above shows that the mechanical system depicted in figure 1B performs signal processing of the sum and difference of the pressures acting on the two tympana. In order to illustrate how the system works, it is instructive to examine an "equivalent" electronic circuit which is shown in figure 2 below. The basic idea behind this "Equivalent Circuit Ormiaphone" is identical to that proposed by Blumlein [6,7] for recording stereo acoustic images using a pair of closely spaced microphones. In effect, the circuit converts very small phase differences at the two sensors, $f_1(t)$ and $f_2(t)$ into amplitude differences at the outputs, $y_1(t)$ and $y_2(t)$. This is a primary goal of most small directionally sensitive receivers.

The circuit first computes the sum and difference of the inputs, as in the numerators in equation (3). The difference signal is low-pass filtered and amplified so that the final outputs become analogous to the right side of equations (4) and (5). Note that the low-pass filter has the same effect as the frequency response of the rocking mode in equation (4) which is $\approx 1/(\omega_1\xi_1\hat{i}\omega)$.

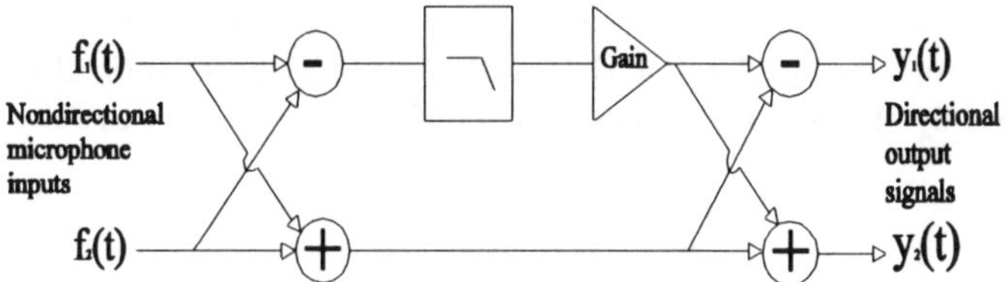

Figure 2. Block Diagram of Equivalent Circuit

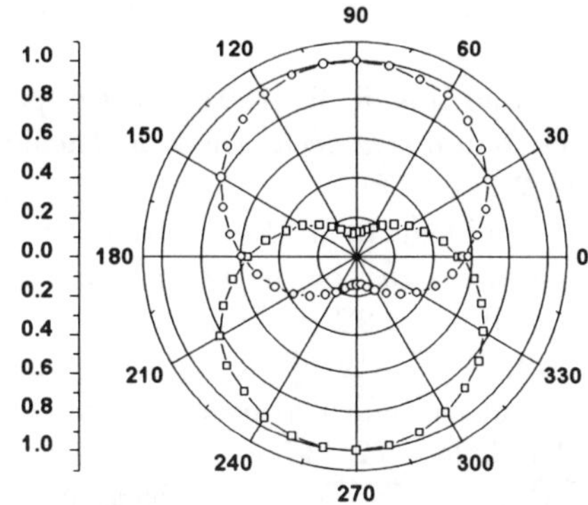

Figure 3. Equivalent Circuit Ormiaphone Directivity at 5kHz

The circuit shown in figure 2 has been built using operational amplifiers. Figure 3 shows measured directivities at 5kHz using this circuit. The omni-directional microphones used to provide the input signals were Brüel & Kjær model 4138 1/8 inch microphones placed .275 inch apart. The directivities are found to be Cardioid patterns which are oriented in opposite directions as predicted in equations (5).

4   Conclusions

A simple analytical model of the response of the ears of the parasitoid fly *Ormia ochracea* has been used to design an analog circuit which mimics the mechanism used by the fly to achieve directional sensitivity in a very small sensor. Measured results obtained using the circuit along with a pair of non-directional microphones are presented which show that the system achieves the desired bi-Cardioid directivity pattern.

5 Acknowledgments

R.N.M., T.T. and R.R.H. are supported by NSF Grant BCS9315854, D.R. and R.R.H. are supported by NINDCD-DC00103 and Hatch NYC191403, and D.R. is supported by the Swiss National Science Foundation and the Janggen-Pöhn Foundation.

References

1. Robert, D., Amoroso, J., and Hoy, R. R. [1992] The evolutionary convergence of hearing in a parasitoid fly and its cricket host. *Science* **258** 1135-1137.
2. Robert, D., Read, M. P., and Hoy, R. R. [1994] The tympanal hearing organ of the parasitoid fly *Ormia ochracea* (Diptera, Tachinidae, Ormiini) *Cell & Tissue Research* **275** 63–78.
3. Miles, R. N., Robert, R., and Hoy, R. R. [1995] Mechanically coupled ears for directional hearing in the parasitoid fly *Ormia ochracea*. *Journal of the Acoustical Society of America* **98** (6) 3059-3070.
4. Fletcher, N. H. and Hill, K. G. [1978] Acoustics of sound production and of hearing in the bladder cicada *Cystosoma saundersii (Westwood)*. *Journal of Experimental Biology* **72** 43-55.
5. Fletcher, N. H. [1992] *Acoustic Systems in Biology*. New York: Oxford University Press.
6. Blumlein, A. D., [1931] British patent 394,325. *Directional Effect in Sound Systems.*
7. Gerzon, M. A. [1994] Applications of Blumlein shuffling to stereo microphone techniques.*Journal of the Audio Engineering Society* **42** 435-453.

FLUID FLOW PROFILES MEASURED IN THE SUPRAORBITAL LATERAL LINE CANAL OF THE RUFF

P.S.K. TSANG, S.M. VAN NETTEN

Department of Biophysics, Nijenborgh 4, University of Groningen,
9747 AG Groningen, The Netherlands.
tsang@bcn.rug.nl

1   Introduction

Fishes detect water motion by means of a lateral line organ. One type of lateral line organ is located in recessed canals on the head of the fish. Water motion outside the fish is passed on via skin membranes[1] to canal fluid which in turn drives a number of dome shaped structures called cupulae. The cupular motion is sensed by stereocilia of hair cells attached to the base of the cupula[2]. The lateral line organ is easily accessible and thus offers the opportunity for the study of a sensitive hair cell organ in a relatively undisturbed natural condition.

Cupular motion in response to an oscillating stimulus sphere placed in the canal has been measured[3], but little data exist regarding the fluid flow within the canal. So far, the analyses of lateral line mechanics have neglected the influence of the canal wall assuming the flow driving the cupula to be spatially uniform[4]. Measurements of fluid motion in the lateral line canal of sprats using seeding particles have been conducted[5], but these were limited to a single point within the canal. Free floating seeding particles suffer from Brownian motion and convection, making them unsuitable for monitoring canal fluid flow at physiological stimulus levels. This led to the development of a sense probe, that follows the fluid motion, with a measuring volume fixed in place and sensitive enough to detect flow velocities down to the order of 1 μm/s.

To further our understanding of the stimulus transduction in the peripheral lateral line organ, the influence of the canal wall on the fluid stimulus, was studied.

2   Methods

The ruff [*Acerina cernua* (L)] used in these experiments were anesthetized by I.P. injection of Saffan (28 mg/kg) (Glaxo)[6] and placed in a small tank where they were fixed in position by head and body clamps.

The cephalic lateral line canals consist of skin covered cartilaginous canals approximately 1 mm deep and 1.8 mm wide with bony bridges covering the cupulae.

For the experiments, a small section of the skin above the supraorbital canal was removed to expose cupula (II) (following the notation of Jakubowski[7]) and the region just behind cupula (I). The experiments described here were performed in empty lateral line canals from which the epithelium and cupula (II) were removed, while the bony bridge above cupula (II) was left intact.

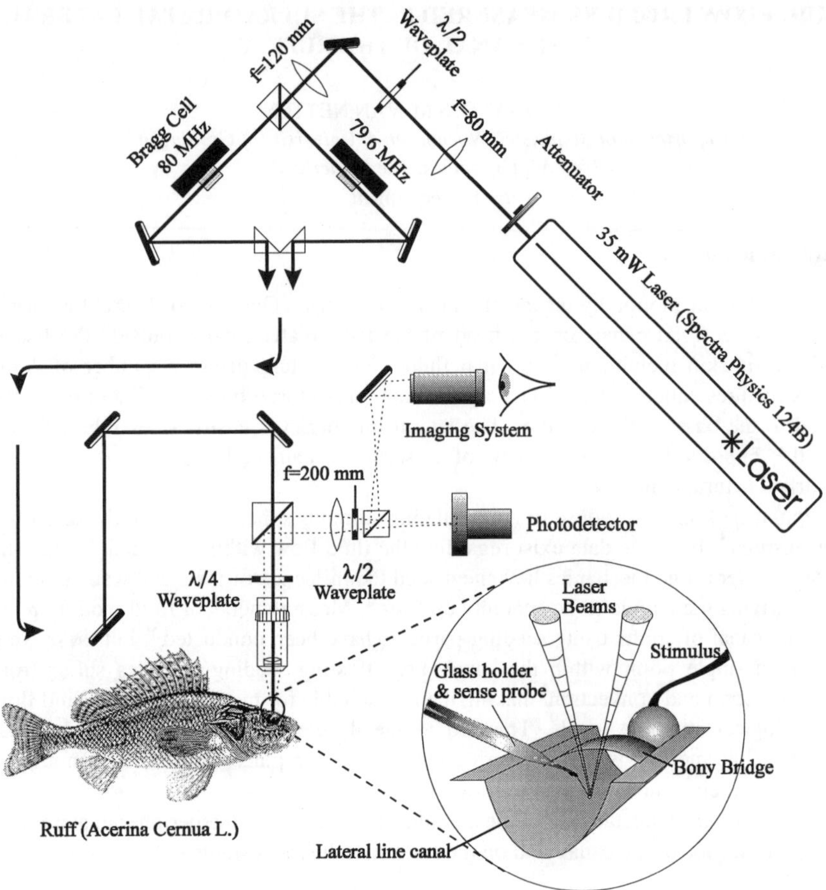

Figure 1: The laser interferometer used for the velocity measurements is very similar to the one described by van Netten[8]. The two laser beams emerge from the Bragg cells with an optical frequency difference of 400 kHz between them. They are directed via a series of mirrors through a polarizing beamsplitter and $\lambda/4$ waveplate before finally being brought to focus upon the surface of the sense probe. The sense probe, driven by the fluid flow, Doppler-shifts the laser light and some of the scattered light travels back along the optical axis and is focused onto the photodetector. An image of the sense probe can be redirected to the imaging system by adjusting the $\lambda/2$ waveplate.

To measure the fluid flow at a selected position within the canal, a sense probe consisting of a small sphere ($\varnothing$ 50 μm) attached to a highly flexible tapered borosilicate glass fibre was used. The glass fibre is around 2.5 mm long and has a diameter of about 4 µm (see Figure 1). The sense probe is mounted on a x,y,z positioner and can be positioned at any location in the fluid.

The positions of the canal walls and the bony bridge were determined by scanning the laser beams from one side to the other. The sense probe was then positioned in the midpoint of the canal at approximately 0.3 mm caudal from the bony bridge. A small stimulus sphere ($\varnothing$ 0.67 mm) driven by a piezoelectric stimulator was then placed on the other side of the bony bridge just behind cupula (I) in order to produce a sinusoidally changing fluid flow in the canal. The magnitude of the stimulus sphere's velocity was kept at 3.14 mm/s over the entire frequency range at which we measured. The velocity of the sense probe moving in response to the evoked fluid motion was measured with a heterodyne laser interferometer at different depths in the canal.

The sense probe was calibrated by measuring its response to a large ($\varnothing$ 4 mm) stimulus ball vibrating sinusoidally in free field, placed a few mm away from it, and found to be frequency independent as expected from theory[4]. In addition, these calibration measurements confirmed that, at the frequencies used, the sense probe's motion is equal to that of the calculated fluid motion to within a few percent (see Figure 2).

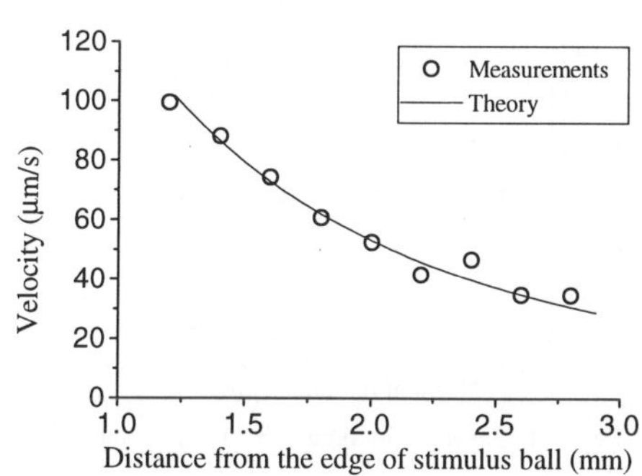

Figure 2. A plot of the free field water flow velocity as a function of horizontal distance away from the edge of the stimulus ball as measured with the sense probe. The stimulus ball has a radius of 2 mm and is vibrating at 10 Hz with an amplitude of 6.75 µm. The solid line is the velocity calculated from theory[4] and shows that the sense probe's motion is reliably following the fluid flow.

The fish was artificially respired with tap water throughout the duration of experiment. The flow of water was stopped during the measurements to avoid unwanted vibrations caused by the flow of water through the gills. The condition of the fish was checked periodically by looking at the blood flowing through the blood vessel inside the eye. The temperature of the surroundings was kept constant at 15°C throughout the duration of the experiment. This slowed the formation of air bubbles in the fish tank and reduced the production of fish slime in the canal.

3   Results

First, measurements were conducted in free field at the same positions with regard to the stimulus sphere and sense probe as to be used in the canal experiments, to be able to isolate the mechanical effects of the lateral line canal. The amplitude and phase of the fluid flow velocity in free field is shown in Figures 3 and 4 and has a fairly flat profile for all frequencies, as expected from calculations on the fluid field caused by a vibrating sphere in large fluid volume[4] for the geometry used.

These characteristics are to be compared with Figures 5 and 6 which show typical measurements in the lateral line canal at various depths and frequencies. For all the fishes investigated, the flow pattern measured in the empty lateral line canal is dependent on the frequency of the stimulus. The smallest separation between the sense probe and the canal floor is approximately 8 μm (allowing room for movement) and together with he radius of the sense probe (25 μm) this means that measurements started at a distance of 33 μm. Clearly, the profiles found in the lateral line canal differ significantly from those measured in free field (Figures 3 and 4), demonstrating that the canal plays an important role in shaping the actual stimulus to the cupula.

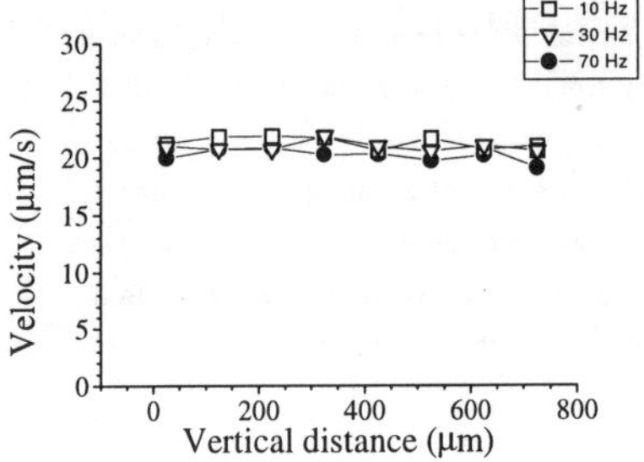

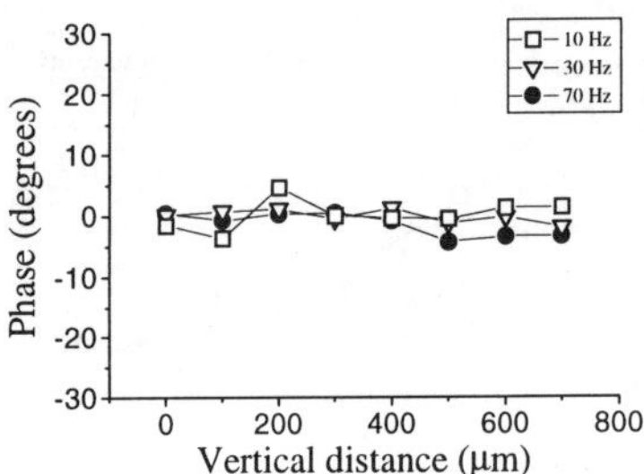

Figure 3. A plot of the velocity as a function of vertical distance from the bottom edge of the stimulus sphere as measured with the sense probe in free field at 2.5 mm away from the stimulus sphere for different stimulus frequencies. The data from 20, 40, 60 Hz were not plotted, since they do not significantly differ from the data plotted above.

Figure 4. Same as in Figure 3 but here the phase is shown.

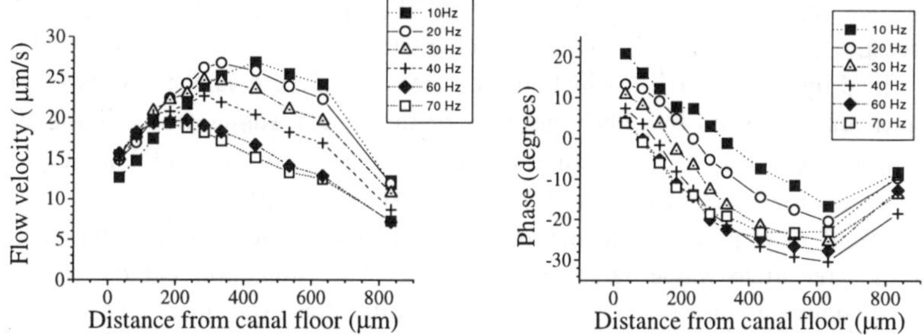

Figure 5. A plot of the velocities measured at different depths in the empty canal for a range of stimulus frequencies. The distance to the edge of the bony bridge is 0.3 mm.

Figure 6. Same as in Figure 5 but here phase is shown.

The maximum of the profile in the canal at 10 Hz is found at approximately 400 μm above the canal floor. As the stimulus frequency increases, the maximum gradually shifts to a value of about 150 μm at the higher frequencies used. When the frequency is increased even more, the profiles do not change significantly anymore from this (not shown).

The phase shown in Figure 6 is very different to that of Figure 4. There is a phase lead near the canal wall but, as the distance away from the floor is increased it changes to a phase lag. From 600 μm onwards, the phase is heading towards zero as the edge of the canal is approached (nearing free field). This was found for all the frequencies at which we measured. An increase in stimulus frequency has the effect of flattening the phase found at the mid region of the canal.

4   Discussion

The experimental results clearly indicate the influence of the lateral line canal's boundary layer. In contrast to measurements made in free field (Figures 3 and 4), the profiles measured in the lateral line canal (Figures 5 and 6) not only show a dependence on vertical distance but also depend on stimulus frequency.

To further characterise the effect of the lateral line canal wall on the fluid flow, the experimental results can be compared with two extreme models that may simulate the canal wall. One model consists of fluid flowing past an (infinite) plate, while the other model considered is fluid flow inside an (infinitely) long tube with radius r. Clearly, the behavior of lateral line canal fluid is expected to behave in an intermediate fashion, since the lateral line canal consists of grooves recessed in bone and is, at least in a hydrodynamic sense, partially open because of the existence of the skin covered openings in the bone. Moreover, during measurements the skin covering these openings was removed.

The fluid velocities in both models can be solved in analytical terms[9] for (spatially) constant pressure gradients and both can be characterised by an a.c. boundary layer thickness defined by $\delta=(2\mu/\omega\rho)^{1/2}$, which gives a measure of the distance over which the fluid is significantly affected by either the plate or the tube's wall. Here, μ is the fluid viscosity (1mPa s for water), ω is the stimulus frequency and ρ is the fluid density (1000 kg/m^3). This yields for δ approximately 180 μm at 10 Hz and 70 μm at 70 Hz.

The a.c. fluid flow past a plate monotonically increases from zero at the plate's surface, to the free field value far from the plate. This transition occurs within a characteristic distance equal to d. This behavior is unlike the experimental results. The profiles measured show maxima over the canal cross-section, similar to the behavior of fluid in tubes. The measured shift of the maximum to the canal floor, as frequency increases, follows the pattern in a long tube in which at low frequencies the profile is parabolic with a maximum in the centre. At high frequencies the profile has a ring-like shape with maxima not in the centre but at a frequency dependent distance from the wall given by[9,10,11]: D_{max} =2.28·δ. Substituting the high stimulus frequency we used (70 Hz), results in 150 μm which is comparable to the position of the maxima found in the lateral line canal at this frequency. Thus, although the canal was open during the measurements, the profiles measured compare favourably with that of a long closed tube.

5   Conclusions

The novel method we employ for *in vivo* flow measurement is sensitive enough to detect velocities down to 1 μm/s at a spatial resolution of 50 microns.

The flow profiles obtained for an empty lateral line canal clearly demonstrate that the cupula receives a stimulus deviating from a flat profile which is also frequency dependent. The fluid flow in the canal is comparable to that in a long tube. The stimulus to the cupula, therefore, is controlled by the boundary layer of the canal. Experiments are now underway to investigate the flow profile and boundary layer generated by the integral structure of canal wall and cupula.

An interesting consequence of the position of the profile maxima found in the lateral line canal, may be that to detect frequencies below 100 Hz, the canal cupulae should extend to at least 150 μm from the canal floor into the fluid to benefit from the maxima in flow velocity. This condition is certainly met in the case of the ruff where the cupulae have an average height of approximately 600 μm.

Acknowledgments

We are very grateful to Prof. H. Duifhuis, P.W.J van Hengel, C. J. Kros, M.P.M.G. van den Raadt and J.E.C Wiersinga-Post for their comments on an earlier version of this manuscript. This research was funded by Netherlands Organisation for Scientific Research (NWO).

References

1. Netten, S.M. van and Maarseveen, J.Th.P.W. van (1994) Mechanophysiological properties of the supraorbital lateral line canal in ruffe (Acerina cernua L.) *Proc. R. Soc. Lond. B* **256,** 239-246.
2. Kroese, A.B.A. and Netten, S.M. van (1989) Hair cell transduction *The mechanosensory lateral line* (Neurobiology and evolution) (ed. by S. Coombs, P. Görner and H. Münz), pp. 265-284 Springer-Verlag.
3. Netten, S.M. van and Kroese, A. B. A. (1987) Laser interferometric measurements on the dynamic behaviour of the cupula in the fish lateral line. *Hearing Res.* **29,** 55-61.
4. Netten, S.M. van (1991). Hydrodynamics of the excitation of the cupula in the fish canal lateral line. *J. Acoust. Soc. Am.* **89,** 310-319.
5. Denton, E.J. and Gray, J.A.B (1983) Mechanical factors in the excitation of clupeid lateral lines. *Proc. R. Soc. Lond. Biol. Sci.,* **218**: 1-26.
6. Oswald, R.L. (1978) Injection anaesthesia for experimental studies in fish. *Comp. Biochem. Physiol.* **60C,** 19-26.
7. Jakubowski, M. (1963). Cutaneous sense organs of fishes. I. The lateral-line organs in the stone-perch (Acerina cernua L.), *Acta Biol. Cracoveniensia, Zool.* **6,** 59-82.
8. Netten, S.M van (1988) Laser interferometer microscope for the measurement of nanometer vibrational displacements of a light-scattering microscopic object. *J. Acoust. Soc. Am.* **83,** 1667-1674.
9. Schlichting, H. (1960). *Boundary-layer theory* (McGraw-Hill Publishing Company, New York).
10. Sexl, T. (1930) Über den von E.G. Richardson entdeckten "Annulareffekt". *Z.Phys.* **61,** 349-362.
11. Womersley, J.R., (1955) Method for the calculation of velocity, rate of flow and viscous drag in arteries when the pressure gradient is known, *J. Physiol.* **127,** 553-563.

DIVERSITY IN HEARING-ORGAN STRUCTURE AND THE CHARACTERISTICS OF SPONTANEOUS OTOACOUSTIC EMISSIONS IN LIZARDS

G. A. MANLEY

Institut für Zoologie der Technischen Universität München, Lichtenbergstr. 4
85747 Garching, Germany.
GAM@cip1.zoo.chemie.tu-muenchen.de

Due to the great diversity of their hearing organs, lizards are perhaps the best group in which to relate SPOAE characteristics to structural patterns. Here, we compare data from 8 species of lizards from 6 families having different evolutionary status. All species regularly show SPOAE in the frequency range from about 1 kHz up to 4 to 7 kHz. We assume these originate in the high-frequency, bidirectionally-oriented segment of the papillae. There are two groups of species with regard to SPOAE characteristics. One group ("unspecialized") is made up of the monitor lizard and the two teiid lizards, the other ("specialized") consists of the remaining species. Both the spectral patterns of SPOAE and the degree of temperature dependence correlate with inner-ear structure: The specialized tectorial structures of geckos and skinks and those papillae lacking a tectorial membrane correlate with smaller SPOAE that show smaller temperature shifts. In contrast, the relatively unspecialized, simpler papillar structure in teiids and varanids, with a continuous tectorial membrane, correlates with fewer, larger SPOAE with greater temperature dependence. This greater dependence may be due to strong coupling through the tectorial membrane of hair cells that represent a greater frequency range.

1 Introduction

Spontaneous otoacoustic emissions (SPOAE) are faint sounds emitted from the inner ear and generated by the sensory hair cells. It is assumed in this paper that the SPOAE in lizards are generated by hair cells whose best acoustic sensitivity lies at the SPOAE frequency.[1,2] The measurement of suppression thresholds in SPOAE in lizards provides the same information about frequency selectivity and sensitivity of the inner ear as single-cell recordings from auditory neurons.[1]

To date, models of SPOAE behavior were tailored to the special features of the mammalian cochlea. However, SPOAE have been described in all classes of terrestrial vertebrates, in spite of great anatomical differences between their inner ears. SPOAE have been described from amphibians,[3] reptiles[1], birds[4] as well as for mammals.[5] As hair cells constitute one of the few common morphological attributes of these different hearing organs, it can be assumed that active force generation by hair cells is an evolutionarily old feature.[6] It is thus legitimate to compare SPOAE across species and larger groupings and ask the question as to the origin of the few differences between them.

At present, it is not clear why SPOAE are only measurable at specific frequencies, and data derived from different animal classes that have anatomically-different hearing organs can help resolve this question. In this respect, lizard hearing organs are the most interesting, as they show both the greatest morphological variation in hearing-organ structure among amniotes and also the consistent presence of SPOAE. The present work was undertaken to investigate whether the patterns of SPOAE in eight species of lizards correlate with peculiarities of the species-specific hearing-organ anatomy.[7-11] Structurally, the basilar papillae of these eight species fall into three classes.

♦ In iguanid and anguid lizards, the presumptive hair-cell area generating SPOAE completely lacks a tectorial membrane.[9,11]

♦ In the two geckos and the bobtail skink, part or all of the high-frequency area is covered by a chain of sallets (small, local pieces of tectorial material).[7-11]

♦ In the teiid lizards and the monitor lizard, the high-frequency area is covered by a continuous tectorial membrane.[9,11]

2 Methods

Data were collected from an iguanid (*Anolis sagrei*, the Bahamas anole), an anguid lizard (*Gerrhonotus leiocephalus*, the Texas alligator lizard), two teiid species (*Callopistes maculatus*, the Chile tegu and *Tupinambis teguixin*, the gold tegu), and a monitor lizard (*Varanus exanthimaticus*). Published data from two gecko species (*Gekko gecko*, the Tokay gecko, and *Eublepharis macularius*, the leopard gecko,[12] and a skink[1,2,13] (*Tiliqua rugosa*, the bobtail lizard) have also been incorporated for comparison, making eight species in all.

Spontaneous otoacoustic emissions (SPOAE) were measured with the animals kept under light anesthesia in a sound-attenuated chamber and using a closed, sensitive microphone system coupled to their external ear canal. The animal's head was gently held using narrow "Velcro" strips. The animals breathed unaided and recovered completely within a few hours following the measurements. The microphone signal was fed to a spectrum analyzer (HP 3561A or Stanford 760) that performed a fast Fourier transformation and an average of 30 - 500 RMS spectra. The frequency range measured was usually from 0.5 to 6.75 kHz. Under these conditions, the noise floor of the system was -6 to -9 dB SPL. All measurements were corrected for the characteristics of the coupler.

Frequency spectra of the sound field in the external auditory meatus were measured at different body temperatures. Body temperature was monitored using a small calibrated temperature sensor in the animal's mouth and was controlled and varied slowly and systematically using a regulated heating blanket and a warming lamp driven via a regulated transformer and placed 35 cm above the animal. Cooling was mostly passive, but occasionally assisted by an ice bag over the animal's back. The range of temperatures used was species-specific, as SPOAE were only present within a certain temperature range.

3 Results

Peaks in the averaged spectra were identified as SPOAE when they were temperature-sensitive and suppressible by external tones. SPOAE were found in a very high percentage of ears, mostly between 1.0 and 5.0 kHz. The two gekkonids, the skink, the iguanid and the anguid lizards averaged between 4 and 15 small SPOAE per ear while the two tegus and the monitor lizards had between two and six SPOAE that were of higher amplitude, in each ear (Fig. 1, Table 1).

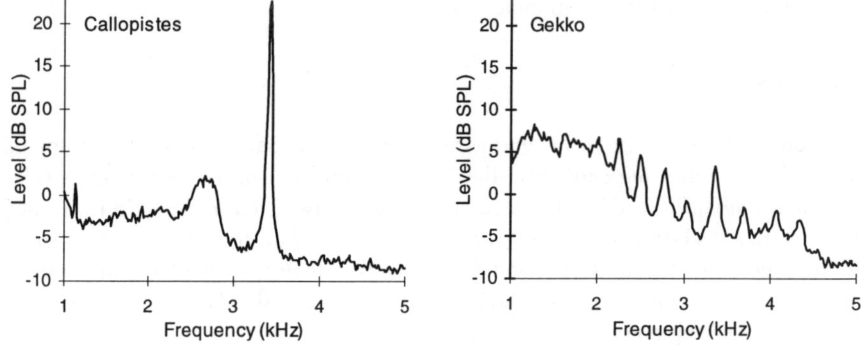

Fig. 1. Representative everaged spectra from the ear canal of (left) the teiid lizard *Callopistes* and (right) the gekkonid lizard *Gekko*.

The SPOAE of all species showed principally the same behavior during a change of temperature, their frequency shifting to higher frequencies when the animals were warmed and to lower frequencies when cooled, but the rate of change was somewhat species-specific (Table 1, Fig. 2).

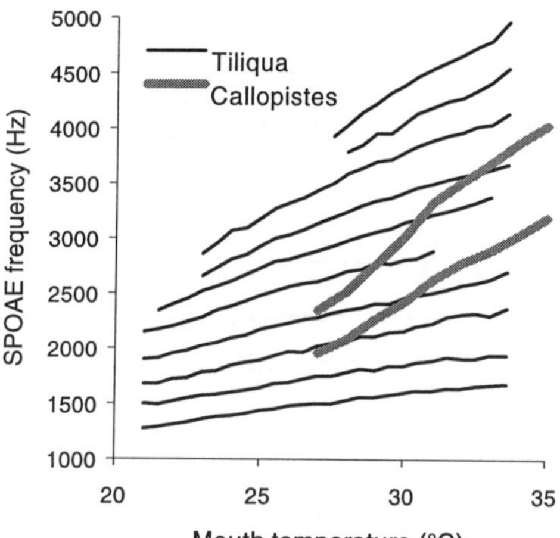

Fig. 2. Change of SPOAE center frequency in (thin continuous lines) one ear canal of the skink *Tiliqua* and (thick continuous lines) an ear canal of the teiid *Callopistes* as a function of temperature.

The spectral patterns, however, of the SPOAE fell into two groups that differed in two main respects: (Table 1)

a) SPOAE amplitudes in the two tegu species and the monitor lizard - the species with an unspecialized papilla - were higher (up to 27 dB SPL).

b) The temperature dependence of the SPOAE frequency was two to three times higher in the tegus and monitor lizard. The average shift of SPOAE frequency in species with specialized papillae was about 60Hz/°C (or 0.015 to 0.06 oct./°C). In unspecialized papillae, however, these values were 100 to 180 Hz/°C, or about 0.055 to 0.1 oct/°C (Fig. 3, Table 1, bottom three - grey - rows).

Table 1: Characteristics of SPOAE in eight species of lizards

Species (number of specimens)	% of ears emitting	Average nr. SPOAE per emitting ear	SPOAE-ampl. [dB SPL] min	max	Frequency shift, oct/°C at 28-30°C
Anolis (6)	100	7	-7.2	4.7	0.02
Gerrhonotus (2)	100	6	-7	3.1	0.035
Gekko (7)	100	12	-6	10.3	0.035
Eublepharis (9)	72	4	-6.6	4.9	0.03
Tiliqua (18)	86	10	-10	9.3	0.03
Varanus (7)	100	5 - 6	-6	27	0.055
Tupinambis (2)	100	7	-7	11.4	0.08
Callopistes (8)	100	2 - 3	-4.5	23.3	0.1

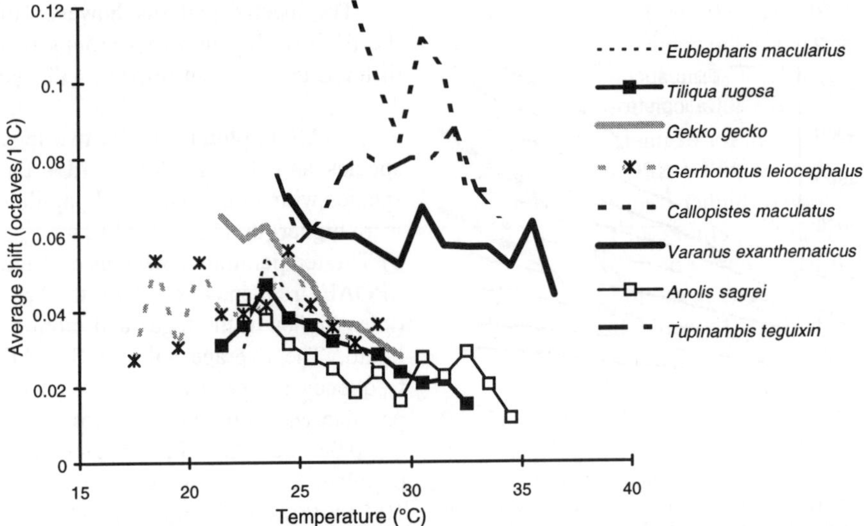

Fig. 3. Average frequency shifts within 1°C temperature steps for all SPOAE in eight species of lizards. The three upper curves are derived from the three most unspecialized papillae (one monitor lizard and two teiid lizards). See also ARO meeting 1996, abstract number 726.

4 Discussion

What might be responsible for the differences in amplitude and in temperature dependence between species? One possibility lies in the structure of the tectorial membrane (TM). In the high-frequency segment of the unspecialized species, a TM is present, continuous and not subdivided. In contrast, the geckos, skinks, iguanids and anguids, while not closely related, show a specialized TM structure, it being either fully or partially divided into a chain of sallets or completely missing. How might this difference in TM structure explain the number and amplitude of SPOAE?

It can be assumed that in hair-cell areas without aTM, but also in areas with sallets, the longitudinal coupling between hair cells is very weak to weak. In such areas, SPOAE would presumably be generated by quite small groups of hair cells. Our calculations in *Anolis* (Gallo and Manley, unpublished) indicate that between 2 and 30 hair cells produce each emission. This implies that in strongly-coupled areas, in contrast, the large SPOAE are produced by a larger group of hair cells. For the same space constant of the distribution of frequencies in the papilla, the natural resonance frequencies of hair-cell groups within strongly-coupled areas would differ more than in groups from less-well-coupled hair-cell areas. This aspect must be considered in the context of the temperature-dependence of SPOAE amplitudes.

In at least some species, higher-frequency emissions can be measured at higher temperatures than can lower-frequency emissions, and vice-versa. In the Bobtail skink *Tiliqua*, for example, the preferred temperature of 2 kHz-SPOAE is 4°C lower than that of 4 kHz-SPOAE.[13] This implies that higher temperatures favour the amplitude of higher-frequency components in emissions and vice-versa. The greater shift with temperature of the strongly-coupled regions found in more unspecialized lizard papillae may be due to the fact that at lower temperatures, the power produced by the hair cells in the lower-frequency part of the coupled hair-cell area producing a given SPOAE would be greater than the power produced by hair cells in the higher-frequency part. The lower-frequency cells would thus determine the center frequency of the SPOAE. At higher temperatures, the reverse would be true. Thus the shift of the center frequency of such SPOAE with temperature would have an added component (over and above the putative viscosity effect seen in the other species) that is due to the shift of dominance among the hair cells within the coupled group. It is also possible that the entire coupled hair-cell group shows a net shift of position along the papilla, accompanied by an equivalent change in frequency.

This idea is compatible with the amplitude differences described above. The greater amplitudes of SPOAE in unspecialized species implies that they are generated by a larger number of hair cells. If the frequency-space constants are the same in equivalently-sized unspecialized and advanced papillae, the coupled hair-cell groups of each SPOAE would cover a larger range of resonance frequencies in species with a continuous TM. Among the three species studied here that belong to the unspecialized group, *Callopistes* has the smallest papilla (0.85 mm in length), and thus the smallest space constant (estimated to be 0.3 mm/octave). The gold Tegu *Tupinambis* has the next larger papilla (1.4 mm; space constant estimated to be 0.6 mm/oct.), and the monitor lizard *Varanus* the largest (2.1 mm; space constant up to 1 mm/oct.[14]). The magnitude of the temperature shifts in unspecialized papillae correlates with this size order; the smallest shift (in *Varanus*) correlates with the largest space constant and thus presumably greater similarity in center frequency of the coupled hair-cell populations producing SPOAE.

Acknowledgements

Supported by the Deutsche Forschungsgemeinschaft within the program of the SFB 204 (Gehör). I thank Christine Köppl, Lothar Gallo, Andrea Pavusa and several undergraduate students for assistance with data collection, for giving me access to unpublished data and for critical comments on an earlier version of the manuscript.

References

1. Köppl, C. and Manley, G.A. (1993) Spontaneous otoacoustic emissions in the bobtail lizard. I. General characteristics, *Hear. Res.* **71** 157-169.
2. Köppl, C. and Manley, G.A. (1994) Spontaneous otoacoustic emissions in the bobtail lizard. II. Interactions with external tones, *Hear. Res.* **72** 159-170.
3. van Dijk, P, Wit, H.P. and Segenhout, J.M. (1989) Spontaneous otoacoustic emissions in the European edible frog (Rana esculenta): Spectral details and temperature dependence, *Hear. Res.* **42** 273-282.
4. Manley, G.A. and Taschenberger, G. (1993) Spontaneous otoacoustic emissions from a bird: A preliminary report, in *Biophysics of hair cell sensory systems*, eds. H. Duifhuis, J.W. Horst, P. van Dijk and S.M. van Netten (World Scientific, Singapore) pp. 33-39.
5. Probst, R, Lonsbury-Martin, B.L. and Martin, G.K. (1991) A review of otoacoustic emissions, *J. Acoust. Soc. Amer.* **89** 2027-2067.
6. Köppl, C. (1995) Otoacoustic emissions as an indicator for active cochlear mechanics: A primitive property of vertebrate auditory organs, in *Advances in Hearing Research*, eds. G.A. Manley, G.M. Klump, C. Köppl, H. Fastl, H. Oeckinghaus (World Scientific, Singapore), pp. 207-216.
7. Köppl, C. (1988) Morphology of the basilar papilla of the bobtail lizard, Tiliqua rugosa, *Hear. Res.* **35** 209-228.
8. Köppl, C. and Authier, S. (1995) Quantitative anatomical basis for a model of micromechanical frequency tuning in the Tokay gecko (Gekko gecko), *Hear. Res.* **82** 1-13.
9. Miller, M. (1973a) Scanning electron microscope studies of some lizard basilar papillae, *Am. J. Anat.* **138** 301-330.
10. Miller, M. (1973b) A scanning electron microscope study of the papilla basilaris of Gekko gecko, *Z. Zellforsch.* **136**, 307-328
11. Wever, E.G., (1978) *The Reptile Ear.* (Princeton Univ Press, Princeton N.J).
12. Manley, G.A, Gallo, L. and Köppl, C. (1996) Spontaneous otoacoustic emissions in two gecko species, Gekko gecko and Eublepharis macularius, *J. Acoust. Soc. Amer.* in press.
13. Manley, G.A. and Köppl, C. (1994)) Spontaneous otoacoustic emissions in the bobtail lizard. III. Temperature effects, *Hear. Res.* **72** 171-180.
14. Manley, G.A. (1990) *Peripheral hearing mechanisms in reptiles and birds*, (Springer Verlag, Berlin, Heidelberg).

COMPARISON OF DISTORTION PRODUCT OTOACOUSTIC EMISSIONS IN HUMANS AND KANGAROO RATS

G.R. LONG, L.A. SHAFFER

Department of Audiology and Speech Sciences

C.L. TALMADGE, P. PISKORSKI

Department of Physics, Purdue University, West Lafayette, IN 47907

The banner-tailed kangaroo rat (Dipodomys spectabilis) and Merriams kangaroo rat (Dipodomys Merriami) are Heteromyid rodents that have evolved in the North American desert and have developed auditory specializations that permit them to detect low frequency sound. Identical paradigms have been used to collect distortion product otoacoustic emissions (DPOAEs) in humans and kangaroo rats. A large number of DPOAEs can be detected in the kangaroo rat and the difference tones (nf2-nf1) can be as large as the more commonly investigated 2f1-f2 DPOAE. In addition to the larger number of DPOAEs in the kangaroo rats, other differences in the DPOAEs have been observed. 1) There is little evidence for DPOAE fine structure in kangaroo rats. 2) The range of f2/f1 ratios producing detectable DPOAEs is much wider in kangaroo rats.

1 Introduction

Models of DPOAE generation should be able to account for inter-species differences in DPOAE levels in the ear canal. In order to ensure that any differences are not due to the experimental paradigms, the data in both species should be obtained using the same paradigms. We present preliminary data from humans and kangaroo rats. Kangaroo rats are members of the genus Dipodomys, the Heteromyid rodents that are native to the deserts of North America. The Heteromyid family encompasses six genera of rodents that are native to North, Central and South America, including the kangaroo rat. Banner-tailed kangaroo rats communicate at a distance by foot drumming, producing low frequency sound.[1] Both kangaroo rat species have developed auditory specializations that permit them to detect low frequency sound.[2]

The middle ear space of the genus Dipodomys is hypertrophied suggesting a reduced stiffness of the middle ear system. Further stiffness reductions include a thinning of the tympanic membrane and the annular ligament, fewer ligaments supporting the ossicular chain, and the reduced size of tendinous attachments to the tensor tympani.[2] Despite the significant size difference, Merriams kangaroo rats and man are sensitive to a similar range of frequencies.[3] In both species, the middle ear transmission of low frequencies is determined primarily by the stiffness of the tympanic membrane and ossicles, in contrast to the gerbil and chinchilla where the major determinant of the low frequency transmission is the volume of the middle ear cavities.[4] Both the kangaroo rat and the gerbil show similar basilar membrane specializations including a thickening of the zona pectinata and hypertrophy of the Hensen's cells[5]. Basilar membrane thickness in Dipodomys is, however, graded with a maximum height of the organ of corti occurring in the second cochlear turn.[5]

2 Method

The stimuli were generated and controlled by a NeXT workstation, attenuated by 2 TDT PA4 programmable attenuators, passed through TDT HB6 headphone buffers and transduced by two Etymotic Research ER-2 tube-phones connected to an ER-10 microphone assembly. The ear canal signals were detected by an ER 10 microphone and filtered (300 Hz - 10 kHz) using a Stanford Research SR-560 amplifier. The output signal from the SR-560 was digitized using a Singular Solutions A/D 64x. Offline analysis of the signals was performed using least-squares-fit (LSF) filters to extract the amplitude and phase of the DPOAEs from the stored signals. An algorithm based on alternating summation and subtraction of data segments separates the signal component from the noise, which is uncorrelated with the signal, and provides an estimate of the noise floor at the frequency of the DPOAE. Overlapping of data segments of 1/6 of the total signal increased the effective number of averages.

The human subjects were seated in a reclining chair in an IAC Booth. The ER10 assembly was positioned in the ear canal using a GSI-33 ear tip. The kangaroo rats were anesthetized by intraperitoneal or subcutaneous injection of ketamine (90 mg/kg) and xylazene (10 mg/kg). The probe assembly was extended into the ear canal using a GSI-33 ear tip and the position of the assembly was stabilized using ear mold material.

3 Results

Representative data are presented in Figure 1 which illustrate the differences in DPOAE levels in kangaroo rats and human subjects. In both species F1 was fixed at 3000Hz and F2 varied (L1=L2=65 dB SPL). DPOAE in both species of kangaroo rats showed the same pattern and were optimal at this frequency. This was also an optimal frequency for this human subject. Only one difference tone was detectable in the human subject and the level was optimal near 800Hz. Many difference tones were discriminable in the kangaroo rat and the level was optimal near the same frequency as the nf1-f2 DPOAE, a similarity not seen with primaries at other frequencies. DPOAE are visible over a more limited frequency range in humans. A similar frequency range is represented on a much shorter basilar membrane in kangaroo rats (9 mm vs 35mm).[6] This may underlie the sharper filtering seen in the human data.

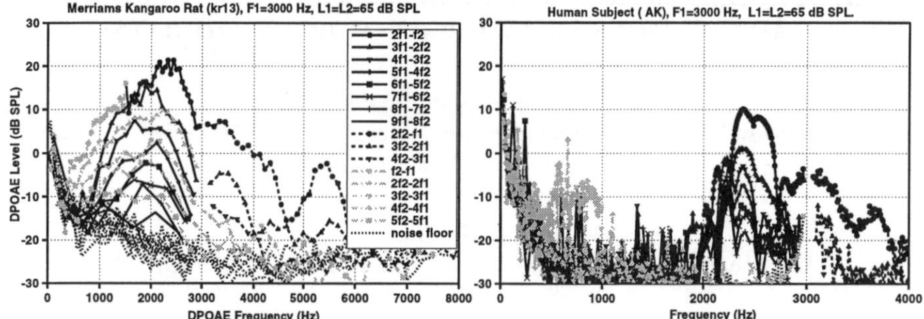

Figure 1: Comparison of DPOAE level in a merriams kangaroo rat and a human subject. Note that the same stimuli were used in both cases and that the abscissa on the human data covers half the frequency range of that used for the kangaroo rat data.

Acknowledgments

Some of the research was supported by NIDCD. We wish to thank Dr.Peter Waser and the Biology Department at Purdue University for the help in obtaining and maintaining the kangaroo rats.

References

1. Randall, J.A. (1993). Behavioural adaptations of desert rodents (heteromyidae), *Anim. Behav.* **45**, 263–287.

2. Webster, D.B. and Webster, M. (1975). Auditory systems of Heteromyidae: functional morphology and evolution of the middle ear, *J. Morph.* **146**, 343–376.

3. Heffner, H.E. and Masterton, B. (1990). Hearing in glires: Domestic rabbit, cotton rat, house mouse, and kangaroo rat, *J. Acoust. Soc. Am.***68**, 1584–1599

4. Rosowski, J.J. (1994). Outer and middle ears, In *Auditory Research, Volume IV – Comparative Mammalian Hearing*, ed. A. Popper and R.R. Fay (Springer-Verlag).

5. Webster, D.B. and Webster, M (1977). Auditory systems of Heteromyidae: cochlear diversity, *J. Morph.* **152**, 153–170, 1977.

6. S.M. Echteler, R.R.Fay, and A.N. Popper. Structure of the mammalian cochlea, In A. Popper and R.R. Fay, editors, *Auditory Research. Volume IV - Comparative Mammalian Hearing.* Springer-Verlag, 1994.

ACOUSTIC DISTORTION-PRODUCTS AS INDICATOR OF COCHLEAR ADAPTATIONS IN JAMAICAN MORMOOPID BATS

M. KÖSSL, G. FRANK, M. FAULSTICH

Zoologisches Institut, Universität München, Luisenstr.14, 80333 München, Germany
email: koessl@zi.biologie.uni-muenchen.de

I.J. RUSSELL

School of Biology, University of Sussex, Falmer, Brighton, BN19QG, U.K.

To study evolutionary adaptations in nonlinear cochlear mechanics, we recorded acoustic distortion-products in three closely related bat species of the mormoopid family. For f2-frequencies between 10-110 kHz, the best frequency ratio f2/f1 and distortion threshold curves were measured. The mustached bat, *Pteronotus parnellii* uses constant frequency (CF) calls with the dominant harmonic (CF2) at about 61 kHz. Just above the 2nd and 3rd CF-component of the call (at 62 and 93 kHz), extremely small best ratios close to 1.0005 and distinct maxima and minima of the distortion thresholds are found. These features that reflect the presence of a sharply tuned cochlear resonator are absent in *Pteronotus quadridens* and *Mormoops blainvillii*, two species that employ broadband frequency-modulated (FM) calls. Instead, they have broad threshold curves with high sensitivity between 30-50 kHz and the best ratios are between 1.08 to 1.4. It appears as if cochlear development towards enhanced frequency tuning in CF-bats has involved major cochlear redesign within a relatively short evolutionary time scale.

1 Introduction

In terms of their echolocation strategy, insectivorous microchiroptera can be divided into FM-bats that use broadband signals and CF-FM-bats whose calls consist of a long pure tone component followed by a short FM signal. The latter type of call is seen as an adaptation for hunting within densely cluttered environment [1]. Slight frequency modulations in the CF-echo, caused by insect wingbeat are used as cue to identify the prey against reflections from surrounding leaves.

The mustached bat, *Pteronotus parnellii* is the only new world CF-FM-bat species known. To resolve the echo-frequency modulations, in the cochlea an expanded region is dedicated to process a small frequency range centered around 62 kHz. A cochlear resonator evident in basilar membrane motion and from strong evoked and spontaneous otoacoustic emissions [2,3] produces enhanced neuronal tuning at 62 kHz with Q10dB values up to 400 [4]. Acoustic distortion-products are characterized by extremely small best ratios f2/f1 at 62 and at 93 kHz [3]. At 93 kHz, enhanced neuronal tuning is also present. Therefore, distortion measurement allows the noninvasive monitoring of high mechanical frequency separation in the cochlea. To address the question how these cochlear filters dedicated to biologically important frequencies have evolved, we measured distortion-products characteristics in two close relatives of the mustached bat.

2   Materials and Methods

Mormoops blainvillii and *Pteronotus quadridens* are fragile bats that would not survive longer transport. We measured the distortion-products in Jamaica using a Notebook PC with a Dockingstation as portable setup. A Microstar DAP 3200e/415 DSP-board with 12 bit A/D and D/A converters was used to generate two sinusoids and to record the microphone signal (sampling rates of 250-500 kHz per channel). For analysis of echolocation calls, several seconds of call sequence, recorded with an Ultra-Sound-Advice S-25 bat detector sensitive up to 200 kHz, were stored to the onboard RAM and displayed online. The program environment was developed in ASYST (Keithley). Two B&K 4135 microphone capsules were used as speakers and a B&K 4133 microphone connected to a B&K 2660 preamplifier recorded the cochlear response. The setup included programmable attenuators and a measuring amplifier that were designed and built by Jim Hartley, University of Sussex. The measuring amplifier proved to have extremely low noise levels and therefore replaced a B&K 2610 amplifier that was used initially. With line-spectra generated by the DSP-board, the sound system was calibrated in situ for constant sound pressure level at the microphone membrane. A coupler was introduced into the ear canal of gently restrained awake bats. Its tip was placed within a few hundred µm distance to the tympanum.

3   Results

Examples of echolocation signals from the three mormoopid bat species, measured from bats resting in a cage, are shown in Fig.1. The calls are similar to those described by Schnitzler et al. [5]. *Mormoops blainvillii*, the antillean ghost-faced bat, emits short downward FM calls containing several harmonics. The FM starting frequencies of the lower harmonics are close to 35, 70, and 105 kHz. *Pteronotus quadridens*, the sooty mustached bat, emits FM-pulses that in about half of the cases were preceded by a short CF-component (Fig.1). The CF/FM starting frequencies were at about 40, 80 and 120 kHz. The call of *Pteronotus parnellii* is much longer and contains a narrow CF component of 20-30 ms duration at about 30, 60, 90 and 120 kHz.

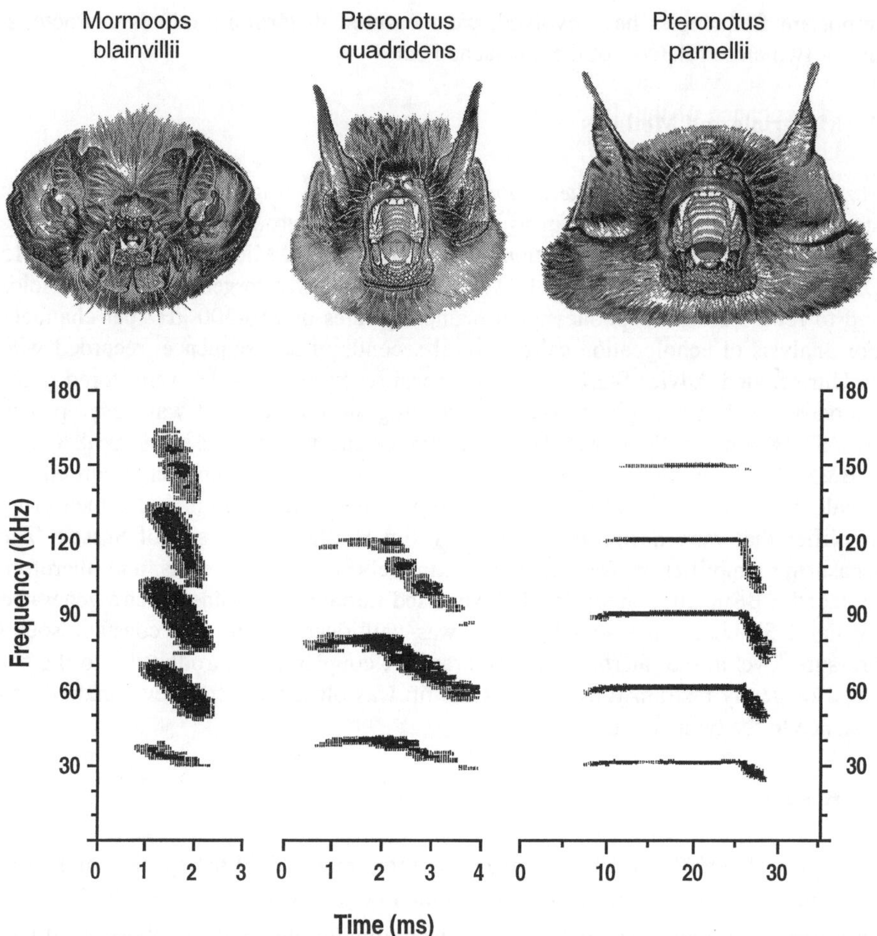

Fig.1   Sonargrams from single echolocation calls of the three mormoopid bat species. The faces were digitized from drawings of Silva Taboada [6].

Acoustic 2f1-f2 distortions were measured during stimulation with two primary pure tone stimuli f1 and f2. The data are referenced to the f2 frequency since it is assumed that the distortions are generated by nonlinear properties of outer hair cells located close to the f2 place in the cochlea [7]. The level of the lower primary f1 was always 10 dB above that of f2. In the mustached bat, this configuration proved to produce maximum 2f1-f2 distortion. For a given f2-frequency, the most critical parameter to evoke large distortion levels is the frequency ratio f2/f1. Fig.2 shows the dependance of the distortion level on the frequency ratio for two different f2 frequencies in the three species. In *Pteronotus parnellii*, close to the individual 2nd harmonic call component at 61 kHz, the best ratio approaches 1 because the first tested ratio of 1.0005 already produces maximum distortion.

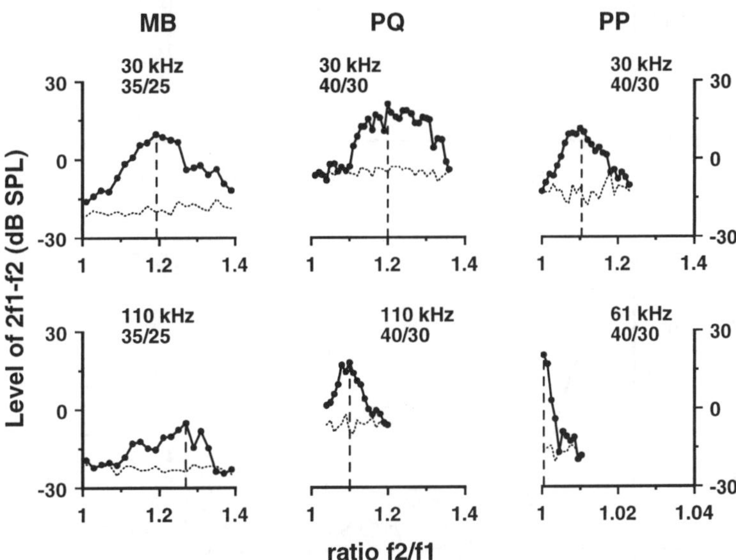

Fig.2 Dependance of 2f1-f2 level on the frequency ratio f2/f1. The f2 frequency was kept constant and is indicated above each curve together with the levels of f1 and f2. The dotted line gives the noise level that for *Mormoops blainvillii* (MB) was lower than for the recordings in *Pteronotus quadridens* (PQ) and *Pteronotus parnellii* (PP) due to a different measuring amplifier used (see methods). Note that for PP at a f2-frequency of 61 kHz, the ratio scale is smaller, the best ratio was at 1.0005. The dashed lines indicate the best ratio.

The best ratios were measured for low primary levels within a wide range of f2 frequencies between 10-110 kHz (Fig.3 top). In *Mormoops blainvillii*, best ratios ranged between 1.12 and 1.42 with maximum values for f2 frequencies around 45 kHz. *Pteronotus quadridens* had best ratios between 1.17 and 1.30 for frequencies below 60 kHz. For higher frequencies the best ratio gradually decreased down to values of about 1.08. In these two species the best ratios are close to those found in other mammals with good high frequency hearing capabilities like the opossum or the gerbil. Preliminary measurements of 2f1-f2 suppression tuning curves also do not indicate that regions of enhanced tuning are present in these two species. In contrast, *Pteronotus parnellii* has best ratios below 1.13 over the whole hearing range with distinct minim of 1.0005 and 1.0018 at 62 and 93 kHz.

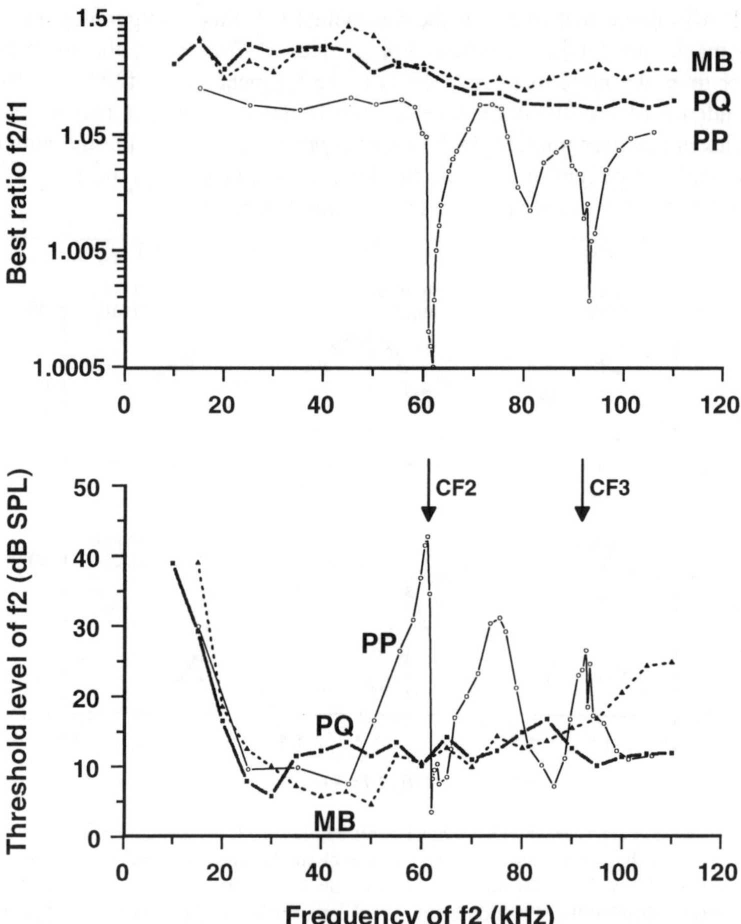

Fig.3 <u>Top:</u> Best ratio f2/f1 for different f2-frequencies in *Mormoops blainvillii* (MB), *Pteronotus quadridens* (PQ) and *Pteronotus parnellii* (PP). <u>Bottom:</u> 2f1-f2 threshold curves. The level of f2 sufficient to elicit a 2f1-f2 distortion of -10 dB SPL (threshold criterion) is plotted. In all cases the level of f1 was 10 dB above that of f2. The data were averaged from two individuals of MB and PQ and 6 individuals of PP [7]. For different individuals of PP, the data were normalized to a cochlear resonance frequency of 62 kHz [7]. The arrows indicate the frequencies of the dominant CF-components of PP.

2f1-f2 I/O curves were obtained at different f2 frequencies after adjusting f1 to the best ratio. Fig.4 shows two sensitive I/O curves from *Mormoops blainvillii* where the 2f1-f2 level reaches that of the f2 stimulus (open symbols, at 10 dB SPL). From I/O functions measured at different f2-frequencies, distortion threshold curves were obtained by plotting the f2 level that was sufficient to induce a distortion of -10 dB obtained by plotting the f2 level that was sufficient to induce a distortion of -10 dB SPL against f2 frequency (Fig.3, bottom). The thresholds of *Pteronotus quadridens* and *Mormoops blainvillii* were most sensitive for frequencies between 30-50 kHz and do not show distinct extrema like the threshold of *Pteronotus parnellii* where maxima appear at the CF2 and CF3 frequency and also at 75 kHz. A few hundred Hz above CF2 there is a sharp minimum.

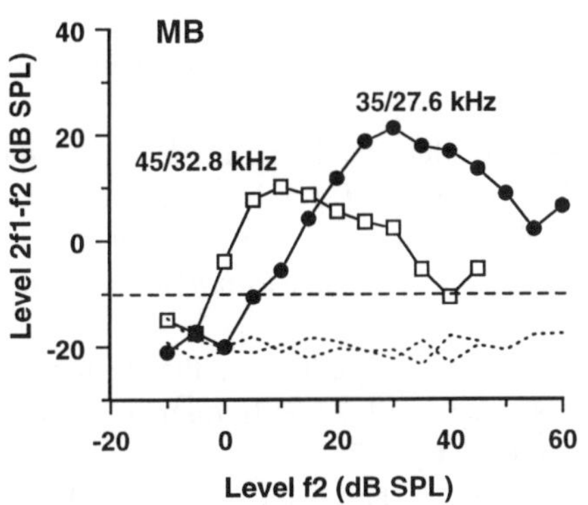

Fig.4
2fl-f2I/O functions for two different primary frequency combinations in *Mor- moops blainvillii*. The level of fl was al- ways 10 dB above that of f2. The dashed line gives the -10 dB SPL distortion thres- hold criterion that was used for calculating the thresholds in Fig.3. The noise level is shown by dotted lines.

4   Conclusions

In terms of best ratios and distortion threshold, *Pteronotus quadridens* and *Mormoops blainvillii* are not particularly adapted to certain frequencies. They show a good high frequency hearing for the overall range of their broadband echolocation signals. There are no significant changes in distortion properties correlated with the short CF-components in the call of *Pteronotus quadridens*. The present data indicate that the evolution towards the specialized cochlea of *Pteronotus parnellii* seems to have occurred rather abruptly and involved three major changes:

(i).. The best ratios are smaller throughout the measured frequency range. This may indicate an improved mechanical frequency separation in the cochlea.

(ii). Just above CF2 and CF3 there are sharp minima in best ratio. If the best ratio reflects the characteristics of a second cochlear filter like the tectorial membrane [8,9] , then close to CF2 and CF3 this filter should be tuned to nearly the same frequency as the primary filter [7,10,11] which could explain the sharp neuronal tuning.

(iii) *Pteronotus parnellii* has pronounced threshold maxima at CF2 and CF3. It may have been of evolutionary advantage to become insensitive for the CF-frequencies of the own call in order to focus on the CF-echoes that, due to Doppler-shifts, are slightly higher in frequency and correlate with threshold minima.

Acknowledgments

We are grateful to the Jamaican Natural Resources Conservation Authority for their support and the Discovery Bay Marine Laboratory for the use of their facilities. This study was supported by the DFG, SFB 204 and the Royal Society.

References

1. Neuweiler, G. (1990) Auditory adaptations for prey capture in echolocating bats, *Physiol. Rev.* **70** 615-641.
2. Kössl, M. and Russell, I.J. (1995) Basilar membrane resonance in the cochlea of the mustached bat, *Proc. Natl. Acad. Sci. USA* **92** 276-279.
3. Kössl, M. (1994) Otoacoustic emissions from the cochlea of the 'constant frequency' bats *Pteronotus parnellii* and *Rhinolophus rouxi*, *Hearing Res.* **72** 69-72.
4. Suga, N. and Jen, P.-H.S. (1977) Further studies on the peripheral auditory system of 'CF-FM' bats specialized for fine frequency analysis of Doppler-shifted echoes, *J. Exp. Biol.* **69** 207-232.
5. Schnitzler, H.U., Kalkov, E., Kaips, I. and Mockdans, J. (1990) Comparative studies of echolocation and hunting behaviour in the four species of mormoopid bats of Jamaica, *5th European Bat Research Conference, Denmark.*
6. Silva Taboada, G. (1979) Los Murcielagos de Cuba, *Editorial Academia, La Habana 2, Cuba.*
7. Kössl, M. and Vater, M. (1996) Further studies on the mechanics of the cochlear partition in the mustached bat. II. A second cochlear frequency map derived from acoustic distortion products, *Hearing Res.* (in press).
8. Brown, A.M., Gaskill, S.A. and Williams, D.M. (1992) Mechanical filtering of sound by the inner ear, *Proc. R. Soc. Lond. B* **250** 29-34.
9. Allen, J.B. and Fahey, P.F. (1993) A second cochlear frequency map that correlates distortion product and neural tuning measurements, *J. Acoust. Soc. Am.* **88** 840-849.
10. Vater, M. and Kössl, M. (1996) Further studies on the mechanics of the cochlear partition in the mustached bat. I. Ultrastructural observations on the tectorial membrane and hair cells, *Hearing Res.* (in press).
11. Kössl, M. and Vater, M. (1996) A tectorial membrane fovea in the cochlea of the mustached bat, *Naturwissenschaften* **83** 89-91.

EVOLUTIONARY PLASTICITY OF COCHLEAR DESIGN IN ECHOLOCATING BATS

M. VATER

Institut für Zoologie, Universität Regensburg, Universitätsstr.31, 93040
Regensburg, germany
email: marianne.vater@biologie.uni-regensburg.de

In order to study adaptations in cochlear design for processing the species characteristic echolocation signals, basoapical gradients in cochlear morphology were analysed in three species of bats. The non-related horseshoe bat (*Rhinolophus rouxi*) and the mustached bat (*Pteronotus parnellii*) share several morphological specializations of the basilar membrane and tectorial membrane that are likely involved in creating exceptionally sharp cochlear tuning to the constant frequency component of the echolocation signal. The smaller relative of the mustached bat, *Pteronotus quadridens* that only emits broadband frequency-modulated calls and exhibits normal cochlear tuning shows a non-specialized cochlear morphology with general adaptations for high frequency hearing.

1 Introduction

Most families of insectivorous microchiropteran bats employ short broadband frequency-modulated (FM)-signals for determination of the direction and distance of the target and discrimination of the nature of the target. Some highly specialized species have evolved a doppler-sensitive sonar system. These CF-FM bats use the long constant frequency (CF) signal component for determination of relative velocity, and detection and identification of flutttering prey insects in heavily echo-cluttered environment [1]. Cochlear structure and function is adapted for processing the species specific echolocation signals. While cochlear tuning in FM-bats is within the standard mammalian range, CF-FM bats have implemented exceptionally sharply tuned cochlear filter mechanisms based on morphological specializations of the passive hydromechanical system. These specialized mechanisms yield neuronal Q 10 dB values of up to 400 within narrow frequency bands around the dominant CF-call component [2].

Dopplersensitive sonar accompanied by enhanced cochlear tuning was created in convergent evolution: in old world horseshoe bats (genus *Rhinolophus* and *Hipposideros*) and in one new world species of the genus *Pteronotus*, the mustached bat (*Pteronotus parnellii*).

The present study adresses two questions: 1. Are there comparable specializations of cochlear morphology in non-related species that possess enhanced cochlear tuning (i.e. the horseshoe bat *Rhinolophus rouxi* and the mustached bat *Pteronotus parnellii*) ? 2. How does cochlear morphology differ in related species that employ broadband and narrowband echolocation systems (i.e. the FM-bat *Pteronotus quadridens* and the CF-FM bat *Pteronotus parnellii*)?

2 Material and Methods

Under deep Ketanest/Rompun anaesthesia, bats were either perfused through the heart with 2.5% glutaraldehyde in 0.1 M phosphate buffer or decapitated and the cochleae were directly perfused through the scalae with the same fixative. Cochleae were decalcified in 7.5% EDTA, dissected into half turns, dehydrated and embedded in epoxide resin. Serial, radial semithin sections (2um) were collected on non-coated glass slides, stained with Richardson blue, and used for quantitative lightmicroscopic analysis. Selected sections from defined cochlear length were remounted, cut ultrathinly and used for TEM-analysis. At least four cochleae obtained from different individuals of each species were analysed. Permission to capture and use the bats for morphological studies was obtained from the Sri lankan Wildlife department (*R. rouxi*) and the Jamaican Natural Resources Conservation Authority (*P. parnellii; P. quadridens*).

3 Results

Schematic illustrations of the organ of Corti in different turns are shown for the three species in Fig. 1. The drawings are made on the same scale to emphazise absolute and relative differences in dimensions.

As a general feature, gradients in dimensions of the receptor cells are far less pronounced than in non-echolocating mammals and in particular the outer hair cells are very small (10-11 um in the hook; maximal length 18-20 um in the apex).

The most dramatic differences among species reside in the morphology of the basilar membrane (BM) and the tectorial membrane (TM). Specializations of cochlear morphology in the two non-related CF-FM bats differ to a certain extent [2], however, they do share some specialized traits. In species specific cochlear positions, there are profound thickenings of the pectinate zone of the BM (Fig. 1 A, 2 C;) that are created by the enlargement of the tympanic BM-compartment due to massive incorporation of radial filaments and the addition of a specialized vestibular BM-compartment that is composed of longitudinal filaments (for Rhinolophus see also [3]). These thickenings are found within a sparsely innervated region of the basal turn (SI-zone) that is located basal to the representation place of the second harmonic CF-signal component (Fig.1). Both CF-FM-bats exhibit specialized gradients in TM morphology: the cross-sectional area of the TM and the extent of its limbal attachment exhibit maxima within the CF2-region that is characterized by sensitive and exceptionally sharp tuning. Preliminary quantitative data for *Rhinolophus* indicate that similar to the mustached bat [4] there is an abrupt change in TM-size and shape at the transition from the SI-zone to the CF2-region (Fig. 2).

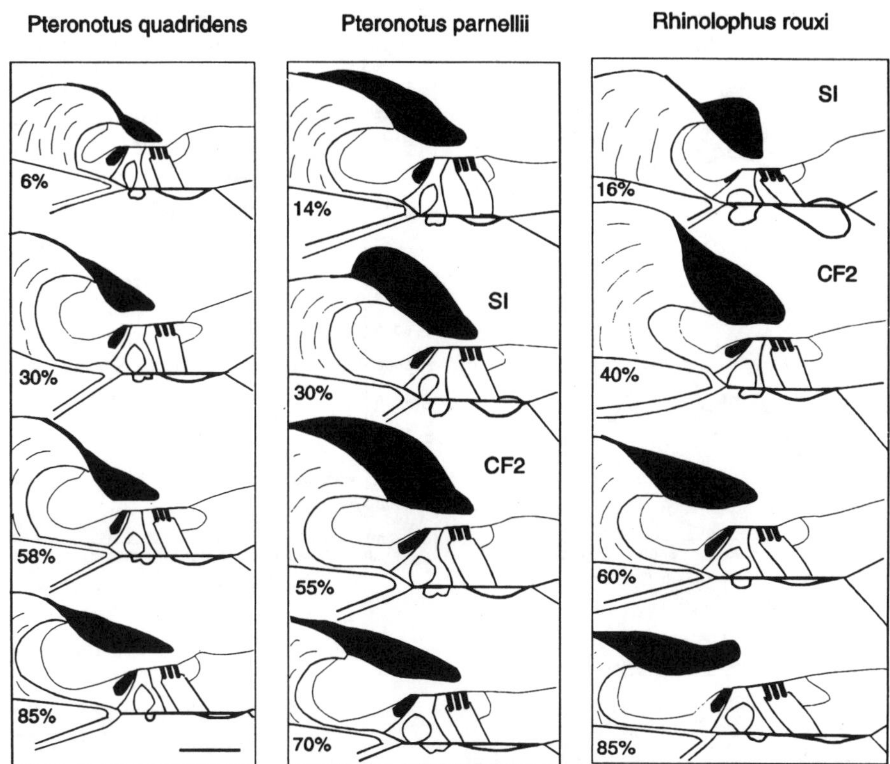

Fig.1. Schematic illustrations of radial sections through the organ of Corti of different bat species. Numbers indicate percent distance from base. SI: sparsely innervated zone of the first half turn; CF2: representation place of the second harmonic constant-frequency signal component. Scale bar: 50 µm.

The FM-bat, *Pteronotus quadridens* that exhibits non-specialized cochlear tuning [5] lacks comparable specializations of cochlear morphology (Fig. 1). Baso-apical gradients in BM-thickness and -width and the size and shape of the TM are gradual (Fig. 2). Except for the most apical cochlear positions, TM-area is much smaller than in the CF-FM bats. Its maximal size corresponds to that seen in the basal turn of the rat cochlea [6]. Significantly, neither TM nor BM nor any other components of the cochlear duct show any feature that can be considered as a preadaptation for the evolution of specialized hydromechanical processing within the genus *Pteronotus*.

52

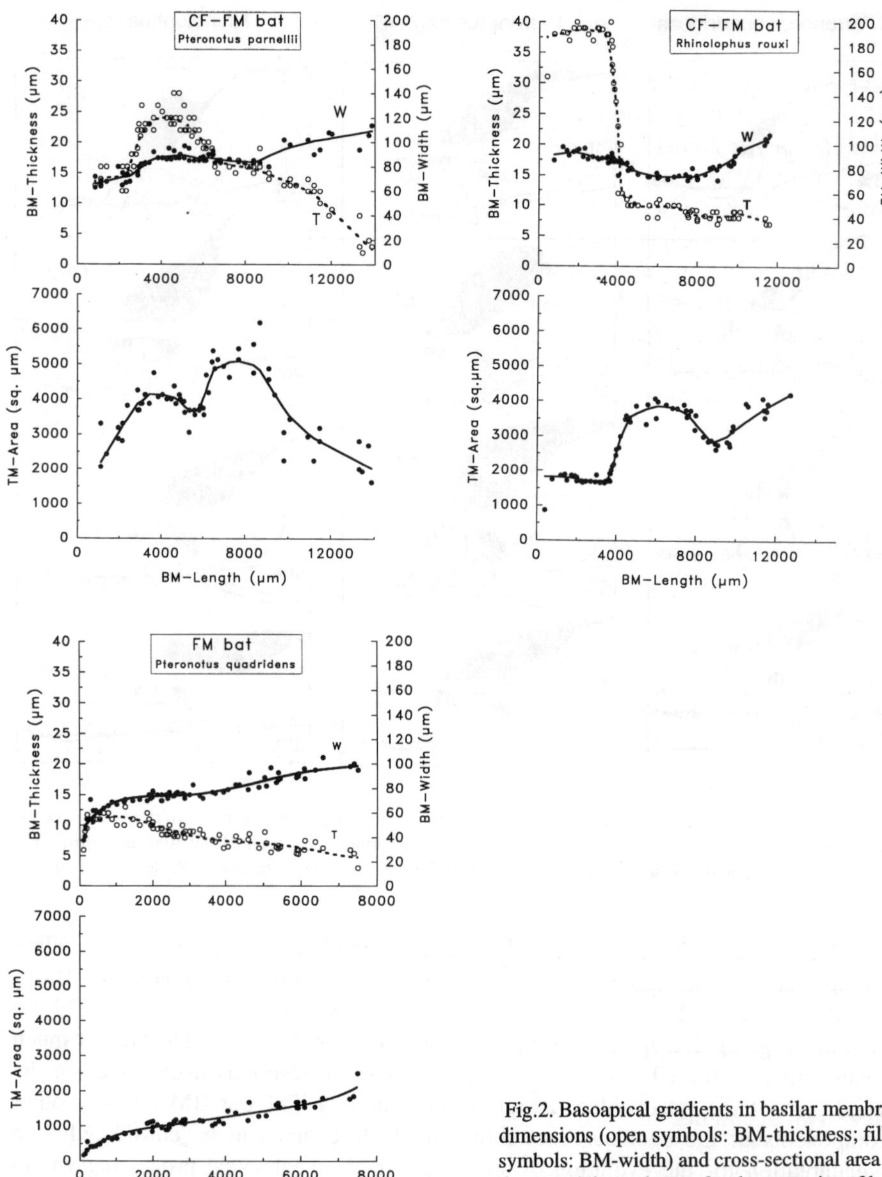

Fig.2. Basoapical gradients in basilar membrane dimensions (open symbols: BM-thickness; filled symbols: BM-width) and cross-sectional area of the tectorial membrane for three species of bats. BM-Length is given in distance from base.

4 Discussion and conclusions

Very clearly both CF-FM bats feature stepwise changes in TM and BM whereas the FM-bat presents a non-specialized cochlea design similar to that of non-echolocating mammals [7] but scaled down for the demands of processing ultrasonic frequencies. The most dramatic evolutionary change in cochlear design among microchiroptera does not occur at the level of the receptor cells but within the accessory mechanical structures.

Similar selection pressures appear to have governed the convergent evolution of stepwise changes in TM and BM morphology in the non-related CF-FM bats. Furthermore, these features likely represent crucial prerequisites to enhance cochlear tuning well beyond the values typically encountered in other mammals. Moreover, the similarities between the two species are indicative of certain constraints in diversity of designing exceptionally sharply tuned cochlear filters: specializations of both TM (see also [8,9]) and BM (see also [3]) appear to be necessary. This emphazises the proposed role of the TM as a resonant structure that influences cochlear tuning [10,11,12] . The specialized cochlear tuning mechanisms in the non-related CF-FM bats probably differ in important detail as indicated by morphological and physiological data. The absolute dimensions of TM and BM differ between both species, the mustached bat cochlea has uniquely specialized gradients in scale volume , and the horseshoe bat has a highly specialized secondary spiral lamina [2] . Strong otoacoustic emissions at the CF2 frequency accompanied by pronounced resonance in the cochlear microphonic are a robust phenomenon of the mustached bat cochlea whereas in horseshoe bats, they are much less pronounced [13] . These differences probably reside in the relative degree of damping of resonant structures [13,14] .

The absence of preadaptations in cochlear morphology of the FM-bat, *Pteronotus quadridens* invites several speculations. First, the change from „broadband" to „narrowband" cochlear processing within the genus *Pteronotus* may have occured rather rapidly on evolutionary time scale. The living relatives of *P.parnellii* studied to date (*P. quadridens*, this study; *Mormoops blainvilli*, Vater unpublished) do not represent transitional stages. Second, the adaptive change in cochlear structure and function is not restricted to a single element but affects multiple components of the passive mechanical system.

Acknowledgements

I thank Prof. Costa (university of Kelaniha), the Sri lankan Wildlife department and the Jamaican Natural Resources Conservation authority for their help, and Gesa Thies for valuable technical assistance. This work was supported by SFB 204 (Gehör, München)

References

1. Neuweiler, G. (1990). Auditory adaptations for prey capture in echolocating bats, *Physiol. Rev.* **70** 615-641.
2. Kössl M. and Vater M.(1995). Cochlear structure and function in bats,.in Hearing by bats, eds. AN Popper and RR Fay (Springer Verlag New York Heidelberg London), pp. 191-235.
3. Bruns, V. (1980). Basilar membrane and its anchoring system in the cochlea of the Greater horseshoe bat, *Anat. Embryol.* **161** 29-50.
4. Vater M. and Kössl M. (1996). Further studies on the mechanics of the cochlear partition in the mustached bat. I. Ultrastructural observations on the tectorial membrane and hair cells, *Hear. Res.* **94** 63-77.
5. Kössl M., Frank, G., Faulstich, M. and Russell, I.J. (1996). Acoustic distortion products as indicator of cochlear adaptations in Jamaican mormoopid bats, this volume
6. Roth, B. and Bruns V. (1992). Postnatal development of the rat organ of Corti. I. General morphology, basilar membrane, tectorial membrane and border cells, *Anat. Embryol.* **185** 559-569.
7. Lim, D.J. (1986). Functional structure of the organ of Corti: a review, *Hear. Res.* **22** 117-146.
8. Henson, M. and Henson, O.W.Jr. (1991). Specializations for sharp tuning in the mustached bat: the tectorial membrane and spiral limbus, *Hear. Res.* **56** 122-132.
9. Kössl, M. and Vater, M. (1996). A tectorial membrane fovea in the cochlea of the mustached bat, *Naturwissenschaften* **83** 89-91.
10. Zwislocki, J.J. and Kletzky, E.J. (1979). Tectorial membrane: a possible effect on frequency analysis in the cochlea. *Science* **204** 639-641.
11. Zwislocki, JJ. and Cefaratti, L.K. (1989). Tectorial membrane. II. Stiffness measurements in vivo. *Hear. Res.* **42** 211-228.
12. Allen, J.B. and Fahey, P.F. (1993). A second cochlear frequency map that correlates distortion product and neural tuning measurements, *J. Acoust. Soc. Amer.* **88** 840-849.
13. Kössl, M. (1994). Otoacoustic emissions from the cochlea of the ′constant frequency′ bats Pteronotus parnellii and Rhinolophus rouxi, *Hear. Res.* **72** 69-72.
14. Henson O.W. Jr., Schuller, G. and Vater, M. (1985). A comparative study of the physiological properties of the inner ear in Dopplershift compensating bats (*Rhinolophus rouxi and Pteronotus parnellii*), *J. Comp. Physiol. A* **157** 587-597.

SUPPRESSION OF EXTERNAL-EAR IMPULSE-RESPONSE SMEARING BY ECHO SIGNAL-PROCESSING IN THE BIG BROWN BAT

J.A. SIMMONS, J. M.WOTTON , P. A. SAILLANT, T. HARESIGN
Department of Neuroscience, Box 1953, Brown University ,Providence, RI 02912
james-simmons@brown.edu

The external ear of the big brown bat receives sonar broadcasts radiating from the bat's mouth and also echoes returning from targets located in different directions. Its impulse response shows 5-6 prominent peaks corresponding to reverberation occurring as sound passes down through the antenna elements of the external ear (pinna with its ridges, and tragus) to the ear-drum. Successive impulse peaks are separated by about 15 μs and together span about 75-90 μs. Moreover, they are followed by 5-6 similar but weaker peaks that stretch the impulse response further, over a total span of 150-180 μs. Behavioral studies document the bat's echo-delay accuracy and resolution in the range of 1-2 μs or better, and even the bat's routine performance requires acuities no worse than 5-10 μs. How does the bat counteract the smearing of echo arrival-times over a span of 150-180 μs to perceive echoes as having unambiguous, discrete arrival-times with errors of less than 1-2 μs? To set up a reference for recognizing echoes, the bat's external ear receives each broadcast sound from the mouth (located about 25° "inboard" relative to the ears and 35-45° below the horizontal plane of the head), while echoes from targets are received more nearly from straight ahead during tracking. The reverberation delays for several of the peaks in the impulse response are direction-dependent, so the broadcast sound and its echoes pass through slightly different impulse responses. When the broadcast sound at the ear-drum is taken as the "input" for determining the external ear's impulse response for *echoes*, the result is less smeared by the external ear, but there still are at least 4 prominent peaks stretched over 60 μs. However, when echo processing is carried out by spectrogram correlation and transformation (SCAT), the resulting abbreviated impulse response contains just 1 prominent peak marking echo arrival time and only 1-2 elevation-dependent side peaks that also appear in the bat's images as measured behaviorally. Thus, the acoustical properties of the external ear interact with the bat's echo signal-processing scheme to produce compact images that define the target's impulse response without smearing, while at the same time incorporating information about target elevation.

1. Introduction

The external ears are the receiving antennas for the sense of hearing. They modify the waveform of sounds arriving at each ear-drum from different directions according to the location of the sound source. Receiving properties have variously been described as direction-dependent changes in the spectrum of sounds (transfer functions) or direction-dependent changes in the time-series waveform (impulse responses). Both monaural and binaural combinations of these descriptive features are implicated in perception of auditory space. However, acoustic stimuli have characteristic spectra and time waveforms due to the identity of the source apart from modifications to the spectrum or the time-series waveform caused by the external ears. How does the auditory system determine the characteristics of sounds if it only observes them through the distorting effects of the external ears? How does the auditory system solve the competing problems of sound recognition, which depends upon determining the characteristics of the sound at its source, and sound localization, which depends upon using the effects of the external ears?

2. Target Images in Bat Sonar

The biological sonar, or echolocation, of bats (Chiroptera) provides a compelling example of the formation of auditory images that depict the characteristics and locations of objects from sounds (Popper and Fay, 1995). Most bats are insectivorous and use their sonar to locate and capture flying prey as well as to avoid obstacles. In echolocation, the features of targets as objects have to be kept distinct from their locations in spite of the fact that the same sounds are used to perceive both the objects and their locations (Simmons, et al., 1995a). The big brown bat, *Eptesicus fuscus*, perceives sonar targets as having specific distances, shapes, and directions (see Popper and Fay, 1995). Underlying the formation of sonar images by *Eptesicus* is representation of the target along the dimension of target range or echo delay (Simmons, 1989). The bat's sonar images consist of a series of echo-delay estimates that depict the locations of different reflecting points and surfaces (glints) at different distances, as well as the horizontal and vertical directions of these glints. This latter point is especially important because the bat often pursues insects that fly into vegetation, and distinguishing prey from clutter entails perceiving the differences between glints that belong to the insect and glints that belong to the vegetation (Simmons, et al., 1995a).

Eptesicus transmits frequency-modulated (FM) sonar signals sweeping from 60 to 25 kHz in the first harmonic and about 100 to 50 kHz in the second harmonic and then uses echoes of these broadcast sounds to determine a kind of impulse response (SCAT image; see Saillant, et al., 1993) for the communication channel consisting of the volume of space out to a maximum operating distance of about 5 m (Kick, 1982). The bat's images portray the arrival-times of the reflected replicas of the broadcast sound that the insect and the vegetation return to its ears. These arrival-times represent the path-lengths associated with the distance to different objects and different parts of the same object. The overall distance to a target is perceived from the time-of-occurrence of echoes in relation to broadcast sounds as registered by the timing of neural responses to different frequencies in the FM sweeps of the bat's sounds and the echoes (Dear, et al., 1993; Simmons, et al.,

1995b). However, *Eptesicus* also perceives the distance to different parts of a target, even when the echoes from the target's glints arrive too close together to be separately registered as different sounds. Echoes are received with an integration time of about 350 μs, so multiple reflections that arrive overlapping each other within the integration-time window are received as just one sound. These overlapping reflections have a complex interference spectrum whose peaks and notches are related to their time separation, and *Eptesicus* transforms the shape of this spectrum into estimates of the time separation of the echoes from individual glints in relation to the overall delay of the entire set of overlapping reflections (Saillant, et al., 1993; Simmons, *et al.*, 1995b). The bat's images thus contain estimates of echo delay that are derived from two distinct processes--a time-domain delay-coding system (Dear, et al., 1993) and a frequency-to-time-domain process equivalent to deconvolution (Saillant, et al., 1993).

3.   Impulse Responses in Echolocation

The sonar images perceived by *Eptesicus* take the form of a series of echo-delay estimates, and the best way to illustrate how the bat uses its external ears and overcomes their effects on echoes is to show the impulse responses for signals passing through different stages of the sonar process (Simmons, 1989).

3.1 Target impulse responses

Fig. 1A shows the impulse response of a single-glint target located at a moderate distance of 0.5-1 m from the bat. Because the target returns only one prominent replica of the incident sound, its impulse response consists of a single prominent peak that registers the arrival-time of the replica (centered at 0 μs in Fig. 1A). This impulse response is not "perfect," however, because the echo is not identical to the broadcast even though there is only one glint to reflect the sound. First, during propagation to and from the target, the spectrum of the echo is modified by atmospheric absorption (Lawrence and Simmons, 1982) to be slightly weaker at higher frequencies of 50-100 kHz than lower frequencies of 20-50 kHz. Second, the reflective strength of the target (its acoustic cross-section) is frequency-dependent, which alters the echo spectrum a bit further. the spectral mismatch between the broadcast sound and the echo results in minor stretching of the impulse response, manifested in Fig. 1A chiefly as a low-amplitude secondary peak. Of course, the glint structure of a complex target would appear as a series of impulse-response peaks--one for each glint, but, for simplicity, only a single-glint target is considered in Fig. 1. From the impulse response in Fig. 1A one can recognize that this target contains just one glint. In fact , the target's most characteristic feature is the presence of the single impulse peak with its one, unambiguous value of delay. This

58

is a "point-target" to the bat, and, to locate the target, the bat has to determine the delay value for the peak.

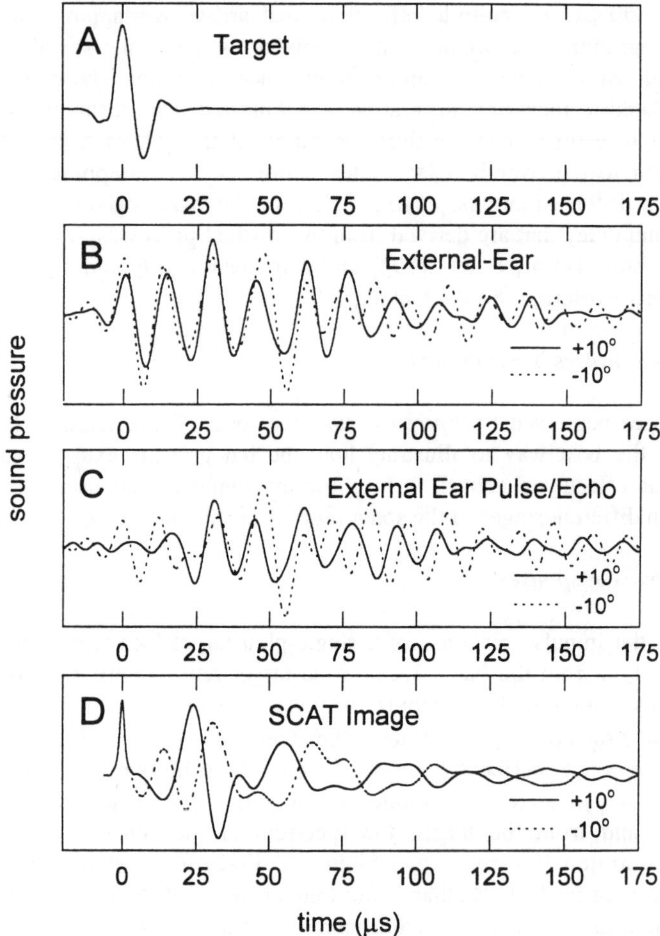

Figure 1. Comparison of impulse responses and the temporal structure of signals at different stages of echo processing. (Time axis refers echo arrival-time to 0 µs.) (A) The impulse response of a single-glint target from echoes arriving at the bat's location. (B) The impulse response of the bat's external ear for sounds arriving from elevations of +10° and -10° at a horizontal direction of straight ahead (impulse responses for passive hearing). (C) The impulse response of the bat's external ear for *echoes* arriving from a target at elevations of +10° and -10° and at a horizontal direction of straight ahead (for sonar). The reference signal for these impulse responses is the bat's broadcast sound arriving from its mouth. (D) SCAT impulse responses for echoes arriving from a target at elevations of +10° and -10° and at a horizontal direction of straight ahead.

3.2 External-ear impulse responses

Echoes returning from objects at different distances are received by the bat's external ears, which have directionally-dependent gain. Each ear is more sensitive to echoes arriving from ipsilateral directions, and the direction of maximum receiving sensitivity is frequency dependent (Jen and Chen, 1988; Wotton, et al., 1995). In *Eptesicus*, the acoustic axis of the external ear is more lateral at low frequencies of 20-30 kHz and migrates systematically towards the front at progressively higher frequencies from 30 kHz to 100 kHz. Moreover, the directional gain of the ear interacts with the directionality of the broadcast sound itself to determine the spectrum of echoes (Simmons, et al., 1995). The combined directionality of the broadcast and of the ears colors the spectrum of echoes beyond what occurs during propagation and scattering, so that, overall, echoes arriving from straight ahead have a nearly uniform spectrum while echoes arriving from off to the side, or above and below the horizontal plane, have progressively weaker contributions at higher frequencies relative to lower frequencies. This effect is gradual, however; echoes arriving from within a cone of space aimed to the front and about 60-80° across have a nearly flat spectrum from directional gain effects.

Besides the overall directionality of gain, the external ear imposes a specific effect that is illustrated by the impulse responses in Fig. 1B for sounds coming from straight ahead in azimuth and +10° or -10° in elevation. While the sound arriving from the target consists of a single replica of the broadcast sound (Fig. 1A), the sound reaching the ear-drum contains a whole series of replicas delayed at intervals of about 15 μs and added to each other. The impulse responses in Fig. 1B show this reverberation as a series of 5-6 prominent peaks stretched across 75-90 μs followed by a similar series of 5-6 lower peaks stretched across an additional 75-90 μs. (The time spacing of adjacent peaks is manifested in the transfer function as prominent interference notches at specific frequencies.) The effect is to stretch or smear the discrete arrival-time of the echo from the single, well-defined peak show in Fig. 1A to the array of multiple peaks shown in Fig. 1B. The width of this whole array is 150-180 μs, which introduces severe ambiguity for specifying the arrival-time of echoes at the ear-drum. The echo-delay acuity predictable from the width of the individual peak in Fig. 1A is replaced by the ambiguity over which peak in Fig. 2B best represents the delay of the echo. An acuity of the order of 50-100 μs would be expected from Fig. 2B, which corresponds roughly to the accuracy of target range discrimination in ordinary experiments with simultaneous or sequential presentation of stimuli. The problem is that *Eptesicus* has an echo-delay accuracy of a fraction of a microsecond and echo-delay resolution of a few microseconds (Simmons, et al.,

1995a), with an intrinsic ambiguity associated with far fewer side-peaks than the impulse responses in Fig. 1B contain.

3.3 External-ear echo impulse responses

The impulse responses in Fig. 1B are for reception of sounds in passive hearing, whereas echolocation is active in nature: To determine echo delay, the bat has to use a reference event to mark the time-of-occurrence of the broadcast sound. Reception of the echo then has to be compared with this earlier time-mark to represent the value of delay. *Eptesicus* and other echolocating bats employ a system of neuronal delay lines which store a short-term replica of the FM sweeps in the broadcast sound for comparison with the FM sweeps in echoes (Dear, et al., 1993; Simmons, et al., 1995b). The problem for determining delay is smearing of the echo by the external ear over a span of 150-180 µs (Fig. 1B), which would seem to rule out specification of echo delay with a precision of better than 1-2 µs. However, the broadcast is not received directly from the bat's larynx but as an airborne sound that radiates from the bat's mouth, which is situated in front of the ears and somewhat below the eye-nostril horizontal plane of the head. Sounds arriving from the bat's mouth encounter the receiving directionality associated with a location 35-45° below the horizontal plane and about 25° towards the middle of the head, or "inboard" for each ear. Thus, both the broadcast sound and each echo go through the complex impulse response of the bat's external ear, just from different directions. That is, the external ear's impulse response for sounds arriving from the mouth is the system's "input" for subsequent delay calculations, while the impulse response associated with the echo is the "output." Fig. 1C shows external-ear impulse responses based on this arrangement of signals. In Fig. 1C, the impulse responses are for echoes rather than just for any sound arriving from +10° or -10° in elevation. (The reference signal for the broadcast sound is assumed to have passed through the external ear from the direction of the bat's mouth.) Echo impulse responses are somewhat shorter in overall duration compared to the impulse responses in Fig. 1B, with perhaps 4-6 major peaks spread over 60-75 µs. This shortening is a consequence of the presence of multiple impulse peaks in both the input and output waveforms together--echo impulse responses accentuate differences between the external ear's characteristics for the broadcast sound and the echo rather than the absolute impulse characteristics for the echo alone. However, although the echo impulse responses in Fig. 1C are marginally shorter than the "regular" or passive-hearing impulse responses for the external ear in Fig. 1B, they still are too reverberant to explain the bat's ability to perceive echo delay with an acuity of no worse than a few microseconds.

3.4 SCAT impulse responses

The bat's echo-processing algorithms do not strictly correspond to impulse response calculations. Instead, the bat employs a spectrogram representation for the FM sweeps in its broadcast sounds and echoes, and the images it perceives are derived from computations carried out on these spectrograms (Saillant, et al., 1993; Simmons, et al., 1995b). Echo processing by *Eptesicus* appears to consist of two parallel pathways--spectrogram correlation and spectrogram transformation. The first pathway is used to determine the arrival-time of echoes from the timing of responses to each frequency in the FM sweep, and the second pathway deconvolves the interference spectrum of echoes to determine delay separations smaller than the integration-time for echo reception, which is roughly 350 µs in *Eptesicus*. The characteristics of SCAT images, or their equivalent, rather than the characteristics of impulse responses have to be used to judge how the bat's external ears influence its perception of echo delay.

Fig. 1D shows SCAT imges computed for the same "input" and "output" signals as were used for the impulse responses in Fig. 1C. These SCAT images (also for target elevations of +10° or -10°) are significantly shorter and more simple in structure than the echo impulse responses. Chiefly, there are fewer peaks. In Fig. 1D there is a single sharp peak (at 0 µs) which registers the arrival-time of the echo from the single-glint target followed by a prominent peak at about 25-30 µs and a lower peak at about 55-65 µs that together replace the whole series of peaks in the impulse responses. The extended series of peaks in the impulse response of the external ear for echoes thus is compressed into these second and third peaks in the SCAT images. That is, the SCAT images usefully concentrate the much-dispersed impulse responses from Fig. 1C into abbreviated "biological" impulse responses that display the arrival-time of echoes with less ambiguity. Moreover, the images that the bat actually perceives resemble the SCAT images rather than the impulse responses. For a single-glint target, *Eptesicus* perceives echo-delay images that correspond approximately to the SCAT images in Fig. 1D, with a single, very sharp peak registering the "first" arrival-time of echoes and another peak 25-35 µs later as a secondary reflection (Simmons, 1989; Simmons, et al., 1995a).

There is considerable elevation-dependence in the timing of peaks in the echo impulse responses shown in Fig. 1C, but this dependence is complicated and spread unevenly across the different peaks. In contrast, the SCAT images in Fig. 1D show a simplified dependence on elevation. The time-intervals between the first and the second peaks and between the first and the third peaks shift to longer times as elevation declines from +10° to -10°. This process concentrates all the information the bat needs to determine delay and elevation into a small number of delay estimates. It specifically removes the smearing of delay estimates contributed by the

62

external ear and uses the elevation dependence of the external ear's impulse response to "insert" a marker for elevation into the delay images.

Acknowledgments

This research was supported by ONR Grant Nos. N00014-89-J-3055 and N00014-95-I-1123, NIMH Grant No. MH00521 (RSDA), NSF Grant No. BCS-9216718, NIMH Training Grant No. MH19118, McDonnell-Pew Grant No. T89-01245-023, and DRF funds.

References

1.   Dear, S.P., Fritz, J., Haresign, T., Ferragamo, M.J., and Simmons, J.A. (1993). Tonotopic and functional organization in the auditory cortex of the big brown bat, *Eptesicus fuscus. J. Neurophysiol.* **70** 1988-2009.

2.   Jen, P.H.S., and Chen, D.M. (1988). Directionality of sound pressure transformation at the pinna of echolocating bats. *Hearing Res.* **34** 101-118.

3.   Kick, S.A. (1982). Target detection by the echolocating bat, *Eptesicus fuscus.* J. *Comp. Physiol.* **145** 431-435.

4.   Lawrence, B.D., and Simmons, J.A. (1982). Measurements of atmospheric attenuation at ultrasonic frequencies and the significance for echolocation by bats. *J. Acoust. Soc. Am.* **71** 585-590.

5.   Popper, A.N., and Fay, R.R. (Eds.) (1995). Hearing by Bats. Springer Handbook of Auditory Research, Springer-Verlag, New York

6.   Saillant, P.A., Simmons, J.A., Dear, S.P., and McMullen, T.A. (1993). A computational model of echo processing and acoustic imaging in frequency-modulated echolocating bats: The spectrogram correlation and transformation receiver. *J. Acoust. Soc. Am.* **94** 2691-2712.

7.   Simmons, J.A. (1989). A view of the world through the bat's ear: The formation of acoustic images in echolocation. *Cognition* **33** 155-199.

8.   Simmons, J.A., Ferragamo, M.J., Saillant, P.A., Haresign, T., Wotton, J.M., Dear, S.P., and Lee, D.N. (1995a). Auditory dimensions of acoustic images in echolocation. In: A.N. Popper and R.R. Fay (Eds.), Hearing by Bats. Springer Handbook of Auditory Research, Springer-Verlag, New York, pp. 146-190.

9.   Simmons, J.A., Saillant, P.A., Ferragamo, M.J., Haresign, T., Dear, S.P., Fritz, J., and McMullen, T.A. (1995b). Auditory computations for biosonar target imaging in bats. In H.L. Hawkins, T.A. McMullen, A.N. Popper, and R.R. Fay (Eds.), Auditory Computation. Springer Handbook of Auditory Research, Springer-Verlag, New York. pp. 401-468.

10.   Wotton, J.M., Haresign, T., and Simmons, J.A. (1995). Spatially dependent acoustic cues generated by the external ear of the big brown bat, *Eptesicus fuscus.* J. Acoust. Soc. Am. 98, 1423-1445.

TYMPANIC RADIATION: AURAL SOUND PRODUCTION IN THE BULLFROG *RANA CATESBEIANA*

A. P. PURGUE

Department of Physiological Science UCLA, CA 90095-1527
apurgue@UCLA.edu

Measurements of the transfer function describing the mechanical coupling of internally generated sound to the enlarged eardrum of male bullfrogs (*Rana catesbeiana*) show distinct energy peaks at 240, 600, 900 and 1220 Hz that are in close agreement with those observed in the spectral envelopes of the release and mating calls. Moreover, when the tympanic membranes are artificially dampened the spectrum of the release call is drastically altered mostly by the disappearance of all components above 300 Hz. As a consequence of this the total power output decreases by 19 dB suggesting that radiation through the ears contributes over 98% of the total power present in the call. The different resonance modes in the tympanic membrane are thus responsible for the characteristic multimodal energy distribution in the bullfrog's calls (i.e., the formants in the call are created by post-glottal filtering). As a corollary of this observation the source spectra (glottal waveform) need to be regarded as extremely broad band, spanning more than 1.5 kHz. These observations point to a previously unsuspected role for the ears in the sound broadcasting process of the bulfrog and possibly other anurans with similarly modified tympanic regions. This is the first reported instance of aural sound production in vertebrate animals and the first evidence for post-glottal filtering in anurans.

EXTRATYMPANIC SOUND SENSITIVITY
OF FROG AUDITORY FIBERS

J. CHRISTENSEN-DALSGAARD, M. KANNEWORFF, M. B. JØRGENSEN
Center for Sound Communication, Institute of Biology, Odense University, Campusvej 55
DK-5230 Odense M, Denmark
E-mail JCD@DOU.DK

The anuran ear is sensitive to sound bypassing the tympanum and this extratympanic input dominates the auditory response at low frequencies. We report on a study of sound sensitivity of the anuran ear using both neurophysiological methods and laser vibrometry measurements of tympanic, columellar footplate and opercular vibrations. The results of the different methods conflict. Single unit recordings of responses to low-frequency sound show both sensitivity and directional characteristics that are not seen in laser vibrometry measurements of tympanic vibrations. In contrast, single unit recordings from detympanated frogs show a marked decline in sensitivity compared to normal frogs also at low frequencies. Measurements from the operculum show very little vibration relative to the otic capsule. These conflicting results suggest that the extratympanic and tympanic pathways are tightly coupled in the frog. This suggests that an explanation for the extratympanic sensitivity could be that the inner ear is stimulated through differential motion of the otic capsule and columella.

Introduction.

Anurans are sensitive to one or more extratympanic inputs that bypass the tympanum and stimulate the inner sensory cells directly. Lombard and Straughan[1] found that the sensitivity to low-frequency free-field sound (in their experiments frequencies below 900 Hz) did not change appreciably when the frogs were detympanated. Later, Wilczynski et al.[2] compared tympanic and extratympanic inputs in *Rana pipiens* and showed that the extratympanic input was more efficient than the tympanic input at frequencies below 300 Hz. Also, an extratympanic input was inferred to explain the discrepancy between Feng's[3] neurophysiological study of directionality (showing high sensitivity and a figure-eight shaped directional characteristic for the low-frequency fibers) and models of the acoustic periphery based on laser vibrometric measurements of the tympanum (showing little vibration and ovoidal directional characteristics at low frequencies)[4]. It is important to note, though, that in this modelling study the extratympanic pathway was purely hypothetical with directional characteristics taken from the neurophysiological data.

The anuran ear contains the same basic structures as other vertebrate ears, i.e. an eardrum (albeit not very modified structurally from normal skin), a single middle ear bone, the columella, and an inner ear containing the labyrinth with both vestibular and auditory sense organs. However, the otic capsule contains a third movable element in addition to the columellar footplate and the round window, the operculum. The operculum covers a portion of the oval window (beside the columellar footplate). It is a structure unique for amphibians and is cartilagenous with a muscle inserted that connects the operculum with the scapula. The operculum may be used for vibration reception[5], but a role in extratympanic sound sensitivity has also been suggested[1,6].

The mechanism of the extratympanic input is still unknown. It has been proposed that sound could be transmitted to the inner ear via bone conduction either through vibrations of the frog's skull transmitted directly to the inner ear fluid or through inertial differential motion of the otic capsule and the columella[2] or the operculum. Alternatively, sound-induced pulsations of the lungs could be coupled to the inner ear via endolymphatic pathways[7]. Finally, sound-induced vibrations of the substrate could contribute, since all low-frequency fibers are sensitive to vibrations[8]. Recently, the latter hypothesis was addressed. It was shown that cancellation of the sound-induced vibrations does not change the sensitivity and, therefore, that the extratympanic sensitivity probably is not mediated through sound-induced vibrations[9].

In the present study we compare results from neurophysiological experiments and laser vibrometry measurements of eardrum, columellar footplate and operculum vibrations in order to elucidate the pathway of extratympanic stimulation.

Neurophysiological experiments.

Details of the experimental methods are described in Christensen-Dalsgaard and Jørgensen[9] and Jørgensen and Christensen-Dalsgaard [10]. Briefly, the VIIIth nerve of grassfrogs (<u>Rana</u> <u>temporaria</u>) were exposed under full anesthesia using a dorsal approach. 1-2 days after recovery the animals were treated with an analgesic and immobilized. The animals were placed in a natural sitting posture on a platform mounted on a vibration exciter. The setup was located in an anechoic room and directional sound stimulation was emitted from 8 loudspeakers. Sound-induced vertical vibrations in the platform were canceled using the vibration exciter. Single unit responses in the VIIIth nerve were recorded using glass microelectrodes. Some of the frogs were detympanated, i.e. approximately 75% of the eardrum was removed bilaterally, leaving the columella suspended by a strip of membrane.

164 fibers found were low-frequency amphibian papilla fibers (best frequency (BF) from 100 to 400 Hz) with sound thresholds between 23 dB SPL and 80 dB SPL at BF. Average sound thresholds decreased from 72 dB SPL at 100 Hz to 50 dB SPL at 400 Hz.

The directional characteristics of the low-frequency fibers was a figure-eight' characteristic, with maximal responses from ipsi- and contralateral stimulus directions and a reduced response at the frontal and posterior angles. When equivalent dB values were calculated for the responses from different directions using the fibers' rate-level functions (see Feng[3]) the maximal difference at different directions was approximately 10 dB. The preferred firing phases of the fibers varied systematically with sound direction .The phase shift between ipsi- and contralateral stimulus direction at 200 Hz averaged 140°.

When the tympana were removed, sound sensitivity decreased by more than 10 dB for fibers with BF's from 150 Hz. In contrast, at 100 Hz there was little effect of removing the tympana. The decrease in sensitivity depended on frequency with the highest decrease in sensitivity at high frequencies. Furthermore, the figure-eight' directionality pattern observed in nerve fibers in intact frogs was not evident in the detympanated frogs.

Laser vibrometry measurements.

The experimental setup for these measurements was similar to that used by Jørgensen[11] except that sound was emitted from eight speakers (placed at 45° intervals).

Eardrum vibrations of <u>Rana</u> <u>temporaria</u> showed a band-pass characteristic with peak vibration amplitudes around 600-1000 Hz. At low frequencies eardrum vibrations were very small. The vibration amplitude increased with frequency at a rate of approximately 16 dB/octave in the low-frequency range. At 400 Hz, maximal amplitude differences (between ipsi- and contralateral stimulus directions) were approximately 3-4 dB, and decreased towards lower frequencies. The directional characteristic at low frequencies was ovoidal.

Preliminary measurements from the columellar footplate showed vibration amplitudes approximately 15-25 dB below the eardrum vibrations with similar frequency responses for footplate and eardrum vibrations. However, the motion of the columellar footplate is complex and other sites may show different vibration amplitudes. In contrast, the frequency response of the operculum was different with a peak at 1200-1500 Hz and less energy at low frequencies. The vibrations were approximately 20 dB below the footplate vibrations.

Discussion

The neurophysiological data on intact frogs show that there is pronounced sensitivity and directionality at low frequencies that does not correlate with the eardrum vibrations. The directional plots are figure-eight shaped for the neural data and ovoidal for the eardrum vibrations and the directionality is much larger in the neurophysiological data. Furthermore, the mean sensitivity of the low-frequency fibers increase with frequency with a rate of approximately 10 dB/octave, whereas eardrum vibration velocities increase with a rate of approximately 16 dB/octave in the low frequency range. Therefore, these results taken together show that the responses of the low-frequency auditory fibers are largely dominated by extratympanic pathways, as concluded by Wilczynski et al[2]. However, it is then surprising that when the tympanum is removed, sensitivity seems to decline, also at the low frequencies. This finding conflicts with the earlier results by Lombard and Straughan[1]. However, in their experiments one of the animals (<u>Hyla</u> <u>versicolor</u>) actually showed a decrease in sensitivity down to below 500 Hz. Also, the curves are based on single individuals and show a large amount of scatter.

The motion of the operculum relative to the otic capsule was very small when stimulated with free-field sound in our experiments. Furthermore, the frequency response of the operculum does not exhibit a pronounced low-frequency resonance. In fact, the vibrations at low frequencies are approximately 20 dB smaller than the vibrations of the columellar footplate in these preliminary experiments. Therefore, it is unlikely that the operculum functions in extratympanic sound reception. Stimulation by sound-induced vibrations in the substrate can probably also be ruled out as an extratympanic pathway[9]. Remaining mechanisms for extratympanic sensitivity are bone conduction or stimulation via the lung pathway. However, lung stimulation is probably most efficient around the resonance frequency of the lung, i.e. around 600 Hz for <u>Rana</u> <u>temporaria</u>). Furthermore, if it is believed that the low-frequency sensitivity is extratympanic the effects seen when the tympana are removed indicates a close connection between tympanic and extratympanic pathways. It is not clear to us why such a close connection should be found for the lung pathway. Therefore, the present results indicate that extratympanic sensitivity is related to bone conduction. Bone conduction can cause direct vibrations of the inner-ear fluid or differential motion of the columella relative to the otic capsule. Removing a part of the tympanum changes the impedance of the columella as seen from the oval window (making it less stiff) and could conceivably also affect these bone conduction pathways. If the low frequency sensitivity is caused by differential motion of the otic capsule and columella, it is interesting to note that a relatively heavy columella would probably increase the low frequency sensitivity because of inertia, while a light columella would increase high-frequency sensitivity because of better impedance match of tympanum and columella to the impedance of air. A compromise between these strategies might effectively limit the high-frequency sensitivity of most frogs.

Finally, the directionality observed for the low-frequency fibers probably can be explained by a simple bone-conduction model proposed by Jørgensen and Christensen-Dalsgaard[12]. Briefly, the inner-ear fluid must have a preferred direction of motion, which is the axis joining the pressure release windows, i.e. the round and oval windows. Probably, vibrations along this axis produces maximal responses in the sensory cells. This axis would proably be almost parallel to the ipsi- and contralateral direction. Stimulation from these directions would then produce maximal responses whereas stimulation from frontal and caudal directions would produce small vibrations in the inner-ear fluid. This model is of course simplistic, and the sound-induced vibrations of the skull remains to be studied.

68

Acknowledgements

The Center for Sound Communication is funded by the Danish National Research Foundation.

References

1. Lombard, R.E., Straughan, I.R. (1974) Functional aspects of anuran middle ear structures. *J. Exp. Biol.* **61** 71-93.
2. Wilczynski, W., Resler, C. and Capranica, R.R. (1987) Tympanic and extratympa nic sound transmission in the leopard frog. *J. Comp. Physiol. A* **161** 659-669.
3. Feng, A.S. (1980) Directional characteristics of the acoustic receiver of the leopard frog (*Rana pipiens*): A study of eighth nerve auditory responses. *J. Acoust. Soc. Am.* **68** 1107-1114.
4. Aertsen, A.M.H.J., Vlaming,M.S.M.G., Eggermont,J.J. and Johannesma, P.I.M. (1986) Directional hearing in the grassfrog (Rana temporaria L.). II. Acoustics and modelling of the auditory periphery. *Hear. Res.* **21** 17-40.
5. Hetherington, T.E. (1988) Biomechanics of vibration reception in the bullfrog, Rana catesbeiana. *J. Comp. Physiol. A* **163** 43-52.
6. Eggermont, J.J. (1988) Mechanism of sound localization in anurans. In B. Fritzsch et al. (eds.) *The evolution of the amphibian auditory periphery*, Wiley Interscience, pp. 307-336
7. Narins, P.M., Ehret, G., Tautz, J. (1988) Accessory pathway for sound transfer in a neotropical frog. *Proc. Natl. Acad. Sci.* **85** 1508-1512.
8. Christensen-Dalsgaard, J., Narins, P.M. (1993) Sound and vibration sensitivity of VIIIth nerve fibers in the frogs Leptodactylus albilabris and Rana pipiens pipiens. *Comp. Physiol. A* **172** 653-662.
9. Christensen-Dalsgaard , J. and Jørgensen, M.B. (1996) Sound and vibration sensitivity of VIIIth nerve fibers in the grassfrog, Rana temporaria. *J. Comp. Physiol. A* **179** (in press).
10. Jørgensen, M.B. and Christensen-Dalsgaard, J. (1996) Directionality of auditory nerve fiber responses to pure tone stimuli in the grassfrog, Rana temporaria. I. Spike rate responses. *J. Comp. Physiol. A*, (submitted).
11. Jørgensen, M.B. (1991) Comparative studies of the biophysics of directional hearing in anurans. *J. Comp. Physiol. A* **169** 591-598.
12. Jørgensen, M.B. and Christensen-Dalsgaard, J. (1996) Directionality of auditory nerve fiber responses to pure tone stimuli in the grassfrog, Rana temporaria. II. Spike timing . *J. Comp. Physiol. A*, (submitted).

FREQUENCY SELECTIVITY OF SACCULAR AFFERENTS OF THE GOLDFISH REVEALED BY REVCOR ANALYSIS

R.R. FAY

Parmly Hearing Institute and Department of Psychology
Loyola University Chicago
6525 North Sheridan Road
Chicago, IL 60626 USA
rfay@luc.edu

Saccular afferents were stimulated by flat-spectrum wideband noise and spike times used to trigger the averaging of the acoustic waveform, creating impulse responses. FFTs of these gave filter functions. Filter functions were easily classified into two groups; low- and high-CF. Filter functions for all afferents have features in common and differ primarily in a 15 dB/octave spectral tilt. The common features may reflect hair cell membrane properties while the spectral tilt may be due to differences in hair bundle stiffness and mode of attachment to the otolithic membrane. These simple mechanisms apparently give rise to a crude peripheral frequency analysis that is considerably elaborated in the central auditory system.

1   Hearing and Frequency Analysis

The saccule is an otolith organ found among all vertebrate classes. While it apparently has an exclusively vestibular function among mammals, it responds to low-frequency seismic vibrations in anurans[1] and acoustic particle motion in fishes[2.] In otophysan fishes (e.g., carp, catfish, minnows, and goldfish), the saccule is the primary hearing organ, responding to sound pressure by virtue of its close mechanical link to the swimbladder via a series of bones, the Weberian ossicles[3]. Saccular afferents project to a set of octavolateral nuclei in the medulla, and their ascending projections make up a central auditory system with elements possibly homologous to those of terrestrial vertebrates at the levels of the mesencephalon, diencephalon, and telencephalon[4].

Physiological properties of mesencephalic[5] and diencephalic[6] cells in goldfish reveal features common to all vertebrates, including frequency selectivity, two-tone inhibition, a diversity of peri-stimulus time histogram profiles, and a progressive loss of phase-locking. Behavioral studies describe a sense of hearing that is also typical for vertebrates. One of its primary features is frequency analysis as revealed in experiments on frequency discrimination[7], masking patterns[8], and behavior consistent with analytic listening[9], and pitch-like and timbre-like[10] perceptions.

Frequency analysis depends, at least in part, on the frequency selectivity of primary saccular afferents. Furukawa and Ishii[11] classified saccular afferents of goldfish into two categories (S1 and S2), in part, based on their characteristic frequencies (CF): S1 CFs are at 600-800 Hz while S2 CFs are at 200-400 Hz .

The origin of this frequency selectivity is not clear. S1 afferents (high-CF) tend to innervate the rostral end of the saccule while S2 afferents (low-CF) innervate the caudal end[11]. There is no evidence that this crude tonotopy arises from a macromechanical frequency analysis. Short hair cells of the rostral saccule show a low-quality resonance (40-220 Hz) to a current step while tall cells of the caudal region show a spike-plateau response[12]. These and other physiological differences suggest that frequency selectivity of primary afferents may arise from membrane properties of hair cells. In addition, it is possible that frequency selectivity arises from micromechanical processes: the rostral hair cells have shorter and presumably stiffer hair bundles than the caudal hair cells.

The present experiments reinvestigate the frequency response functions of saccular afferents in the goldfish using the reverse-correlation, or REVCOR method[13]. These experiments follow up a recent observation[14] that the REVCOR filter shapes of low- and high-CF afferents have common features in fine structure. The present study focuses on these common features and reveal what appears to be a single dimension that determines CF. This dimension is a simple "spectral tilt" that could arise from micromechanical processes at the level of hair cell stereociliary bundles and their mode of stimulation.

2   Methods

Responses of 53 single saccular afferents were recorded extracellularly in 3 common goldfish (*Carassius auratus*). The recording tank (Plexiglas cylinder, 23 cm in diameter and 28 cm high) rested on a Micro-G vibration-isolation table inside a sound attenuating chamber. Sound was generated by a University Sound UW-30 underwater loudspeaker buried in water-saturated sand at the bottom of the cylinder.

Goldfish were anesthetized in a 1:5000 solution of MS-222, immobilized with an intramuscular injection of Pavulon (1 µg/g body weight), and respirated. The skull was glued to a brass post that pressed the upper palate onto a respirator tube. The fish was positioned in the tank's center with the tail angled down and the top of the skull above the surface. After removing bone overlying the brainstem, the cerebellum was retracted to expose the saccular nerve. The cranial cavity was filled with a fluoroinert liquid (3M Inc., FC-77) to help maintain a view of the nerve. Spikes were recorded using KCl-filled pipettes and were time-stamped with 0.1 msec accuracy.

A response area was obtained using 500 msec tone bursts (20 msec rise/fall times) presented at frequencies between 100 to 1200 Hz at various levels within the fiber's dynamic range. A fiber was stimulated with 10, 2.5 sec noise samples (10 kHz sample rate). Noises were synthesized in a 100 to 2k Hz band with a flat (+/- 3 dB) spectrum measured using a CH-17 Clevite hydrophone replacing the fish in the tank.

REVCOR functions were computed by averaging hydrophone recordings of the noise samples triggered by spike times, for 51.2 msec before and after each spike. This estimates the impulse response of the linear filtering that precedes spike generation[13]. An FFT of the impulse responses estimated an afferent's filter shape between 100 and 2500 Hz within a dynamic range of about 20 dB. REVCORS were obtained for several noise levels spanning each fiber's dynamic range.

3   Results with Discussion

Figure 1A shows results for four afferents that are typical of the 53 afferents studied. Each panel shows a representative impulse response function, REVCOR filter functions obtained at three sound pressure levels, and frequency response area functions (RAs) in response to iso-level tone bursts at several levels. Figure 1B illustrates that impulse responses for both low- and high-CF afferents can be generally classified into two groups based on their polarity. Afferents in the top two rows have major upward peaks while those in the bottom two rows have downward peaks. The times of the peaks are 2.1 msec +/- 0.4 msec preceding the falling phase of each spike. These polarity differences probably arise from the hair cell orientation patterns of the goldfish saccule; hair cells in the dorsal half have their kinocilia oriented dorsally while those in the ventral half are oriented ventrally[15].

The RAs for the two high-CF afferents are typical of those reported earlier[16]. Afferent B22 (top left) has a CF near 600 Hz, and CF threshold of 15 dB re:1 dyne cm^{-2}. The most excitatory frequency (or best frequency - BF) remains at CF throughout the dynamic range. The RA for afferent C10 (top right) shows a CF at about 900 Hz, and a CF threshold of about 10 dB. Note that the BF for this afferent shifts downward to about 600 Hz as level is raised. This is common among high-CF saccular afferents[5].

The impulse responses for B22 and C10 are brief and nearly symmetrical with at most three observable oscillations. The FFTs of these and other impulse responses show a peak at about 600 Hz with roll-offs toward lower and higher frequencies. Thin vertical lines approximately locate features (peaks or corners) of the filter functions. In general, these features include a major peak at 600 Hz, and minor peaks at about 170 Hz and 900 Hz. Note that for afferent C10, the 900 Hz peak in the filter functions corresponds to the CF determined from the RA. For B22, the 600 Hz peak in the filter functions corresponds to CF.

The RAs for the two low-CF afferents (bottom panels) show CFs in the region of 200 Hz, and CF thresholds at about 5 dB. For afferent C15 (bottom left), the BF remains at CF as level increases. For afferent C17, however, the BF shifts upward as level increases. At frequencies above BF, both afferents show a relatively steep decline in tone-evoked activity that converges at the spontaneous rate between 500 Hz (C15) and 700 Hz (C17), and falls below spontaneous at higher frequencies. This single-tone suppression is common among low-CF saccular afferents in goldfish[5].

Impulse responses and filter functions for C15 and C17 show relatively broad tuning with corners at about 150-200 Hz and 600 Hz. Although the REVCOR features near 200 Hz tend to correspond with CF determined from the RAs, the corner features at 600 Hz do not. For C15, 600 Hz tones are suppressive rather than excitatory, and for C17, all iso-level functions decline steeply at 600 Hz. Thus, REVCOR filter functions present a somewhat different view of tuning than do the RAs. On the other hand, the effects of level on BF for the RAs tend to correspond to level effects seen in the REVCORS: filter shape remains relatively independent of level for C15 but is tilted toward the 600 Hz feature at higher levels for C17. Note also that for C10, increasing the level from -20 dB to -10 dB causes a small change in the relative heights of the features at 900 and 600 Hz that parallels the downward shift in BF seen in the RA.

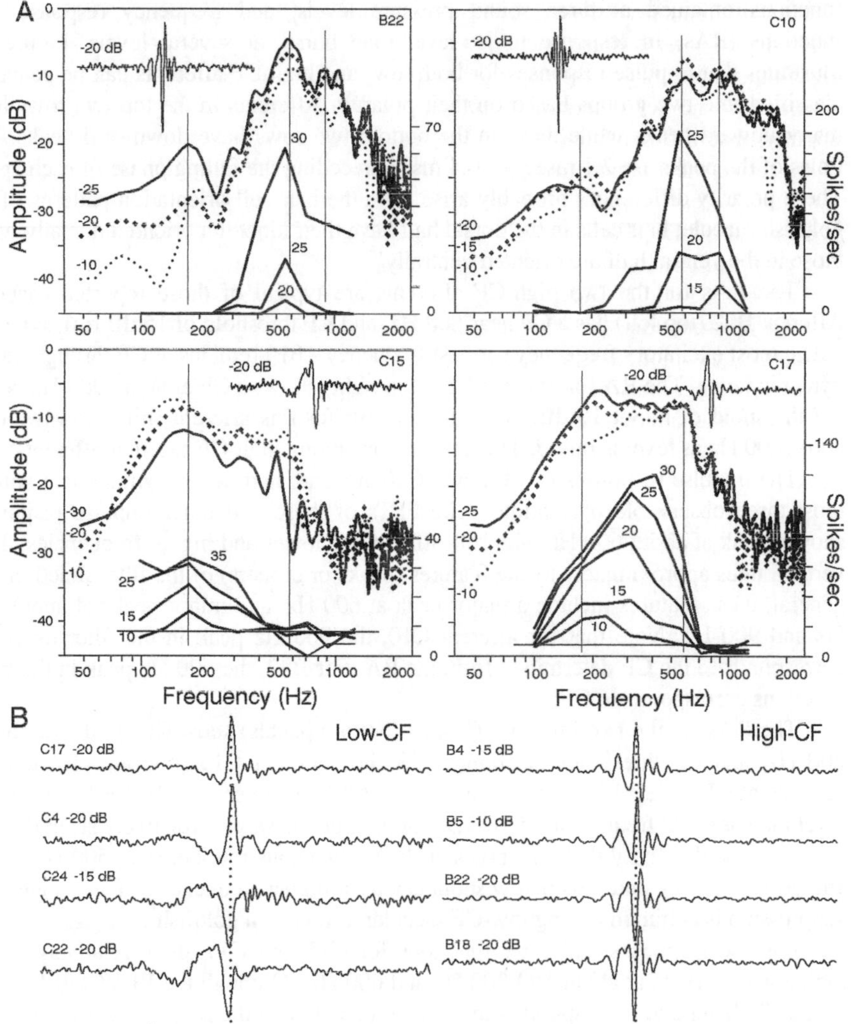

Figure 1: (A) Frequency response data for four representative afferents. The impulse response (40 msec in duration) is shown as an inset, smoothed by a 5-point moving average (0.1 msec/point). The filter shapes (smooth curves) are FFTs of impulse responses after subtracting the averaged, smoothed acoustic spectrum, and then smoothing using a 5-point moving average (9.77 Hz/point). The left ordinate applies to the REVCOR filters and is in dB with an arbitrary reference. The dotted and dashed lines serve to visually separate the functions. Noise spectrum levels in dB re: 1 dyne cm^{-2} are given for each impulse response and filter function. Iso-level spike rate functions of tone burst frequency (RAs) are shown as lines connecting data points, referred to the right ordinate. Numbers are sound pressure levels in dB re: 1 dyne cm^{-2}. Spontaneous rates are: 0 for B22 and C10, 16 spikes/sec for C15, and 4.4 spikes/sec for C17. (B) Representative impulse responses for eight afferents illustrating their classification according to polarity.

All afferents investigated are similar in having at least two of the three REVCOR filter shape features illustrated in Figure 1 (in the regions of 170-220, 600, and 900 Hz). It thus appears that there may be two sets of mechanisms that determine frequency selectivity; one set determining the shared features in spectral fine structure and another that differentiates the low- and high-CF groups. In an effort to further characterize the fundamental similarities and differences between CF groups, filter functions were averaged across afferents within each group (Figure 2). These averages highlight the three shared features in spectral fine structure, but also suggest that the two groups differ in one simple way; the high-CF filter seems to be a spectrally tilted version of the low-CF filter, and vice versa.

To illustrate this, the low-CF average was rotated around the 400 Hz point by 15 dB/octave and plotted as a dotted line that overlies the high-CF filter. Similarly, the high-CF average was rotated by 15 dB/octave in the opposite direction. These rotations reproduce the alternative filter accurately between about 170 and 1100 Hz. One mechanism that could explain these correspondences is that low-CF afferents innervate

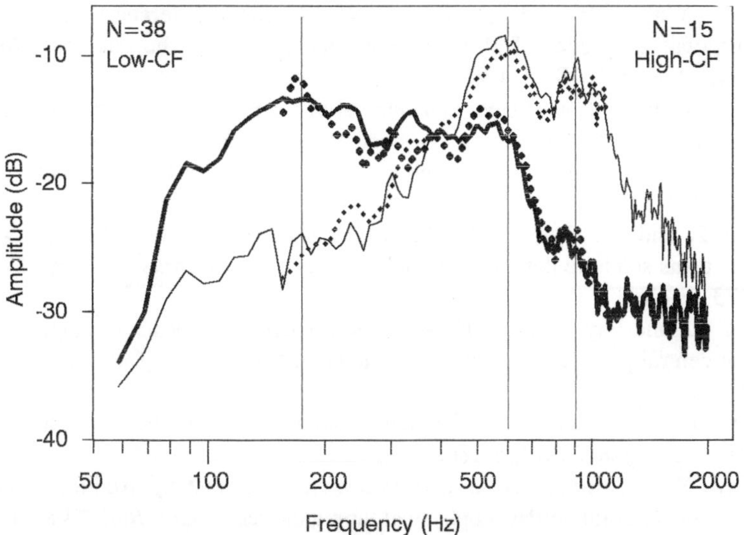

Figure 2: Averaged filter functions for low- and high-CF afferents. The dashed lines are the result of tilting the alternative filter function by 15 dB/octave. See text.

hair cells responding to otolith displacement while high-CF afferents contact hair cells responding to otolith acceleration. These differences could arise from differences between hair cells in hair bundle stiffness[12] and the friction of coupling between the hair bundle and the otolithic membrane[17]. It has been noted that a similar spectral tilt operates in the mechanosensory lateral line system to give the acceleration-coupled canal neuromasts a response to higher frequencies of hydrodynamic flow than the velocity-coupled superficial neuromasts[18]. However, in the present case this scheme predicts a 12 dB/octave difference in frequency response, not the 15 dB/octave observed.

In any case, a simple spectral tilt that differentiates low- and high-CF primary afferents appears to provide the brain with information used to create the kind of tetrapod-like frequency analysis we have observed among midbrain neurons[5], and the typically "vertebrate" sense of hearing exhibited by goldfish[19].

Acknowledgments

This research was supported by an NIH NIDCD grant 2 P01 DC00293-09. Thanks to Sheryl Coombs, Bill Yost, Bill Shofner, and Roy Patterson for helpful discussions.

References

1. Narins, P.M. and Lewis, E.R. (1984) The vertebrate ear as an exquisite seismic sensor. *J. Acoust. Soc. Amer.* **76** 1384-1387.
2. Edds-Walton, P., and Fay, R.R. (1995) Regional differences in directional response properties of afferents along the saccule of the toadfish (*Opsanus tau*). *Biol. Bull.* **189** 211-212.
3. von Frisch, K. (1936) Über den Gehörsinn der Fische. *Biol. Rev.* **11** 210-246.
4. Streidter, G. (1991) Auditory, electrosensory, and mechanosensory lateral line pathways through the forebrain in channel catfishes. *J. Comp. Neurol.* **312** 311-331.
5. Lu, Z. and Fay, R.R. (1993) Acoustic response properties of single units in the torus semicircularis of the goldfish, *Carassius auratus. J. Comp. Physiol*, **173** 33-48.
6. Lu, Z., and Fay, R.R. (1995) Acoustic response properties of single units of the central posterior nucleus of the thalamus in goldfish (*Carassius auratus*). *J. Comp. Physiol.*, **176** 747-760.
7. Fay, R.R. (1970) Auditory frequency discrimination in the goldfish. *J.Comp. Physiol. Psychol.* **73** 175-180.
8. Fay, R.R. Ahroon, W.A. and Orawski, A.T. (1978) Auditory masking patterns in goldfish:Psychophysical tuning curves. *J. Exp. Biol.* **74** 83-100.
9. Fay, R. (1992) Analytic listening by the goldfish. *Hear. Res.* **59** 101-107.
10. Fay, R.R. (1995) Perception of spectrally and temporally complex sounds by the goldfish (*Carassius auratus*). *Hear. Res.* **89** 146-154.
11. Furukawa, T., and Ishii, Y. (1967). Neurophysiological studies on hearing in goldfish. *J. Neurophysiol.* **30** 1377-1403.
12. Sugihara, I. and Furukawa, T. (1989) Morphological and functional aspects of two different types of hair cells in the goldfish sacculus. *J. Neurophysiol.* **62** 1330-1343.
13. de Boer, E, and de Jongh, H.R. (1978) On cochlear coding: Potentialities and limitations of the reverse correlation technique. *J. Acoust. Soc. Amer.* **63** 115-135.

14. Fay, R.R., Chronopoulos, M., Patterson, R. (1996) The sound of a sinusoid: Perception and neural representations in the goldfish (*Carassius auratus*). *Auditory Neuroscience* (in press).
15. Platt, C. (1977). Hair cell distribution and orientation in goldfish otolith organs. *J. Comp. Neurol.* **172** 283-297.
16. Fay, R.R. (1990) Suppression and excitation in auditory nerve fibers of the goldfish, *Hear. Res.* **48** 93-110.
17. Rogers, P. H. and M. Cox (1988) Underwater sound as a biological stimulus, in *Sensory Biology of Aquatic Animals*, eds. J. Atema, R. R. Fay, A. N. Popper, W. N. Tavolga (Springer, New York) pp. 131-149.
18. Coombs, S, Janssen, J, and Mongomery, J. (1992) Functional and evolutionary implications of peripheral diversity in lateral line systems, in *The Evolutionary Biology of Hearing*, eds. D.B. Webster, R. R. Fay, A. N. Popper (Springer, New York) pp. 267-294.
19. Fay, R.R. (1988) *Hearing in Vertebrates: A Psychophysics Databook* (Hill-Fay Associates, Winnetka, IL).

THE MECHANICS OF THE AVIAN COCHLEA: RATE-INTENSITY FUNCTIONS OF AUDITORY-NERVE FIBRES IN THE EMU

C. KÖPPL[*#], G. K. YATES[*] AND G. A. MANLEY[*#]

*Department of Physiology, The University of Western Australia
Nedlands 6907 Western Australia
#Institut für Zoologie der Technischen Universität München
Lichtenbergstraße 4, 85747 Garching, Germany
CK@cip1.zoo.chemie.tu-muenchen.de

Measurements of rate-level functions in high-frequency (>1.5 kHz) single auditory-nerve afferents of the emu indicate that at CF, almost all fibres show a sloping saturation. Below CF, their responses are closer to a saturating type. This is conistent with the presence of a compressive non-linearity at CF, as has been shown for the guinea pig. In the emu, however, for fibres at any given CF, the break point in the intensity function of each fibre co-varies with the neural sensitivity, suggesting that the cochlear amplifier is not global but is local to each region of the papilla. This finding is consistent with previous theories on the function of the avian hearing organ.

1 Introduction

Excitatory rate-level (I/O) functions of auditory-nerve fibres are not always of a simple saturating type. In mammals, it has been established that there are 3 intergrading types, characterized by different slope patterns of their I/O function at CF:[1] saturating (sigmoidal, with a clear rate plateau), sloping-saturating (with a break between a steeper slope at low levels and a shallow slope at higher levels) and straight (with an overall shallow slope showing no indication of saturation). Those 3 types are correlated with the 3 spontaneous rate classes (high, medium, low, respectively) and the different threshold sensitivities commonly recognized in mammals (low, medium and high, respectively). Rate-intensity functions far below CF, in the tail region of the tuning curve, are always saturating. By correcting the I/O functions at CF by an off-CF function, a nonlinear, highly compressive function can be derived that strongly resembles the I/O functions typically measured for basilar membrane (BM) motion.[2,3] It was therefore suggested that the different shapes of I/O function in auditory-nerve fibres result from their different sensitivities relative to the uniform mechanical input from the BM, whose nonlinearity is a consequence of the saturation of the active feedback process commonly termed the cochlear amplifier. According to this hypothesis, sensitive fibres begin to respond in the low-level, linear region of the BM and show a clear saturation. The I/O functions of fibres of medium sensitivity contain a portion of the linear region, but then show a break in their slope where the BM displacement starts to become compressive. Insensitive fibres do not begin to respond until the BM displacement has reached the upper, nonlinear region; their I/O functions are therefore of relatively low slope and are straight.

Comparatively little is known about the micromechanics of the avian inner ear. Like mammals, birds show a differentiation of their hair cells into two types, tall hair cells and short hair cells, that are, however, not sharply differentiated.[4] In their extreme forms they are characterized by an innervation pattern which bears a resemblance to that typical of mammals: Tall hair cells are contacted by several afferent as well as small efferent terminals, whereas short hair cells receive no afferent but large efferent terminals.[5] Bird hair cells are not arranged in rows, many more than in mammals are found in any one cross-section of the cochlea[6] and active afferents innervate more than just the most neural row. A potentially important difference between birds and mammals with respect to cochlear mechanics is that in birds, a significant proportion of hair cells is situated not on the BM but on the cartilagenous neural limbus. The BM supports a travelling wave and its input-output function appears to be linear, whereas the neural limbus hardly moves at all.[7] However, fibre-tracing studies in the starling and pigeon have shown that it is the hair cells on the neural limbus which provide the most sensitive input to afferent fibers.[8,9] This suggests an important micromechanical role for the tectorial membrane in birds.[10]

Despite the linear behavior of BM motion,[7] some sort of active feedback or cochlear amplification may also be assumed for birds. Compelling indirect evidence is the presence of several types of otoacoustic emissions.[11] In mammals, otoacoustic emissions are commonly believed to reflect outer hair cell motility, which is assumed to be the physical basis of the cochlear amplifier.[12] A mechanism similar to outer hair cell motility appears unlikely in birds.[11] However, the sparse afferent innervation or even complete lack thereof on avian short hair cells also suggests some local role for those hair cells, perhaps in another form of an amplification mechanism.[10]

We chose to investigate the I/O behaviour of auditory-nerve fibres in a bird, the young Australian emu. Our aims were: a) to look for evidence of non-linear behavior at CF compared with off-CF and b) to compare the properties of any such nonlinearity with that found in the guinea pig.[1]

2 Methods

Data were collected from 19 emus (*Dromaius novaehollandiae*) aged from 1 to 14 days post-hatching. They were anaesthetized with a combination of pentobarbital („Nembutal") and chloral hydrate („Chlorthesin"), artificially respirated and held at $38.7 \pm 0.7°C$ in a sound-attenuating chamber. Their condition was monitored using the electrocardiogram and muscle-potential recordings. Stimuli were delivered in a calibrated, closed sound system. The cochlear ganglion was exposed using a dorsolateral approach, and access to the entire length of the ganglion was possible in some preparations. Glass microelectrodes were advanced into the ganglion using a custom-built motor drive while presenting noise bursts as a search stimulus. Custom hardware and software were used to control the frequency synthesizer, attenuator and tone gate by a PC, as well as to record the spike responses digitized through a custom-built window discriminator.

Frequency tuning curves for individual afferent fibres were derived using two programs, one a threshold hunting routine, the other via interpolation of responses to pseudo-random stimuli within a pre-defined matrix of frequencies and sound-pressure levels centred at the unit's CF. The matrix was generally repeated three times for tuning curves and the discharge rate for each combination of frequency and sound pressure averaged. For I/O functions, the matrix was reduced to fewer frequencies and the stimuli presented up to ten times. Complete sets of 10 repeats of raster data were analyzed from 42 afferents. In addition, the I/O functions derived using the tuning-curve matrix data were analyzed for a further 18 afferents.

Using an iterative procedure, I/O function parameters were curve fitted as a group (all frequencies) for any one fibre, assuming that the spontaneous rate (parameter A_0 in Fig. 1) and the slope of the compressive region of the cochlear amplifier (parameter A_4) were invariant across all frequencies, and that the saturation firing rate was constant for all frequencies above 1 kHz. The parameters A_2 (a measure of the low-intensity sensitivity of the fibre) and A_3 (the break point in the slope) were permitted to vary with stimulus frequency.

3 Results

At their respective CF, virtually all afferents were classified as having a 'sloping saturation' (after[1]). Only one fibre in a very young chick qualified as 'saturating', and it had a very high threshold. A few I/O functions could be classified as being 'straight'. Below CF, however, the responses were closer to the saturating type. These responses are consistent with a highly compressive non-linearity in the cochlear amplifier, as seen in mammalian fibres.

As for conventional neural threshold measures, our parameter A_2 was found

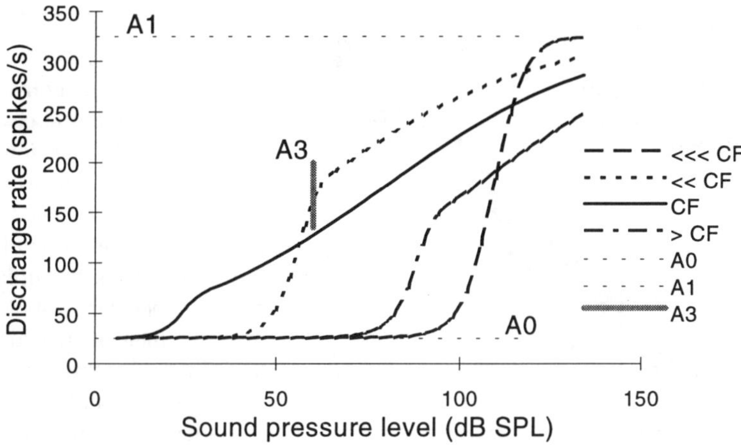

Fig.1: The parameters used in fitting the I/O functions to auditory-nerve experimental data. The four curves are typical for the following frequencies: very much below CF, a little below CF, at CF and above CF. The spontaneous rate, A0, the maximum firing rate, A1, and the slope of the compressive nonlinear drive to the system, A4 (not shown), are constrained to be the same for all frequencies. The sensitivity parameter, A2, and the intensity at which the break occurs, A3, are permitted to vary with frequency. A3 is only shown for one frequency. A2 is the intensity at which the AP rate would reach half its maximum driven rate (i.e., A0 + (A1 - A0) / 2) if the function were saturating.

to be much more sharply tuned than the presumed BM tuning curve (Fig. 2; BM assumed to be the same as in the pigeon). The breakpoint in the slope of the I/O functions (A3) was found not to be constant between fibres having the same CF, but to co-vary with sensitivity (A2). In other words, the break of the slope of the I/O function at CF occured at a higher sound pressure in neurons whose sensitivity was poorer.

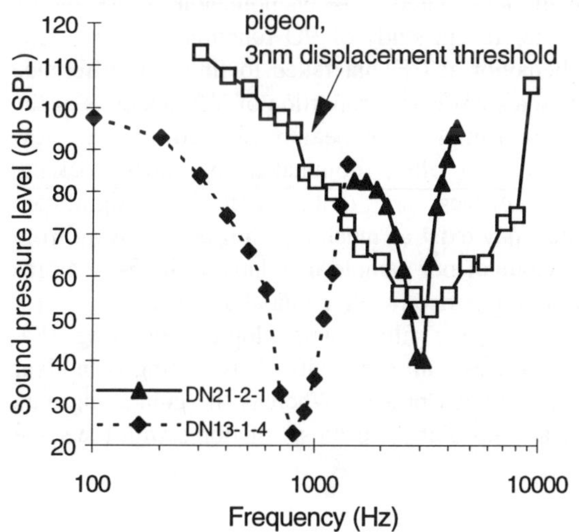

Fig 2. A comparison of the frequency tuning of the parameter A2 for two auditory-nerve fibres of the emu and basilar membrane tuning (for the pigeon).[7]

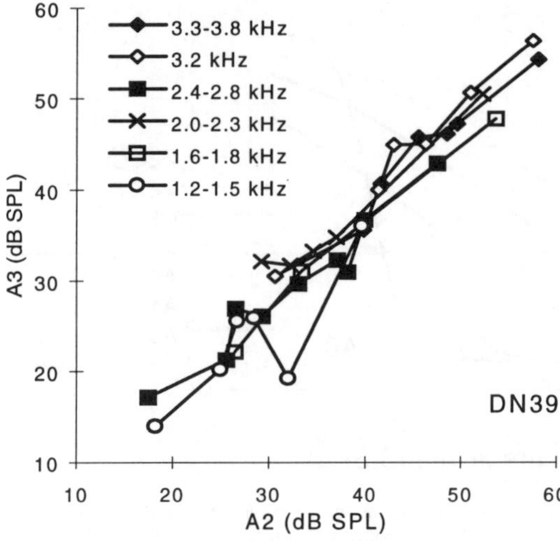

In fact, on average, these parameters followed each other closely in a 1:1 fashion over a range of more than 30 dB (Fig. 3). If it can be assumed that the breakpoint in the slope of the I/O function reflects the upper limit of a cochlear amplification process, then it would appear that, in birds, this amplifier is very localized, either to individual hair cells or to small groups of hair cells.

Fig. 3. Diagram to illustrate the co-variation of the parameters A2 and A3 for six sets of nerve-fibre data, each centred on a different range of CFs.

4 Discussion

Our results are consistent with the presence of a compressive non-linearity at CF, comparable to the situation in mammals, where this phenomenon is commonly termed the cochlear amplifier. Another recent study of I/O functions in a bird, the pigeon, also described non-linear behavior at CF, but failed to find any difference from off-CF functions, and also found a significant proportion of I/O functions of the saturating type.[13] However, the data sample was heavily skewed towards low frequencies, where discharge rates are often dominated by phase-locking. Furthermore, low-frequency tuning curves are quite broad and significant nonlinearity of the cochlear amplifier may exist as much as a full octave away from CF. We believe the discharge behaviour of our sample of relatively high-CF fibres (1.5-4 kHz) provides a better basis for comparison with mammalian data.

Both bird studies, however, agree that for fibres with sloping-saturating I/O-functions, the breakpoint strongly correlates with sensitivity. This finding is in clear contrast to equivalent results from the guinea pig[1,14]. Whereas the guinea-pig data indicate that there is a global cochlear amplifier for each set of fibres with the same

CF, the emu data suggest that the cochlear amplifier is local and its operational range is reflected in the local neural thresholds.

This difference is not entirely unexpected considering the known differences in morphology and innervation of the mammalian and bird cochlea. In mammals, all recorded cochlear afferents originate on a single row of inner hair cells; afferents at the same CF but with different thresholds will therefore reflect the activity of that same inner hair cell at different sound-pressure levels. In birds, by contrast, afferent contacts are made on hair cells that are placed either across the entire width, in the apical papillar region (30 to 50 hair-cells wide), or across about half of the width in the basal cochlear region (10 to 15 hair cells wide). These afferent fibres mostly contact only one hair cell and individual hair cells are contacted by one or two afferent fibres.[5] At any one CF, afferents with different thresholds will therefore reflect the activity of different hair cells.

Previous work tracing physiologically-characterized afferent fibres even suggests a *systematic* change of threshold with the position of the innervated hair cell across the papilla.[8,9] If we assume that in birds, the break in the slope of nerve-fibre I/O functions results from the onset of saturation of a cochlear amplification process (probably in the mechanical-to-electrical transduction stage as in the guinea pig), then this systematic distribution of thresholds suggests that the amplification process has a different threshold for different positions across the papilla for the same CF. The amplification process would thus be localised to individual hair cells or to small groups of hair cells.

Since the avian cochlea is as sensitive as the mammalian cochlea, the frequency selectivity is, if anything, even higher,[6] and otoacoustic emissions can be measured [11], there seems little doubt that a cochlear amplifier of some sort exists in birds. As many or most of the short hair cells at least of the basal region lack afferent synapses[5], it has been suggested that over the higher-frequency region of the cochlea, these hair cells are in some way involved in amplification.[10] Some of these cells are, however, very small (3-4 µm tall), so that cell-shape changes as suggested for mammals can hardly be important.[11] Instead, rapid movements of the hair-cell bundles are more likely.[10] Such movements would be oriented across the papilla and not perpendicular to it, and thus not be fully manifest in measurements of BM movement. Instead, the energy would be fed into the tectorial membrane.[10] This can explain why the most sensitive hair cells of birds are not over the free BM, but are rather placed over the cartilage-like neural limbus.

Acknowledgements

Supported by the Deutsche Forschungsgemeinschaft within the SFB 204 (Gehör), a grant from the Australian NH&MRC to the Perth group and a Visiting International Exchange Fellowship to GAM from the Australian ARC.

References

1. Winter, I.M, Robertson, D. and Yates, G.M. (1990) Diversity of characteristic frequency rate-intensity functions in guinea-pig auditory nerve fibres, *Hear. Res.* **45** 191-202
2. Sellick, P.M, Patuzzi, R. and Johnstone, B.M. (1982). Measurement of basilar membrane motion in the guinea pig using the Mossbauer technique, *J. Acoust. Soc. Am.* **72** 131-141.
3. Robles, L, Ruggero, M.A. and Rich, N.C. (1986). Basilar membrane mechanics at the base of the chinchilla cochlea. I. Input-output functions, tuning curves, and phase responses, *J. Acoust. Soc. Am.* **80** 1364-1374.
4. Manley, G.A, Gleich, O, Kaiser, A. and Brix, J. (1989) Functional differentiation of sensory cells in the avian auditory periphery, *J. Comp. Physiol. A* **164** 289-296
5. Fischer, F.P. (1994) General pattern and morphological specializations of the avian cochlea, *Scan. Electr. Micros.* **8** 351-364.
6. Manley G.A. (1990) *Peripheral hearing mechanisms in reptiles and birds.* Springer-Verlag, Berlin, Heidelberg, N.Y.
7. Gummer, A.W, Smolders, J.W.T. and Klinke, R. (1987) Basilar-membrane motion in the pigeon measured with the Mössbauer technique, *Hear. Res.* **29** 63-92.
8. Gleich O. (1989) Auditory primary afferents in the starling: correlation of function and morphology, *Hear. Res.* **37** 255-267
9. Smolders, J., Ding-Pfennigdorff, D. and Klinke, R. (1995) A functional map of the pigeon basilar papilla: correlation of the properties of single auditory nerve fibres and their peripheral origin, *Hear. Res.* **92** 151-169.
10. Manley, G.A. (1995) The avian hearing organ: a status report. in *Advances in Hearing Research*, eds Manley, G.A., Klump, G.M., Köppl, C, Fastl, H., Oeckinghaus, H. (World Scientific, Singapore) pp. 219-229
11. Köppl, C. (1995) Otoacoustic emissions as an indicator for active cochlear mechanics: A primitive property of vertebrate auditory organs. In: *Advances in Hearing Research*, eds. G., Manley, G. Klump, C. Köppl, H. Fastl, H. Oeckinghaus (World Scientific, Singapore) pp. 207-216.
12. Brownell, W.E, Bader, C.R., Bertrand, D. and Ribaupierre, Y. (1985). Evoked mechanical responses of isolated cochlear outer hair cells, *Science* **227** 194-196.
13. Richter, C.-P, Heynert, S. and Klinke, R. (1995) Rate-intensity functions of pigeon auditory-nerve afferents, *Hear. Res.* **83** 19-25.
14. Müller, M., Robertson, D. (1991) Shapes of rate-versus-level functions of primary auditory-nerve fibres: Test of basilar membrane mechanical hypothesis. *Hear. Res.* **57** 71-78.

DOES STOCHASTIC RESONANCE PLAY A ROLE IN HEARING?

P. M. NARINS

Dept. of Physiological Science, UCLA, Los Angeles, CA 90095-1527 USA
e-mail: pnarins@ucla.edu

J. H. BENEDIX, JR.

Department of Biological Sciences, DePauw University,
Greencastle, IN 46135 USA
e-mail: jbenedix@depauw.edu

F. MOSS

Department of Physics, Univ. of Missouri at St. Louis, St. Louis, MO 63121 USA
e-mail: c4646@slvaxa.umsl.edu

This study was motivated by the notion that the internal noise in the anuran auditory system might play a role in improving information transmission in nerve fibers. Internal noise is ubiquitous in all sensory systems, suggesting there may be some selective advantage for this phenomenon. One mechanism that could take advantage of noise to enhance signal transmission is known as *stochastic resonance* (SR). SR is a strictly nonlinear effect, driven by noise and a weak (subthreshold) coherent signal. The goal of the present study was to determine the change in the signal-to-noise ratio (S/N) of the encoded stimulus at the level of the eighth nerve with changes in the internal noise, controlled indirectly by manipulating body temperature. Thus, core temperature shifts were induced experimentally and the resulting changes in S/N were quantified. Single fiber recordings were made from the eighth nerve of 24 anesthetized adult northern leopard frogs, *Rana pipiens pipiens*, while the body temperature was shifted within a range of 8 - 29 °C. We found that the S/N of stimulus encoding in both saccular and in low-frequency amphibian papilla (AP) fibers increased with temperature, whereas the S/N from mid-frequency AP fibers did so to a lesser extent. Although our results do not demonstrate SR in the sense that the S/N did not pass through a maximum at a particular internal noise intensity, they do demonstrate the profound influence of the internal noise on the S/N derived from the neural spike trains.

1 Introduction

Ectotherms such as anuran amphibians may experience daily temperature changes in their natural habitats of more than 10-15_C; thus it is of considerable biological interest to characterize the temperature-dependence of auditory function in these animals and the consequent alteration of the internal noise level of the auditory system. The goal of the present study was to determine the effect of internal noise on information transmission in the frog auditory periphery. To achieve this, we experimentally shifted core temperature to manipulate the internal noise level, and examined the resulting changes in signal-to-noise ratio (S/N) of the auditory nerve spikes. Thus, we measured how the S/N of the encoded stimulus at the level of the auditory nerve was affected by temperature-induced changes in the internal noise level.

This study was motivated by the possibility that the internal noise in the anuran auditory system may play a role in enhancing information transmission in auditory nerve fibers. One possible mechanism that could take advantage of noise to enhance signal transmission is a physical phenomenon known as *stochastic resonance* (SR).[1,2] Stochastic resonance is a strictly nonlinear effect, most often observed in systems with bistable energy potentials, driven by noise and a weak (subthreshold) coherent signal. It is also evident in threshold systems similar to the earliest models for the stochastic behavior of sensory neurons[3] and in subthreshold operation of the Fitzhugh-Nagumo model neuron.[4,5] The noise, which may be either internal to the system, as in certain noisy sensory neurons, or externally-applied, for example in the process of weak signal detection in a noisy environment, adds to the signal to produce superthreshold "spikes" which occur at more-or-less random times, but are to some degree coherent with the signal. Measures of the information content of the spike train, such as the signal-to-noise ratio derived from power spectra, quantitatively show the degree of coherence. SR is characterized by maximum information transfer at some optimal level of the noise intensity, and usually falls off above and below this optimum. Here we present a preliminary report of our attempt to observe SR or related nonlinear effects in a vertebrate auditory system by manipulating the internal noise via core temperature shifts.

2 Materials and Methods

Northern leopard frogs, *Rana pipiens pipiens,* (n=24), were used in our experiments. Frogs were anesthetized 1 h prior to surgery with sodium pentobarbital; injections of tubocurarine chloride were administered every 3-4 h to maintain immobility. A headphone (Beyer DT 48) mounted in a specially-constructed brass housing delivered the calibrated stimulus to the animal. The body temperature of the frog was manipulated in steps of 0.1 °C with a Peltier plate and a matching control unit. During experiments, body temperatures were kept within a range of 8-29 °C, and most of the data were collected at temperatures ranging between 14-24 °C. For each isolated auditory axon a frequency threshold curve was produced using the standard automated up-down tracking method.[6,7] Fibers originating from the sacculus were distinguished from AP fibers using three criteria: (1) CF < 150 Hz, (2) high spontaneous rate, and (3) extreme sensitivity to vibration.

Using an IBM compatible personal computer equipped with Asyst 3.1 software, S/Ns for individual auditory neurons were determined by first presenting a constant tone to the frog and collecting the spike times. Each spike in the train was converted (by the window discriminator) to a standard rectangular pulse of width Δt = 0.59 ms. The train of standard pulses was then sampled at a rate of 10 points/cycle of the stimulus tone, for a sample time equal to 2048 points (1 sweep). An FFT was computed for these 2048 points, and a power spectrum was obtained; ten such spectra were averaged.

Examples of power spectra measured at four different temperatures indicate that the general shape is a sincx function (Fig. 1). For a random sequence of identical pulses, the amplitude of the sincx function in the limit of low frequency is proportional to the r.m.s. pulse repetition rate, i.e. to the noise intensity. The resulting mean power spectrum typically exhibited a narrow peak located at the tone frequency that stood out above the broadband background 'noise' (Fig. 1). The noise level was measured directly from the power spectrum as the noise amplitude at the base of the signal peak, while the signal strength (area above the noise but beneath the signal peak) was determined by integrating the power spectrum in the vicinity of the stimulus frequency and measuring the change in this plot at the signal frequency (Fig. 1, inset). The resultant S/N was calculated from a standard definition[8]: $10\log_{10}(S/N)$ dB, where S is the signal strength and N is the noise amplitude. Power spectra were collected at as many temperatures as possible during the time the electrode was in contact with a fiber. Linear regression slopes for the relationship of S/N to temperature, S/N to noise, and noise to temperature were calculated for each fiber.

3 Results

Fifty-eight fibers from those frogs (n=24) that were exposed to at least four temperatures were included in the analysis. In a fiber that originated in the caudal portion of the AP (CF=1.05 kHz) and tested with a continuous tone of 0.5 kHz at 89 dB SPL (Fig. 1), the signal peaks became progressively larger with increasing temperature. However, not all fibers illustrated this behavior. Data from representative fibers from the sacculus, rostral AP and caudal AP are shown in Figure 2, where in the left column the S/Ns are plotted versus temperature, and in the right column the S/Ns are replotted versus the internal noise measured from the power spectra at the base of the signal feature.

For example, although 16/19 saccular fibers showed significant positive slopes in the linear regression of S/N on temperature (median slope: $0.479 \text{ dB} \cdot {}^{\circ}\text{C}^{-1}$), only 5/15 rostral AP fibers (median slope: $-0.044 \text{ dB} \cdot {}^{\circ}\text{C}^{-1}$) and 6/15 caudal AP fibers (median slope: $0.695 \text{ dB} \cdot {}^{\circ}\text{C}^{-1}$) did so. There were no significant differences between the regression slopes of any pair of fiber groups (K=4.53, P=0.105).

Best-fit linear regressions of S/N on noise level were significant for 15/19 saccular fibers (median slope: $0.231 \text{ dB} \cdot \text{V}^{-2}$), 9/15 rostral AP fibers (median slope: $0.090 \text{ dB} \cdot \text{V}^{-2}$) and 8/15 caudal AP fibers (median slope: $0.056 \text{ dB} \cdot \text{V}^{-2}$). Multiple comparisons revealed that regression slopes for the saccular fibers were significantly greater than those for the rostral AP fibers, which in turn were significantly greater than the slopes for the caudal AP fibers (K=14.01, P=0.001).

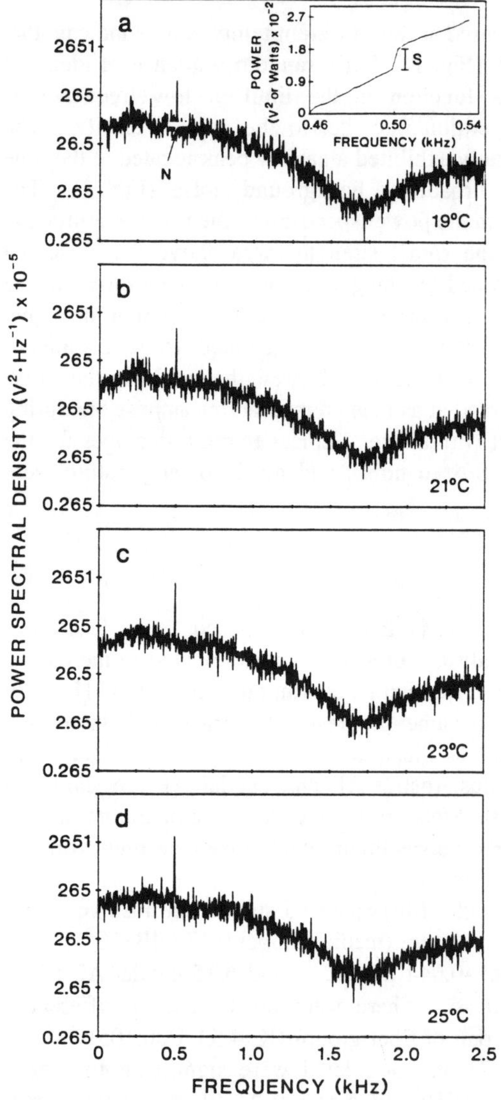

Fig 1
Averaged power spectra (n=10) for a representative auditory fiber innervating the caudal end of the amphibian papilla (CF=1.05 kHz) of the northern leopard frog. Each spectrum was produced by stimulating with a constant tone of 500 Hz at 89 dB SPL and sampling the resulting spike train at 10 points per stimulus cycle for 20,480 cycles. Noise level was determined by measuring the height of the curve [labeled 'N' in (a)], below each signal 'spike', while signal level was determined by integrating the spectrum around the signal frequency and measuring the height of the 'step' labeled 'S' in the inset of (a). The temperature of the dorsal surface of the frog's oral cavity is given in the lower right of each plot.

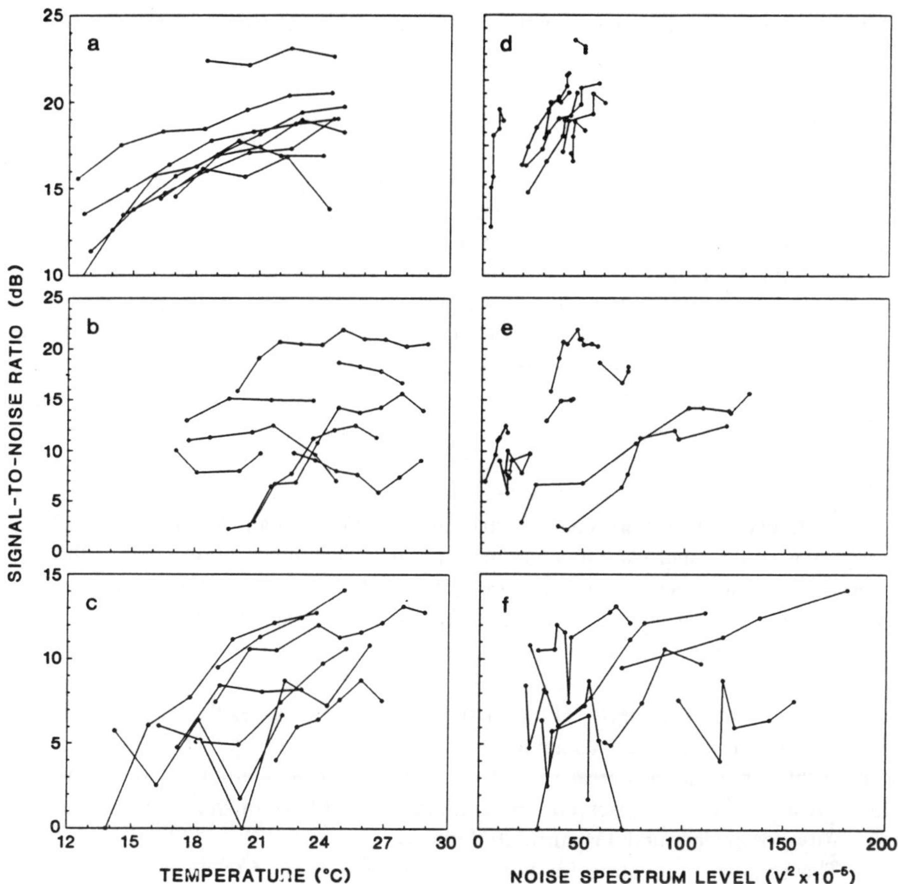

Fig. 2. Signal-to-noise ratios plotted against temperature for 24 randomly chosen fibers innervating (a) the sacculus, (b) the rostral (low frequency) region of the amphibian papilla, (c) the caudal (mid frequency) extension of the amphibian papilla, and against internal noise for the same fibers (d, e, and f, respectively). Each signal-to-noise ratio was calculated as $10\log_{10}(S/N)$ in dB, where S is the signal power and N is the noise power measured as shown in Figure 1. Temperature was incremented in steps of 1 or 2 °C.

Regression slopes of noise on temperature were significant for 14/19 saccular fibers (median slope: 1.91 $V^2 \cdot {}^{\circ}C^{-1}$), 7/15 rostral AP fibers (median slope: 1.40 $V^2 \cdot {}^{\circ}C^{-1}$) and 6/15 caudal AP fibers (median slope: 4.00 $V^2 \cdot {}^{\circ}C^{-1}$). Multiple comparison tests showed that the slopes for the caudal AP fibers are significantly greater than those for the saccular fibers (K=6.48, P=0.04), while the rostral AP fibers had intermediate slopes, not significantly different from either of the other two fiber groups.

4 Discussion

Our results demonstrate (in most cases) S/Ns do not pass through maxima when plotted either against temperature or against internal noise intensity, and hence we do not claim to have observed SR in a sensory system by manipulating the internal noise. They do, however, demonstrate the profound influence of the internal noise on the S/N derived from the neural spike trains: in contrast to the behavior of many physical systems or systems driven by external noise which show stochastic resonance, the S/N for frog auditory neurons appears to be an increasing function of internal temperature. This observation implies that in our experiments the signal intensity increased faster than the internal noise as the temperature was raised. Recently, very similar results have been observed for the temperature dependence of the crayfish mechanoreceptor system.[9]

In theory, temperature changes may affect both mechanical and electrical properties of the inner ear. It is assumed that mechanical structures such as the tectorial membrane would be less temperature dependent than would electrical properties of the ear, such as kinetics of the hair cell channels. The effects of temperature changes on the tectorial membrane in the frog that may lead to the observed CF-shifts have been discussed.[10] These changes may be summarized using two different models: (1) a stiffness-dominated model that predicts an increase in CF with decreasing temperature, and (2) a viscosity-dominated model that predicts an increase in CF with increasing temperature. Since the latter result is in fact observed for auditory nerve fibers in the frog,[11,12] the viscosity-dominated model is currently favored.

The original motivation for this study was the attempt to understand the effect of temperature on information transmission in the frog auditory nerve. Since increasing the body temperature of an ectotherm such as an amphibian is known to affect auditory processing in multiple ways, we assumed that the S/N for spike encoding in the auditory periphery is also temperature dependent since increased temperature is correlated with increased internal noise. This should result in lower S/Ns as temperature is increased. In fact, we found that in nearly all fibers tested, higher temperatures nearly always were correlated with increased S/Ns. This counterintuitive result implies that temperature changes in the inner ear affect the signal and the noise magnitudes differently. We are now carrying out (Smotherman and Narins, in preparation) direct measurements of the temperature dependence of noise in K^+- and Ca^{++}-dependent K^+ channels in sensory hair cells from the amphibian papilla of *Rana pipiens pipiens* to estimate the contribution of the electrical noise to the auditory nerve phenomenon we have described herein.

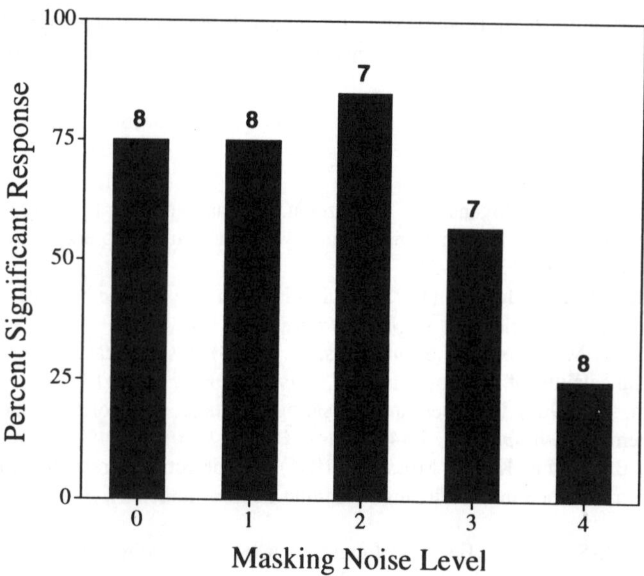

Fig. 3. Mean percentage of significant responses (calls) given by males of the Puerto Rican coqui in response to tones presented alone or in simultaneous masking noise. Above each bar is the number of frogs tested at each level of masking noise. Masking noise levels 1-4 are derived from octave band measurements and correspond to 32.0, 40.9, 47.5 and 50.6 dB/Hz mean spectrum level, respectively.

Preliminary evidence from acoustic playback experiments with calling male frogs in their natural habitat suggest a possible role of background noise for improving behavioral responses. Synthetic call notes were broadcast both alone and embedded in progressively higher levels of broadband masking noise to individual calling males of the Puerto Rican arboreal frog, *Eleutherodactylus coqui*.

Surprisingly, low-to-intermediate levels of masking noise resulted in the highest calling rate from the males tested (Fig. 3). This result could be interpreted as a manifestation of the "capture" effect whereby attention is focused on the call notes being broadcasted, since neighboring males' calls are being masked by the broadband masking noise. Additional experiments are needed to test this hypothesis.

90

Acknowledgments

We thank Margaret Kowalczyk for help with the figure preparations and W. Huang for assisting with the data analysis. This research was supported by a NIDCD grant DC-00222 to PMN and by ONR grants N00014-92-J-1235 and N00014-90-J-1327 to FM.

References

1. Douglass, J. K., Wilkens, L. Pantazelou, E. and Moss, F. (1993) Noise enhancement of information transfer in crayfish mechanoreceptors by stochastic resonance. *Nature* **365** 337-340.
2. Wiesenfeld, K. and Moss, F. (1995) Stochastic resonance and the benefits of noise: from ice ages to crayfish and SQUIDs. *Nature* **373** 33-36.
3. Landahl, H., McCulloch, W.S. and Pitts, W. (1943) A statistical consequence of the logical calculus of nervous nets. *Bull. Math. Biophys.*, **5** 135-137.
4. Fitzhugh, R. (1961) Impulses and physiological states in theoretical models of nerve membrane. *Biophys. J.*, **1** 445-466.
5. Pei, X., Bachmann, K. and Moss, F. (1995) The detection threshold, noise and stochasic resonance in the Fitzhugh-Nagumo neuron model. *Phys. Letters A*, **206** 61-65.
6. Kiang, N.Y.-S., Moxon, E.C. and Levine, R.A. (1970) Auditory nerve activity in cats with normal and abnormal cochleas, in *Sensorineural Hearing Loss*, eds. G.E.W. Wolstenholme, J. Knight (Churchill, London), pp. 241-273.
7. Evans, E.F. (1979) Single unit studies on the mammalian cochlear nerve, in *Auditory Investigation: The Scientific and Technological Basis,* ed. H.A. Beagley (Clarendon Press, Oxford), pp. 324-367.
8. Stremler, F.G. (1990). *Introduction to Communication Systems.* Addison-Wesley, New York, Chapts 3 and 8.
9. Pantazelou, E., Dames, C., Moss, F., Douglass, J. and Wilkens, L. (1995) Temperature dependence and the role of internal noise in signal transduction efficiency of crayfish mechanoreceptors. *Intern. J. Bifurc. and Chaos*, **5** 101-108.
10. Benedix, J.B. Jr., Pedemonte, M., Velluti, R.A. and Narins, P.M. (1994) Temperature dependence of two-tone suppression in the auditory nerve of the frog. *J. Acoust. Soc. Am.*, **95** 2738-2745.
11. Stiebler, I.B.and Narins, P. M. (1990) Temperature-dependence of auditory nerve response properties in the frog. *Hear. Res.*, **46** 63-82.
12. van Dijk, P., Lewis, E.R. and Wit, H.P. (1990) Temperature effects on auditory nerve fiber response in the American bullfrog. *Hearing Res.* **44** 231-240.

PIGEON SPONTANEOUS AND EVOKED ACTIVITIES:
A RENEWAL PROCESS?

C.-P. RICHTER, M. KLUGE, R. KLINKE

*Zentrum der Physiologie, J.W. Goethe - Universität, Theodor-Stern-Kai 7,
60590 Frankfurt / Main, Germany*

S. JOEKEN

*Institut für Theoretische Neurophysik, Universität Bremen,
Postfach 330 440, 28334 Bremen, Germany.*

Abstract: Spontaneous activities of pigeon auditory nerve fibers were tested for a renewal process. The experiments falsified mutually statistically independent lengths of time intervals between successive actions potentials. However, the generation of action potentials on the eighth nerve by a complex system as the inner ear might not be described by a simple renewal process. The superposition of many different stochastic processes are conceivable in composed systems as the ear. Therefore, spontaneous activities have been described in the present experiments by a doubly embedded stochastic model, the Hidden Markov Model. The model is composed of hidden and observable states. These different hidden states generate with different probabilities the action potentials (observable states) on the auditory nerve. In addition to spontaneous activities, responses of pigeon auditory nerve fibers to white noise stimuli have been evaluated to investigate signal transduction. Wiener kernels have been identified by fast orthogonal search. The results suggest that nonlinearities are only instantaneous and that the investigated acoustically evoked neuronal activities might be described by cascades of linear and static nonlinear devices. Considerable improvements are possible by generalization of the ordinary Wiener series, so that prior neuronal activity can be taken into account. Recorded inter-spike-interval distributions and rate-intensity functions can be described by a stochastic model derived from extended functional series.

1 Introduction

Neuronal activities of single auditory nerve fibers in birds have been studied in different species.[1-9] Spontaneous and evoked activities have been described by the mean number of action potentials (APs) within a given time interval and the distribution of the APs following the onset of an acoustic stimulus.[1-9] Histograms of the probability for inter-spike-time-intervals with a certain length have shown a decreasing probability for time intervals with increasing length of the interval. On the first sight, the probability of the interval lengths in the inter-spike-time-interval-histograms (INTHs) decayed exponentially. Nevertheless, closer inspection of the INTHs showed a greater number of short time intervals between successive APs.[4]

Modeling of the spontaneous activities in pigeon auditory nerve fibers failed if an exponential (Poisson-) or gamma distribution of the inter spike time intervals was assumed[4]. However, the distribution of the INTHs which is almost a Poisson distribution[4,5] suggest that a stochastic process might well describe the INTHs found in pigeon auditory nerve fibers.

As the inner ear is a complex system the encoding of mechanical energy in action potentials on the eight nerve includes many steps. For example: an acoustic stimulus applied to the tympanon causes vibration of the papilla basilaris which bends the stereovilli of the hair cells. For the hair cell the bending of the stereovilli is the adequate stimulus which depolarizes the hair cell. Subsequently transmitter is released which results in the generation of action potentials on the nerve. Each of these steps might be described by a stochastic process, finally leading to stochastic neuronal activity. In the present experiments, more complex models were used to describe neuronal activities obtained from pigeon auditory nerve fibers.

2   Data collection

The methods of recording single fiber activities from the avian cochlear ganglion have been published previously[5,3] and are only reviewed briefly.

Animals: Pigeons (Columba livia) of both sexes age 0.5 to 3 years were used. The animals were anaesthetized with sodium pentobarbital; initial dose 50 mg/kg, maintenance dose 6-8 mg/kg every hour. After tracheotomy, a plastic tube was inserted into the trachea and the abdominal air sacs were opened for continuous ventilation. In order to clamp the P_{CO_2}, high flow rates (200-350 ml/min) of a 96% O_2 and 4% CO_2 mixture saturated with H_2O vapor were used[3]. ECG and body temperature were monitored continuously. The body temperature was kept constant at 40.5°C with a heating blanket. Additional anesthetic was given if the heart rate rose above 180/min. Following the fixation of the head to a custom-made head holder with dental acrylic, scala tympani and the cochlear ganglion were exposed. A dorso-lateral approach was used for access to the inner ear.

Stimulation: A noisy stimulus was generated by an arbitrary wave form generator (Model 75, Wavetek) by superimposing of 4096 random telegraph processes resulting in a pseudo-Gaussian white noise sequence. The latter was band limited to 0.62-2500 Hz. The signals were fed into a custom-made attenuator followed by a Cyrus amplifier. The stimulus was delivered by a Beyer DT48 headphone in a closed field. The sound pressure level at the ear canal was monitored with a Sennheiser KE4-211 probe microphone calibrated with a B&K (type 4134) condenser microphone.

Data recording: Single fiber activity recorded by micro pipettes from the cochlear ganglion was preamplified by a Dagan 8000 and fed into a custom-made window discriminator. Action potentials were transformed into technical spikes (pulses of 220 μs duration), which were sampled by a CED 1401+/PC system with a temporal resolution of 10 μs.

3   Renewal process

A test to falsify a renewal process was performed in 235 spontaneously active auditory afferents. This was achieved by comparing two autocorrelograms calculated from the same time series of APs by two different methods. The first, method is to calculate the autocorrelogram $\hat{C}(\tau)$ directly from the time series of APs as shown in Eq. 1.

$$\hat{C}(\tau) = \lim_{N \to \infty} \frac{1}{N} \sum_{k=1}^{N} x_k(t) x_k(t+\tau) \tag{1}$$

where N denotes the number of APs and $x(t)$ the times an AP is observed ($x(t) = 1$ for an AP and $x(t) = 0$ for no AP). With the INTH of the given time series of APs and the integral equation of the renewal theory[10] the autocorrelogram might also be calculated reversely by Eq. 2 [11]. This method is based on the condition that the time series can be described by a renewal process[10,11]. Thus, the second method only reveals the same autocorrelogram compared with the results obtained by the first method if the neuronal activity can be described by a renewal process.

$$\hat{C}(\tau) = \sum_{\phi_i \leq \tau} \hat{h}(\phi_i) \hat{C}(\tau - \phi_i) \tag{2}$$

Differences in the autocorrelograms calculated with the two different methods introduced, yields as a test to falsify a renewal process.

For 188 of the 235 pairs of autocorrelograms calculated from the time series obtained from pigeon auditory nerve fibers were significantly different. Consequently, for 80% of the fibers recorded, spontaneous activities cannot be described by a renewal process.

A renewal process states mutually statistically independent lengths of time intervals between successive actions potentials. For the case that the length of inter spike intervals is dependent on the length of a previous time interval, spontaneous activities cannot be described by a renewal process. However, the neuronal activity may be stochastic. For this reason a more complex description with a stochastic model, the Hidden Markov Model, was used to describe spontaneous activities of pigeon auditory nerve fibers.

94

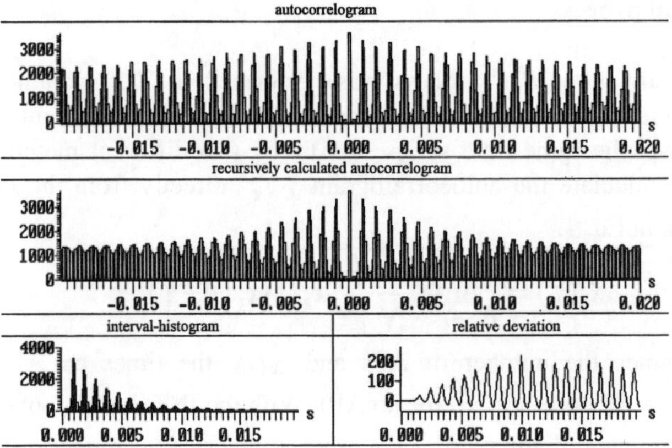

Figure 1: Autocorrelograms calculated using Eq 1 (upper trace) and Eq. 2 (middle trace). Interval-histogram and relative deviation between both autocorrelograms (lower trace). Differences between the both autocorrelograms are significant (Kolmogorov-Smirnov-test, p=0.05).

4   Hidden Markov Model

In general, the Hidden Markov Model (HMM) assumes that the probability of an observable event is dependent on different hidden states of the system[14]. For the inner ear the hidden states include all possible components of the system between the stimulus and the action potential. The observable events are the action potentials and the time intervals between successive APs. For every hidden state a different probability to generate an AP is assumed. This doubly embedded stochastic model was used to describe spontaneous activities of the pigeon auditory afferents. For this model the autocorrelogram was calculated from the time series of the APs and reversely according to Eq. 3:

$$\hat{C}_{HMM}(\tau > 0) = \sum_i \sum_j P_{obs}(\phi_i)(M^\tau)_{ij} P_{obs}(\phi_i)\rho_s(\phi_j) \tag{3}$$

where P_{obs} denotes the probability for an AP, $\phi_i = i\Delta t$ the phase of the system, M the transition matrix of the internal states and ρ_s the transition matrix of the

A selection of 10 auditory nerve fibers for which a renewal process was falsified were tested whether neuronal activities might be described by a HMM. For the neurons tested, no significant differences were found for the HMM (Figure 2).

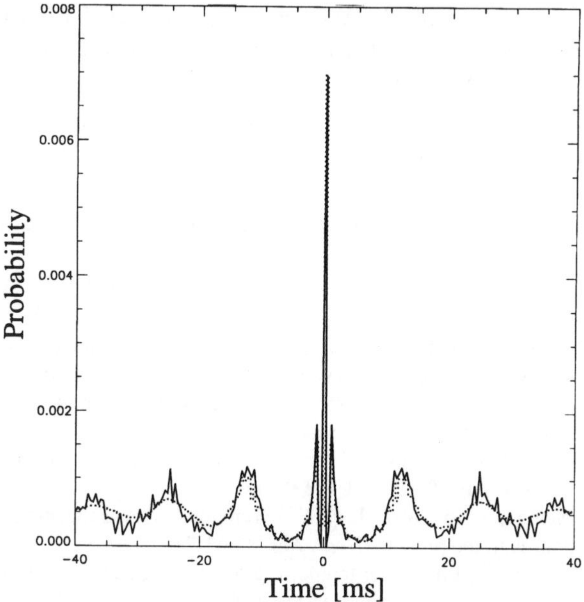

Figure 2: Dotted line: Model, solid line: autocorrelogram calculated directly from the time series. Differences between the both autocorrelograms are not significant (Kolmogorov-Smirnov-test, p=0.05).

5 Advanced Modeling

In a subsequent series of experiments pigeon ears were stimulated with a noisy stimulus. Response patterns of the auditory nerve were investigated by means of extended functional series expansions. In order to determine Wiener series representations of the investigated neurons the fast orthogonal search algorithm was used.[12] The results suggest that nonlinearities are only instantaneous and the signal transduction in the pigeon inner ear can be described by a cascade of linear and static nonlinear devices.[13] Only slight improvements in describing the system result from the nonlinear terms of the series expansion. Again, if neuronal activity prior to an AP is taken into account considerable improvements in approximation of the system have been observed. Evoked activities than can be described by means of

$$y_{1,1}(t) = k_0 + \int_0^\infty k_1(\tau)x(t-\tau)d\tau + \int_{\varepsilon>0}^\infty g(\tau)y(t-\tau)d\tau \qquad (4)$$

where $x(t)$ is the Gaussian white noise stimulus and $y(t)$ is the time series of action potentials of the neuron. The kernels k_0, $k_1(\tau)$ and $g(\tau)$ were identified by application of the fast orthogonal search[12,13], such that the mean square error $\overline{(y(t) - y_{1,1}(t))^2}$ was minimized. It has to be emphasized that the kernel $k_1(\tau)$

generally does not agree with the Wiener kernel calculated from the same time series of APs. However, for all neurons investigated in the present experiments, the kernels did not differ significantly.

Acknowledgments

Supported by the DFG Ri 699/2-3 and the Dr. Paul und Cilli Weill Stiftung

References

1. Sachs, M.B., Woolf,N. and Sinnott, J.M. (1980) Response properties of neurons in the avian auditory system: Comparisons with mammalian homologues of the neural encoding of complex stimuli. In: Comparative studies of hearing in Vertebrates, Popper, A.N. and Fay, R.R. Eds. Springer Verlag. 323-353.

2. Temchin, A.N. (1988) Unusual discharge patterns of single fibers in the pigeons auditory nerve. *J. Comp. Physiol. A* **163** 99-116

3. Hill, K.G., Stange,G. and Mo, J. (1989) Temporal synchronization in the primary auditory responses in the pigeon. *Hear. Res.* **39** 63-74

4. Gummer, A.W. (1991) First order temporal properties of spontaneous and tone-evoked activity of auditory afferent neurones in the cochlear ganglion of the pigeon. *Hear. Res.* **55** 143-166

5. Klinke ,R., Muller, M., Richter, C.-P and Smolders, J.W.T. (1994) Preferred intervals in birds and mammlas: a fliter response to noise? *Hear. Res.* **74** 238-246.

6. Manley, G.A. (1979) Preferred intervals in the spontaneous activity of primary auditory neurons. *Naturwissenschaften* **66** 582-584.

7. Manley ,G.A., Gleich, O., Leppelsack, H.-J. and Oeckinghaus, H. (1985) Activity patterns of cochlear ganglion neurones in the starling. *J. Comp. Physiol A* **157** 161-182.

8. Manley, G.A., Kaiser, A., Brix, J. and Gleich, O. (1991) Activity patterns of primary auditory-nerve fibres in chickens: development of fundamental properties. *Hear. Res* **57** 1-15.

9. Smolders, J.W.T., Ding-Pfenningdorff, D. and Klinke, R. (1995) A functional map of the pigeon basilar papilla: correlation of the properties of single auditory nerve fibres and their peripheral origin. *Hear. Res.* **92**, 151-169.

10. Cox, D.R. (1962) *Renewal Theory* (J. Wiley & Sons, New York,

11. Deppisch, J. (1993) *PhD Thesis, Theoretische Physik Frankfurt*

12. Joeken, S., Schwegler, H. and Richter, C.-P. (1996) Modeling stochastic spike train responses of neurons: an extended Wiener series analysis of pigeon auditory nerve fibers. *Biol. Cybern.* (in press)

13. Korenberg, M.J. (1988) Identifying nonlinear difference equation and functional expansion representations: the fast orthogonal algorithm. *Ann. Biomed. Eng.* **16**, 123.

14. Rabiner, L.R. (1989) A tutorial on Hidden Markov Models and selected applications in speech recognition. *Proceedings of the IEEE* **Vol 77**(**2**) 257

TEMPERATURE DEPENDENCE OF VARIOUS COMPONENTS IN THE FROG INNER EAR

P. VAN DIJK, H.P. WIT

ENT Department, Audiology, P.O. Box 30.001
9700 RB Groningen, The Netherlands
P.van.Dijk@med.rug.nl

The response of primary auditory nerve fibers to acoustic noise stimulation of the tympanic membrane was measured, while slowly changing the animals body temperature. Both the stimulus signal and the nerve fiber response were stored on DAT tape. Offline we computed the second-order Wiener kernel, and the first five polynomial correlation functions for each fiber as function of temperature. The computed kernel and functions implied a simple 'sandwich' model, which consists of the cascade of a bandpass filter, a static nonlinearity, and a lowpass filter. Our analysis indicated that the characteristic frequency of the first filter changed with temperature for 18 out of 20 low frequency (CF<1 kHz, amphibian papilla) fibers and 1 out of 11 high frequency fibers (CF>1 kHz, basilar papilla). For the remainder of fibers, the characteristic frequency did not depend on temperature. For the second (low pass) filter, cutoff frequency increased in all fibers, with a thermal Q10 of between 2 and 4. In addition, the shape of the input-output function of the nonlinear element did not change with temperature. This suggests that the shape of the input-output function of the transduction nonlinearity in hair cells does not depend on temperature.

1 Introduction

The physiology of the frog inner ear shows conspicuous dependence on body temperature. With increasing temperature, [1] the threshold of auditory nerve fibers decreases[1,2], [2] the characteristic frequency of auditory nerve fibers in the amphibian papilla (AP) increases, while frequency tuning of the basilar papilla (BP) does not depend on temperature[1-3], [3] otoacoustic emission frequencies increase[4], while emission peak level displays a complicated pattern[5], and [4] the opening and closing rates of transduction channels in the sacculus increase[6]. All these effects are reversible. With the exception of the last result mentioned, the other data were obtained from experiments where the inner ear was left intact. Although in those preparations the damage to the inner ear is supposedly minimal, it is hard to relate the observed temperature dependence to specific mechanisms in the inner ear. This problem can not be overcome completely, but here, we describe a method which enables localization of the temperature effects. The nerve fiber responses are described with the simple cascade system shown in Figure 1. We will show the dependence of bandpass and lowpass filter functions on temperature. In addition, it is found that the shape of the

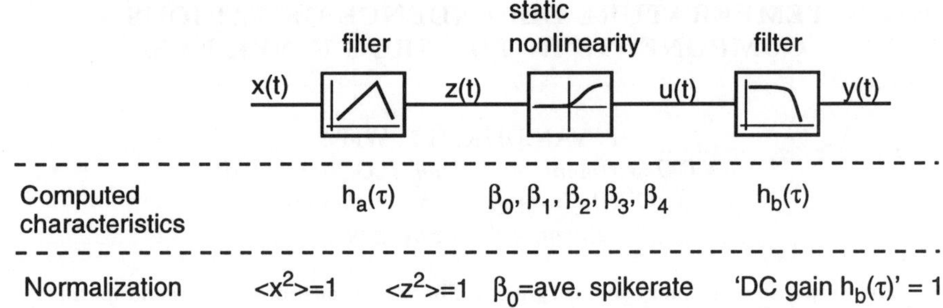

Figure 1: The 'sandwich' model

(transduction) nonlinearity does not change with temperature.

2 Material and Methods

The response of individual auditory nerve fibers in response to continuous white Gaussian noise was recorded as function of body temperature, in the European edible frog, *Rana esculenta*. Details on the anethetics, the stimulus presentation, and the nerve fiber recording are described by Van Dijk *et al.*[7]. The body temperature of the animal was controlled with Peltier devices, and was monitored with a thermocouple placed in the frog's eustachian tube. While recording from a particular fiber, the frog's body temperature was slowly changed.

Offline, the recorded signals were analyzed on a computer. Each recording was sectioned in consecutive intervals. These intervals were typically between 200 and 300 seconds in duration. Since body temperature changed during the recording, each interval corresponds to a particular temperature range. Within one time interval, the body temperature of the frog typically changed between 1 and 2 °C.

We applied Wiener kernel analysis[8] to each record section. In the spike signal, the action potentials were identified with a level crossing algorithm. The second-order Wiener kernel was computed by 'reversely' correlating the spike moments t_i with the stimulus signal $x(t_i - \tau)$ at $\tau = \tau_1$ and τ_2 seconds prior to the occurrence of the spike[7]:

$$k_2(\tau_1, \tau_2) \quad = \quad \frac{1}{2A^2T} \sum_{i=1}^{N} [x(t_i - \tau_1)x(t_i - \tau_2) - \phi_{xx}(\tau_2 - \tau_1)], \qquad (1)$$

where N is the total number of spikes in the record, T is the length of the record section, A is the spectral density of the input signal, and ϕ_{xx} is the autocorrelation function of the input noise. In all computations we normalized the variance of the input noise $x(t)$ to $\phi_{xx}(0) = \langle x^2 \rangle = 1$.

In addition to the entire second-order kernel, we computed the diagonals of the first five kernels. With the normalization $\phi_{xx}(0) = 1$, these diagonals are identical to the polynomial correlation functions[9], *e.g.*

$$P_n(\tau) \equiv k_n \underbrace{(\tau, \tau, \cdots, \tau)}_{n} = \frac{1}{n! A^n T} \sum_{i=1}^{N} He_n[x(t_i - \tau)], \qquad (2)$$

where He_n is a Hermite polynomial, *e.g.* $He_0 = 1$, $He_1(x) = x$, $He_2(x) = x^2 - 1$, $He_3(x) = x^3 - 3x$, $He_4(x) = x^4 - 6x^2 + 3$.

The computed Wiener kernels were fitted with the sandwich model (Figure 1). The model consists of two filters, with impulse responses $h_a(\tau)$ and $h_b(\tau)$ respectively, and a static nonlinearity with input-output function

$$u = \beta_0 + \beta_1 He_1(z) + \beta_2 He_2(z) + \beta_3 He_3(z) + \beta_4 He_4(z) + \cdots. \qquad (3)$$

For the sandwich model, the second-order Wiener kernel is given by[7]:

$$k_2(\tau_1, \tau_2) = \beta_2 \int_0^\infty h_b(\sigma) h_a(\tau_1 - \sigma) h_a(\tau_2 - \sigma) d\sigma. \qquad (4)$$

This formula was fitted to the computed second-order kernel (Eq. 1), using a χ^2 minimalization procedure. Given the filter functions h_a and h_b, which resulted from this procedure, the parameters of the nonlinearity can be computed from the polynomial correlation functions. It can be shown[9] that the polynomial correlation functions of the sandwich model are given by

$$P_n(\tau) = \beta_n h_a^n * h_b, \qquad (5)$$

where '*' indicates convolution. We computed the convolution $h_a^n * h_b$ using the filter function h_a and h_b, and then scaled the parameters β_n using a least squares fit of the model function

$$|\mathcal{F}[P_n|_{model}]| = \beta_n |\mathcal{F}[h_a^n * h_b]| + c \qquad (6)$$

to the Fourier transform $\mathcal{F}[P_n]$ of the measured polynomial correlation function (Eq. 2). In this equation, $\mathcal{F}$ represents Fourier transform, and the constant c reflects the fact that the predicted and measured polynomial correlation functions usually have different noise levels.

The procedure described above was performed for each recorded section. Thus, for each fiber, we obtained the filter functions h_a and h_b as function of temperature, along with the parameters β_0 through β_4 of the nonlinear element.

3 Results

The left column of panels in Figure 2 shows the second-order Wiener kernel and the first- through fourth-order polynomial correlation functions for an amphibian papilla nerve fiber[a]. The center column shows the results of the fit procedure (see Eq. 6), used to compute the coefficient β_i of the nonlinearity Eq. 3. The right column gives the characteristics of the three elements in the sandwich model (figure 1). The first filter is a bandpass filter, while the second filter is a low pass filter. Close to DC, the second filter displays a highpass characteristic (see panel m). The nonlinear input-output function (panel l) resembles a rectifier characteristic.

With increasing temperature, were observed an upward shift of the characteristic frequency of the first filter for 18 out of the 20 AP fibers, and 1 out of the 11 BP fibers. No shift was observed for the remainder of the fibers. The majority of BP fibers were tuned to approximately 2 kHz. The single BP fiber for which the characteristic frequency displayed temperature dependence was tuned to 3.2 kHz (at 20 °C).

With increasing temperature, the highpass characteristic close to DC, which was observed in the second filter, becomes more pronounced. This highpass portion may be interpreted as an adaptation effect. Thus, with increasing temperature, adaption becomes stronger. In addition, the low pass cutoff frequency of the second filter increases (see Fig. 2m) corresponding to a thermal Q_{10} of 2 to 4.

The coefficients of β_0 through β_4 increased at similar rate, when body temperature was raised. This is illustrated in Fig. 3, which shows the quadratic coefficient β_2 versus the linear coefficient β_1. The fact that all coefficients change at the same rate, indicates that the shape of the input-output function of the nonlinearity in the sandwich model does not depend on temperature.

---

[a]In figure 2, the polynomial correlation functions were normalized with the constant $1/N$ (N is the number of spikes), instead of the constant $1/(n!A^nT)$ shown in Eq. 2. For example, the first-order function P_1 shown in panel (b) simply is the average of the noise prior to the spikes. Recall that the variance of the noise is $\langle x^2 \rangle = 1$.

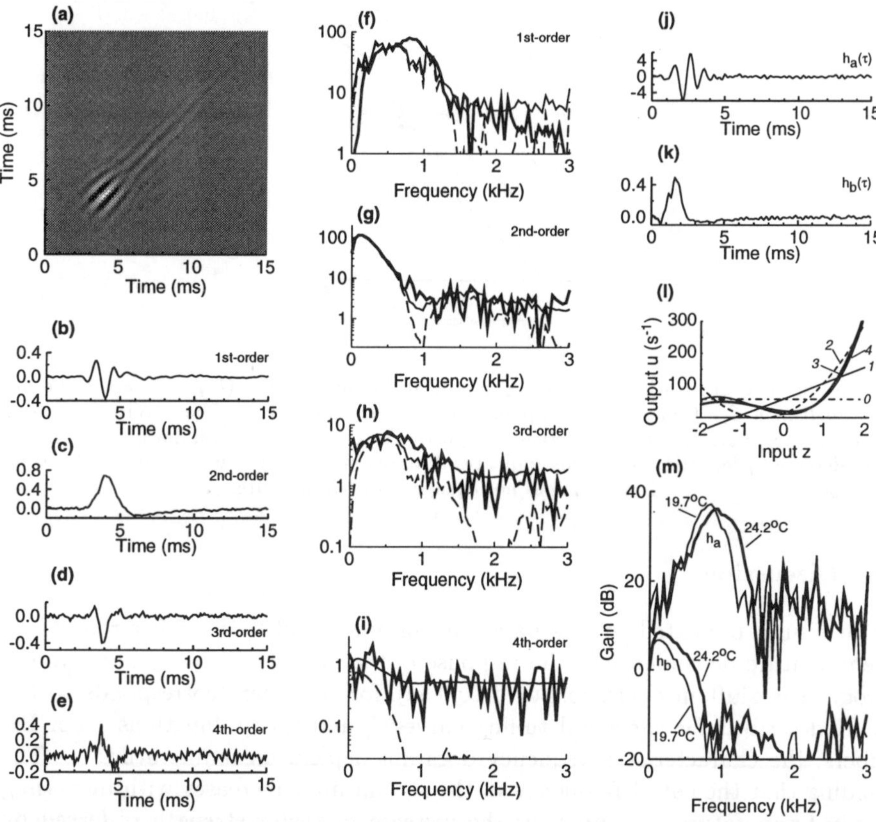

Figure 2: (a) Grayscale plot of the second-order Wiener kernel. (b)-(e) First- through fourth-order polynomial correlation function. (f)-(i) Fast Fourier transforms of polynomial correlation functions (heavy solid lines). The fitted function Eq. 6 (thin solid line) and the same function without the background level c (dashed curve) are also shown. (j) Impulse response h_a. (k) Impulse response h_b. (l) Input-output function of the static nonlinearity. The heavy solid curve shows the I/O function Eq. 3, truncated after the fourth order term $\beta_4 He_4$. The same function is shown, but truncated after the 0th-, 1st-, 2nd-, and 3rd-order term, respectively (corresponding numbers are shown in the panel). (m) Fourier transform of the impulse responses in (j) and (k) (heavy solid line, and see below). Stimulus: 80 dB SPL Gaussian noise, low pass filtered with cutoff frequency 5 kHz; record length: 230 seconds; total number of spikes: 13268; average spike rate: 57.7 s^{-1}; temperature 24.2 ^{o}C. The thin solid lines in panel (m) also show results at 19.7 ^{o}C where the average spike rate was 47.6 s^{-1}.

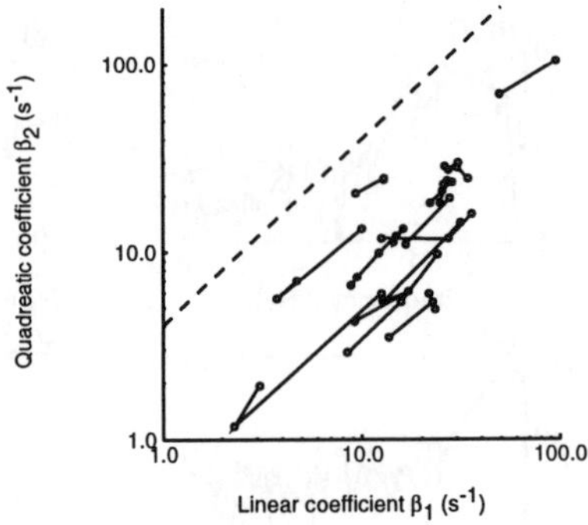

Figure 3: The quadratic coefficient β_2 of the static nonlinearity (Eq. 3) versus the linear coefficient β_1. Connected data points are from the same nerve fiber. With increasing temperature, both β_1 and β_2 increase proportional to each other. Similarly, β_0, β_3, and β_4 increased proportionally. This indicates that the shape of the nonlinear input-output function does not change with temperature.

4 Discussion

The results presented in this paper are in agreement with earlier reports on temperature dependence of the response of the primary auditory nerve in the frog. The shift in characteristic frequency for AP fibers corresponds to the shift described for threshold tuning curves[1,2], and revcor functions[3]. For BP fibers, the characteristic frequency does not depend on temperature[1-3]. The finding that the cutoff frequency of the second filter increases with increasing body temperature, accounts for the increase of vector strength observed by Stiebler and Narins[2].

Seemingly not in agreement with earlier reports is that in 4 AP fibers the characteristic frequency did *not* change with temperature. However, for these fibers, the temperature dependence of the second filter may account for the behavior of revcor function[3], and possibly of threshold tuning curves[1,2].

In one BP fiber the characteristic frequency did change with temperature. No such result has been described before for basilar papilla fibers. This particular BP fiber was unusual in an other aspect too: it's characteristic frequency (3.2 kHz) was significantly higher than for other BP fibers (2 kHz).

The most important finding is that the shape of the input-output function of the nonlinearity in the sandwich model does not depend on temperature. We assume that the nonlinear element represents the static properties of the transduction mechanism in hair cells. Our results suggest that these properties do not depend on temperature. Similar results were obtain by Corey and

Hudspeth[6]. In an in vitro preparation of the bullfrog sacculus, they found that the shape of the static I/O-function of the hair cell transduction apparatus does not change with temperature. In terms of their model for the transduction channels, this means that the energy difference between open and closed states of the channels does not depend on temperature.

Acknowledgments

The research of Pim van Dijk is supported by the Royal Netherlands Academy of Sciences and Arts. The ENT department in Groningen is part of and supported by the Groningen Graduate School for Behavioral and Cognitive Neurosciences (BCN).

References

1. Moffat, A. J. M. and Capranica R. R. (1976) Effects of temperature on the response of the auditory nerve in the American toad (*Bufo americanus*), *J.Acoust.Soc.Am.*, **60** Suppl1. S80.
2. Stiebler, I. B. and Narins, P. M. (1990) Temperature-dependence of auditory nerve properties in the frog, *Hear. Res.* **46** 63–82.
3. Van Dijk, P., Lewis, E. R. and Wit, H. P. (1990) Temperature effects on auditory nerve fiber response in the American bullfrog, *Hear. Res.* **44** 231–240.
4. Van Dijk, P., Wit, H. P., and Segenhout, J. M. (1989) Spontaneous otoacoustic emissions in the European edible frog (*rana esculenta*): Spectral details and temperature dependence, *Hear. Res.*, **42** 273–282.
5. Long, G. R., Van Dijk, P., and Wit, H. P. (1996) Temperature dependence of spontaneous otoacoustic emissions in the edible frog (*Rana esculenta*), *Hear. Res.*, accepted.
6. Corey, D. P. and Hudspeth A. J. (1983) Kinetics of the receptor current in bullfrog saccular hair cells, *J. Neurosci.* **3** 962–976.
7. Van Dijk, P., Wit, H. P., Segenhout, J. M. and Tubis, A. (1994) Wiener kernel analysis of inner ear function in the American bullfrog, *J. Acoust. Soc. Am.* **95** 904–919.
8. Schetzen, M. (1989) *The Volterra and Wiener Theories of Nonlinear Systems* (Krieger, Malabar, Florida).
9. Eggermont, J. J., Johannesma, P. I. M. and Aertsen, A. M. H. J. (1983) Reverse-correlation methods in auditory research, *Q. Rev. Biophys.* **16** 341–414.

SPIKE RATE MODELS FOR AUDITORY FIBERS

G. WOLODKIN, W .M. YAMADA AND E. R. LEWIS
Department of Electrical Engineering, University of California
Berkeley, CA 94720, USA

K. R. HENRY
Department of Psychology, University of California,
Davis, CA 95616, USA

In this paper we examine the response of primary auditory afferents in the bullfrog *Rana catesbeiana* and in the Mongolian gerbil *Merionis unguiculatis*, and attempt to model the input–output behavior in terms of a spike rate model. The model, consisting of a linear time–invariant filter in cascade with a static nonlinearity (a Wiener model), is constructed using a white noise stimulus. Having constructed the model, a periodic stimulus is applied to the ear and the predicted spike rate is compared to the post–stimulus spike histogram (PSTH). Our results demonstrate the ability to model tuning properties of low frequency auditory fibers via linear filters in state space form. The state space parameterization is advantageous as it has fewer parameters and allows for the possibility of gain scheduled or parameter–varying models to account for changes in tuning with *e.g.* stimulus power.

1 Introduction

The study of tuning in auditory fibers has a rich history [1,2,3]. There are many ways to study tuning, however, and the relationship between the various so-called tuning curves is unclear. In this paper we shall focus on the white noise or reverse correlation technique [2,4,5], in which the tuning properties have a systems–based interpretation. The resulting tuning curves or REVCOR functions have the interpretation of linear filters, and can be connected to an underlying model. The model can be used in a simulation or prediction setting, and its output compared to experimental data. Here we show by such a comparison that a linear filter in cascade with a static nonlinearity results in a reasonable model for the spike rate in low frequency auditory units.

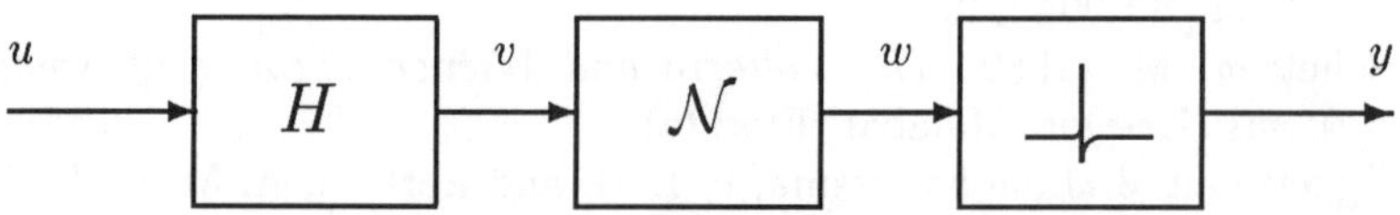

Figure 1: The Wiener Model with Poisson spike generator.

2 The Wiener Model

In low frequency auditory fibers where phase locking occurs, one candidate model is the Wiener model. This model consists of a linear time–invariant filter in cascade with a static nonlinearity. We point out the possible confusion between the *Wiener model*, a simple block–structured system as depicted in Figure 1, and *Wiener kernels* in general [6]. We shall use the latter to obtain estimates for our model parameters.

To account for the spike train output of auditory fibers, we must add to the standard Wiener model a spike generator. In this paper we shall assume the spike generator to be Poisson, in which case the nonlinear output has the interpretation of spike rate. Under such circumstances, one can easily show that the REVCOR estimate or first order Wiener kernel for such a system results in an unbiased estimate for impulse response of the linear block [7,8].

In terms of higher order Wiener kernels, one can show that the second order kernel for a system as shown in Figure 1 is a rank one matrix, described by the outer product of the impulse response with itself. A Wiener system may have higher order kernels as well. For this reason it may be preferable to identify the structured system consisting of only two sub–blocks, rather than to attempt a kernel expansion which ignores any knowledge of the underlying structure. Note that the Wiener model of Figure 1 is a special case of the more general Korenberg or Sandwich model [9,10], in which a second linear filter follows the nonlinearity.

3 Parametric vs. Non–parametric estimates

One problem with REVCOR and cross correlation estimates in general stems from the fact that they are *non–parametric* estimates [11], requiring hundreds if not thousands of points to accurately represent the true impulse response waveform. The estimates are often noisy, and may in practice need to be truncated outside a finite time window. To avoid these problems, we apply state space identification techniques [12] to the REVCOR estimate and obtain the least mean square error fit in terms of the impulse response. The state space model has far fewer parameters than the REVCOR estimate, allowing one to look for trends between fibers in terms of a few parameters. In addition, one can use the results of the identification process to estimate dynamic order of the underlying system.

4 Model Validation

Once the model is obtained, the next step is to validate the model by testing its predictive power on new data. For the case of a linear model, de Boer and de Jongh have shown positive results in the cat [7]. We show similar results here for the frog and the gerbil, examining not only the linear model but also the static nonlinearity [13]. As would be expected, the nonlinearities in general provide rectification. For the gerbil, a higher background firing rate can be seen in the nonlinear graph.

Model validation was done using a periodic noise stimulus. A trigger pulse marked the start of this stimulus, so that a PSTH could be computed to estimate the spike rate. To compensate for the essentially zero background firing rate in the frog, an additional random Gaussian noise was added to the input. Without this noise, units tended to phase lock to some features in the stimulus, missing others due to refractory periods.

Using the PSTH over many presentations of the same stimulus, we are able to essentially "average" past the spike generator and obtain the spike rate. We can then compare this rate to the output of our Wiener model and examine our ability to predict the rise and fall of firing rate vs. time.

5 Experimental Results

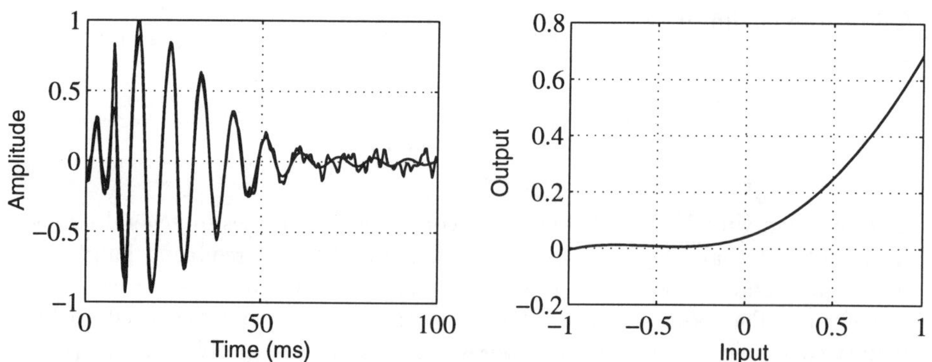

Figure 2: Frog unit, Wiener model (linear filter and nonlinear graph).

We show data here for two units. The first is from a low frequency auditory unit in the frog, with CF just above 100 Hz. Model estimates were obtained using a band limited white noise (flat to 10 kHz). Enough data was collected

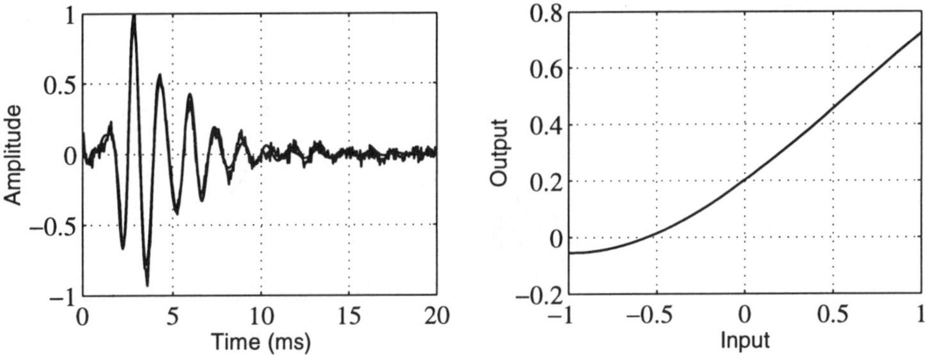

Figure 3: Gerbil unit, Wiener model (linear filter and nonlinear graph).

in order to obtain several thousand spikes, three minutes for the frog and one minute for the gerbil. Experimental procedures have been outlined in previous work [14].

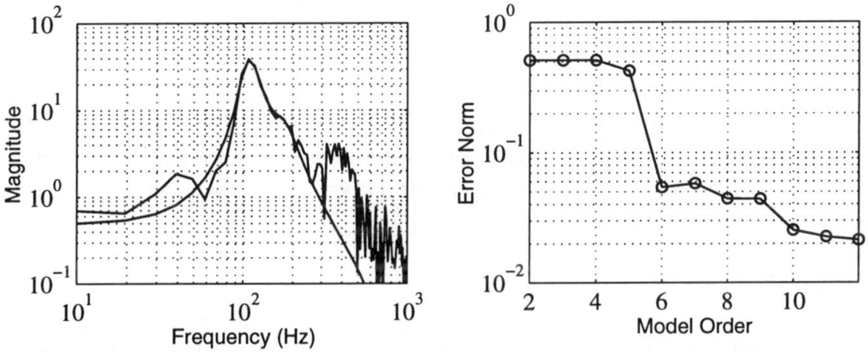

Figure 4: Frog, A. Linear model (frequency domain), B. Error norm versus model order.

After collecting the white noise data, the stimulus was switched to a periodic stimulus. For the frog, this stimulus consisted of a 200 ms waveform, band limited between 20–500 Hz and played repeatedly with no gaps. For the gerbil, the stimulus was a 40 ms waveform, band limited to between 20–1000 Hz and played with a period of 101 ms. For the frog, a small amount of noise was added to the input stimulus, enough to produce a reasonable background firing rate. Stimuli were played for three and one minutes, respectively, again

108

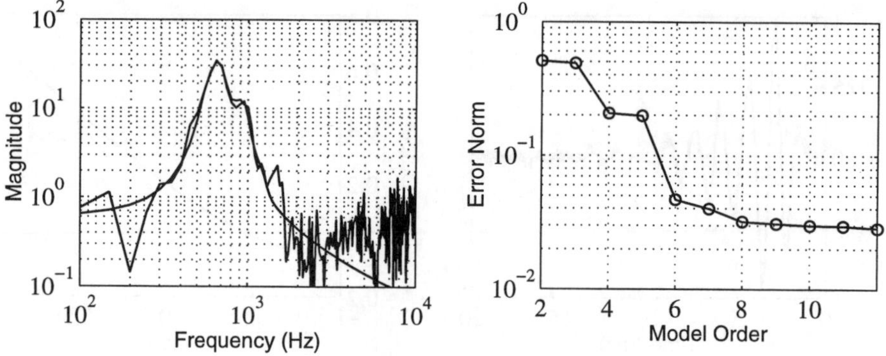

Figure 5: Gerbil, A. Linear model (frequency domain), B. Error norm versus model order.

to obtain several thousand spikes. For each unit, a PSTH was generated from the spike data to obtain an estimate of the spike rate.

From the white noise data, the non–parametric REVCOR model was approximated by a low order state space model. The order of this model is a free parameter, and various orders from 2 to 12 were tried. For the units investigated, a significant drop is seen in the mean square error between orders 5 and 6. Beyond order 12, no improvement was seen. A plot of error versus order is shown in Figure 5 for the frog unit, and in Figure 5 for the gerbil.

Plots of the linear model output are compared with PSTH data in Figure 5 and Fig 6. Comparing with the output of the nonlinearity is not so interesting, as it merely removes the bottom half of the curve and in fact makes visual comparison somewhat more difficult.

6 Discussion

Ideally one would like to compare model output with recorded output. Such a comparison is complicated by the spike process, however, and in this work we make do by comparing our estimate for the spike rate with an estimate of the true spike rate, obtained via the PSTH. Direct comparison of spike trains is an open problem, one which is worthy of further discussion.

Since the Wiener model is a special case of the Sandwich model, we conclude that the Sandwich model can indeed be used to describe low frequency units as well as high frequency units. This is not in contradiction with van Dijk *et al* [10], but rather stems from assumptions made with regard to non–overlapping passbands. Indeed for the low frequency fibers, the same second

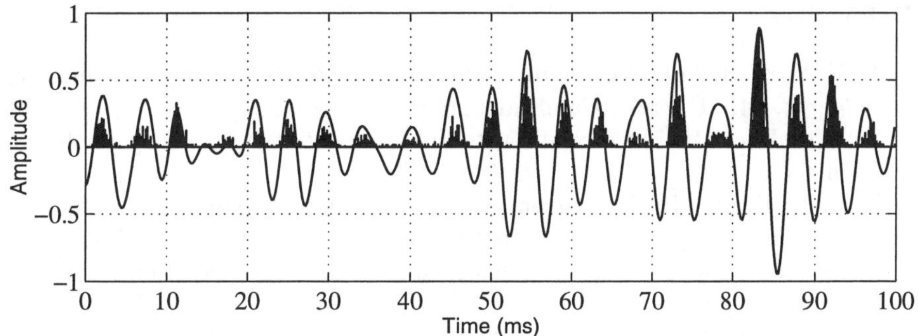

Figure 6: Frog unit, linear model predictions.

filter most likely is there, but is well approximated by an identity operator at the frequencies passed by the first filter.

One future goal of this work is to use the state space reduction techniques to build parameter–varying models for auditory fibers, both in terms of center frequency and in terms of stimulus power.

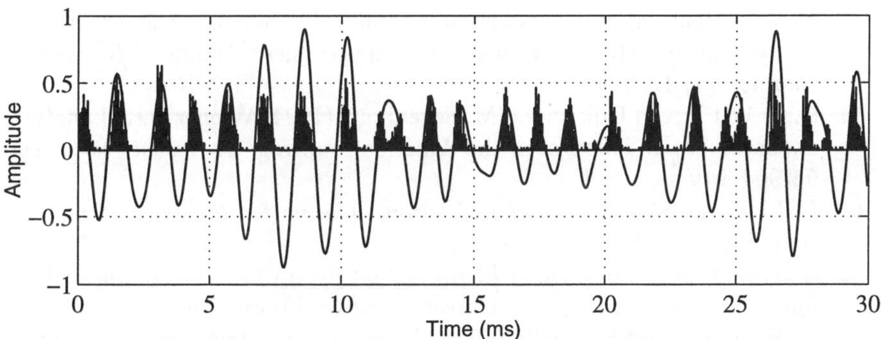

Figure 7: Gerbil unit, linear model predictions.

References

1. N. Y. Kiang (1965) *Discharge patterns of single fibers in the cat's auditory nerve.* M.I.T. Press, Cambridge, Mass.
2. E. de Boer (1967) Correlation studies applied to the frequency resolution of the cochlea. *J. Aud. Res.* **7** 209–217.
3. E. F. Evans (1977) Frequency selectivity at high signal levels of single units in cochlear nerve and nucleus. In E.F. Evans and J.P. Wilson, editors, *Psychophysics and Physiology of Hearing*, pages 185–196. Academic Press, London.
4. P. Z. Marmarelis and K. I. Naka (1972) White-noise analysis of a neuron chain: An application of the Wiener theory. *Science* **175** 1276–1278.
5. J. J. Eggermont (1993) Wiener and volterra analyses applied to the auditory system. *Hear. Res.* **66** 177–201.
6. S. A. Billings (1980) Identification of non-linear systems – a survey. *IEE Proceedings* **127** 272–285.
7. E. de Boer and H. R. de Jongh (1978) On cochlear modeling: Potentialities and limitations of the reverse-correlation technique. *J. Acoust. Soc. Am.* **63** 115–135.
8. X. L. Yu (1991) *Signal Processing Mechanics in Bullfrog Ear Inferred from Neural Spike Trains.* PhD thesis, University of California, Berkeley.
9. M. J. Korenberg and I. W. Hunter (1990) The identification of nonlinear biological systems: Wiener kernel approaches. *Annals of Biomedical Engineering* **18** 629–654.
10. H. P. Wit P. van Dijk and J. M. Segenhout (1994) Wiener kernel analysis of the inner ear function in the Americal bullfrog. *J. Acoust. Soc. Am.* **95** 904–919.
11. L. Ljung (1987) *System Identification, Theory for the User.* Prentice-Hall, Englewood Cliffs, New Jersey.
12. G. Wolodkin (1996) *System Identification for a Class of Structured Nonlinear Systems.* PhD thesis, University of California, Berkeley.
13. G. Wolodkin and K. Poolla (1995) A least-squares technique for identification of biological nonlinearities. In *Proceedings of the 1995 American Control Conference*, Seattle.
14. E. R. Lewis and K. R. Henry (1989) Cochlear nerve responses to waveform singularities and envelope corners. *Hear. Res.* **39** 209–224.

WIENER KERNEL ANALYSIS AND THE SINGULAR VALUE DECOMPOSITION

W. M. YAMADA, G. WOLODKIN and E. R. LEWIS

Department of Electrical Engineering, University of California
Berkeley, CA 94720, USA
yamada@bandit.eecs.berkeley.edu

K. R. HENRY

Department of Psychology, University of California,
Davis, CA 95616, USA

The first and second order Wiener kernels, K_1 and K_2, are used to examine the tuning properties of auditory units in the bullfrog, *Rana catesbeiana*, and the Mongolian gerbil, *Merionis unguiculatis* . The structure of these kernels (matrices) is examined using the singular value decomposition. The SVD allows us to replace the two-dimensional convolution associated with K_2 by a parallel combination of first-order kernels, each followed by a square-law device. We find that typical K_2 are well-approximated by low-rank matrices. Under these conditions, we are able to extract tuning properties using broad-band noise stimuli, even in the case of units that do not phase lock to stimuli and therefore have no K_1, i.e. no REVCOR function.

1 Acoustic Tuning and the Wiener Kernels

A set of Wiener kernels, $(K_1, K_2, K_3, \cdots, K_n)$, composes a linear description of a nonlinear transformation in terms of a parrallel set of input convolutions of increasing order. The Wiener kernels of a system describe the operation of that system. This was clearly shown to the auditory community by de Boer [1] who demonstrated that the PSTH in response to a repeated acoustic waveform can be predicted by convolution of K_1 with that waveform.

One property of Wiener kernels is that they are mutually orthogonal. This property implies that the best first order model of a system's operation, in terms of linear convolution, is K_1, and the best second order model of the operation of a system is the combination of K_1 and K_2. In our analysis we truncate the Wiener kernels at the second order.

$K_1[i]$ describes the magnitude of the effect that the stimulus value at delay, i, from the present time, $x(i)$, has on the response at the present time, p. $K_2[i, j]$ describes the effect that the stimulus at two delay times has on the response at the present time. The actual response of the system may be approximated by the sum of these two contributions.

$$p = y_1 + y_2 = \sum_i \mathrm{K}_1(i)\mathrm{x}(i) + \sum_{i,j} \mathrm{K}_2(i,j)\mathrm{x}(i)\mathrm{x}(j). \tag{1}$$

The response p is the probability of a spike occurance, and y_1 and y_2 are respectively, the contributions to the response of K_1 and K_2. Note that digitizing our data requires that all math be carried out discretely, so that the delay times, i and j, are integers.

Wiener kernels may be calculated by correlating the output spike train in response to a Gaussian distributed wide band noise input [2,3,4]. K_1 has been used to describe both the temporal and tuning properties of phase locked peripheral acoustic sensors and central acoustically sensitive neurons. However, K_1 does not exist for non-phase locked neurons. For this reason, interest in K_2 has grown. Unfortunately, the structural difference between K_1 and K_2 makes it difficult to compare tuning and temporal descriptions implied by K_1 to those implied by K_2. This comparison is necessary in studies that compare the tuning properties of phaselocked to non-phaselocked units and in studies that compare the AC and DC components of phase locked units.

First order cross correlation results in a vector equal to the average of all the stimulus waveforms that immediately precede spikes. In other words, K_1 describes correlations in time between a spike and the stimulus.

$$\mathrm{K}_1[i] \quad \propto \quad \mathrm{E}\left[x(t_n - i)\right]; \text{ where, } t_n = \text{time of } n^{th} \text{ spike}$$

Second order cross correlation results in a matrix that equals the average cross product of stimuli preceding a spike, corrected for the average cross product of noise expected regardless of the presence of a spike (a covariance matrix). K_2 has been dubbed the lagged product function or the time-dependant autocorrelation before a spike: terms that are descriptive of the information found in K_2 .[5]

$$\begin{aligned} \mathrm{K}_2[i,j] \quad &\propto \quad \mathrm{E}\left[x(t_n - i)x(t_n - j)\right] - \mathrm{E}\left[x(t - i)x(t - j)\right] \\ &= \quad \mathrm{E}\left[x(t_n - i)x(t_n - i - \Delta)\right] - \mathrm{E}\left[x(t - i)x(t - i - \Delta)\right]. \end{aligned}$$

Here i is a delay after which the autocorrelation is calculated, $\Delta = j - i$.

From the preceding expectations, it is seen (for a white noise input) that the Fourier transform of K_1 is the expected average 'mix' of frequencies (and phase of those frequencies) that precede a spike. Likewise, the Fourier transform of K_2 is the average power of the stimulus frequencies that precede a spike and the delay at which that power occurs (sometimes called the Spectro-Temporal Receptive Field). Tuning derived in this way is interesting because when one takes the FFT of the Wiener kernels one has described in terms of frequency the process by which the auditory unit transforms an arbitrary acoustic signal into a neural signal. However, we are now left with the quandry of comparing a single dimensional FFT to a 2 dimensional FFT.

2 The Singular Value Decomposition

The singular value decomposition (SVD) is a standard tool in linear algebra.[6,7] Here we state one form for the SVD. Details can be found in any standard text on matrix computations[8].

Theorem 2.1 *Let A be a symmetric matrix in $\mathbf{R}^{m \times m}$. There exists a unitary matrix*

$$U = \left[\begin{array}{ccc} u_1 & \cdots & u_m \end{array} \right] \in \mathbf{R}^{m \times m}$$

such that

$$U^T A U = diag(\sigma_1, \ldots, \sigma_p) \in \mathbf{R}^{m \times m}$$

with $\sigma_1 \geq \sigma_2 \geq \cdots \geq \sigma_p \geq 0$.

The σ_i are the *singular values* of A, and the columns of U, u_k, are the *singular vectors* of A. A convenient fact that stems from the above result is that A can be written as the sum of rank-one matrices. Furthermore, for a matrix with rank $r < p$, it is easy to show that only the first r singular values are non-zero. A common practice when one carries out numerical computations with large matrices, is to examine the singular values and choose a threshold below which the singular values can be ignored, thus assigning a "numerical rank" to the matrix. The resulting truncated sum

$$\hat{A} = \sum_{k=1}^{q} u_k \sigma_k v_k^T \tag{2}$$

where q is the assigned rank is optimal in the two-norm sense.

The use of equation 2 is illustrated in figure 1 which pictures K_2 of a basillar papilla unit in the bullfrog (A), and the recomposition of K_2 from it's singular value/vector pairs truncated at rank 5 (B), 10 (D) and 100 (C). This unit is well above the frequency range of phase locking units and has no K_1. Frames E and F show respectively the first singular vector, u_1, and the $FFT(u_1)$, demonstrating that tuning can be derived for a non-phase locked auditory unit from the svd(K_2).

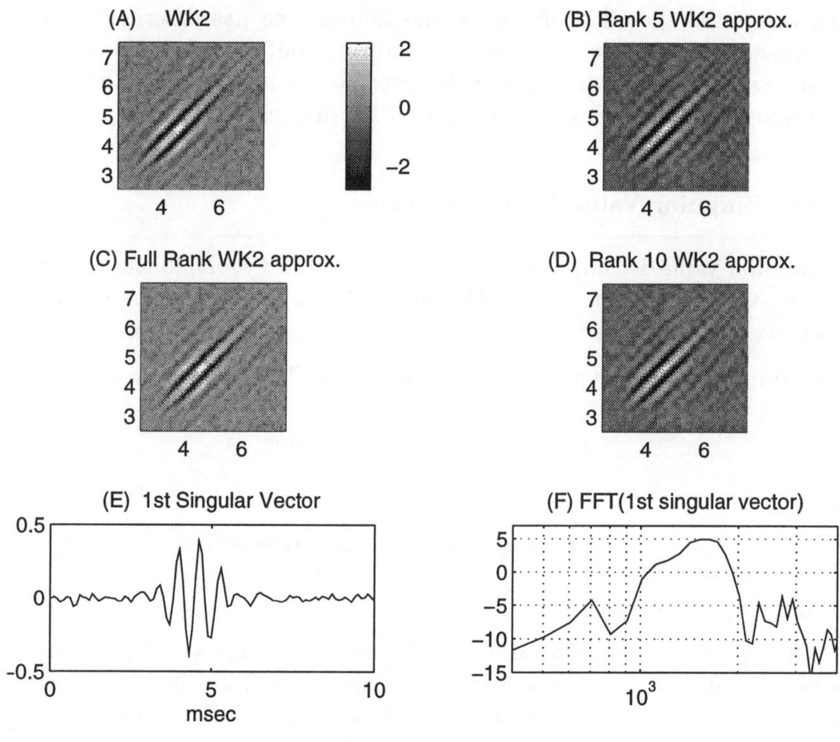

Figure 1: Singular Vector Recomposition.

By plugging the result of 2 into 1 we may describe the contribution to the output of K_2 as

$$
\begin{aligned}
y_2 &= \sum_{i,j} \left[\sum_{k=1}^{q} u_k \sigma_k u_k^T \right]_{(i,j)} x(i)x(j) = \sum_{k=1}^{q} \sigma_k \sum_{i,j} \left[u_k u_k^T \right]_{(i,j)} x(i)x(j) \\
&= \sum_{k=1}^{q} \sigma_k \sum_{i,j} u_k(i) u_k(j) x(i) x(j) = \sum_{k=1}^{q} \sigma_k \sum_{i} u_k(i) x(i) \sum_{j} u_k(j) x(j) \\
&= \sum_{k=1}^{q} \sigma_k \left(\sum_{i} u_k(i) x(i) \right)^2 .
\end{aligned}
$$

The final equality describes a first order operation similiar to the operation of K_1, but whose result is squared. This result is interesting because most kernels analysed to date are of rank lower than 5. This implies that the operation of the second order Wiener kernel may be approximated by less than five such first order convolution operations. This significantly reduces the computational burden of K_2 while at the same time illuminating the operation of K_2 on the acoustic signal in terms that are easily grasped.

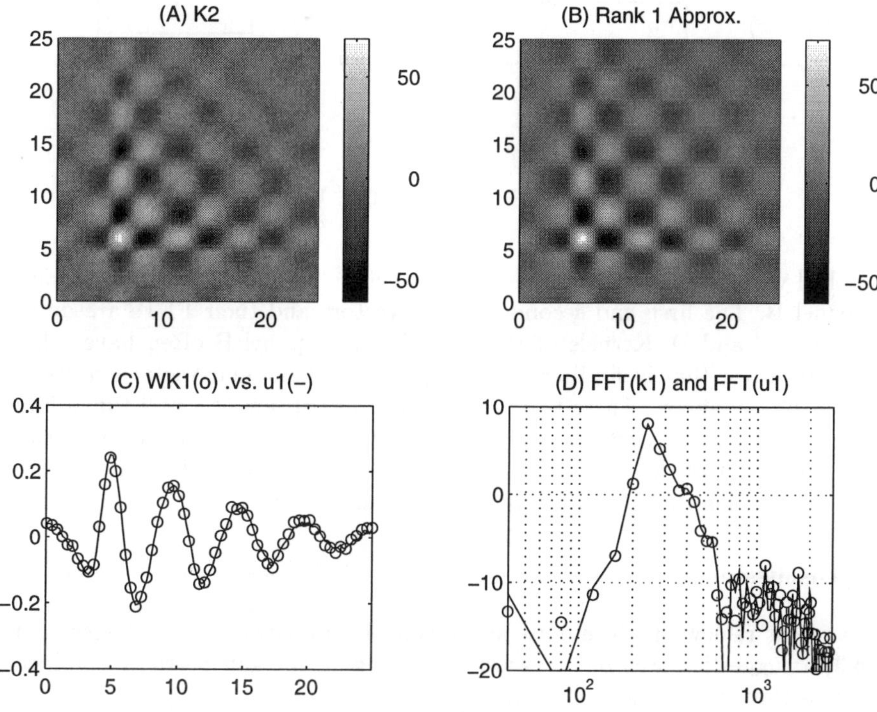

Figure 2: Amphibian Papilla.

The K_2 of an amphibian papilla unit is shown in figure 2 panel A. This kernel is rank one (see reconstructed kernel in frame B). The first singular vector AND the K_1 are graphed in frame C, where the K_1 has been normalized to be unitary. In frame D the $FFT(K_1)$ and $FFT(u_1)$ are graphed, they are nearly identical. Because K_2 for this unit is rank 1, it's operation can be described by a single first order convolution, the output of which is squared. This operation is pictured in figure 3 using box model notation.

Our third example of the SVD is presented in figure 4. This figure shows the SVD of K_2 in a gerbil mid-frequency cochlear unit. The K_1 of this unit is

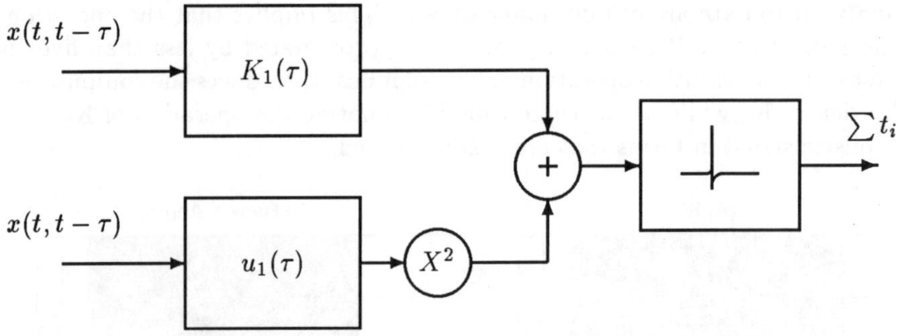

Figure 3: Block Model of AP Unit.

graphed with the first singular vector in panel A. The K_2 of this unit is drawn in panel B. The first and second singular vectors and their FFTs are drawn in panels C and D. Kernels of the form shown in panel B often have a first singular vector that is similiar to K_1, and a second singular vector similiar to K_1 but phase lagged. These two vectors are a description of a well-tuned filter that lacks phase locking, i.e. they yield a DC response but no AC response. The magnitude of these vectors can be directly compared to the magnitude of K_1 to determine the AC/DC balance of the unit's tuning.

3   Discussion

In a recent review of white noise analysis in the auditory system (Eggermont; 1993) a suggestion was put forward that bridging the gap between nonlinear systems theory and auditory physiology would require that more effort be applied first to the application of kernels to prediction of the response to unknown stimuli (modelling) and second to the interpretation of the kernels in such a way as to illuminate the system and it's function under study.

We feel that the result in this paper addresses the second of these goals. An intuitive understanding of first order convolution (the operation of K_1) is easily grasped. By explaining the operation of K_2 in terms of several first order convolutions, an intuitive understanding of K_2 is easily grasped. This is especially significant when lack of phase lock precludes calculation of K_1.

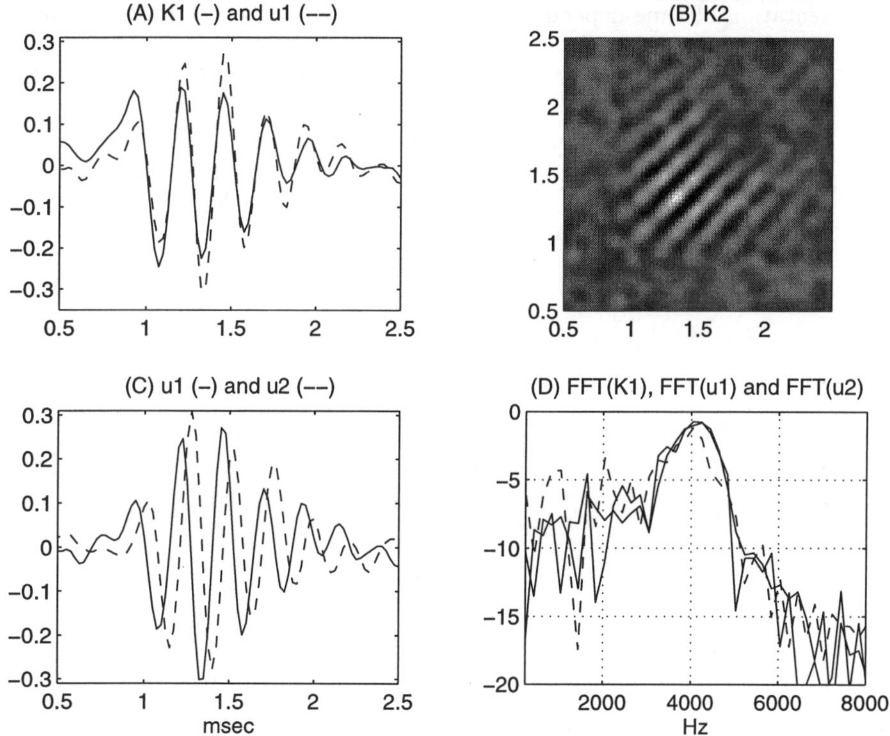

Figure 4: Gerbil Cochlear Unit.

References

1. E. de Boer and H. R. de Jongh (1978) On cochlear modeling: Potentialities and limitations of the reverse-correlation technique. *J. Acoust. Soc. Am.* **63** 115–135.
2. J. J. Eggermont (1993) Wiener and volterra analyses applied to the auditory system. *Hear. Res.* **66** 177–201.
3. Martin Schetzen (1980) The volterra and wiener theories of nonlinear systems. John Wiley and Sons, New York.
4. E. de Boer and P. Kuyper (1968) Triggered correlation. *IEEE Trans. BME* **15** 115–135.
5. P.I.M. Johannesma J.J. Eggermont van Stokkum, I.H.M. (1986) Repre-

sentation of time-dependant correlation and recurrence time functions. *Biol. Cybernet.* **55** 17–24.

6. E. Beltrami (1893) Sulle funzioni bilineari. *Gionale di Mathematiche* **11** 98–106.

7. C. Eckhart and G. Young (1939) A principal axis transformation for non-hermitian matrices. *Bull. Amer. Math. Soc.* **45** 118–121.

8. G. H. Golub and C. F. Van Loan (1989) *Matrix Computation.* John Hopkins University Press, Baltimore, MD.

STUDIES OF MECHANOELECTRIC TRANSDUCTION IN CONCENTRIC HAIR BUNDLES OF INVERTEBRATES

U. THURM, M. BRINKMANN, R. GOLZ, P. LAWONN, D. OLIVER

Institut für Neuro- und Verhaltensbiologie, University of Münster
Badestr. 9, D48149 Münster, Germany

In most invertebrate phyla epithelial mechanoreceptor cells sensitive to water movements carry a concentric hair bundle that consists of a single cilium which is surrounded by a stiff conical cylinder of interconnected stereovilli (collar configuration). A similar arrangement makes up the cnidocil apparatus of hydrozoan nematocytes (stinging cells). Intracellular voltage and current clamp measurements in nematocytes of marine polyps *(Corynidae)* revealed depolarizing receptor responses when force was applied to the cnidocil. Characteristics of transduction were similar to those of vertebrate hair cells, with the exception of an absence of directional sensitivity. By electronmicroscopy of sensory and stinging cells, the cilium or cnidocil was found to be linked to the surrounding stereovilli by radial chains of intra- and extracellular structures that are mounted between the ciliary microtubules and the actin-skeleton of the stereovilli. Monoclonal antibodies directed against the extracellular chain-component of *Hydra* abolished mechanosensitivity if they were present during the formation of the connection. Results are compared with findings on related insect and vertebrate mechanoreceptors and are discussed with respect to the location of mechanically gated ion channels.

1   What are and where occur Concentric Hair Bundles?

In *lower* chordates like the lancelet *Branchiostoma*, epithelial mechanoreceptors carry a hair bundle that consists of a single, long cilium and a number of shorter, stiff microvilli (stereovilli=stereocilia) as is also the case in most epithelial mechanoreceptors of the *higher* chordates, i.e. the vertebrates. In contrast to the latter, the hair bundle of the lower chordates has a concentric configuration: the cilium is surrounded by the stereovilli in one or a few rings (Fig. 1). This *collar* configuration is the very standard for epithelial mechanoreceptors in most invertebrate phyla, except the arthropods[1]; it may be the predecessor of the excentric hair bundle of the vertebrates, and exists already in cnidarian polyps and medusae[2].

Each stereovillus of such a bundle is connected to its neighbours by horizontal filamentous links[3,4]. Thus a stiff tube or cone results which is anchored by root structures in the cytoplasm. A basal tapering of stereovilli that allows their deflection in vertebrate hair cells does not exist in these concentric hair bundles. The cilium, often stiffened by additional skeletal elements, is suspended in the center of this tube by radial, horizontal filamentous connectors which link it to the surrounding stereovilli (contact region ≤1 μm long). No analog of the obliquely arranged tip links of vertebrate hair bundles has been found in these concentric bundles.

Physiological studies of collar receptor cells were hampered so far by the slender form of their cell soma and by their sparse occurence. The *cnidocil apparatus* of the stinging cells of hydropolyps and medusae, however, follows the same organizational scheme of concentric hair bundles[5] and these cells are

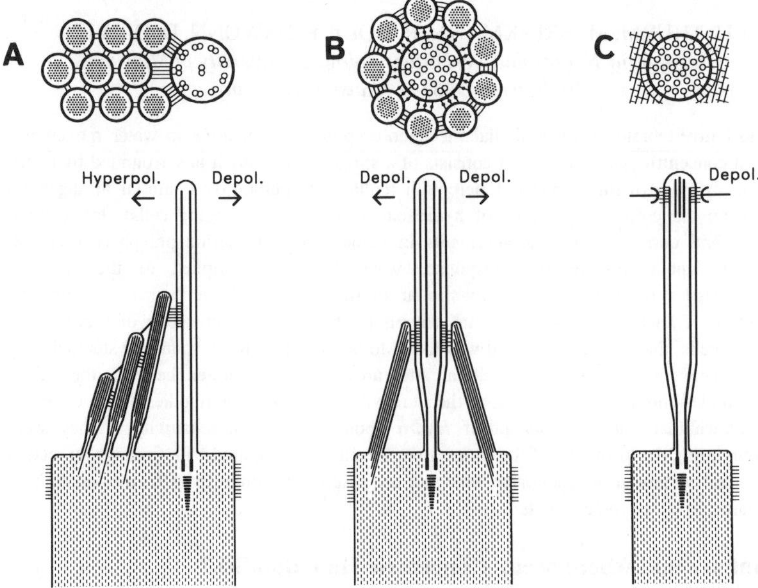

Figure 1: Configurations of cilia epithelial mechanoreceptor cells. A: vertebrate hair cell; B: concentric hair bundle of invertebrates (collar receptor); C: insect mechanoreceptor. Arrows indicate directions of force. Above: cross sections at the level of membrane connections (A: composite section).

present in large numbers in the tentacles of the animals. Stinging cells, also called *nematocytes*, since long have been assumed to be mechanosensitive. Their hair bundles are freely accessible and represent an advantageous paradigm for molecular analysis of signal transduction.The familiar function of the nematocytes is the exocytotic discharge of their stinging capsule, which ejects an evaginating long tubule that serves in catching and killing of prey. This discharge is triggered by mechanical stimulation of the cnidocil apparatus, mostly if the cell has been sensitized by adequate *chemical* stimulation *preceding* the mechanical stimulus. Therefore mechanosensitivity can be studied in nematocytes like in sensory cells. Mechanical stimulation of nematocytes induces postsynaptic responses in other cells of the tentacle, thus proving that nematocytes also act as true mechanoreceptor cells[6].

2 Electrophysiology

2.1 Methods

We studied mechanoelectric transduction of large nematocytes (stenoteles) in isolated non contractile tentacular spheres of marine Corynidae polyps (mostly *Stauridiosarsia producta*). Locally defined mechanical stimuli were applied by a glass probe of 1-4 µm diameter. The probe was moved by a two-dimensional piezo-electric driver controlled by optoelectronic devices in two feed-back circuits. Conventional intracellular microelectrodes were used for recording in voltage or current clamp mode[7].

2.2 Characteristics of mechanoelectric transduction in concentric hair bundles

Local force applied to the tip of the cnidocil apparatus (as explained below) caused depolarizing responses of phasic-tonic time course similar to those of vertebrate hair cells. The response is an increase in an unspecific cation conductance, up to 30 nS at maximal amplitude. The corresponding inward current was carried mainly by the prevalent outside-sodium and could be blocked by streptomycin. The increase in conductance started with a delay of < 50 µs compared to the start of deformation (charging of capacities taken into account). Thus, the characteristics of mechanoelectric transduction at the concentric hair bundle of the nematocytes studied indicate a direct mechanical control of ion channels with properties similar to those of vertebrate hair cells. (For purely sensoric concentric hair cells see[8]).

The mechanosensitivity of the nematocytes was strictly limited to deformations within the hair bundles. At oblique displacements of the probe against the tip of the cnidocil apparatus, excursions of 0.5 - 1.0 µm produced saturating responses. They were reached along a sigmoid stimulus-response curve. All receptor potentials were of depolarizing sign, independently of the direction of a deflection of the hair bundle. This absence of directional sensitivity corresponds to the rotational symmetry of the hair bundles. Displacements of the base of the cnidocil apparatus within the epithelial plane did not stimulate. Maximal voltage changes, up to 50 mV, were obtained by displacements of the cnidocil in its longitudinal direction. Stress between the cnidocil and the stereovilli appeared to be the most efficient stimulus. In cells which have a cilium that is much longer than the stereovilli it is the only natural stimulus; while in the nematocytes studied, having a short cnidocil, the tips of the stereovilli can get touched. In these cells a second mechanism became evident when the cnidocil was lost. Then, smaller depolarizations could still be elicited by pushing against the tips of the stereovilli. Pushing against the side of the ring of stereovilli, in contrast, did not stimulate. Thus, some local sensitivity for a pressure gradient may exist in the tips of the stereovilli.

3 Structural Basis of Transduction

The usual stimulatory force which acts laterally or obliquely on the cilium or cnidocil is transmitted along the stiff rod to the supporting ring of stereovilli and to the ciliary base. From the cilium to the stereovilli, the force can be expected to get transmitted at least partially by stress along the intermembrane connectors. We tested the role of this component of force for the mechanical control of the transduction channels by raising antibodies against these connectors.

3.1 Blocking of mechanosensitivity by monoclonal antibodies raised against intermembrane connectors

Cnidocils of *Hydra* can easily be induced to be shed ("autotomized") and can thus be isolated[9]. They are regenerated by the nematocytes within 3 hours. During the absence of the cnidocils no discharge of the nematocytes can be induced mechanically; this capability returns with the regeneration of the cnidocils. (In *Hydra*, fortunately, discharge can be induced purely mechanically when animals have starved > 3 days.) We raised monoclonal antibodies (Bd 2.2.) against the intermembrane connectors of the cnidocils of *Hydra vulgaris*[10]. When the cnidocils were isolated, the antibody marked connectors in the former contact region at both, the cnidocil and the stereovilli, indicating a homophilic mechanism of connection. The antibody did not interfere with the mechanosensitivity of the nematocytes of *Hydra* when it was added in the normal state of the cells. But if present during regeneration of the cnidocils, the antibody Bd 2.2 abolished the restoration of the mechanosensitivity irreversibly[11]. (The ability to discharge remained unchanged, as electrical stimulation revealed.) The strict association of this loss of mechanosensitivity with the regeneration of the cnidocils indicates that the binding of the antibody interferes with the restoration of connector coupling. The mechanosensitivity-abolishing consequence of this interference suggests that the intermembrane connectors are essential for the transmission of stimulatory force to the mechanosensitive channels. Based on the following findings, we hypothesize that the connectors do so by being connected to these channels.

3.2 Intermembrane connectors are part of transmembranous chains mounted between cytoskeletons

Within the cilium of the concentric hair bundles, we regularly found radially arranged bridges, about 20 nm long, connecting the membrane to the microtubule doublets[3,4]. In the longitudinal direction of the cilium, the bridges occur limited to the region of the stereovillus-cilium contact; in this area they are regularly spaced with about 20 nm periodicity. In the circumference, the bridges are located opposite to the rows of extracellular connectors. Freeze edging exposed intramembrane particles in the spacial arrangement of the connectors, i.e. in a somewhat larger number than that of the intracellular bridges. Inside the stereovilli, their total membrane is connected to the actin core by regularly spaced bridges, as is known also from other microvilli.

Dissolving the lipids of the membranes by application of detergent during fixation revealed that the intermembrane connectors indeed are the central element of chains that connect the microtubule-based skeleton of the cilium to the actin-based skeleton of the stereovilli, thereby traversing both the membranes (Fig. 2A).

3.3   Are ion channels constituents of the transmembranous connector chains?

The organization found is appropriate to conduct and to concentrate a considerable proportion of the stimulatory force to a limited number of molecules that penetrate the membranes. Such molecules are best candidates for the force-dependent gating of ion channels. The finding that mechanosensitivity is abolished when antibodies interfere with the regeneration of the intermembrane connectors is a strong indication for these channels to be a constituent of the transmembranous chains. The question, whether the channels are located at the side of the cnidocil

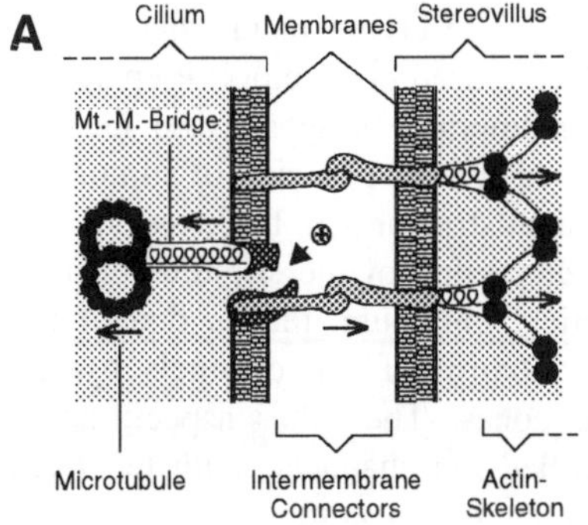

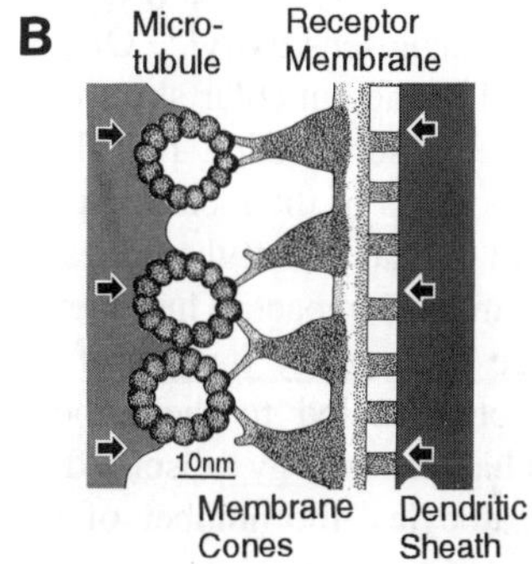

Figure 2 A: Model of the chain that connects ciliary microtubules and stereovillar actin skeleton and controls ion channel gating in a concentric hair bundle. Topograhic details and organization of ion channel are hypothetic. Arrows indicate stimulatory tension with reference to the channel. B: Slightly schematized drawing of microtubule-membrane complex in insect mechanoreceptor at the site of impact of stimulatory force (arrows). From freeze substitution preparation[13,14].

or the stereovilli or at both sides cannot be decisively answered at present. Some help may be the maximal number of channels that can simultaneously be activated, since the number of chain-elements is higher in the membrane of the stereovilli than of the cnidocil. If one assumes a single channel conductance similar to that of large vertebrate hair cells - 100 nS - one arrives at about 300 channels for the amplitude of saturating receptor currents in large nematocytes of *S. producta*[7]. This number is quite similar to the number of microtubule-membrane bridges which can be calculated for nematocytes of *Tubularia larynx*[3] and is also about 300. This similarity is certainly somewhat accidental, but it indicates that the connector chains traversing the membrane of the cnidocil are conceivable to include the receptor channels (Fig.2A). Essential support for this conclusion derives from the following results on mechanoreceptors of insects.

3.4 Correspondence between the collared cilium and the ciliary outer segment of insect mechanoreceptors

In epithelial mechanoreceptors of arthropods no stereovilli exist. A single, modified cilium is exposed to the stimulatory force which is transmitted by a part of the cuticle. The cilium also finds its support in the arthropod-characterizing cuticle (Fig. 1C). The solid-character of the cuticle allows in favorite objects a very precise localisation of the force impact and a determination of the stimulatory path length (minimum <1 Å)[12,13]. The adequate stimulus is local monoaxial pressure directed vertically to the plain of the membrane. In the region of stimulus impact, and only in this region, the membrane is connected to the peripheral layer of microtubules by cone-shaped bridges of very similar size and periodicity as found in the cilium of concentric hair bundles (Fig. 2B). Disaggregration of these microtubules causes loss of mechanosensitivity[14]. On its outside, the stimulus-receiving membrane area is linked to the cuticular sheath by short, more tightly spaced connectors. Preparation by freeze-substitution revealed the microtubule-membrane bridges to be integral components of the membrane: "membrane integrated cones". Freezing of stimulated states indicated that the cones are the most compliant structures in the cross section of stimulus impact. Thus they absorb an essential portion of the stimulus energy. Since this energy itself was near to the theoretical minimum, this is one of the aspects that led to the hypothesis of a gating control of ion channels by the mechanical energy absorbed in the membrane cones. The other aspect: as in nematocytes, the number of mechanically controlled ion channels estimated from saturating receptor currents was found to be similar to the number of membrane cones in the same type of cell. In the most sensitive insect receptors no other membrane area exists that could perform direct control of ion channels than this ciliary area which contains the membrane cones. Therefore we propose that the microtubule-membrane bridges are associated with mechanosensitive ion channels most probably in a 1:1 manner, also in concentric hair bundles. In these hair bundles an opening by tension is most likely, in contrast to the insect receptors studied (Fig. 2).

5   Perspectives towards Vertebrate Hair Cells

Our results revealed the contact region between the cilium and the stereovilli as a structural basis of transduction. This connection has been conserved in evolution for the transmission of stimulatory force at a bottleneck-position in nearly all vertebrate hair cells except the mammalian organ of Corti. Its structure in the vertebrate kinocilium is similar to that in collared cilia, though not identical[15]. In the kinocilium a contribution of this connection to mechanoelectric transduction has not been excluded so far[16]. This contribution may add transducer properties which are different from those of the stereovilli, e.g. in adaptive behavior.

The association of the "horizontal" intermembrane connectors with mechanical gating of channels supports the suggestion that the gating performed by vertebrate stereovilli may be associated with their horizontal links (as we suggested earlier[17,18]) because of their closer analogy compared with the "tip links". But this consideration does not exclude an evolutionary new construction.

Acknowledgments

This research was supported by the Deutsche Forschungsgemeinschaft, particularly SFB 310, and Fonds der Chemischen Industrie.

References

1. Budelmann, B.U. (1989) Hydrodynamic receptor systems in invertebrates, in *The Mechanosensory Lateral Line*, eds. S. Coombs, P. Görner, H. Münz (Springer-Verlag, Berlin) p. 607–631.
2. Golz, R., Thurm, U. (1994) The ciliated sensory cell of *Stauridiosarsia producta* (Cnidaria, Hydrozoa) - a nematocyst-free nematocyte? *Zoomorphology*, **114** 185–194.
3. Golz, R., Thurm, U. (1991) Cytoskeleton-membrane interactions in the cnidocil complex of hydrozoan nematocytes, *Cell Tissue Res* **263** 573–583.
4. Hüesker L, Thurm U (1994) Ultrastructure of the cilium-stereovilli complex of sensory-collar cells, in *Sensory Transduction*, eds. N. Elsner, H. Breer, (Thieme-Verlag, Stuttgart) Abstr. Nr. 66.
5. Slautterback, D.B. (1967) The cnidoblast-musculoepithelial cell complex in the tentacles of *Hydra*, *Z Zellforsch* **79** 296–318.
6. Brinkmann, M., Thurm, U. (1995) Interaction of mechano- and chemosensory signals within the same sensory cell, *Pflügers Arch-Eur J Physiol* **429** R153.
7. Brinkmann, M., Oliver, D., Thurm, U. (1996) Mechanoelectric transduction in nematocytes of a hydropolyp (Corynidae), *J Comp Physiol A* **178** 125–138.
8. Oliver, D., Thurm, U. (1996) Mechanoreception by concentric hair cells of hydropolyps, *Göttingen Neurobiol Report* (Thieme-Verlag, Stuttgart) 92.
9. Golz, R., Thurm, U. (1990) Cnidocil regeneration in nematocytes of *Hydra*, *Protoplasma* **155** 95–105.
10. Golz, R., Thurm, U. (1992) Monoclonal antibodies against surface components of the mechano- and chemosensitive cnidocil-complex of *Hydra vulgaris*, *Cell Tissue Res* **268** 327–333.

11. Lawonn, P., Golz, R., Thurm, U. (1995) Blocking of mechanosensitivity in hydrozoan nematocytes by a monoclonal antibody, *in Göttingen Neurobiol. Report 1995*, eds. N. Elsner, R. Menzel (Thieme-Verlag, Stuttgart) 703.

12. Thurm, U. (1983) Mechano-electric transduction, in *Biophysics*, eds. W. Hoppe, W. Lohmann, H. Markl, H. Ziegler (Springer-Verlag, Berlin, Heidelberg) p. 666–671.

13. Thurm, U., Erler, G., Gödde, J., Kastrup, H., Keil, T.A., Völker, W., Vohwinkel, B. (1983) Cilia specialized for mechanoreception, *J Submicroscopic Cytology* **15** 151–155.

14. Erler, G. (1983) Sensitivity of an insect mechanoreceptor after destruction of free dendritic microtubules by means of vinblastine, *Cell Tissue Res* **229** 673–684

15. Ernstson, S., Smith, C. A. (1986) Stereo-kinociliar bonds in mammalian vestibular organs, *Acta Otolaryngol (Stockh)* **101** 395–402.

16 Hudspeth, AJ., Jacobs, R. (1979) Stereocilia mediate transduction in vertebrate hair cells. *Proc Natl Acad Sci USA* **76** 1506–1509

17 Thurm, U. (1981) Mechano-electric transduction, *Biophysics of Structure and Mechanism.* **7** 245–246.

18 Schmidt, B., Thurm, U. (1984) Structures transmitting stimulatory force to the sensory hairs (stereovilli) of the frog sacculus, *Verh Dtsch Zool Ges* **77** 326.

Descriptive models of middle and outer Ear

The reader will find that advances in descriptions of middle and outer ear operation have required instrumentation that pushes the state of the art at least as severely as that required for observations of mechanics at the cellular level. Among the papers in Part Two, one finds applications of confocal microscopy, laser velocimetry, and extraordinarily carefully executed microacoustic measurements.

THE EFFECT OF THE *PARS FLACCIDA* OF THE TYMPANIC MEMBRANE ON THE EAR'S SENSITIVITY TO SOUND

J.J. ROSOWSKI, S.W. TEOH, D.T. FLANDERMEYER

Eaton-Peabody Laboratory, Massachusetts Eye and Ear Infirmary
243 Charles Street, Boston, MA 02114, USA
jjr@epl.meei.harvard.edu

This paper is part of a series of studies on the acoustic function of the *pars flaccida*. Here we report laser measurements of the motion of the *pars tensa* and *pars flaccida* components of the gerbil tympanic membrane. The measurements demonstrate that the *flaccida* and the *tensa* have greatly different mechanical characteristics and that motions of the *flaccida* and umbo are independent. The new data are consistent with both a model of *flaccida* function put forth by Kohllöffel[1] and previous input impedance and middle-ear sound-pressure measurements in this species[2-4]. The data clearly demonstrate that the ear's response to low-frequency sounds is reduced by a *flaccida*-induced increase in middle-ear cavity sound pressure and a concomitant decrease in the pressure difference across the *pars tensa*. The results associate the presence of a significant *pars flaccida* and small middle-ear cavity with decreased sensitivity to low-frequency sounds.

1. Introduction

1.1 Pars Flaccida and Pars Tensa

The tympanic membrane of the Mongolian gerbil (and many other mammals[1]) is made up of two components (Figure 1). The *pars tensa* is attached to the malleus and appears tautly stretched between the manubrium of the malleus and the tympanic ring. The *pars flaccida* is a loose membrane lying posterior and dorsal to the *tensa*. The boundary between the two portions of the membrane is near the lateral process of the malleus.

The original descriptions of the *flaccida*[5,6] suggested that the membrane played a role in regulating middle-ear static pressures. Kohllöffel[1], however, suggested an acoustic function. In his model (Fig. 2) the *flaccida* acts as an independent path for sound volume velocity to flow from the ear canal into the middle-ear cavity.

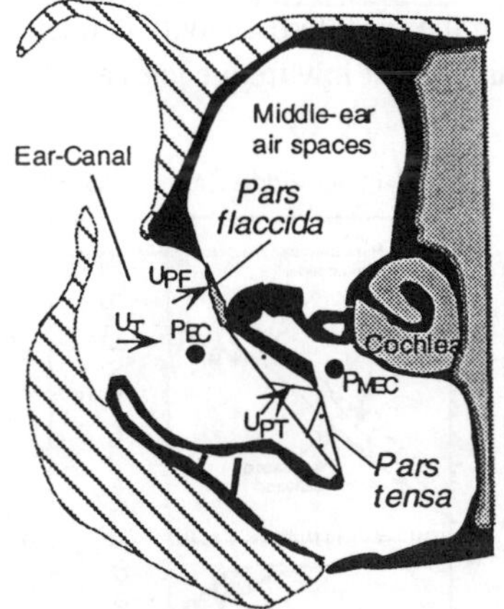

Figure 1:
The Middle Ear of the Mongolian Gerbil
(*Meriones unguiculatus*)

The volume velocity U_T in the ear canal and the associated sound pressure P_{EC} act as inputs in the model analog. The ratio of these inputs is the middle-ear input admittance $Y_T = U_T/P_{EC}$. Part of the volume velocity U_{PF} moves the *flaccida*, while the rest U_{PT} moves the *tensa*. The sum of the two currents is the volume-velocity input to the middle-ear cavity. The pressure in the cavity is the ratio of the summed currents and the cavity's acoustic admittance: $P_{MEC} = U_T/Y_{CAV}$. The volume velocity of the *tensa*, which acts on the ossicles and cochlea, is the product of the admittance of that path and the pressure difference across the tympanic membrane:

$$U_{PT} = (P_{EC} - P_{MEC}) Y_{TOC}. \qquad (1)$$

Figure 2: A circuit diagram of the hypothetical function of *pars flaccida*

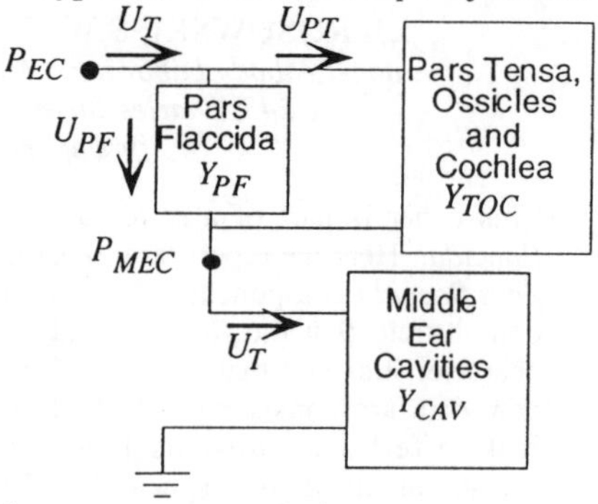

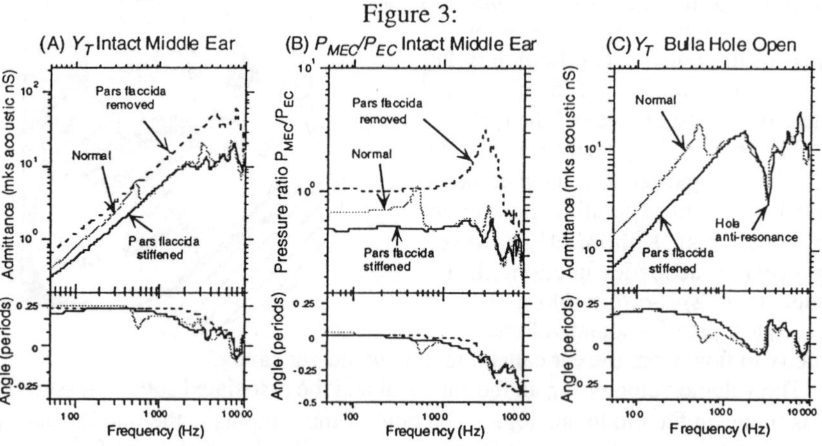

The pressure difference is a function of the three component admittances:

$$\frac{P_{EC} - P_{MEC}}{P_{EC}} = \frac{1}{\dfrac{Y_{PF} + Y_{TOC}}{Y_{CAV}} + 1}. \qquad (2)$$

According to Eqn. 2, if $|Y_{PF}| \ll |Y_{TOC}|$ the pressure difference is relatively insensitive to Y_{Pf}, while if $|Y_{PF}| \geq |Y_{TOC}|$, the pressure difference across the tympanic membrane and the motion of the *tensa* and ossicles is reduced.

1.2 Measures of Middle-Ear Input Admittance and Cavity Sound Pressures.

We have previously shown[2-4] that stiffening or removing the *pars flaccida* affect middle-ear input admittance and middle-ear sound pressure in the gerbil (Figure 3). When the middle-ear cavity is intact (3A), stiffening the *flaccida* decreases the input admittance at low frequencies and has little effect at frequencies above 1 kHz.

Figure 3:

Removing the *flaccida* results in an admittance which is dominated by the cavity compliance at frequencies less than 3 kHz. (At higher frequencies, the resistance and inertance introduced by the constriction of the *flaccida* rim become important.) Some of the stiffening-induced changes in Y_T are echoed in measurements of middle-ear cavity sound pressure (3B). Stiffening the *flaccida* reduces the low-frequency plateau in $|P_{MEC}|$, but has little effect at higher frequencies. Furthermore, the frequency region where stiffening reduces $|P_{MEC}|$ is the same region in which $|Y_T|$ is reduced. Removing the *flaccida* equalizes P_{EC} and P_{MEC} at frequencies below 2 kHz; at higher frequencies a resonance exists between the cavity compliance and the inertance of the bony rim around the removed *flaccida*.

The contribution of the middle-ear cavity to Y_T at frequencies below 2 kHz was greatly reduced by opening a 1 mm diameter hole in the bulla wall (Fig. 3C). The hole greatly increased the cavity admittance at those low frequencies and introduced an anti-resonance (a sharp decrease) in Y_{CAV} at 3 kHz[7]. When the hole is open, the low-frequency input admittance is dominated by the stiffness of the membrane components and we see a sizable increase in the low frequency $|Y_T|$ measured both before and after stiffening the *flaccida*. We also see a larger difference between the pre- and post-stiffening admittances when the bullar hole is open.

The admittances and pressures of Fig. 3 are well fit by the model structure of Fig. 2 using model parameters defined from the measurements (Fig. 4), where (a) Y_{CAV} is the admittance of a 0.2 cc volume, (b) Y_{TOC} is the admittance measured when the *flaccida* is stiffened with the series admittance of the cavities removed, and (c) Y_{PF} is calculated from the measurement of the total admittance and the values of the other two components. Eqns. 1 & 2 and the block admittance values suggest that the *flaccida* will reduce the motion of the ossicles in the region where $|Y_{PF}| \geq |Y_{TOC}|$, i.e. at frequencies below about 500 Hz.

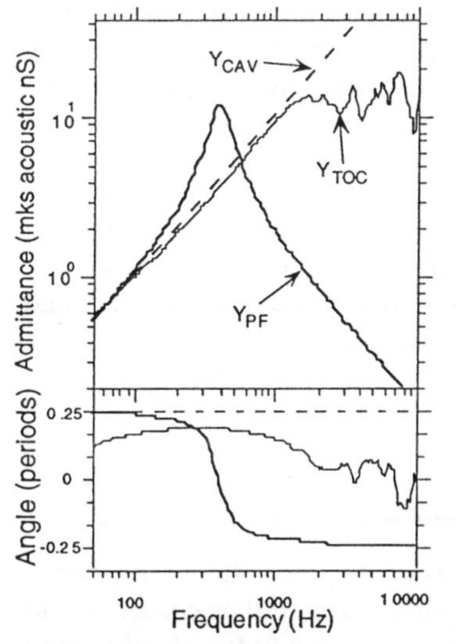

Figure 4: Estimates of Model Ys

1.3 The Goal of this Study

We further investigate *flaccida* function with direct measurements of the motion of the *flaccida* and *tensa*. Such measurements 1) directly determine the frequency response and relative motions of the *flaccida* and *tensa*, 2) investigate whether the two membrane components move independently from each other, and 3) directly test the hypothesis that the *flaccida* reduces the motion of the *tensa* when the cavities are intact. We also investigate the role of the *flaccida* in hearing in other mammals.

2. Methods

Young mature gerbils were anesthetized and surgically prepared.[a,2-4,7] The auditory bulla was exposed, and a vent tube was sealed in the bullar wall. A second bullar hole was opened. To allow better access to the umbo, part of the bony lateral ear-canal wall was removed, taking care not to open the middle-ear cavity. Triangles of reflective tape ($\approx$500 μm per side) were placed on the *tensa* at the umbo and in the center of the *flaccida*. A small brass tube ($\approx$6 mm id) with a side-mounted microphone and sound tube was sealed to the ear canal. The lateral opening of this brass tube was sealed with a glass coverslip. A Polytec® fiber-optic laser velocimeter was focused through the glass on either the umbo or *flaccida* reflector. The angle between the plane of the umbo and the laser beam was $\approx 60°$. The angle between the plane of the *flaccida* and the beam was 80°. The angles introduce small, $\approx$15%, errors into the velocity data which are not corrected in the figures we show.

Repeated measurements were made of *flaccida* and umbo motion, with the bullar hole open and sealed. The *flaccida* was then stiffened with a circular sheet of hardened dental acrylic (≈ 200 μm thick; the diameter of the acrylic sheet ≈ 3 mm was slightly smaller than that of the *flaccida*).[2-4] A new reflector was placed on the acrylic, and measurements were made of the motion of the acrylic and the umbo.

Velocity-to-ear-canal-sound-pressure transfer functions were measured using an Ariel® DSP-16+ board and Sysid® software. Measurements (Fig. 5) were made with chirp stimuli of 50 to 25000 Hz bandwidth (results illustrated by lines without symbols), and with pure tones of frequencies between 25 and 800 Hz (illustrated by circles). The latter stimulus type led to superior signal to noise ratios but required more time. All of the measurements we show are from one ear; similar results were found in five others.

3. Results

3.1 Relative motion of the Flaccida and Umbo: Bullar Hole open

A comparison (Figure 5A) of the relative velocities of the *flaccida* and the umbo, measured with the bullar hole open demonstrates differences in the sensitivity and frequency response of the two structures. The *flaccida* velocity transfer function V_F/P_{EC} is roughly consistent with that of a series RLC circuit: the velocity is compliance dominated at frequencies less than 300 Hz, mass dominated at frequencies above 700 Hz with a clear resonance at 350 Hz. By comparison, the umbo velocity V_U shows a broader, higher frequency peak and a less-clear mass dominance above the peak. Part of the complicated velocity responses at higher-frequencies can be attributed to the 3 kHz antiresonace produced by the interaction of

---

[a] The experimental protocol was approved by the Institutional Animal Care and Use Committee of the Mass. Eye and Ear Infirmary.

the open bullar hole and the bullar air space. At low-frequencies the velocity of the *flaccida* is 8 to 10 times larger than the umbo velocity. At higher frequencies, the umbo velocity is of larger magnitude.

Figure 5: Measures of *Flaccida* and *Tensa* Velocity with Bullar Hole Open

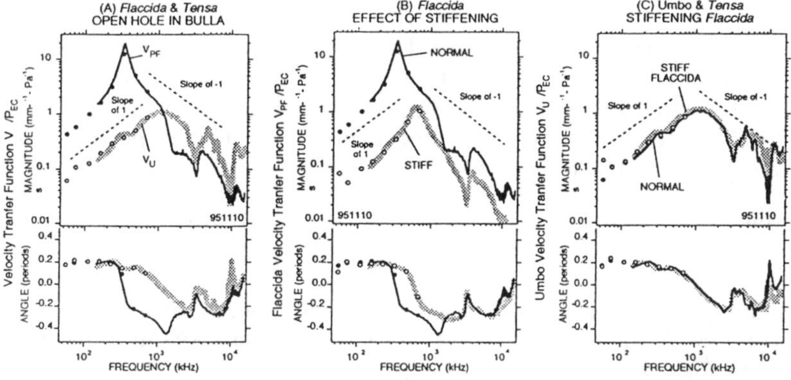

3.2 The effect of Flaccida Stiffening

Placement of the acrylic sheet on the *flaccida* (Fig. 5B) reduces *flaccida* velocity at low frequencies by more than a factor of ten, increases the resonant frequency by about a factor of two and decreases *flaccida* velocity at high frequencies by about a factor of two. These changes are consistent with an increase in *flaccida* stiffness and mass. The sheet has little effect on the velocity of the umbo (Fig. 5C), suggesting that the umbo moves independently of the *flaccida*.

3.3 Relative motion of the Flaccida and Umbo: Bullar Hole closed

Closing the hole in the bulla, while maintaining the vent causes a decrease in the velocity of both the *tensa* and *flaccida* at low-frequencies, and removes the effects of the 3 kHz bullar-hole anti-resonance (Fig. 6). Similar cavity-hole induced changes have been observed in the mechanics of gerbil and other mammalian middle ears[7,8] and have been associated with the addition of the cavity comp-

Figure 6: Effect of Closing the Bulla Hole

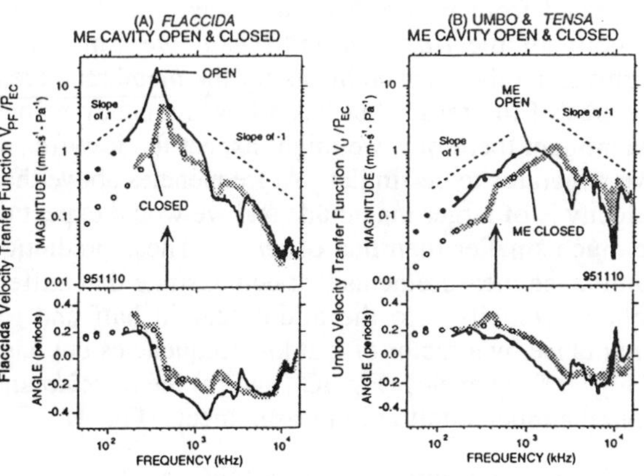

liance and the removal of the inertance of the bullar hole.

134

Some of the changes in low-frequency umbo velocity produced by closing the bullar hole – particularly the rapid change in magnitude and angle near 450 Hz and the increased reduction in velocity at lower frequencies – cannot be explained by a simple change in the cavity admittance, but is perfectly consistent with Eqns. 1&2 and the component admittances of Figure 4. With the cavity closed, the force that drives the motion of the umbo and *tensa* (Eqn. 1) depends on the relative magnitude of Y_{PF} and Y_{TOC} (Eqn. 2). At f < 600 Hz, when $|Y_{PF}| > |Y_{TOC}|$ (Fig. 4), P_{EC}-P_{MEC} is decreased as is the motion of the umbo. At f > 600 Hz, $|Y_{PF}| < |Y_{TOC}|$ and the umbo velocity should be less affected by the presence of the *flaccida*. The hypothetical 600 Hz break frequency is close to that of the observed rapid decrease in umbo velocity at 450 Hz (the arrow in Figure 6B).

4. Discussion

4.1 Comparisons of the Motion of the Flaccida and Tensa

The data we have gathered point out several differences between the acoustic function of *flaccida* and *tensa,* and lead to a prediction about the utility of the *flaccida* in the mammalian ear.

The *flaccida* is a resonant structure ($Q_{10} \approx$ 1-2) with a peak frequency near 400 Hz. The *flaccida* velocity is compliance dominated at lower frequencies and roughly mass dominated at higher frequencies. Umbo velocity shows a higher ($\approx$ 1 kHz) , more damped ($Q_{10} \approx 0.25$-0.5) best frequency with a slower high-frequency roll-off. These differences are consistent with the observation that increasing the *flaccida* impedance only affects low-frequency middle-ear input admittance.

The point-velocity data we present are consistent with the independence of the *flaccida* and *tensa* sound paths, in that the shield clearly reduces the velocity of the *flaccida* without affecting umbo motion (Figs 5B&C). The data suggest, but do not prove that the entire *tensa* moves independently from *flaccida*.

The relative amplitudes of the *flaccida* and *tensa* volume velocities can be estimated from Figure 5A. If we assume the measurements reflect the average velocity of the *flaccida* and *tensa*, we can compare volume velocities after normalizing the measurements for the membrane areas. The *flaccida* is about 1/10 the area of the *tensa*, but has a low-frequency velocity that is 10 times greater in magnitude; therefore, we might expect the low-frequency volume-velocities of the two structures to be similar. At frequencies above the *flaccida* resonance, the umbo velocity is of larger magnitude and we would expect the *flaccida* volume velocity to be much smaller than that of *tensa*. These predictions are consistent with (a) the admittance measurements that demonstrate that stiffening the *flaccida* cuts the total volume velocity into the middle ear in half and reduces the open cavity input admittance by a factor of 2 at low frequencies but has little effect on the admittance at higher frequencies (Fig 3C), and (b) the *flaccida* and *tensa* admittances computed from the input admittance measurements (Fig. 4).

4.2 The Relationship between Flaccida and Low-Frequency Hearing Sensitivity.

Our mechanical and acoustic data suggest a relationship between the presence of

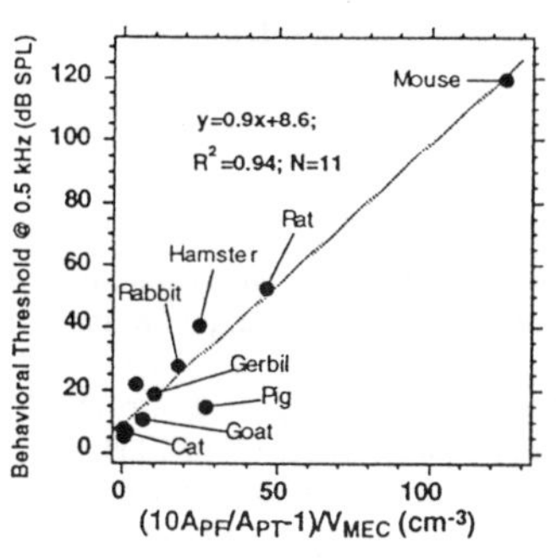

Figure 7: Low-Frequency Hearing Limits and a parameter related to V_{PT}/P_{EC}

the *flaccida* and decreased low-frequency hearing ability. While some animals with large *flaccida/tensa* area ratios have poor low-frequency hearing (e.g., rat and mouse), others (e.g., pig and goat) have good low-frequency sensitivity.[1,9,10] A complication in such comparisons is the middle-ear air volume; the circuit of Fig. 2 suggests that large volumes reduce the influence of *flaccida* motions on P_{MEC}. Strong interspecific correlations (Fig. 7) can be obtained between behavioral thresholds at low-frequencies and a parameter that normalizes variations in *flaccida/tensa* area ratio by variations in middle-ear cavity volume.

Acknowledgments

This work was supported by a grant from the National Institute of Health, NIH RO1-DC00194. Mr. Teoh is supported by NIH training grant T32-DC-00038. We would also like to thank Bill Peake and Mike Ravicz for their input.

References

1. Kohllöffel, L. (1984) Notes on the comparative mechanics of hearing. III. On Shrapnell's membrane, Hearing Research, 13 83-88.
2. Teoh, S.W. (1996) The roles of *pars flaccida* in middle-ear acoustic transmission. S.M. Thesis, MIT, Cambridge MA.
3. Teoh, S.W., Flandermeyer, D.T. and Rosowski, J.J. (1996) The effect of *pars flaccida* of the tympanic membrane on hearing function, Abstracts of the 19th Midwinter Meeting of the Association for Research in Otolaryngology p 196.
4. Teoh, S.W., Flandermeyer, D.T. and Rosowski, J.J. (1996) The effect of *pars flaccida* of the tympanic membrane on hearing function, in prep.
5. Shrapnell, H. (1832) On the form and structure of the membrana tympani, Lond. Med. Gazette 10: 120-124.
6. Stenfors, L.-E., Salén, B. and Windblad, B. (1979) The role of the *pars flaccida* in the mechanics of the middle ear, Acta oto-laryngol. 88: 395-400.
7. Ravicz, M.E., Rosowski, J.J. and Voigt, H.F. (1992) Sound-power collection by the auditory periphery of the Mongolian gerbil *Meriones unguiculatus*: I. Middle-ear input impedance. J. Acoust. Soc. Am. 92: 157-177.
8. Guinan, J. J., & Peake, W. T.(1967) Middle-ear characteristics of anesthetized cats. J. Acoust. Soc. Am. 41: 1237-1261.
9. Fay, R. (1988). Hearing in Vertebrates: a Psychophysics Databook, (Hill-Fay Associates, Winnetka IL).
10. Heffner, R., & Heffner, H. (1990) Hearing in domestic pigs (*Sus scrofa*) and goats (*Capra hircus*). Hearing Research, 48: 231-240.

EVOKED OTOACOUSTIC EMISSIONS, A NEW TOOL FOR NON-INVASIVE ANALYSIS OF MIDDLE-EAR NETWORK IN MAN.

P.AVAN, B.BÜKI*, M.DORDAIN, J.J.LEMAIRE, J.CHAZAL.

*Biophysics and Neurosurgery Departments, University Medical School, PO Box 38
63001 Clermont-Ferrand, France
*ENT Department, Semmelweis University, Budapest, Hungary
e-mail : Paul.Avan@u-clermont1.fr*

Otoacoustic emissions travel directly from the cochlea where they are generated to the external auditory meatus through the middle-ear network, hence their phase and amplitude characteristics are particularly sensitive to any change in the ear's impedance. Cubic distortion tones -CDT- at 2f1-f2 in response to a pair of primary tones at f1 and f2 were detected in humans in a broad frequency range (.7 to 4 kHz). The goal of this work was to assess the effect of various changes in the stiffness of stapes' annular ligament on CDT characteristics. The sensitivity of otoacoustic emission phases to intracranial pressure increase due to posture changes was evaluated and another experiment during invasive surgery allowed to disclose a linear relationship between the phase of low-frequency emissions and intracranial pressure changes : Df (°) = 0.20 x DICP (daPa). Quantitatively similar effects were obtained when triggering the contralateral acoustic reflex in humans. The reflex-induced attenuation barely exceeded 5 dB at about 20 dB above reflex threshold, despite a large phase shift effect on CDTs. A computational middle ear model allowed to fit the experimental data with theoretical predictions. Furthermore, dynamical aspects of CDT changes during posture changes or stapedius muscle contraction could be recorded.

1 Introduction

Standard middle-ear impedance analyzers only provide indirect and qualitative information about impedance changes of the various parts of the middle ear network, such as middle-ear pressure changes, intralabyrinthine pressure variations or middle ear muscle contractions. Their limitation is due to the shunt impedance of the eardrum which dominates the overall recorded signal. In contrast, otoacoustic emissions are generated inside the cochlea then they propagate to the external ear canal through the middle ear. Thus, their phase and amplitude characteristics should be sensitive to any change in the ear's impedance, and especially to the stiffness of the stapes subsystem.

Cubic distortion tone -CDT- otoacoustic emissions at $2f_1$-f_2 in response to a pair of primary tones at f_1 and f_2 are particularly convenient tools for such purposes because they can be detected in a broad frequency range (i.e. .7 to 8 kHz in humans) and individual measurements can be collected after averaging only 1 to 4 s.[1] Firstly, new data concerning the relationship between intracranial pressure and CDTs will be presented and compared to middle-ear muscle reflex data as well as to theoretical predictions of a computerized standard middle-ear model. Dynamical aspects of these middle ear changes will be discussed. In comparison, middle-ear pressure alterations lead to completely different patterns of CDT changes.

2   Methods

Three different paradigms were used to elicit middle-ear impedance changes. They aimed at altering only the stiffness of the stapes'annular ligament, namely posture change likely associated with variations of intracranial pressure -ICP- (n=20 ears), direct change of the hydrostatic pressure of cerebrospinal fluid through lumbar puncture[2,3] (n=18 ears) and stapedius muscle contraction induced by loud contralateral broadband-noise stimulation[3] (n= 8 ears). Middle-ear pressure was systematically derived from the peak on the tympanogram before and after emission measurements and had to be stable within 10 daPa otherwise results were discarded.

In all cases but those with lumbar puncture, CDTs were monitored with f_2 varying from 4 to .7 kHz (10 steps /octave). The primary tone levels were 60 dB SPL at f_2 and 70 dB SPL at f_1. Around these levels, the mean slope of CDT amplitude growth function was 0.7 dB/dB increase of both primaries. CDT were obtained with a Cubdis system using 1 to 4 s time averaging.[1] In the case of direct ICP increase, the experiments were performed in an operating theater during a surgical procedure for chronic hydrocephalus detection. Such a procedure is carried out in awake patients but requires minimal external sensory stimulations so as to avoid spurious ICP elevations due to patient's restlessness. CDT primary tones would have been disturbing so that click-evoked otoacoustic emissions were recorded instead (ILO88 Otodynamics, clicks presented at 10 dB above subjective hearing level).

Data analysis consisted in plotting the phase and amplitude of CDTs -or click-evoked emissions- as a function of the external parameter of interest (sitting or supine posture - 0° or 20° head-down with respect to horizontal-, ICP, contralateral sound level). Eventually, a computational model of middle-ear network was implemented using Zwislocki's proposal,[4] Lutman and Martin's values[5] and Kemp's analysis of backward propagation.[6] Its results accounting for alterations of primary tones due to forward propagation and of backward-propagated CDTs were fitted to experimental data using reasonable values for parameter adjustments.

3 Results and interpretation

3.1 Intracranial pressure

Posture changes induced typical CDT alterations that mainly involved a phase lead at frequencies below 2 kHz. The phase lead tended to be maximum around the resonance frequency of the middle ear. In contrast, amplitude changes were negligible except perhaps below 1 kHz. Fig.1 shows the mean variations of phase and amplitude, and an individual example. Interindividual variations concerning the position of maximum phase shift were about 0.5 kHz but the pattern of CDT changes was remarkably constant. The results of the experiment with direct ICP measurements were fully consistent with posture results (fig.1, open squares). A highly significant linear regression relating CDT phase shift Df to ICP increase was disclosed : Df (°) = 0.20 x DICP (daPa). The whole experiment is described in details in a recent paper.[7] The presence of a phase shift of otoacoustic emissions in all patients with increased ICP, whatever their age, may provide a non invasive tool for ICP monitoring in patients with hydrocephalus treated with a ventriculo-peritoneal shunt. This method could be complementary with respect to those based upon tympanic membrane displacement measurements.[2,8]

The middle ear computer model fully confirmed the pattern and size of the observed effects (fig.2). The phase lead when the stiffness of stapes' annular ligament presumably increases is easily predictable, as well as its frequency characteristics with a maximum effect below the resonance frequency of the concerned subsystem. It was less straightforward to anticipate the small size of the amplitude effect.

3.2 Stapedius muscle contractions

The effect of stapedius muscle contractions induced by a loud contralateral broadband sound was expected to affect stapes stiffness in a quite similar manner.[3] This was confirmed by intraindividual comparisons of stapedius reflex vs posture (fig.3). In addition, it was possible to evaluate directly the efficacy of stapedius muscle contractions (2 dB amplitude change between 0.6 and 1 kHz for the typical example of fig.3, with a contralateral noise stimulus presented 20 dB above reflex threshold, corresponding to adding up forward and backward attenuations).

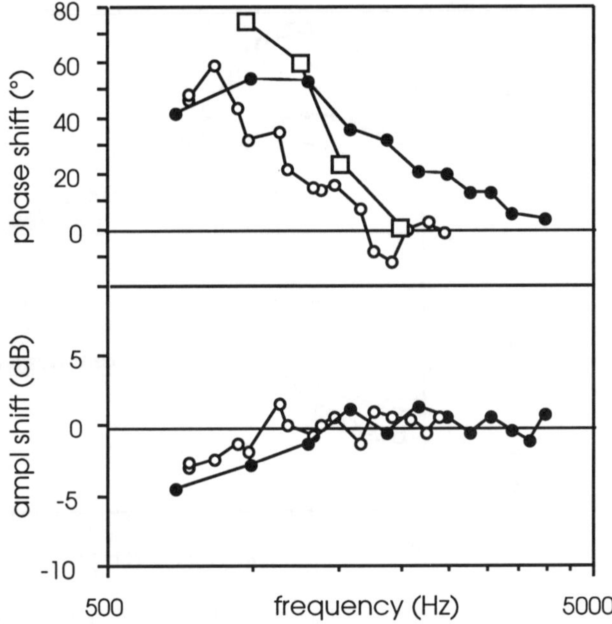

Figure 1 : CDT changes in phase and amplitude due to posture change (sitting/supine). Open circles: individual result; closed circles: mean shifts (n=20; SD was about 25° for phase and 3 dB for amplitude shifts); open squares: phase shifts of click-evoked emission components for DICP = 290 daPa (directly measured through lumbar puncture).

3.3   Dynamical aspects of stapes stiffness changes

CDTs were elicited by a pair of primary tones with fixed frequencies (1.2 and 1 kHz), and measurements were repeated every 4 s. Figure 4 displays an example of continuous CDT phase recording when a subject moves from sitting to recumbent position, then to sitting position again, then to head-down posture (20° with respect to horizontal). It takes 20 to 30 s to reach plateau phase shift when ICP increases, whereas it seems that the phase decays to its initial value more rapidly when ICP decreases. The maximum phase shift may be proportional to ICP increase, according to Davson's estimations of ICP changes with posture.[9]

140

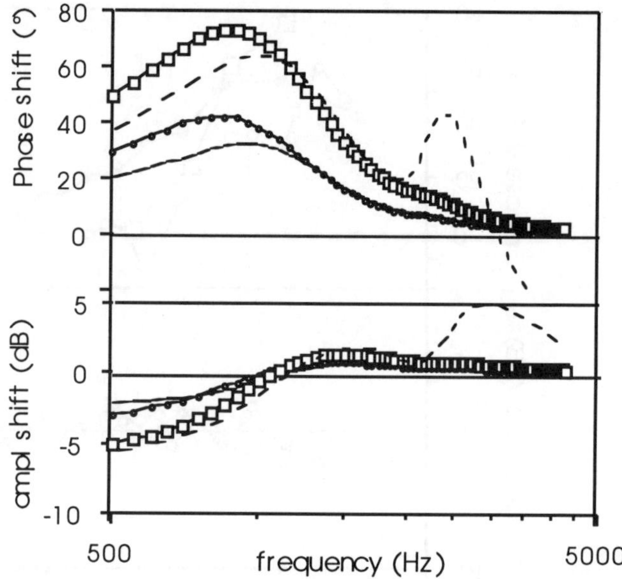

Figure 2 : CDT phase and amplitude shifts due to increase of stapes stiffness computed from a classical middle ear model (open circles: forward transmission changes; solid line: backward transmission effect; open squares: total changes reflected by CDTs. Dashed lines: for comparison, distinctive shifts due to middle-ear pressure change)

Contralateral acoustic reflex effects on CDT phase and amplitude could also be monitored continuously (fig.4, bottom). Reflex threshold detected on CDT changes was similar to the one obtained with standard impedance bridge measurements using a probe tone at 226 Hz, namely 85 dB SPL on this example. Comparison of CDT changes induced by continuous vs. intermittent contralateral noise allowed to check that acoustic reflex strength began to decay when the stimulus duration exceeded 4 to 8 s. In the absence of decay, reflex induced attenuation around 1 kHz was small (maximum 5 dB for forward plus backward attenuation, whose strength is similar according to the model- fig.2). In the meantime, the phase shift of sounds getting through the middle ear was conspicuously large around 1 kHz, and even up to 2 kHz according to fig.3. From these observations, it is tempting to speculate that the middle -ear muscle reflex might play an important role in sound localization, rather than in protective attenuation of loud sounds.[10,11]

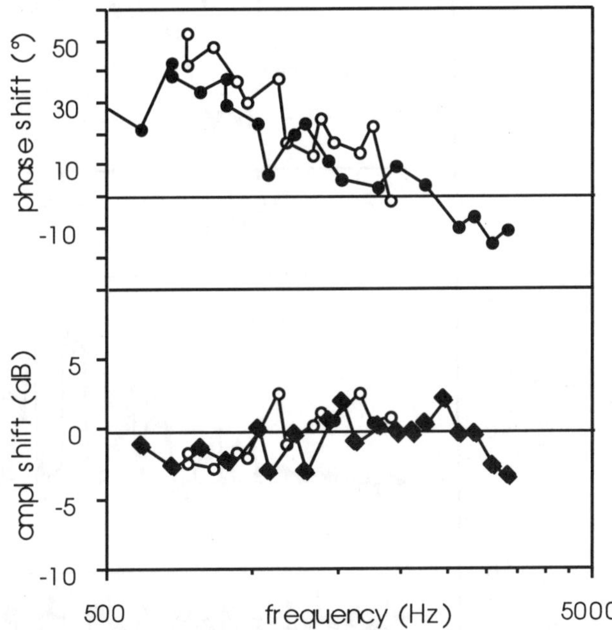

Figure 3: Contralateral stapedius reflex was triggered by broadband noise (20 dB above reflex threshold determined with an impedance bridge using a probe at 226 Hz). Broadband noise was presented during 4 s synchronous with CDT recording, then interrupted 1 s and presented again for the next CDT measurement so as to avoid any reflex decay due to prolonged noise stimulation. (closed symbols: CDT shifts due to stapedius muscle contraction; open symbols: CDT shifts due to posture change -sitting vs. recumbent- in the same ear)

Finally, control measurements were carried out with middle-ear pressure. Definitely different patterns of CDT changes were obtained for pressure variations ranging from -100 to +100 daPa and partial agreement with the model's predictions (thick lines, fig. 2) could be obtained for negative middle ear pressures. However positive middle ear pressure results were not symmetrical, suggesting a more complex behavior than the one predicted from simple lumped middle ear models.

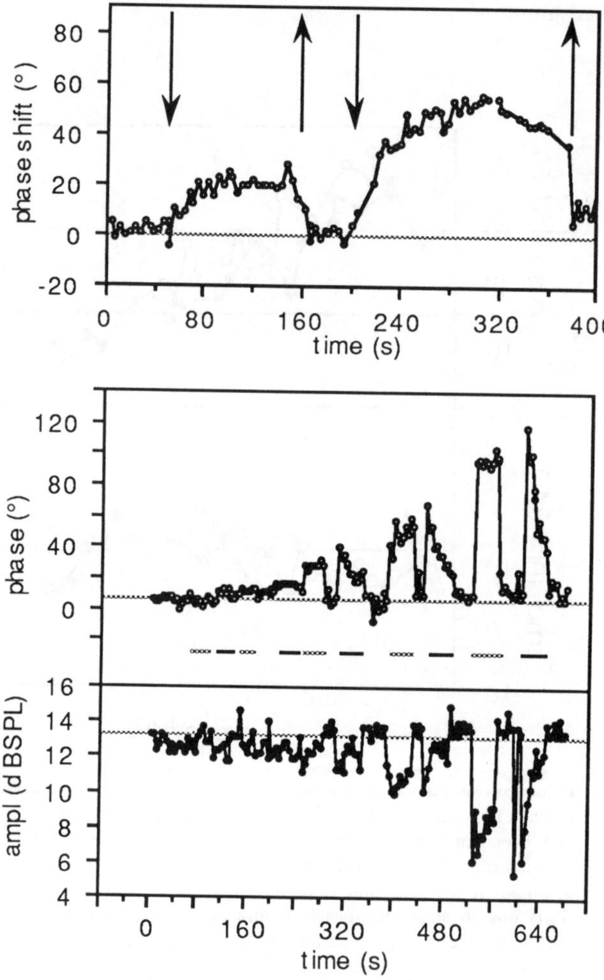

Figure 4: Top: continuous monitoring of CDT phase (4s sampling period) around 1 kHz during posture changes (arrows pointing downwards: recumbent posture, 0° then -20° with respect to horizontal; upward arrows: back to sitting posture). Bottom: CDT phase and amplitude during contralateral ear stimulation with broadband noise. Noise level increased from 85 to 105 dB SPL i.e. 0 to 20 dB above impedancemetric threshold. Noise was presented twice at the same level, once with intermittent presentation synchronous to CDT acquisition (dotted lines), and another time with continuous presentation allowing reflex decay after about 10 s(solid lines).

Acknowledgments

Parts of this work greatly benefited from discussions and experiments with Drs Hero Wit, Pim van Dijk and Bert Maat and a paper is currently in preparation with these authors about other similar aspects of middle-ear mechanics. Fundings were obtained from a French-Hungarian Balaton PAI grant, APAPE / OMFB (1995-97), and from grant CNAM/TS INSERM #4AIC04.

References

1. Allen, J.B. (1990) In: *Cubdis user manual* (Bell Labs).
2. Casselbrant, M. *Acta Otolaryngol. (Stockh)*, suppl.**362** 7-57 (1979).
3. Pang ,X.D.and W.T. Peake,W T. (1985) In: J.B. Allen et al (eds) (Springer-Verlag, Berlin,).
4. Zwislocki, J.J. (1962) *J.Acoust.Soc.Am.* **34** 1514-1523.
5. Lutman, M.E. and Martin, A.M. *J.Sound Vibr.* (1979) **64** 133-157.
6. Kemp, D.T. (1980) *Hear.Res.* **2** 533-548.
7. Büki, B., Avan, P., Lemaire, J.J., Dordain, M., Chazal, J. and Ribari, O. (1996) *Hear.Res.* **94** 125-139
8. Marchbanks, R.J. and Reid, A. (1990) *British J. Audiol.* 24, 179-187.
9. Davson , H. (1960) In: *Handbook of physiology*, ed. J. Field, H.W. Magoun and V.E. Hall (American Physiological Society, Washington DC.).
10. Borg, E., Counter, S.A. and Rosler, G. (1984) In: *The acoustic reflex*, ed. S.Silman (Academic Press, Orlando,).
11. Kobler, J.B., Vacher, S.R. and Guinan Jr, J.J. (1987) *Brain Res.* **425** 372-375.

DIRECT MEASUREMENT OF THE REVERSE TRANSFER FUNCTION OF THE GUINEA PIG MIDDLE EAR

P. MAGNAN, R. PROBST, J. SMURZYNSKI

HNO-Universitätsklinik, Kantonsspital
4031 Basel, Switzerland
magnan@ubaclu.unibas.ch

P. AVAN

Laboratoire de Biophysique, Université d'Auvergne
63001 Clermont Ferrand, France
paul.avan@u-clermont1.fr

A. DANCER

French-German Research Institute of Saint-Louis
68301 Saint-Louis, France
dancer@nucleus.fr

Intracochlear acoustic pressure measurements allow to determine both the forward and the reverse middle-ear transfer functions. In the guinea pig with open bulla, for a given signal at the base of scala vestibuli (either delivered by an external sound source or corresponding to the cubic distortion products) the acoustic pressure recorded in the occluded ear canal is lower by 30–35 dB (from 100 Hz to 10,000 Hz), and in phase with the intracochlear signal.

1 Introduction

The forward middle-ear transfer function (fMETF) can be measured by applying a signal to the tympanic membrane and recording the intracochlear acoustic pressure in scala vestibuli close to the stapes with miniature pressure transducers and tiny probe tubes. The fMETF has been measured in this way in the cat, the chinchilla and the guinea pig[1–5].

To measure the reverse middle-ear transfer function (rMETF) with the same technique, an intracochlear sound source is necessary. In the guinea pig we used two different methods. First, a pure tone was applied directly to the perilymph and the acoustic pressure signals measured at the base of scala vestibuli and in front of the tympanum were compared. In the second place we used as an intracochlear sound source the cubic distortion product (CDP) generated by two primaries applied in front of the tympanum, and we compared the CDP measured in the ear canal to the CDP measured at the base of scala vestibuli.

All measurements were performed on deeply anaesthetized pigmented guinea pigs with open bulla. Precise information referring to the intracochlear pressure measurement techniques has been reported elsewhere[1,4]. Sound pressure in front of the tympanic membrane was measured either with a B&K microphonic probe (when a sound was applied at the apex of the cochlea), or with the help of the microphone (ER–10B) of the acoustic probe (Etymotic Research) used in connection with the CDP measurement system: CUBDIS[6].

2   Results

2.1   Pure Tones Directly Applied to the Cochlear Fluids

We apply a pure tone to the apex of the cochlea or in the first turn of scala vestibuli with the help of a miniature loudspeaker fitted to a small tube sealed to the cochlea. This sound propagates into the cochlear fluids and an acoustic pressure can be measured at the base of scala vestibuli, close to the oval window, by a miniature pressure probe[4]. This pressure acts on the stapedius footplate and represents the input (reference) of the rMETF. Simultaneous measurements of the acoustic signal in front of the tympanic membrane with the help of a microphonic probe allowed to determine the rMETF in 4 guinea pigs from 20 Hz to 5,000 Hz (Figure1).

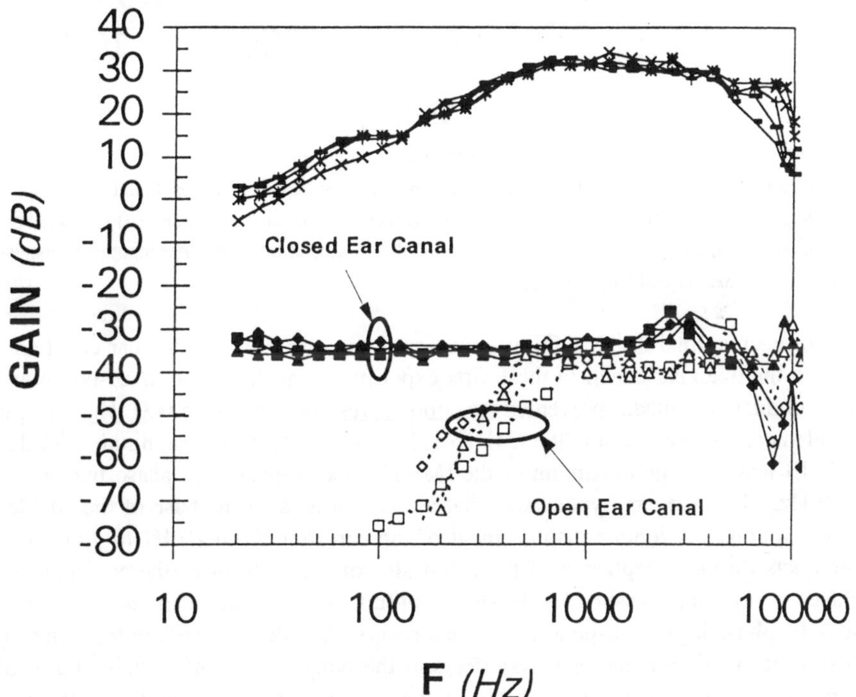

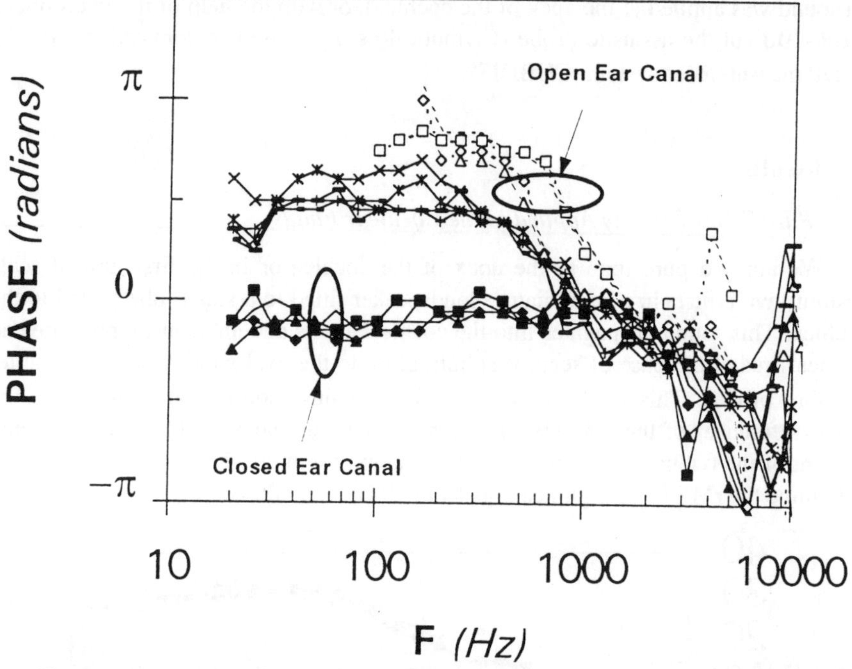

Figure 1: Reverse middle-ear transfer functions in 4 guinea pigs with open bulla. Amplitude and phase measured in the ear canal refer to the signal recorded at the base of scala vestibuli and correspond to the rMETF (geometrical symbols - continuous lines: occluded ear canal condition, dashed lines: open ear canal condition). Upper curves with crossed symbols correspond to the forward middle-ear transfer function in 5 guinea pigs with open bulla.

For each animal the rMETF was measured: (i) with the occluded ear canal and, (ii) with the open ear canal. In these first experiments, artifacts due to air-borne and bone-conducted sounds prevented to obtain results beyond 5,000 Hz. In the occluded ear canal condition, the rMETF is flat, both in terms of magnitude (-35 dB, i.e. 5 dB less than the maximum of the fMETF) and of phase (0° phase lag), up to 2,000 Hz. Thus, we can hypothesize that a constant level at the base of the cochlea induces a constant volume displacement of the eardrum (from 20 Hz to 2,000 Hz) which acts on the compliance of the small air volume in front of the eardrum and induces a constant pressure level. The amplitude and the phase of the rMETF (-35dB, 0° phase lag) correspond to an ideal reverse middle-ear pressure transformer. No significant friction and/or mass effects of the tympano-ossicular chain and/or of the middle-ear ligaments is observable. In these measurements the bulla is left open. Opening the bulla (volume ≈ 0.25 cm^3) is known to increase the amplitude of the forward METF at low frequencies ($< 1,500$ Hz) because the stiffness of the normal guinea pig middle ear is dominated by the air enclosed in the bulla[5]. In the reverse direction (rMETF), if the ear canal is occluded (for example by the measuring probe), the small volume of air between the probe and the tympanic membrane ($v_1 \approx 0.05$ cm^3) supersedes the stiffness of the middle ear itself. Therefore, opening the bulla has only a minor effect on the rMETF in this condition. Moreover, in our experiments, small experimental changes of the air volume in front of the eardrum did not induce significant changes of the rMETF amplitude. This result can be explained if we consider the behavior of an ideal reverse middle-ear pressure transformer. A pressure p_2 applied to the stapedius footplate is equilibrated by a pressure p_1 in front of the tympanic membrane. If p_2 is constant, p_1 must remains constant and a (small) change of volume in front of the tympanic membrane does not induce a change of p_1 (a smaller volume corresponds to a smaller volume displacement of the stapes and of the eardrum).

In the open ear canal condition, the rMETF decreases by about 12 dB/octave below ≈ 600 Hz and exhibits a corresponding phase lead. The volume displacement of the eardrum is then loaded by the radiation impedance of the outer ear (and no longer by the compliance of a small air volume)[5,7].

2.2 *CDP as an Intracochlear Acoustic Source*

The cubic distortion product (CDP) is generated in the cochlea at the frequency of $2f_1-f_2$ by stimulating it with two pure tones (primaries) at f_1 and f_2. The intracochlear CDP originates near the f_2 place from where it is propagated both to its apical characteristic frequency place and towards the base of the cochlea, leading to a tone at $2f_1-f_2$ within the ear canal[6,8,9]. The intracochlear CDP can be considered as an acoustic source placed inside the cochlea and the rMETF can be calculated by measuring simultaneously the intracochlear CDP acoustic pressure near the stapes and in front of the tympanic membrane as an otoacoustic emission.

In our experiments the f_2/f_1 ratio was kept close to 1.2 and f_2 was varied from 1,562 Hz to 12,451 Hz in 20 steps per octave. The target levels of the primary tones set by the CUBDIS system were $L_1 = 60$ dB SPL and $L_2 = 50$ dB SPL. Due to the characteristics of the probe in the guinea pig ear canal, actual levels measured in front of the tympanum were different. Because of the background noise, reliable detection of CDP was possible only above 1,500 Hz.

Results obtained in a typical guinea pig are presented on Figure 2. The level of the CDP measured in the ear canal is approximately 36 dB below the level of f_2 at the same location which is in agreement with previous data[10]. The level of the CDP measured in the scala vestibuli is approximately 26 dB below the level of f_2 at the same location. The difference between the level of the primaries measured in the

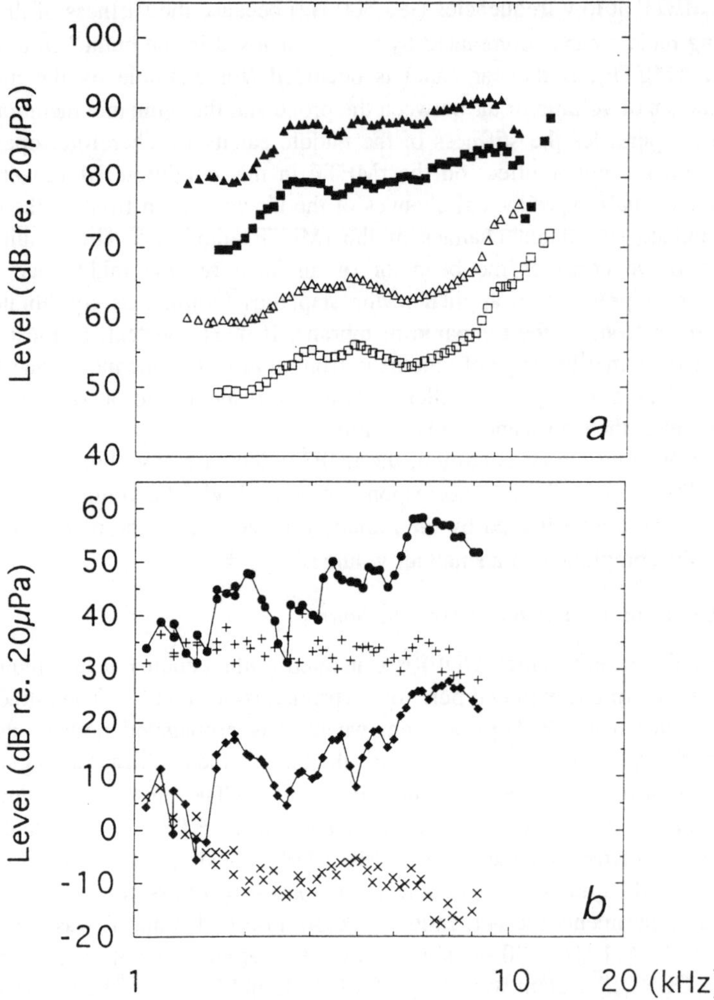

Figure 2: Results for a typical guinea pig: (a) level of primary tones measured in the ear canal (open symbols) and at the base of scala vestibuli (filled symbols) as a function of frequency, (b) level of CDP at the base of scala vestibuli (filled circles) and in the ear canal (filled diamonds) as a function of frequency (crosses: +, x indicate the background noise levels).

scala vestibuli and in the ear canal represents the fMETF gain with open bulla (Figure 2a). The difference between the CDP measured in the ear canal and in the scala vestibuli corresponds to the rMETF gain (Figure 2b). The rMETF gains measured on four animals in the same experimental conditions are very comparable and almost constant from 1,500 Hz to 8,300 Hz (between -30 and -35 dB) which is in agreement with other data[11,12]. Although precise phase measurements were not performed on the CDP signals in these preliminary experiments, it looks like the rMETF exhibits the same behavior from 20 Hz to 8,000 Hz. Up to this frequency, no significant mass effect of the tympano-ossicular chain is observable[5] and the probable vibration modes of the tympanic membrane do not limit the efficiency of the rMETF.

3 Conclusion

To our knowledge, this is the first study reporting direct measurements of the reverse middle-ear transfer function in vivo. Experiments in progress using a new sound source applied to the guinea pig cochlea and a more sensitive detection of the signal should allow to determine the rMETF in amplitude and in phase at least up to 10,000 Hz. These results will help to quantify (for example) the CDP within the cochlea by measuring noninvasively the CDPs in the ear canal. Because CDPs (as well as SOAEs and EOAEs) are an expression of the intracochlear mechanical processes, it will be possible to describe better the active mechanisms within the cochlea both in physiological and experimentally changed conditions.

More work is needed to know how to extrapolate the results obtained in the guinea pig to the man. The different characteristics of the human middle ear (i.e., relative contribution of the middle ear elements to its global stiffness, vibration modes and "effective area" of the tympanic membrane[5]...) prevent direct extrapolation of our results[13].

References

1. Dancer, A. and Franke, R. (1980) Intracochlear sound pressure measurements in guinea pigs, *Hear. Res.* **2** 191–205.
2. Nedzelnitsky, V. (1980) Sound pressures in the basal turn of the cat cochlea, *J. Acoust. Soc. Am.* **68** 1676–1689.
3. Décory, L., Guilhaume, A., Dancer, A. and Aran, J-M. (1989) On the origin of interspecific differences in auditory susceptibility, in *Cochlear Mechanisms,* eds. J.P. Wilson and D.T. Kemp, NATO ASI Series A: Life Sciences Vol. 164 (Plenum Press, New York and London) pp. 225–234.
4. Magnan, P., Dancer, A., Evrard, G., Vassout, P. and Avan, P. (1995) Etude de la propagation et de la dissipation du signal acoustique au niveau de l'oreille interne du cobaye, *French-German Research Institute of Saint-Louis, Saint-Louis, France,* Rpt. R 116/95.
5. Rosowski, J.J. (1994) Outer and Middle Ears, in *Comparative Hearing: Mammals,* eds. R.R. Fay and A.N. Popper (Springer-Verlag, New York, Berlin) pp. 172–247.
6. Allen, J.B. and Fahey, P.F. (1992) Using acoustic distortion products to measure the cochlear amplifier gain on the basilar membrane, *J. Acoust. Soc. Am.* **92** 178–188.
7. Rosowski, J.J., Carney, L.H. and Peake, W.T. (1988) The radiation impedance of the external ear of cat: Measurements and applications, *J. Acoust. Soc. Am.* **84** 1695–1708.

8. Kim, D.O. (1980) Cochlear mechanics: implications of electrophysiological and acoustical observations, *Hear. Res.* **2** 297–317.

9. Martin, G.K., Lonsbury-Martin, B.L., Probst, R., Scheinin, S.A. and Coats, A.C. (1987) Acoustic distortion products in rabbit ear canal. II. Sites of origin revealed by suppression contours and pure-tone exposures, *Hear. Res.* **28** 191–208.

10. Brown, A.M. (1987) Acoustic distortion from rodent ears: A comparison of responses from rats, guinea pigs and gerbils, *Hear. Res.* **31** 25–38.

11. Powers, N.L., Salvi, R.J., Wang, J., Spongr, V. and Chun Xiao Qiu (1995) Elevation of auditory thresholds by spontaneous cochlear oscillations, *Nature* **375** 585–587.

12. Zwicker, E. and Harris, F.P. (1990) Psychoacoustical and ear canal cancellation of $(2f_1\text{-}f_2)$ distortion products, *J. Acoust. Soc. Am.* **87** 2583–2591.

13. Puria, S. and Rosowski, J.J. (1996) Measurement of reverse transmission in human middle-ear, *ibidem.*

MEASUREMENT OF REVERSE TRANSMISSION IN THE HUMAN MIDDLE EAR: PRELIMINARY RESULTS

SUNIL PURIA AND J.J. ROSOWSKI

Eaton-Peabody Laboratory, Massachusetts Eye and Ear Infirmary,
243 Charles Street
Boston, MA 02114, USA
(sunil@epl.meei.harvard.edu, jjr@epl.meei.harvard.edu)

The transmission of emissions from the inner ear to the ear canal depends on the reverse-middle-ear pressure gain $G_R(\omega)$. This gain was determined from the ratio of the ear-canal pressure to vestibule pressure in response to sound introduced into the inner ear of a human cadaver temporal bone. The reverse gain magnitude $|G_R|$ has a maximum of approximately -22 dB at 0.8 kHz. The forward pressure gain $G_F(\omega)$ in the same ear shows a maximum of 16 dB at 0.7 kHz. The reverse gain is affected by the acoustic load in the ear canal. The effect of this load can be removed by calculating the open-circuit or Thévenin equivalent G_R. At their peaks G_F and G_R are consistent with the anatomical transformer idea. However, away from their peaks both G_F and G_R exhibit quite different frequency dependencies and our measurements suggest that G_R is not a simple transformation of G_F.

1. Introduction

The middle-ear forward pressure gain $G_F(\omega)$ is the ratio of the vestibule pressure $P_v^F(\omega)$ to ear-canal pressure $P_{ec}^F(\omega)$ in response to sound in the ear canal (Fig. 1A). The reverse pressure gain $G_R(\omega)$ is the ratio of the ear-canal pressure $P_{ec}^R(\omega)$ to vestibule pressure $P_v^R(\omega)$ in response to sound in the inner ear (Fig. 1B). (The superscripts "F" and "R" refer to measurements made in the forward and reverse directions.) In Figure 1 the ear-canal, tympanic membrane (TM) and ossicles are represented by a two-port model[1,2].

Otoacoustic emissions (OAEs) propagate from the inner ear through the middle ear and into the ear canal where they are measured[3] (Fig. 1B). It is known that changes in middle-ear stiffness alter OAEs[4], mass loading of the cat tympanic membrane reduces distortion product otoacoustic emissions (DPOAEs) to a greater extent than that predicted by changes in forward transmission[5], and severe middle-ear pathologies greatly diminish OAEs[3,6]. However, there are no direct measurements of the reverse pressure gain in the human middle ear and thus the reverse gain remains unknown. Our goal is to measure both reverse pressure gain and forward pressure gain and to deduce the role of the middle ear in measurements of OAEs. The role of the ear-canal transducer impedance on measurements of OAEs is also examined.

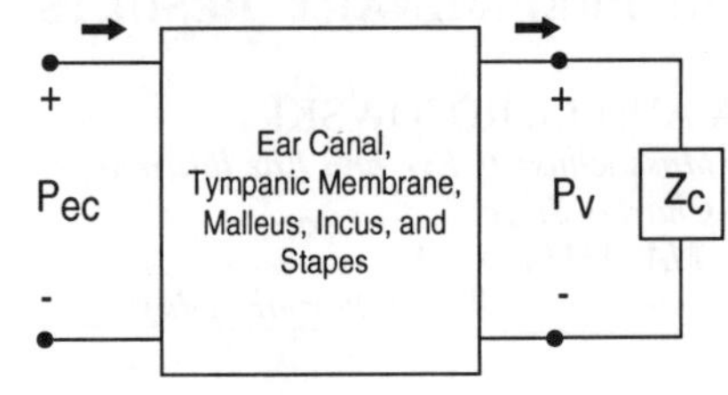

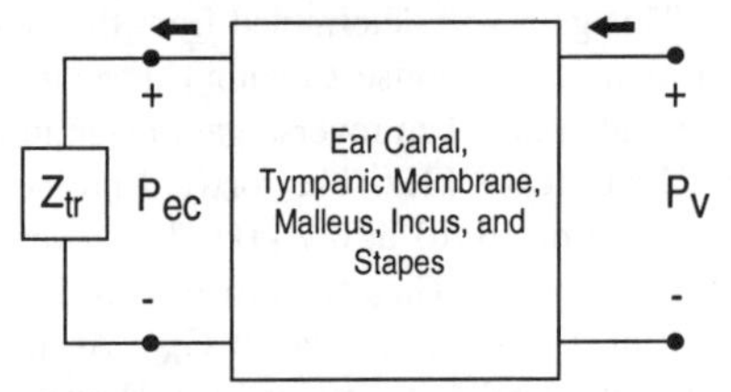

Figure 1: Two-port model representation of the middle ear with cavities wide open. P_{ec} is the ear-canal pressure and P_V is the vestibule pressure. (A) Forward pressure gain $G_F(\omega)$ through the middle-ear is measured with an acoustic stimulus in the ear canal. For this case the middle-ear load is the cochlear input impedance Z_C. (B) Reverse pressure gain $G_R(\omega)$ through the middle ear is measured with a stimulus in the inner ear. For this case the middle-ear load is the impedance of the transducer Z_{tr} used to make ear-canal measurements.

2. Methods

Forward and reverse measurements made in one normal temporal-bone ear are reported. Figure 2 illustrates the preparation developed for these measurements which is a modification of an earlier preparation[7,8]. Frozen human temporal bones are thawed, the bony ear canal shortened by drilling and a brass coupling ring attached to the ear opening with dental cement. The ring allows reproducible coupling of the different ear-canal sound sources used in this study. The middle-ear cavity is widely exposed by opening and enlarging the hypotympanum.

The inner-ear pressure transducer is placed in the vestibule by way of an enlarged internal auditory canal and a hole drilled through the fundus of the canal inferior to the transverse crest and just anterior to the singular canal, and sealed in place with Jeltrate. A hole is drilled through the utricle wall and a steel tube cemented in place. The inner-ear sound source (IESS) is coupled to the steel tube via a polyethylene tube to minimize transfer of mechanical vibrations to the bone. Measurements shown here were made after degassing the temporal bone and while slowly flushing the inner ear with degassed saline as was previously shown to be important for removing bubbles from the inner ear[8].

Measurements were made with chirp stimuli containing frequencies from 50 Hz to 25 kHz with the SYSid© system (SYSid Labs, Berkeley, CA). All three microphones were calibrated and electrical outputs converted to absolute sound pressures. The custom ear-canal transducer system was also calibrated for acoustic impedance measurements.

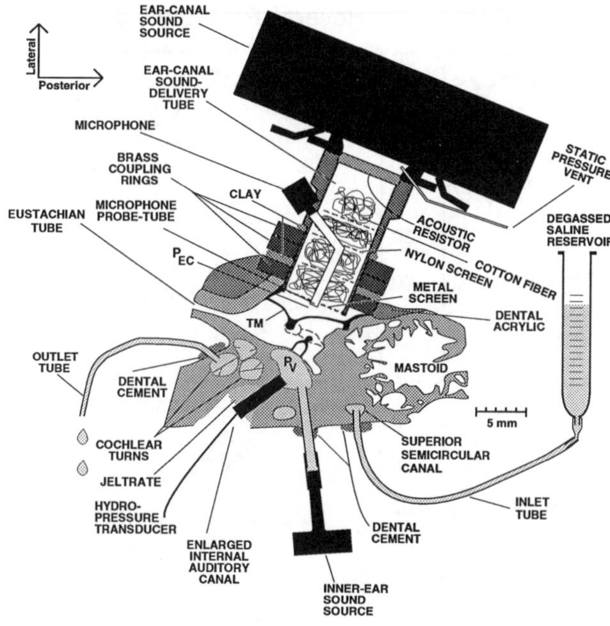

Figure 2: Human temporal bone preparation developed to measure forward and reverse pressure gains. The ear-canal sound source (either DT-48 or ER10c) is used to generate sounds for measurements of forward pressure gain, while the inner-ear sound source is used to generate sounds in the cochlea for measurements of reverse pressure gain. The inner-ear pressure P_V is measured with the hydro pressure transducer placed in the vestibule facing the footplate. The ear-canal pressure P_{ec} is measured with the probe-tube microphone that is an integral part of either ear-canal sound system.

The RMS sound pressure level in the vestibule $|P_v^R|$ produced by the IESS was approximately 115 dB SPL, while the ear-canal pressure $|P_{ec}^F|$ produced by the custom system was approximately 105 dB SPL. Levels of DPOAEs in the ear canal are typically less than 20 dB SPL for primary levels below 75 dB SPL suggesting that intracochlear DPOAE pressures are significantly less than the levels produced by the IESS. Characteristics of the human middle-ear are linear[8] for ear-canal pressures below 120 dB SPL suggesting that measurements of G_R can be extrapolated to physiologic levels.

3. Results

3.1 Forward pressure gain

Measurements of forward gain $G_F(\omega)$ from one ear are shown in Fig. 3A,B. The maximum gain is approximately 16 dB at 0.7 kHz. These measurements are typically lower than the mean but within the range of measurements made in four other temporal bone ears[8].

3.2 Reverse pressure gain

The reverse gain $G_R(\omega)$ for the same ear is shown in Fig. 3C,D (right column). The maximum gain is approximately -22 dB at 0.8 kHz. $|G_F|$ and $|G_R|$ show greatly different frequency dependencies. However, as is shown in section

154

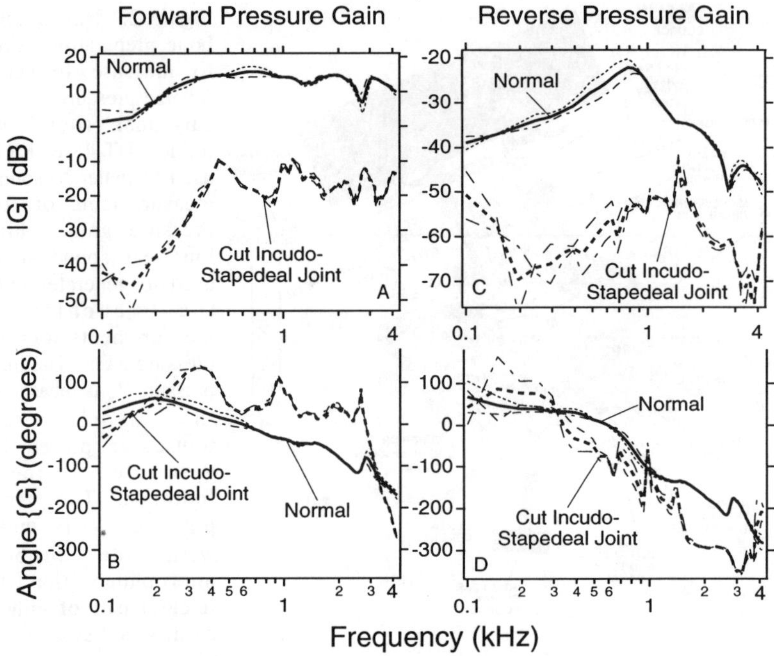

Figure 3: Left column (panels A and B) shows the forward pressure gain G_F while the right column (panels C and D) shows the reverse pressure gain G_R in the same ear for the 0.1 kHz to 4.2 kHz range. The normal measurements are the averages of two measurements made on two separate sessions (4 days apart). Two measurements after cutting the incudo-stapedial joint from the same session are also shown. The thin lines show individual measurements while thick lines show averages. Cut ossicles phase (panel D) was shifted up by 200 degrees for ease of comparison.

3.4 the influence of the ear-canal transducer on the frequency dependence of G_R must also be taken into account before comparing forward and reverse transmission.

3.3 Non-ossicular sound transmission

Our goal is to measure the forward and reverse sound transmission through the ossicles. However, there are additional paths of sound from the source to the measurement site that can confound measurements. First, the sound sources radiate acoustic energy from their enclosures into the atmosphere and can thus provide a direct path for sound to the measurement location. Second, the sources also produce vibrations that may be transferred to the bone. In reverse transmission, such vibrations can result in motions of the ear-canal walls that produce pressures not originating from the inner ear.

We estimated the effect of these non-ossicular sound transmission paths by measuring the reverse and forward pressure gain after cutting the incudo-stapedial joint. These measurements are also shown in Fig. 3. Cutting the ossicles reduces the forward gain by approximately 25 dB or more, and reduces the reverse gain by approximately 10 dB or more. The signal-to-noise ratio for all measurements was typically greater than 15 dB in the 0.3 - 4.2 kHz range, and less in the 0.1 - 0.3 kHz range. At frequencies above 4.2 kHz non-ossicular sound transmission was measured to be within 10 dB of the ossicular component, therefore, we limit the data we show to the 0.1 to 4.2 kHz frequency range.

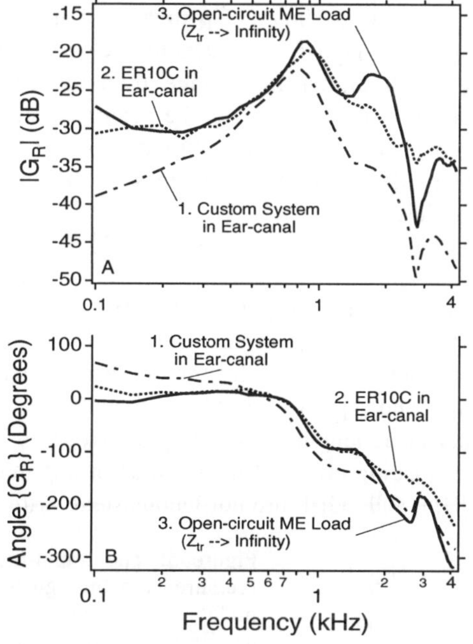

Figure 4: The reverse pressure gain G_R was measured with the custom ear-canal system (1) and the ER10C system (2). The impedance looking into the middle ear is Z_{me}. To remove the load of the custom transducer Z_{tr} from the middle ear, G_R was multiplied by $1+Z_{me}(Z_{tr})^{-1}$. The resulting reverse gain corresponds to the open circuit condition G_R^{OC}. The vestibule pressure for the custom system and the ER10C systems were not very different. Thus it is assumed that the vestibule pressure is the same for the open-circuit and normal conditions.

3.4 Effect of the transducer on measurements of otoacoustic emissions

Measurements of $G_R(\omega)$ can be influenced by the impedance of the transducer used to measure ear-canal pressure[9,10]. To quantify the effect of the transducer on G_R the custom ear-canal system shown in Fig. 2 was removed and replaced with an ER10C system which is physically very different and thus its acoustic impedance is very different. Measurements of G_F with the ER10C system and the custom-built system were indistinguishable. However, Fig. 4 shows that the ear-canal load has a significant effect on both the magnitude and phase of $G_R(\omega)$ suggesting that the ear-canal transducer has a significant effect on reverse transmission. For stimulus frequencies below 0.25 kHz and above 1.5 kHz, $|G_R|$ is higher by 6-10 dB when measured with the ER10C in comparison with the custom system.

The effect of the ear-canal terminating impedance can be removed by computing the Thévenin ear-canal pressure[11] and normalizing by the vestibule pressure. Such a transfer function corresponds to the open-circuit reverse gain G_R^{OC}, or the reverse gain measured with a transducer with an infinite input impedance. The impedance of the calibrated custom sound system Z_{tr}, the input impedance of the middle-ear, the ear-canal pressure and the vestibule pressure were used to compute G_R^{OC} shown in Fig. 4.

The reverse gain magnitude measured with the custom sound system is less than the open circuit gain for all frequencies shown. G_R measured using the ER10C is more similar to the open-circuit gain for frequencies below 1.2 kHz suggesting that the ER10C has a much higher impedance than the custom system. This is not surprising given the large diameter of the custom system in comparison to the ER10C system consisting of a foam plug with small tubes. Above 1.2 kHz the ER10C impedance dampens the resonances of G_R^{OC} which are due to the ear-canal, TM, and ossicles.

4. Discussion

If we assume that the measured (Fig 4) peak (-19 dB) of $|G_R^{OC}|$ approximately corresponds to the reciprocal of the transformer ratio $(N_{tr})^{-1} = (A_{fp}/A_{tm})(L_i/L_m)$, then the transformer ratio N_{tr}, for the one ear shown in Fig. 3, is approximately 19 dB (A_{tm} and A_{fp} are the TM and footplate areas while L_m and L_i are the malleus and incus lengths). Peak $|G_F|$ of 16 dB is 3 dB lower than N_{tr} and this is due to the loading effect of the cochlea on the middle ear[8]. Thus, measured peaks of $|G_F|$ and $|G_R|$ are not inconsistent with the

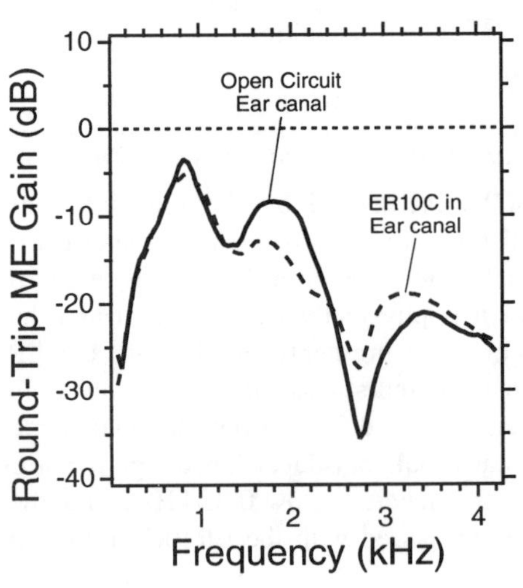

Figure 5: The round-trip pressure gain through the middle-ear measured with an ER10C and for the open circuit condition. The magnitude of the forward gain (Fig. 3A) and the two reverse gains (Fig. 4A) were added. This figure shows the frequency response of an ear to a click stimulus under the assumption that the inner-ear reflects the same amount of energy at all frequencies. (Note the linear frequency axis.)

anatomical transformer ratio[12]. However, the different frequency dependencies of G_R (Fig 4) and G_F (Fig. 3A,B) suggests that the reverse pressure gain is not simply the reciprocal of the forward pressure gain at all frequencies.

To what extent does the middle ear shape the frequency dependence of evoked OAEs? Figure 5 shows the sum of the forward and reverse gains which is the round-trip middle-ear pressure gain. The round-trip gain has a maximum in the 1-2 kHz region. The frequency dependence of the middle ear shown in Figure 5 has a remarkable similarity to the frequency dependence of click evoked OAEs and of DPOAEs in individual ears[13] suggesting that the characteristics of the middle-ear dominate the spectrum of ear-canal emission measurements.

Acknowledgments

We thank C. Quinten Davis and D. M. Freeman for sharing their designs of inner-ear sound sources, Michael E. Ravicz for construction of acoustic assemblies and W.T. Peake and C.A. Shera for suggestions. This work supported by research grants R03 DC 02677 and PO1 DC 00119 from NIDCD of NIH.

References

1. C. A. Shera and G. Zweig, *J. Acoust. Soc. of Am.* **92**:1356-1370 (1992).
2. W. T. Peake, J.J. Rosowski, and T.J. Lynch, *Hearing Research* **57**:245 (1992).
3. D. T. Kemp, *J. Acoust. Soc. of Am.* **64**:1386-1391 (1978).
4. D. T. Kemp, in *Tinnutus, Ciba Found. Symp.*, ed. by D. Evered and G. Lawrenson (Pitman, London, 1981).
5. M. Wiederhold, in *The Mechanics and Biophysics of Hearing,* ed. by P. Dallos, C. Geisler, J. Matthews, M. Ruggero, and C. Steele (Springer-Verlag, Berlin, 1990).
6. J. P. Wilson, *Hearing Research* **2**:233-252 (1980).
7. S. Puria, J. J. Rosowski and W.T. Peake, in *Biophysics of hair cell sensory systems,* ed. by H. Duifhuis, J. W. Horst, P. van Dijk and S. M. van Netten (World Scientific, Singapore, 1993).
8. S. Puria, J. J. Rosowski and W.T. Peake, "Sound-pressure measurements in the cochlear vestibule of human-cadaver ears," Submitted to *J. Acoust. Soc. of Am.*, (1996).
9. D. T. Kemp, *Hearing Research,* **2**:533-548 (1980).
10. J. W. Matthews, in *Mechanics of Hearing,* ed. by E. de Boer and M. Viergever (Martinus Nijhoff, Delft, 1983).
11. P. F. Fahey and J. B. Allen, in *Peripheral Auditory Mechanisms*, ed. by J.B. Allen, J. L. Hall, A. Hubbard, S. T. Neely, and A. Tubis (Springer-Verlag, 1986).
12. E. G. Wever and M. Lawrence, *Physiological Acoustics* (Princeton University, N.J., 1954).
13. J. Smurzynski and D. O. Kim, *Hearing Research,* **58**:227-240 (1992).

MALLEUS VIBRATIONS IN THE CAT EAR ARE THREE DIMENSIONAL

W.F. DECRAEMER
Universtity of Antwerp, Ruca, 171 Groenenborgerlaan
Antwerpen, B-2020 Belgium
wimdec@ruca.ua.ac.be

S.M. KHANNA
Columbia University, 630 West 168th Street
New York, NY 10032 USA
smk3@cunixf.cc.columbia.edu

Classically the motion of the malleus is described as rotation around its suspension axis. When malleus motion was measured at many points along its length, it was found that the amplitude was not proportional to the distance of the rotation axis and that all points did not vibrate in phase contradicting the classical hypothesis. To characterize the malleus motion fully vibration was measured at a set of points on the manubrium in the cat ear with a laser heterodyne interferometer. To obtain the 3D components of the motion of a given point the preparation was rotated by means of two orthogonal goniometers around the observed point. From the 3D motion of a set of points the motion of the malleus was calculated assuming rigid body motion.

1 Introduction

The motion of the malleus is generally described as rotation around a fixed axis[1]. In cat this axis runs through the cranial anchorage of the anterior mallear process and the end of the posterior incudal ligament. When malleus vibration was measured at many points along its length, it was found that the amplitude was not related to the distance of the point to the rotation axis[2]. Further experiments showed that equally large vibrations were present in the other two dimensions[3,4]. The motion of the malleus is therefore three dimensional.

To characterize this motion malleus vibrations in the cat ear were measured from different viewing directions with a laser heterodyne interferometer. By measuring vibration at a large set of points distributed over the entire manubrium surface a complete description of the rigid body motion of the malleus could be obtained.

2 Material

The experiments were performed on anesthetized cats (3 in total, at this time we can only show results for 1 animal) . The external ear was completely removed up to the cartilagenous part of the ear canal to optimize visual access to the entire manubrium surface. The bulla was vented through a capillary to prevent the building-up of static middle ear pressure. The animal's head was immobilized with respect to the interferometer.

3   Methods

The malleus was visualized through the external ear canal with a confocal microscope. With this approach the greater part of the manubrium is strongly slanted with respect to the observation direction and because the ear canal is so narrow the possible change in viewing angle is very restricted.

First the coordinates of the outline of the manubrium are determined using the optical scales that are part of the X, Y, and Z positioning system of this microscope-interferometer. On a plot of the manubrium outline 4 observation points were selected (Fig.1).

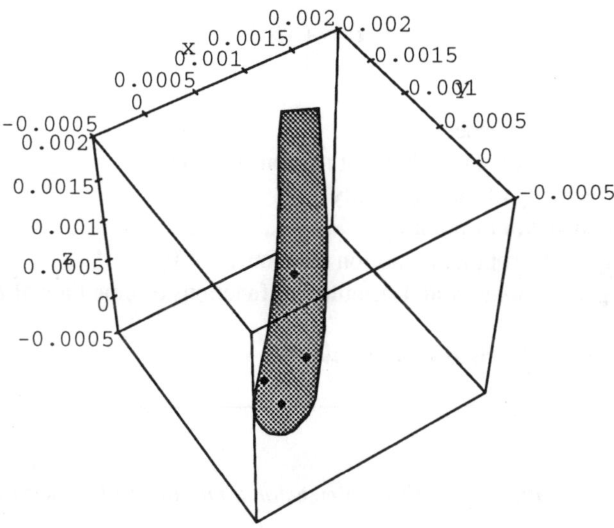

Fig. 1

Position of the observation points on the manubrium

The axis of the ear canal is along the vertical z-axis

The motion of these points was measured from different viewing directions. Two nested goniometers are used to rotate the preparation needed to change the viewing angle. The axis of rotation of the two goniometers is precisely adjusted to be at the focal point of the microscope objective, so that the motion of any selected point can be measured from different viewing angles. Amplitude and phase of vibration of each point was measured over a wide frequency range (100 to 22,000 Hz) at five viewing angles (-15,-10,0,10,15 deg) along the vertical plane and five in the horizontal plane.

4   Rigid body motion

The general motion of a rigid body may be decomposed in a rotation followed by a global translation of the body. Consequently the velocity of a point P_i of the malleus can be written as

$$\mathbf{v}_i(t) = \mathbf{v}_t + \mathbf{\Omega}(t) \times \mathbf{r}_i \tag{1}$$

$\mathbf{v}_i$: velocity of P_i with respect to O_{xyz}
$\mathbf{v}_t$: velocity of the global translational motion component
$\mathbf{\Omega}$: angular velocity of the rigid body
$\mathbf{r}_i$: rest-position vector of point P_i
$\mathbf{\Omega} \times \mathbf{r}_i$: velocity of the rotational motion component of P_i
With the present harmonic sound stimulus all functions of time t are also harmonic.

5   Calculation of the rigid body motion

5.1 Step 1 : Calculation of the three-dimensional motion of all observation points

For each point P_i - and at each frequency - the vibration was measured at different viewing angles by changing the goniometers positions in small increments. We have previously shown[2] how these measurements can be used to compute the amplitude and phase for the x, y and z component of the displacement of the given point.

5.2 Step 2 : Three-dimensional rigid body motion of the malleus

The 3-D motion components for all points P_i at a given frequency are then utilized in a subsequent numerical fitting procedure to reconstruct the 3-D rigid body motion of the malleus. This fit determines the parameters v_t en Ω that describe the rigid body motion as shown in Eq. 1. This is repeated for each experimental frequency.

6   Results

The 3D rigid body motion of the malleus can be specified by the parameters v_t en Ω within Eq. 1. Unless the motion is very simple, f.i. a pure rotation about a fixed axis or a pure translation a table with numerical values of the motion parameters v_t en Ω does not tell how the body is moving.

A much more illustrative way is to calculate the motion of a part of the rigid body, here we chose the outline of the manubrium - once we have v_t en Ω we can use Eq. 1 to calculate the motion of an arbitrary point of the object with coordinates x,y,z - and to animate the motion of the manubrium by displaying it as a moving body in a 3D color shaded projection on a TV or computer screen.

In this paper we will use an intermediate way by plotting the position of the body at a given number of equally spaced phases during one cycle of its vibrational motion. The rest position of the manubrium outline is indicated with the dots, the displacements along the outline with the line segments extending from these dots.

The malleus motion is strongly frequency dependent. In this context we can only illustrate the wide variety of vibration modes by showing two typical examples. The very small displacements (of the order of 10^{-8} m) are multiplied by a scale factor to make them visible on the 3D plots. Eight phases are shown for each frequency, starting at the left with the manubrium position when the pressure stimulus is at its maximum, and each subsequent position T/8 spaced in time. Two views are shown, one showing the manubrium in a frontal view, the other in a view from the side.

On the plots showing the motion at 585 Hz we see how that the manubrium performs an in-plane rotation, a small rotation about an axis almost perpendicular to the manubrium surface (Fig. 2, upper panel), while in the side view we see an almost pure lateral translation (Fig. 2, lower panel).

The high frequency plots show in the frontal view a quite strong in-plane rotation and in-plane, sideways, translation (Fig. 3 upper panel). The sideways view reveals how the manubrium slides up and down in its own plane while at the same time it has an out-of-plane rotation and translation (Fig. 3 lower panel).

6.1 *Low frequency*

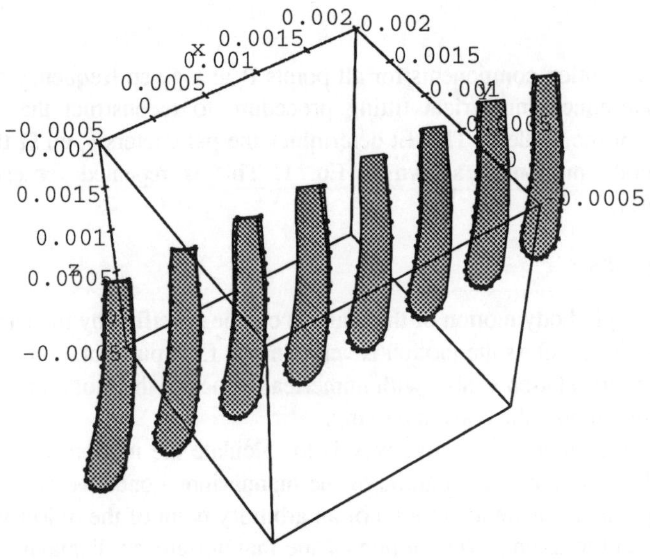

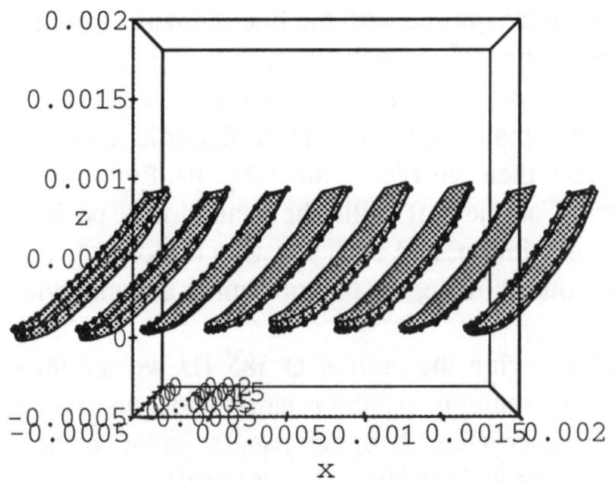

Fig. 2
A frontal (upper panel) and a side view (lower panel) of the motion of the manubrium at 580 Hz.

6.2 High frequency

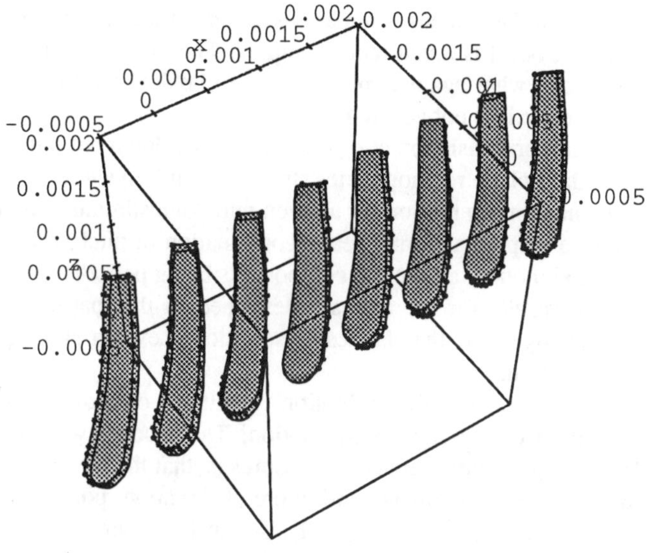

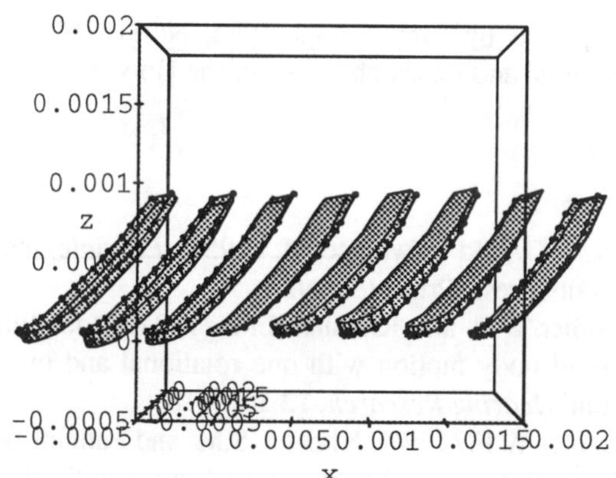

Fig.3
A frontal (upper panel) and a side view (lower panel) of the motion at 13.8 kHz.

164

7 Discussion

The motion of the malleus is not as described classically a rotational vibration about a fixed axis, but it is much more complex. The motion is different from frequency to frequency what again implies that the classical description of a pure rotation about a fixed axis is not verified.

Rotation or translation components may be dominant but mostly they are both present. Their phase relation varies strongly with frequency.

The manubrium motion for a given pure tone stimulus may be compared to the motion of a ship on a stormy sea, a combination of pitch, roll and yaw on top of a translational motion, all motion components being periodic.

In the results for the animal described in this paper there seems to be no frequency range were the classical description is even a good approximation of the observed motion.

Uncertainties on the vibration results of course influence the final determination of the rigid body motion, The gradual way in which the malleus mode is changing with frequency reassures us that the present results are genuine.

More recent experiments with more observation points on the manubrium are now available, a preliminary analysis confirms our present findings. The full analysis will learn us also about interanimal variation.

Acknowledgments

Research supported by Emil Capita Fund, NOSH, National Fund for Scientific Research, Belgium and Research Funds of the University of Antwerp (RUCA).

References

1   Wever, E.G. and Lawrence M. (1954) *Physiological Acoustics,* Princeton University Press, Princeton, NJ.

2   Decraemer W.F. and Khanna, S.M. (1994) Modelling the malleus vibration as a rigid body motion with one rotational and one translational degree of freedom, *Hearing Research,* **72 1/2** 1-18.

3   Decraemer W.F. (1994), Khanna, S.M. and Funnell, W.R.J. (1994) A method for determining three dimensional vibration in the ear, *Hearing Research* **77,** 19-37.

4   Decraemer W.F. and Khanna S.M. (1995) Malleus vibration modelled as rigid body motion, *Acta Otolaryngol. Belg.,* **49**(2) 139-145,

Part Three

Descriptive Models of cochlear function

The descriptive models in Parts Three and Five set the stage for the synthetic models in Parts Four and Six. The reader will find that all of the quantitative synthetic modeling described in Parts Four and Six conforms to what is perhaps the most widely employed metamodel in biophysics—namely general circuit theory (along with its distributed-parameter and stochastic counterparts). There is a concept that arises in the circuit-theory metamodel that should deeply concern those of us who are reductionists by inclination—it is the concept of irreducibility. It applies to all models belonging to the class of general circuit models-- including electric circuit models, fluid circuit models, and rigid-body mechanical circuit models, and their stochastic counterparts (e.g., Markov chains). Because it applies to such models, it applies as well to real systems when we attempt to represent or understand those systems in terms of those models.

In the theory of Markov chains, irreducibility is a fundamental element in various ergodic theorems. For both deterministic and stochastic models, it is related to another theorem—the one that should be of deep concern to reductionist biologists: In an irreducible circuit model, properties of the circuit as a whole generally are attributable to all of its elements (not attributable to an individual element or to a proper subset of the elements). Among the circuit properties that fall in this category are the circuit's natural frequencies (or eigenfrequencies)—which are key ingredients in descriptions of the behavior of linear models and in Wiener- or Volterra-series descriptions of nonlinear models. In an irreducible circuit model, no eigenfrequency is entirely attributable to an individual element or to a proper subset of the elements. Thus, reductionist analysis of a real system in terms of such properties, using a circuit model as a vehicle for understanding, would require either identification, isolation, and complete characterization (descriptive model) of every element, or conjectures about the properties and connections of all elements that cannot be isolated and characterized.

An irreducible circuit model is one in which the direction of causality is blurred by interaction, every state variable affects directly or indirectly every other state variable-- there are no buffers. To make hierarchical modeling possible, the biophysicist must seek either putative buffers in the system under investigation, or else must use descriptive models (such as two-port or multiport models) that transcend need for buffers. In the nervous system, spiking axons presumably provide buffering-- to the extent that the triggering properties of the axon and the subthreshold processes leading up to triggering are not affected by what is connected to the other end of the axon. Synapses also might provide buffering-- in the sense that postsynaptic events might not affect presynaptic processes. In Parts Four through Six, one finds a wide range of choices regarding where stimuli are applied and where responses are measured, each choice reflecting, tacitly, a different view of where buffered boundaries might be found in the auditory periphery.

OHCs SHIFT THE EXCITATION PATTERN VIA BM TENSION

J.B. ALLEN

AT&T Research Laboratory,
Murray Hill, NJ 07974,
jba@research.att.com

We now know that outer hair cells (OHC) nonlinearly compress the dynamic range of basilar membrane motion [26,27] and the neural response,[31] extending the otherwise limited dynamic range of the inner hair cell (IHC) response.[21,2] This role of the OHC may be quantified using many objective measures. *Loudness*, measured by Fletcher and Munson's [18] loudness balance method, shows a 1/3 power law compressive function of intensity (i.e., Stevens' Law). This dynamic loudness compression is provided by normal OHC function.[7] *Recruitment* results when there is loss of this compression, as when OHCs are damaged.[29,10,2,3,4] *Masking patterns* provide a psychoacoustic measure of cochlear nonlinearity. The OHC compression show up in the 1923–1924 masking growth curves of Fletcher [14] and Wegel and Lane [30] as the *upward spread of masking*. The elevated tails of tuning curves are also evident in the upward spread of masking data as the elevated threshold. These masking data also seem very similar to *two–tone suppression* results.[1,13] Otoacoustic emissions (*SFOAEs* and *DPOAEs*) are an objective measure of the OHC nonlinear compression.[9] I shall connect these physical and psychoacoustic measures using a cochlear model whose basilar membrane (BM) stiffness is signal dependent as a result of a dynamic change in BM radial tension by the outer hair cells.[20] According to this nonlinear model, as the signal intensity increases, the BM radial tension decreases, resulting in a decreased local BM stiffness, and therefore a basal shift of the BM and neural excitation patterns (EP) by up to $\approx 1/2$ octave.[6] This EP shift shows up in basilar membrane velocity data, cochlear microphonics, neural "revcor" functions, simultaneous and forward masking patterns, two–tone suppression data, and noise trauma studies. When the steep apical (low-pass) slope of the low–loss BM traveling wave shifts across the basal (high–pass) response of the tectorial membrane transfer function,[5,6,8] a narrow–band neural-like compressed tuning results. The resulting CF sensitivity is compressive, with a power–bandwidth (ERB) that is approximately independent of intensity, consistent with the *critical ratio* measure of Fletcher (1938), Egan and Hake (1950),[16,17,12,4] as well as some more recent animal data. Thus OHCs play an important and quantifiable role in loudness, neurosensory hearing loss, masking, two–tone suppression, and OAEs.

1 Introduction

Our understanding of the auditory system's large 120 dB dynamic range is fundamentally incomplete. For example, *recruitment*, the most common form of neurosensory hearing loss, is best characterized as the loss of dynamic range.[29,3,4] Recruitment results from outer hair cell damage.[10] To successfully design hearing aids that deal with the problem of recruitment, we need models that improve our understanding of *how* the cochlea achieves this dynamic range.

I shall begin by showing that the dynamic range of the IHC must be less than 65 dB (in fact it is probably less than 50 dB, but I can not prove this). This raises the question: *How can the basic cochlear detectors (the IHCs) have a dynamic range of less than 65 dB, and yet the auditory system has a dynamic range of 120 dB?* A great deal of indirect evidence shows that this extra dynamic range results from mechanical nonlinear signal compression provided by outer hair cells. This compression shows up in auditory psychophysics and in cochlear physiology in many ways. In this paper we summarize some of the basic relationships between the OHC and various psychophysical measures to explore *how* OHCs extend the IHC dynamic range.

2 The Dynamic Range Problem

The question of dynamic range in the auditory system is a long standing problem. Previously this question has been raised in the context of both the nerve cell and the synapse. I am raising the same question, but presynaptically, with respect to the IHC's transmembrane voltage, which is limited at the high end by the open circuit voltage seen by the cell, and at the low end by the membrane Johnson noise and cilia Brownian motion.

It is argued here that the main function of the OHCs is to solve this cochlear dynamic range problem. This argument consists of showing that the inner hair cell transmembrane voltage dynamic range (i.e., the cell's functional range) is less than 65 dB. From estimates of (a) the RMS Johnson (thermal) noise voltage, and (b) the maximum available signal voltage across the hair cell membrane, we may bound the IHC transmembrane voltage dynamic range. If the dynamic range in acoustic intensity is greater than the dynamic range of the IHC detectors, one must conclude that the signal driving the IHC detectors is compressed. Many studies have identified the OHC as the source of the this compression, starting with the speculations of Lorente de No in 1937 [22] following the discovery of loudness recruitment.

The RMS transmembrane thermal Johnson noise voltage V_c of the IHC is given by

$$V_c^2 = 2kTR \int_{-\infty}^{\infty} \frac{1}{1 + (2\pi f RC)^2} df = \frac{kT}{C}. \tag{1}$$

where R is the membrane leakage resistance and C the membrane capacitance. The IHC capacitance has been found to be about 9.6 pF by Kros and Crawford.[19] From Eq. 1, $V_c = 21.1$ μV at body temperature ($k = 1.38 \times 10^{-23}$ Joule/degree-Kelvin, $T = 310°$ K).

Table 1: Estimates of various cochlear measures at 0, 60, and 120 dB SPL at 1 kHz. The BM displacement data is from Nuttall[25] and is at 18 kHz. Column "SLOPE (dB)" shows the dB ratio of the dynamic range of the "MEASURE" to the dynamic range of the sound intensity.

MEASURE (UNITS)	THRESHOLD	—	MAXIMUM	SLOPE (dB)
Power (Watts/cm^2)	10^{-16}	10^{-10}	10^{-4}	
Intensity (dB-SPL)	0	60	120	
Stapes displacement (nm)	0.001	1	1000	1
BM displacement (nm)	0.2	7	?	0.61
Cilia displacement (nm)	0.05	1.1	$<50\,(1°)$	0.5
IHC voltage (mV)	0.02	0.67	30	0.53

The maximum open circuit DC voltage across the cilia is about 120 mV. The maximum change in cell voltage that has been observed is 30 mV RMS. The ratio of 30 mV to the noise floor voltage (e.g., 21.1 μV), expressed in dB, is 63 dB. The maximum dynamic range in signal intensity of the auditory system is approximately 120 dB. This leaves about 57 dB of dynamic range unexplained. We conclude that *there must be nonlinear compression (level dependent gain) built into the mechanics of the cochlea* to account for the large acoustic dynamic range. Since the discovery of loudness recruitment it has been suspected that it is the job of the OHCs to provide this compression.[22,10] The real question before us is: *What is the chain of events that leads to the stimulus compression seen by the IHCs?*

Estimate of the Cilia Displacement at the Hearing Threshold. Russell *et al.* have estimated the *in vitro* sensitivity of the mouse culture hair cell as 0.4 mV/nm, or 30 mV/degree of angular rotation of stereo cilia.[28] Assuming a thermal noise floor of 20 μV RMS, the IHC displacement sensitivity of the cell at the thermal-noise threshold is 0.05 nm. Given that 1 degree of cilia displacement corresponds to 30 mV, a cilia displacement of more than a degree would drive the cell into saturation, and would likely rupture the delicate structures of the cilia transduction channels. A summary of dynamic level estimates of the stapes, basilar membrane, cilia displacements, and IHC RMS voltage levels, is provided in Table 1.

The conclusion that the OHCs must be compressing the dynamic range of the IHC's excitation signal (e.g., the TM–RL shear) is further supported by basilar membrane velocity measurements which show a nonlinear growth of response. However there are several problems. While the BM data show compression, this compression is different in many ways from that of the IHC excitation signal. For example, recent two–tone BM suppression results have been found to be quite different from the corresponding neural measures.[11] Furthermore the bandwidth (ERB) of the BM signal is not in agreement with detection experiments of tones in wide band noise, namely critical ratio experiments of Fletcher and others. In this paper we shall explore old psychophysical data with new insights.

3 Tone–on–Tone Masking

In 1923 Fletcher [14] and 1924 Wegel and Lane [30] described the first detailed *narrow–band* tone masker, tone maskee (*tone–on–tone masking*) simultaneous masking data for masker frequencies f_m between 0.25 and 4 kHz and intensities between 0 and 85 dB SL. These data provided a very basic measure of the hearing process that, while frequently verified, is not understood to this day. When we explain these masking data, we will better understand the role of the OHC compression. Figure 1 shows *masking level curves* $M(f_p, f_m, I_m)$ for a $f_m = 400$ Hz masker, with f_p as the parameter. The masking is defined as $M \equiv I_p^*/I_{\text{ref}}$. The $*$ on I_p^* indicates that I_p is at the detection threshold. The intensity $I_{\text{ref}} = I_p^*$ is the threshold intensity of the probe when the masker is off ($I_m = 0$). These data follow a power–law intensity dependence of the threshold probe intensity on the masker intensity, namely

$$\frac{I_p^*}{I_{\text{ref}}} = \left(\beta \frac{I_m}{I_{\text{ref}}}\right)^{\kappa}, \tag{2}$$

with an exponent κ that systematically depends on the relative frequency between the masker and the probe. There are three basic regions of masking patterns corresponding to *critical–band masking* ($f_p \approx f_m$), the *downward spread of masking* ($f_p < f_m$), and the *upward spread of masking* ($f_p > f_m$). For probes higher in frequency than the masker frequency, the exponent κ is much greater than 1. For probes lower in frequency than the masker frequency, the exponent is less than 1. When the probe and masker are within the critical band, the exponent is close to 1.

Critical–Band Masking. For probe frequencies near the masker frequency of 400 Hz the masking is approximately characterized as *linear in intensity.*[30] . For example, at $f_p = 0.45$ kHz (dash-dot line in Fig. 1) the masking curve is well approximated by the linear relation ($\kappa = 1$, $\beta = 1/40$)

$$\frac{I_p^*(f_p, I_m)}{I_m} = \frac{1}{40} \tag{3}$$

for I_m greater than about 25 dB SL, as indicated by the dotted line superimposed on the 0.45 kHz masking curve. Equation 3 is similar to Weber's Law for JNDs, extended to the case of masking (i.e., $\Delta I \equiv I_p^*$).

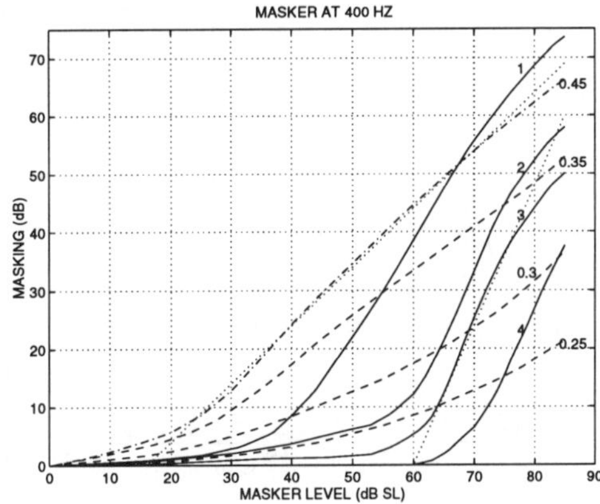

Figure 1: Tone–masking–tone data from Fletcher (1923) and Wegel and Lane (1924) for a masker at 400 Hz. The dashed lines correspond to probe frequencies between 0.25–0.45 kHz, while the solid lines correspond to probe frequencies of 1–4 kHz. The masking between 0.4 and 0.45 kHz is proportional to the masker level (i.e., the slope is close to 1). For 2, 3, and 4 kHz there is a threshold effect between 55–65 dB SL. For these frequencies the slope is greater than 1. For probe frequencies below the masker the slopes change with level, but is always less than 1.

While the "linearity of masking" seems to be a trivial empirical observation, it is a surprising result. It is not obvious, at first glance, why the masking should be proportional to intensity. When the probe is added to the masker within a critical–bandwidth, the basilar membrane motion signals add (e.g., two sin waves beat). However, the response level of the basilar membrane motion, the neural response, and the resulting loudness are all compressive–nonlinear functions of level. In fact the observation summarized by Eq. 3 inspired the famous JND experiments of Riesz (1928) which were the first to show that, for tones, the exponent is not exactly 1 (the "near miss" to Weber's law).

Below about 60 dB-SL the masking is greatest near the masker frequency. At 67 dB-SL the masking curve corresponding to the 1000 Hz probe frequency crosses the 450 Hz curve, as the frequency of maximum masking shifts to higher frequencies. At 80 dB-SL the probe frequency corresponding to the maximum masking is about 1.5 octaves above the masker frequency. This is more easily seen in Fig. 2 where the data of Fig. 1 have been plotted as iso-intensity contours (i.e., *masking patterns*).

We conclude that *the excitation pattern (EP) shifts toward the base as the intensity is raised.* Based on model studies, the most likely explanation for the EP shift is a BM stiffness change with level.[6,5] These studies showed that the IHC compressive nonlinearity can be also be explained by a dynamic BM stiffness, assuming the tectorial membrane acts as a high–pass filter. We extend this model by adding LePage's assumption that the dynamic radial BM

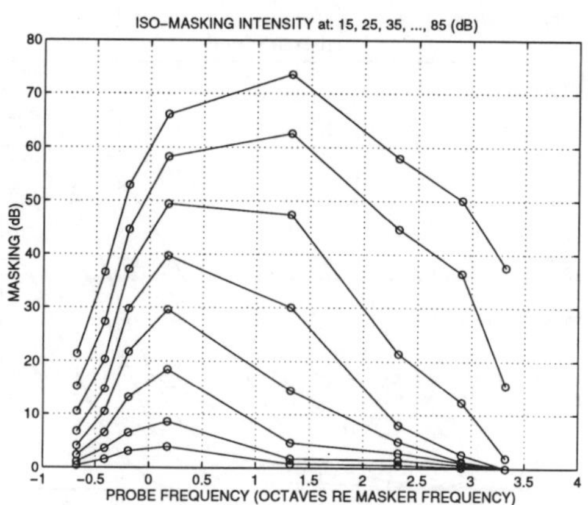

Figure 2: When the data of Fig. 1 is plotted as masking patterns, we see the upward spread of masking as well as the 1/2 octave shift in the frequency of greatest masking.

tension controls the BM stiffness,[20] due to a signal dependent dynamic OHC stiffness or length change.

The Spread of Masking. As may be seen from Fig. 1 (solid lines) for the *upward spread of masking* case ($f_p = 2$–4 kHz $> f_m$), the onset of masking is abrupt at about 55–65 dB ($\beta = 10^{-6}$) and has a slope (on log–log scales) of $\kappa = 2.4$, that is

$$\frac{I_p^*(f_p, I_m)}{I_{\text{ref}}} = \left(10^{-6}\frac{I_m}{I_{\text{ref}}}\right)^{2.4}.$$

This expression is shown in Fig. 1 as the dotted line, superimposed on the 3 kHz probe curve. This steep slope is loosely referred to as the *upward spread of masking.* The expansive power–law exponent of $\kappa = 2.4$ must depend on the the basilar membrane compression at the masker frequency, independent of the probe frequency f_p, because the high frequency probe excites the basal "tail" region of the EP where the basilar membrane response is approximately linear. It logically follows that the exponent $\kappa = 2.4$ must be the reciprocal of the basilar membrane compression exponent ($0.42 \approx 1/2.4$) at the masking frequency's characteristic place.

For the *downward spread of masking* case ($f_p < f_m$) (dashed lines), the growth of masking is a compressive power law ($\kappa < 1$) with an exponent κ that depends on intensity as well as probe frequency. In this case there is no clear "threshold" effect, as there is in the $f_p > f_m$ case. For this case Eq. 2 is not as useful a representation since κ depends on all the variables. The amount of masking depends on the steep apical slope of the masker excitation pattern and its spreading into the region of the probe. From Fig. 1, as the masker level is raised, the masking is less than would be predicted by a linear ($\kappa = 1$) growth of masking. From Fig. 2, as the intensity of the masker is increased, the masker excitation pattern shifts away from the low intensity probe masking pattern, reducing the relative masking. As the probe intensity reaches higher levels, its masking pattern also begins to shift toward the base, leading asymptotically to a linear growth of masking at higher levels.

Forward Masking and Two–Tone Suppression. The shift in the excitation pattern is confounded by the fact that both the probe and masker are on simultaneously. Is the basal shift in the EP still seen at high levels for forward masking? The answer to this is yes, as was first shown by Munson and Gardner in 1950,[24] and later by Lutfi.[23] Data from these papers clearly show that the 1/2 octave shift in the EP does not depend on the probe and masker being present simultaneously and provide data that may allow us to estimate the release time of the BM stiffness change.

Two–tone suppression has many properties in common with the masking data of Fig. 1. For example, when the suppressor is *higher* in frequency than the suppressed (CF) probe, the suppression growth is shallow (i.e., weak), and is present at low levels. This case is similar to the low frequency probes of Fig. 1. When the suppressor is *lower* in frequency, the suppression growth is steep (i.e., strong) and has a threshold at about 55-65 dB SPL.[13,1] It seems that the explanation given in this paper for masking also applies to two–tone suppression.

Summary. It appears that cochlear compression and the shifting excitation pattern are both related to normal OHC function. To shift the EP, the OHC stiffness or length change must change the BM stiffness. If the BM stiffness is determined by the radial tension in the BM, as proposed by Fletcher,[15] and LePage,[20] then a local change in the BM tension would change the local BM stiffness, and therefore the BM tuning.[6] This would result in a shift of the excitation patterns with intensity, as observed in the masking pattern data.

References

1. Abbas, P. and Sachs, M. (1976) Two–tone suppression in auditory–nerve fibers: Extension of a stimulus–response relationship. *Journal of the Acoustical Society of America* **59(1)** 112–122.
2. Allen, J. (1996) DeRecruitment by multiband compression in hearing aids. In: W. Jesteadt and *et al.*, editors, *Modeling Sensorineural Hearing Loss.* Lawrence Erlbaum, Inc., Hillsdale, NJ.
3. J. Allen (1996) DeRecruitment by multiband compression in hearing aids. In: Kollmeier, B., editor, *Psychoacoustics, speech, and hearing*

aids. World Scientific, Singapore.

4. Allen, J. (1996) Harvey Fletcher's role in the creation of communication acoustics. *Journal of the Acoustical Society of America* **99(4)** 1825–1839. Reprint of material from preface of Fletcher's 53 book, with some important additions on the critical band.

5. Allen, J.B. (1980) Cochlear micromechanics: A physical model of transduction. *Journal of the Acoustical Society of America* **68(6)**1660–1670.

6. Allen, J.B. (1990) Modeling the noise damaged cochlea. In: Dallos, P., Geisler, C.D., Matthews, J.W., Ruggero, M.A., and Steele, C.R., editors *The Mechanics and Biophysics of Hearing* Springer-Verlag, New York.

7. Allen, J.B. (1995) Harvey Fletcher 1884–1981. In: Allen, J.B., editor, *The ASA edition of* Speech, Hearing in Communication. Acoustical Society of America, Woodbury, New York.

8. Allen, J.B. and Fahey, P.F. (1993) A second cochlear-frequency map that correlates distortion product, neural tuning measurements. *J. Acoust. Soc. Am.* **94(2, Pt. 1)** 809–816.

9. Allen, J.B., and Lonsbury-Martin, B.L. (1993) Otoacoustic emissions. *Journal of the Acoustical Society of America* **93(1)** 568–569.

10. Carver, W.F. (1978) Loudness balance procedures. In: Katz, J., editor, *Handbook of clinical audiolgy, 2^{d} edition*, Williams and Wilkins, Baltimore MD.

11. Copper, N., and Rhode, W. (1996) Two tone suppression and two tone distortion in apical and basal cochlear mechanics. In: *The Nineteenth ARO midwinter meeting*, number 220 in 19, page 55.

12. Egan, J., and Hake, H. On the masking pattern of a simple auditory stimulus. *Journal of the Acoustical Society of America* **22** 662–630.

13. Fahey, P.F. and Allen, J.B. (1985) Nonlinear phenomena as observed in the ear canal, at the auditory nerve. *Journal of the Acoustical Society of America* **Feb** 599–612.

14. Fletcher, H. (1923) Physical measurements of audition and their bearing on the theory of hearing. *Journal of the Franklin Institute* **196(3)** 289–326.

15. Fletcher, H. (1930) A space-time pattern theory of hearing. *Journal of the Acoustical Society of America* **1** 311–343.

16. Fletcher, H. (1938) Loudness, masking and their relation to the hearing process and the problem of noise measurement. *Journal of the Acoustical Society of America* **9** 275–293.

17. Fletcher, H. (1938) The mechanism of hearing as revealed through experiments on the masking effect of thermal noise. *Proceedings National Academy Science* **24** 265–274.

18. Fletcher, H., and Munson, W. (1933) Loudness, its definition, measurement, and calculation. *Journal of the Acoustical Society of America* **5** 82–108.

19. Kros, C., and Crawford, A. (1990) Potassium currents in inner hair cells isolated from the guinea–pig cochlea. *Journal of Physiology* **421** 263–291.

20. LePage, E. (1990) Helmholtz revisited: Direct mechanical data suggest a physical model for dynamic control of mapping frequency to place along the cochlear partition. In: Dallos, P., Geisler, C.D., Matthews, J.W., Ruggero, M.A., and Steele, C.R., editors, *The Mechanics and Biophysics of Hearing*, Springer-Verlag, New York.

21. Liberman, M. (1984) Single-neuron labeling and chronic cochlear pathology III. Stereocilia damage and alterations of tuning curve thresholds. *Hearing Research* **16** 55–74.

22. Lorente de No, R. (1937) The diagnosis of diseases of the neural mechanism of hearing by the aid of sounds well above threshold. *Trans. Am. Otol. Soc.* **27** 219–220. Discussion of E. P. Fowler's paper on recruitment.

23. Lutfi, R. (1988) Complex interactions between pairs of forward maskers. *Hearing Research* **35** 71–78.

24. Munson, W. and Gardner, M. (1950) Loudness patterns – a new approach. *Journal of the Acoustical Society of America* **22(2)** 177–190.

25. Nuttall, A, and Dolan, D. (1996) Steady–state sinusoidal velocity responses of the basilar membrane in guinea pig. *Journal of the Acoustical Society of America* **99(3)** 1556–1565.

26. Rhode, W. (1971) Observations of the vibration of the basilar membrane in squirrel monkeys using the Mössbauer technique. *Journal of the Acoustical Society of America* **49**.

27. Ruggero, M., Robles, L., and Rich, N. (1990) Middle-ear response in the chinchilla and its relationship to mechanics at the base of the cochlea. *Journal of the Acoustical Society of America* **87** 1612–1629.

28. Russell, I., Richardson, and Cody (1986) Mechanosensitivity of mammalian auditory hair cells *in vitro*. *Nature* **321(29)** 517–519.

29. Steinberg, J., and Gardner, M. (1937) Dependence of hearing impairment on sound intensity. *Journal of the Acoustical Society of America* **9** 11–23.

30. Wegel, R., and Lane, C. (1924) The auditory masking of one pure tone by another and its probable relation to the dynamics of the inner ear. *Physical Review* **23** 266–285.

31. Yates, G., Winter, I., and Robertson, D. (1989) Basilar membrane nonlinearity determines auditory nerve rate–intensity functions and cochlear dynamic range. *Hearing Research* **45** 203–220.

MAMMALIAN COCHLEAR RESPONSES TO THE ACUTE APPLICATION OF THE TAURINE ANALOGUE, ß-ALANINE

A.R. CODY

Department of Physiology and Pharmacology
The University of Queensland, Queensland, 4072, Australia
a.cody@mailbox.uq.oz.au

Application of ß-Alanine to the round window of the guinea pig cochlea, while recording responses to gated tones produced frequency selective losses of up to 40dB in the threshold sensitivity of the eighth nerve. Sensitivity recovered completely within a period of 50-80 minutes. Changes in the cochlear microphonic were also recorded but in contrast, these were seen as a level and time dependent enhancement of up to 24dB in the input-output function for low frequency stimuli. Complete recovery was also recorded. Application of taurine and the osmotic diuretic mannitol, did not alter either the eighth nerve thresholds or significantly alter the cochlear microphonic. This suggests that the action of ß-Alanine is *not* non-specific and it may directly affect the functional properties of cellular elements in the cochlea.

1 Introduction

Taurine is an amino acid that is found in high concentrations in the central nervous system (CNS), particularly the glial cells, and is thought to have at least two major roles as a presumptive inhibitory neuromodulator and as an osmoregulator.[1] ß-Alanine is the carboxylic analogue of taurine but in contrast to taurine is found in very low concentrations in the CNS. This amino acid appears to form a specific substrate for g-aminobutyrate acid (GABA) and like taurine is also found in glial cells. There is also evidence that ß-Alanine competitively inhibits taurine uptake.[1] In the mammalian cochlea taurine is predominantly restricted to the support cells[2] particularly the Deiters cell, and as a result these cells have been proposed as the cochlear equivalent of the glial cells of the CNS. The Deiters cell forms a close contact with the outer hair cell and could play an important metabolic and mechanical role in cochlear function. In view of the potential "glial-like" function of the Deiters cell it was proposed that the acute application of the taurine analogue ß-Alanine could modify the functional properties of the Deiters cell and therefore help to elucidate the role of this cell in cochlear function.

2 Methods

2.1 Experimental

Guinea pigs (3-500g) were anaesthetised with an intra peritoneal injection of ketamine hydrochloride (60mg/Kg) and xylazine hydrochloride (8mg/Kg) and mounted in hollow earbars in a sound shielded room. The pinna was then removed and entrance to the middle ear gained by a small hole in the bulla. A silver wire electrode was placed on the round window and cochlear sensitivity assessed by monitoring the just noticeable response of the first negative (N_1) component of the compound action potential (CAP) to gated tones (1ms rise time, 50ms duration). The growth of the cochlear microphonic (CM) and the CAP was then determined for stimulus frequencies ranging from 0.265 - 23.99 kHz and stimulus levels ranging from 0 to + 80 dB sound pressure level (dB SPL re 20 µPa) with respect to CAP threshold. Following this initial stimulus paradigm a continuous low frequency tone (530 Hz, 30dB above CAP threshold) was delivered to the animal and the magnitude and phase of the resultant CM monitored by a lock-in-amplifier (Stanford Research Systems SR530). The analogue output from this device was continuously digitised for off-line analysis. Following a suitable recording time (1-2 min) a small volume of 50 mM solution of ß-Alanine, taurine or the osmotic diuretic mannitol, was placed on the round window and changes in the cochlear potentials to the 530 Hz tone tracked for up to 70 minutes. During this period the CAP threshold sensitivity of the cochlea was monitored at 10 minute intervals and cochlear function assessed using the frequency and intensity combinations described previously. The cochlear potentials were digitised and the data stored on a personal computer.

2.2 Analysis

Digitised CM records (bandwidth dc - 37 kHz) were analysed using a Fast Fourier transform (FFT) and the magnitudes of the steady state (dc) and the phasic components (ac) determined for all the frequency and intensity combinations of the stimuli used in the experimental series. This data was then used to reconstruct input-output functions for the CM following the application of the specific pharmacological agent to the round window.

2 Results

Application of ß-Alanine to the round window of the anaesthetised guinea pig results in an increase in the magnitude of the ac cochlear voltages recorded in response to a continuous 530 Hz tone and a decrease in the phase. This is clearly seen in the example shown in the upper portion of figure 1. These changes are recorded approximately 1 - 1.25 minutes following application of the amino acid to the round window. The voltage increase in the CM is relatively rapid over a short time period changing at a rate of 7-8 µV/min before reaching a plateau. The voltage response to the fixed level stimuli then recovers to reach pre ß-Alanine application levels over a period of approximately 60 - 80 minutes. Time dependent changes are also recorded in the phase but in this case the phase decreases with time following the application of ß-Alanine. When the diuretic, mannitol is applied to the round window there is no significant change in either the magnitude or the phase of the CM monitored at the round window. This is seen in the bottom panel of figure 1. In this case the fundamental component of the CM changed by less than 1µV over a period of 5 minutes while there was no apparent alteration in the phase. A similar result was seen for taurine and also if ß-Alanine application was preceded by strychnine hydrochloride. It would appear that only ß-Alanine directly modifies cochlear function for this experimental paradigm.

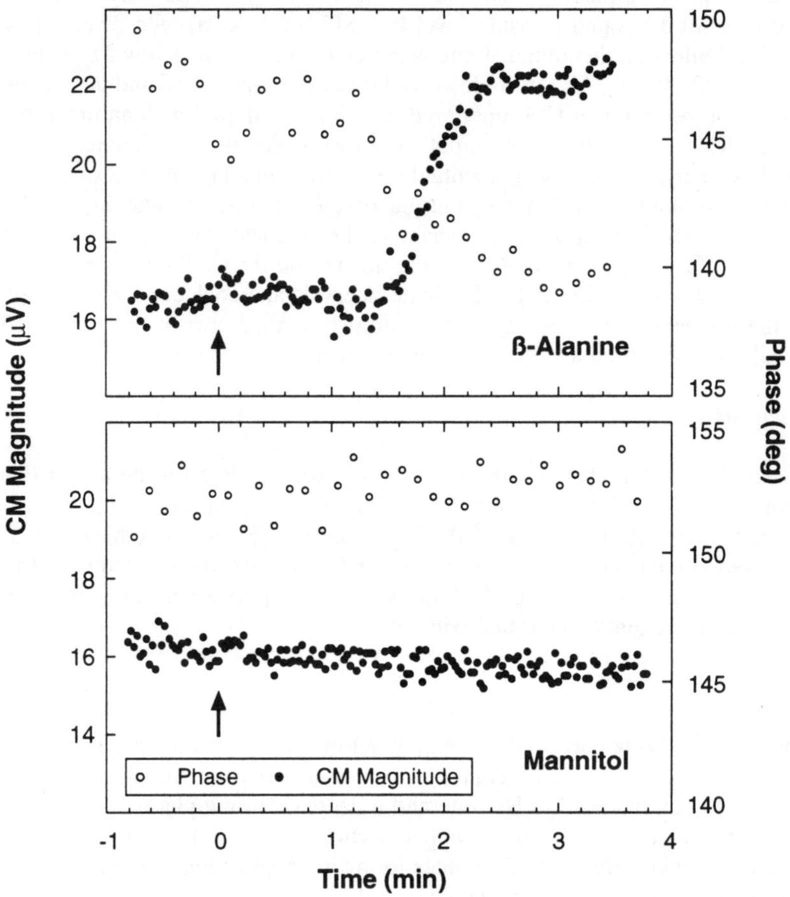

Figure 1. Magnitude and phase of the round window cochlear microphonic in response to a continuous 530 Hz sinusoid presented at a level 30 dB above the 530 Hz CAP threshold. The arrow represents the point at which the amino acid was placed on the round window (time zero).

When cochlear sensitivity and the CM is analysed as a function of level and stimulus frequency then it is obvious that ß-Alanine can alter both the CAP thresholds and the CM growth functions. Figure 2 shows two different animals where either ß-Alanine or mannitol was applied to the round window.

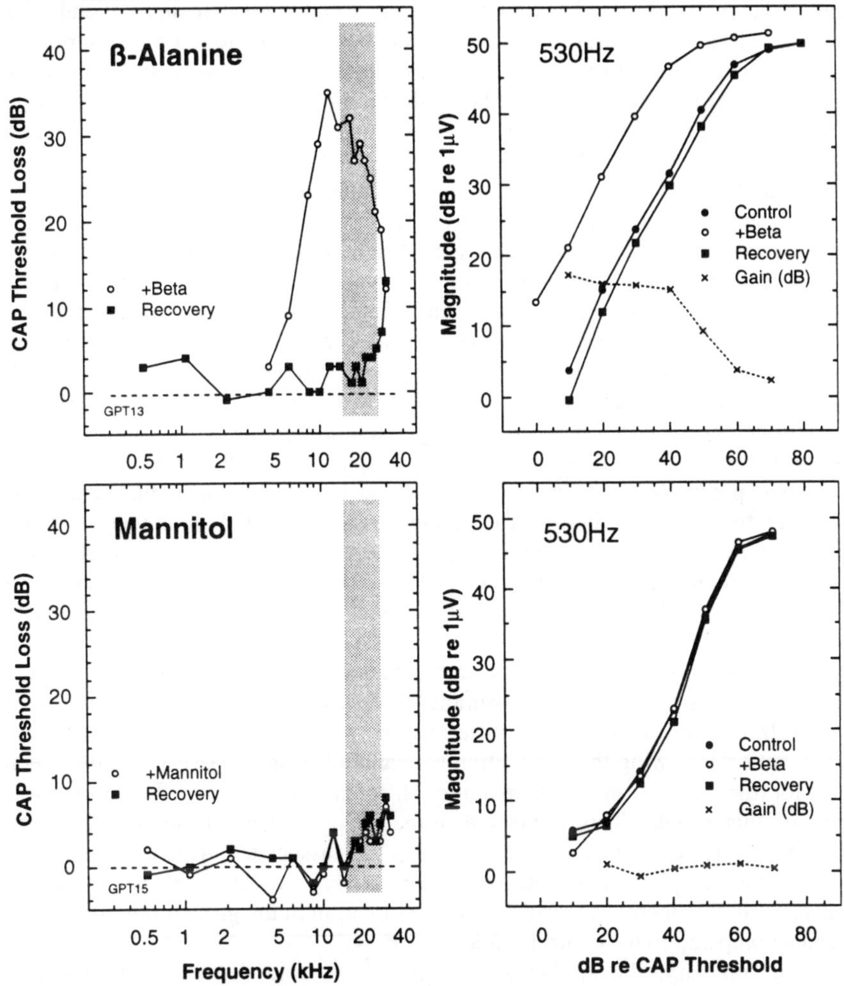

Figure 2. Compound action potential threshold losses (left panels) and the cochlear microphonic magnitude (right panels) following the application of ß-Alanine and Mannitol to the round window. The stippled areas in the left panel represent the estimated length constant (in frequency terms) for CM decay from its source for an electrode placed on the round window.[3]

For this figure the CAP, N_1 threshold sensitivity changes are shown in the left panels and the CM input-output functions in the right panels. In the first instance application of ß-Alanine results in a loss of CAP threshold that is large (25 - 44 dB) and distributed over a wide frequency range that generally extended from

180

around 4 kHz up to 30 kHz. Maximum loss were seen over the frequency band from 10-20 kHz. These large threshold losses recovered over a period of 50 - 80 minutes so that for most animals (4 of 5), the CAP threshold sensitivity was almost identical to that first recorded. In the case of the application of mannitol or taurine, losses in CAP threshold sensitivity are minimal (4-6 dB) and mainly restricted to the highest frequencies (22-30 kHz) as shown in figure 2.

For the CM, the application of ß-Alanine has profound effects on the growth of the magnitude with stimulus level. For the fundamental component of the CM in response to a 530 Hz stimulus (figure 2 right panels), the control input-output function demonstrates a typical saturating curve (filled circles). Following the application of ß-Alanine the magnitude of the fundamental demonstrates a significant and level dependent gain, which effectively moves the curve to the left (open circles). The gain is maximised at the lowest stimulus levels as shown by the dashed curve. For this curve the difference in CM magnitude of the post ß-Alanine curve and the control curve is plotted as a function of stimulus level. Following the recovery of the CAP threshold the CM input-output curve (filled squares) recovers to mirror the pre-application curve. When the specific glycine antagonist strychnine was applied to the round window prior to the application of ß-alanine there were no obvious differences between the control, post ß-alanine or the recovery input-output functions for frequencies less than about 1 kHz. Above this frequency, in contrast to the ß-Alanine alone data, the input-output functions demonstrate a loss of sensitivity at low stimulus levels.

Application of the osmotic diuretic mannitol had no obvious effect on the growth of the CM magnitude with stimulus level as shown in the lower panel of figure 2. In this case there is little difference between the control curve the input-output function following the application of mannitol or the recovery curve as seen clearly for the control and post mannitol difference curve plotted in the lower portion of this panel. This implies that the changes seen in cochlear function following ß-Alanine application, are probably not associated with a non-specific osmotic action. Application of taurine resulted in very similar results to that shown for mannitol in that there was virtually no modification in the growth function of the CM when compared to the control or recovery curves.

In summary, the application of the amino acid ß-Alanine results in a substantial decrease in CAP threshold and a frequency and level dependent enhancement of the magnitude of the CM recorded as a field potential at the round window. The alteration in both cochlear sensitivity and the CM magnitude is reversible over a time period of 60-80 minutes and its effect appears to be modified in a complex manner by the specific glycine antagonist, strychnine. For the osmotic diuretic mannitol, or the amino acid taurine, there were no obvious changes to either the CAP sensitivity or the CM magnitude within the experimental time frame.

3. Discussion

An explanation for the alteration in cochlear function following the application of ß-Alanine is that this amino acid mimics a cholinergic agonist in its action leading to a hyperpolarization of the outer hair cell (OHC). Prior application of the specific glycine antagonist strychnine appears to substantially modify, if not block, the influence of ß-Alanine which suggests that ß-Alanine may be acting as a non specific glycine agonist. This could account for the loss in CAP threshold and also in the increase in the magnitude of the CM for low frequency stimuli.

If it is assumed that ß-Alanine is acting as an inhibitory agonist then the loss of CAP threshold following ß-Alanine application may have a dual origin. In the first instance the agonist may act at the axodendritic synapse of the type I radial afferents and the lateral olivocochlear neurones. There is some evidence that this is a cholinergic pathway.[4] Secondly, the loss and recovery of the CAP sensitivity may mirror a decrease and recovery of the mechanical stimulus to the IHC. By implication this suggests that the micromechanical properties of the organ of Corti are modified and that the OHC may be the protagonist. There is direct in vitro evidence, that application of cholinergic agonists to the OHC lead to a hyperpolarization of the cell and an increase in the length.[5,6] These changes can be blocked by curare and strychnine. There is also evidence for acetylcholine receptor epitopes on mammalian OHCs[7] and that the intra cochlear perfusion of strychnine can block the acoustically activated action of the medial olivocochlear efferents.[8] In this case it is hypothesised that activation of these crossed pathways leads to activation of nicotinic-like receptors on the OHC.

In terms of the increase in the CM that was observed with ß-Alanine application a simple hyperpolarization that increases the diving potential across the apical pole of the OHC cannot account for the magnitude change. Shifts of up to 24 dB were recorded but a gain of this size would require an increase of an order of magnitude in the driving potential.

The more likely scenario is that the increase in the low frequency CM is a combination of an increase in the driving potential, through activation of basolateral K^+ conductances, coupled with a change in the mechanical properties of the organ of Corti so that the OHC transducer channel is biased towards a more sensitive portion of its input-output curve. Given the morphological evidence that the OHC stereocilia are firmly embedded in the tectorial membrane a sustained, but reversible, length change in the OHC could mean that the angular relationship between the OHC stereocilia and the apical surface of the OHC is modified leading to a bias of the transducer towards the open state. This is supported by the change in the CM input-output curve shown in figure 2 which, following the application of ß-Alanine, is seen as a shift to the left rather than as a vertical displacement.

Based on this study it would appear that the acute application of ß-Alanine has profound effects on cochlear function. These effects are probably the result of ß-Alanine acting as an inhibitory cholinergic agonist which would dominate any changes potential or actual, associated with modifying the osmoregulatory role of taurine. The mostly likely cochlear target for the action of ß-Alanine is the OHCs rather than the Deiters cell.

182

Acknowledgments

Funds for this work were provided by the Garnett Passe and Rodney Williams Memorial Foundation.

References

1. Huxtable ,R.J. (1992) Physiological actions of taurine *Physiological Rev.* **72** 101-163.
2. Usami, S. and Ottersen, O.P. (1995) The localisation of taurine-like immunoreactivity in the organ of Corti: a semiquantitative, post-embedding immuno-electron microscope analysis in the rat with some observations in the guinea pig, *Brain Res.* **676** 277–284.
3. Patuzzi, R.B., Yates, G.K., Johnstone, B.M. (1989). The origin of thelow-frequency microphonic in the first cochlear turn of the guinea-pig *Hear. Res.* **39** 177-88.
4. Abou-Madi, L., Pontarotti, P. Tramu, G., Cupo, A., Eybalin, M. (1987). Coexistence of putative neuroactive substances in lateral olivocochlear neurons of rat and guinea pig, *Hear. Res.* **30** 135–146.
5. Housley, G.D. and Ashmore, J.F. (1991). Direct measurement of the action of acetylcholine on isolated outer hair cells of the guinea pig cochlea *Proc. Roy. Soc. Lond. B. Biol. Sci.* **244** 161–167.
6. Santos-Sacchi, J. (1989) Asymmetry in voltage-dependent movements of isolated outer hair cells from the organ of Corti *J. Neurosci.* **9** 2954–2962.
7. Pinkert, P.K., Gitter, A.H., Zimmerman, U., Kirchner, T., Tzartos, Zenner, H–P. (1990). Visualisation and functional testing of acetylcholine receptor–like molecules in cochlear outer hair cells, *Hear. Res.* **44** 2533.
8. Kujawa, S.G., Glattke, T.J., Fallon, M., Bobbin, R.P. (1994). A nicotinic–like receptor mediates suppression of distortion product otoacoustic emissions by contralateral sound, *Hear. Res.* **74** 122–134.

THE SIGNIFICANCE OF THE COCHLEAR TRAVELING WAVE FOR THEORIES OF FREQUENCY ANALYSIS AND PITCH

STEVEN GREENBERG

University of California, Berkeley and
International Computer Science Institute
1947 Center Street, Berkeley, CA 94704
steveng@icsi.berkeley.edu

Auditory theory has traditionally pitted "place" (the tonotopically organized spatial pattern of excitation) versus "time" (the temporal pattern of discharge) with respect to the neural representation underlying specific attributes of acoustic sensation. This long-standing controversy has been of particular significance for models of pitch and frequency analysis, but casts its theoretical shadow over the discipline as a whole. A potential resolution of this historical opposition is proposed, in which place and time are viewed as flip sides of a complex representational matrix of neural activity, bound together through the mechanics of the cochlear traveling wave and its interaction with central loci of coincidence detection and inhibition. Frequency analysis is viewed as possessing two operational components. One is excitatory, based on spatially circumscribed patterns of temporally coherent peripheral activity and processed by central coincidence-sensitive neural elements. The other involves central inhibitory elements driven by non-synchronous activity distributed over a broad tonotopic domain. Together, these two mechanisms can account for the preservation of frequency selectivity across a wide range of frequencies and sound pressure levels, despite dramatic changes in the average-rate-based profile of neural activity. The traveling wave is also of importance in formatting the peripheral spatio-temporal response pattern germane to periodicity analysis and the perception of pitch. The present framework resolves the long-standing schism between spectral and temporal theories by virtue of a formulation in which pitch is viewed as resulting from the interplay of place and temporal information bound together into a coherent representation through the operation of central coincidence-sensitive neural populations. Within this perspective, both frequency resolution and neural synchrony are required for a robust sensation of pitch to occur.

1 Introduction

The displacement pattern of basilar membrane vibration is tonotopically organized, with high frequencies reaching their apogee towards the base of the cochlea and low frequencies achieving their maximum near the apex.[1] This systematic relationship between peak displacement and cochlear location serves as the linchpin of the "place" model of spectral representation and of auditory theory in general.

In recent years this "classic" place model has come under increasing scrutiny in light of experimental observations demonstrating that this spatial organization of excitatory activity is largely discernible only under a restricted set of conditions in the auditory periphery, thus calling into question its ability to subserve frequency coding at sound pressure levels typical of speech communication and musical performance.

184

In place of classic tonotopy many recent models of pitch and frequency analysis focus on the temporal properties of peripheral activity, principally the phase-locking behavior of single neural elements in the auditory nerve and ventral cochlear nucleus.[2,3]

However, neither the temporal nor place approaches specify the operations through which the peripheral patterns are transformed into constellations of excitatory and inhibitory activity characteristic of the upper reaches of the auditory pathway, nor do they provide a principled account of the physiological basis for the perceptual stability of spectral representation and pitch extraction characteristic of human listening experience.

2 Cochlear Traveling Wave Delay

The motion of the basilar membrane proceeds in an orderly fashion from base to the point of maximum displacement, beyond which the wave damps outs relatively quickly. The velocity of this traveling wave is very fast in the base, being nearly instantaneous (i.e., in the range of tens to hundreds of microseconds [μs]) for frequencies above 4 kHz, but slowing dramatically for peak displacements in the apex. The transit time from base to apex requires 10 ms or greater.[4,5]

The travel time for the cochlear traveling wave can be estimated from the latency of initial excitation of single auditory-nerve (AN) fibers to sinusoidal signals as illustrated in Figure 1. The cochlear delay (d_i) at a given frequency (f_i), can be modeled with a simple equation of the form:

$$d_i = f_i^{-1} + k$$

where k represents a delay constant of 0.002 s. This cochlear latency behavior represents the predicted response time of a minimum phase filter (f_i^{-1}) plus a 2-ms transmission time from transducer to the base of the cochlea. Although many properties of basilar membrane motion and filtering are non-linear, in terms of the cochlear traveling wave delay, the partition appears to act like a linear transducer.

There are two functional consequences of this latency behavior.

3 Latency Representation of Spectrum and Pitch

First, the shape of the delay function allows one to estimate the latency disparity between any two spectral components. For example, the initial spike latency for a 1-kHz signal is 3 ms, while that for a 0.5-kHz component is 4 ms, resulting in a latency disparity of 1 ms. Although this latency disparity is negligible for high-frequency signals, it can be considerable for low-frequency components within the core of the speech and musical range. It is also of significance that the initial latency of excitation remains stable as a function of sound pressure level for auditory-nerve fibers whose characteristic frequencies are in close proximity to that of the signal. This important property of cochlear latency behavior is considered below (Section 4).

Such latency behavior provides a means of encoding low-frequency spectral information using a parameter of the peripheral excitation pattern distinct from, and yet still very much associated with the classical place mechanism. A given frequency produces a specific time signature that remains essentially stable over a circumscribed population of neurons. This latency signature is not only preserved, but appears to be enhanced at the level of the auditory cortex, where the latency disparities are magnified by a factor of three.[6] There is some evidence that this latency behavior applies not only to the spectrum but also to encoding pitch-relevant information,[7] as discussed below (Section 8).

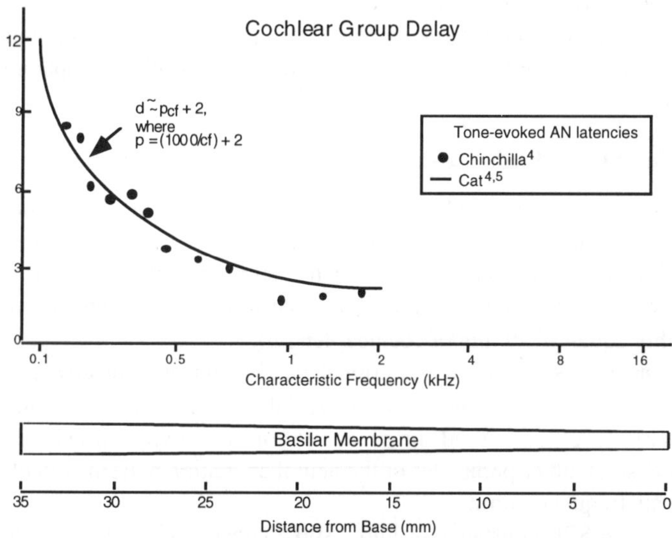

Figure 1 Latency of auditory-nerve fiber excitation as a function of sinusoidal signal frequency. Data derived from references 4 and 5. Solid curve fit to the equation indicated.

4 Stability of Spectral and Pitch Representation

The delay properties of the cochlear traveling wave also provide a potential means of stabilizing spectral information across a wide dynamic range of sound pressure levels and acoustic environmental conditions.

At the point of cochlear resonance, the initial latency of auditory-nerve-fiber excitation remains constant across sound pressure level.[8] In consequence, a certain proportion of fibers will fire synchronously at onset in such a fashion as to potentially serve as a reliable frequency cue, particularly in concert with the latency gradient properties described above (Section 2).

Many neurons in the auditory brainstem and cortex appear to function as "coincidence" detectors, in that their probability of firing increases when multiple afferent input arrives within a narrow time window (typically on the order of tens or a few hundreds of microseconds). For example, at the level of the primary auditory cortex, cells typically discharge reliably only in response to stimulus onset and to certain forms of amplitude and frequency modulation, with firing rates rarely in excess of 20-30 spikes/s.[9] The initial latency variance of such units is typically small (often less than 100 μs).[10] Although such cells are excitable by a relatively broad range of frequencies, the tuning of cortical neurons remains remarkably stable across sound pressure levels when measured in terms of discharge "doubtlets" and "triplets," which likely reflect large numbers of synchronous thalamic input.[11] The bandwidth of such multiple-onset tuning functions is roughly comparable to the critical band.

5 A Possible Latency Basis for the Critical Band

The critical band is a well-established limit of frequency selectivity that plays a central role in many perceptual attributes of sound.[12] Its physiological and anatomical bases remain obscure, although there appears to be a consistent relationship with distance along the cochlear partition (in the human, one critical band is roughly equal to 0.9 mm of cochlear length).[13]

A defining characteristic of the critical band is its relative constancy across sound pressure level.[12] In view of the appreciable broadening of tuning at high sound pressure levels observed in measures of selectivity based on average discharge rate, some other parameter of the neural excitation pattern is likely to form the basis of this frequency limit.

In view of the SPL-constancy of initial spike latency at cochlear resonance and the activation properties of coincidence-detector neurons, it appears likely that one important physiological component subserving frequency selectivity is the temporal coherence of peripheral neural discharge. Although the tonotopic extent of neural excitation increases with sound pressure level, the width of highly onset-synchronized activity is unlikely to enlarge significantly. And since it is this highly synchronized activity that is particularly effective in exciting higher-level auditory coincidence detector neurons, it could readily serve as a reliable basis for encoding both frequency information and defining its limits of resolution. Thus, it may be that the physiological basis of the critical band may rest on the synchronicity of neural activity across a contiguous extent of a tonotopically organized gradient.

6 Possible Origins of Lateral Inhibition

Lateral inhibition serves to sharpen the spectral profile of excitatory neural activity.[14] The origins of this important form of automatic gain control remains unclear. The magnitude and bandwidth of lateral suppression observed in the auditory nerve is considerably smaller than their counterparts driven by inhibition in many units (particularly choppers and pauser-buildups) of the cochlear nucleus.[15]

Both the bandwidth and magnitude of lateral inhibition among choppers and pauser-buildups increases with gain in signal intensity in a manner consistent with the tonotopic expansion of auditory-nerve activity as measured in terms of average rate.

The response properties of both choppers and pauser-buildups resemble integrators with relatively long time constants (for choppers, on the order of 2 to 10 ms, and for pauser-buildups, on the order of 20 to 100 ms).[15] The precise timing of afferent input does not appear to be an important variable in determining their level of excitation.

The intensity-dependent nature of lateral inhibition suggests that its origins lie in the activity of neural elements relatively insensitive to input latency and which respond to the magnitude of activity largely irrespective of its temporal characteristic. Lateral inhibition thus appears to serve as a rough metric of integrated activity across a wide bandwidth of the tonotopic axis and to preserve a dynamic range of response for spectral coding.

7 Interplay between Synchronized Excitatory and Inhibitory Activity

The spectral representation of a sound may thus represent a combination of highly synchronous activity distributed over circumscribed tonotopic regions, signaling detailed information pertaining to aurally resolved components, along with a much more broadly distributed non-synchronized activity pattern associated with the overall energy level of the signal, and which serves as input to an automatic gain control mediated by neural inhibition.

8 Synchronous Activity as a Possible Basis for Pitch

Auditory-nerve fibers are capable of synchronizing their activity on a sustained basis to frequencies below 3 kHz.[16] Circumscribed AN-fiber populations, synchronized to aurally resolved spectral components, provide a potential mechanism for encoding low pitch in the auditory periphery on the basis of "spectral" information associated with aurally resolved harmonics.

As a consequence of the temporal characteristics of the cochlear traveling wave described above (Section 2), the latency disparity among neighboring harmonics are such that the times of discharge associated with each spectral band are statistically correlated with those of its neighbors. As a consequence, it is possible to derive a periodicity analysis based on the correlation of synchronous activity across the spectrum in a manner resembling a running autocorrelation. The delay line, as it were, is derived from the cochlear traveling wave. The differential delays associated with specific periodicities appear to be magnified in primary auditory cortex, similar to the pattern observed for encoding spectral information[8] (Section 3).

9 The Significance of the Cochlear Traveling Wave

There is much in our listening experience that cannot readily be accommodated within the current theoretical framework for auditory analysis of sound. Neither the classical place nor temporal models can, by themselves, account for many of the important properties of acoustic perception, such as the stability and apparent continuity of sound sources under a wide range of environmental conditions. A broader physiological and computational perspective is required to provide a more complete account of how such signals as speech and music are represented and processed in the auditory pathway.

Towards this end, it is suggested that the fine interplay between excitatory and inhibitory auditory processes may originate in the latency behavior of the cochlear traveling wave, providing the means through which different components of the acoustic signal are placed into appropriate temporal register for the central brainstem and cortex to operate on. In this sense the cochlear traveling wave may serve to temporally "preformat" the peripheral activity pattern entering the cochlear nuclei in such a fashion as to provide for fast, accurate and efficient extraction of features pertaining to pitch, intensity and spectral information. Thus, at least some portion of the transduction properties of the periphery (particularly those pertaining to spectral selectivity and filtering) are likely to be sculptured by requirements of the central auditory pathway.

References

1.   Békésy, G. von (1960) *Experiments in Hearing* (McGraw Hill, New York).
2.   Meddis, R. and Hewitt, M. (1991) Virtual pitch and phase sensitivity of a computer model of the auditory periphery. I. Pitch identification, *J. Acoust. Soc. Am.* **98** 2866-2882.
3.   Slaney, M. and Lyon, R. (1993) On the importance of time - a temporal representation of sound, in *Visual Representations of Speech Signals*, ed. M. Cooke, S. Beet, and M. Crawford (Wiley, Chicester) pp. 95-118.
4.   Ruggero, M. and Rich, N. (1987) Timing of spike initiation in cochlear afferents: dependence on site of innervation, *J. Neurophys.* **58** 379-403.

5. Goldstein, J., Baer, T. and Kiang, N.Y-S. (1971) A theoretical treatment of latency, group delay and tuning characteristics for auditory nerve responses to clicks and tones, in *The Physiology of the Auditory System,* ed. M.B. Sachs (National Educational Consultants, Baltimore) pp. 133-141.

6. Roberts, T. and Poepple, D. (1996) Latency of auditory evoked M100 as a function of tone frequency, *NeuroReport* **7** in press.

7. Ragot, R. and Lepaul-Ercole, R. (1996) Brain potentials as objective indexes of auditory pitch extraction from harmonics, *NeuroReport* **7** 905-909.

8. Kiang, N.Y-S. (1965) *Discharge Patterns of Single Fibers in the Cat's Auditory Nerve* (MIT Press, Cambridge).

9. Schreiner, C. E. and Urbas, J. V. (1986) Representation of amplitude modulation in the auditory cortex of the cat. I. The anterior auditory field (AAF), *Hearing Res.* **21** 227-241.

10. Clarey, J. C., Barone, P. and Imig, T. (1992) Physiology of thalamus and cortex, in *The Mammalian Auditory Pathway: Neurophysiology,* ed. A.N. Popper and R. R. Fay (Springer, New York) pp. 232-334.

11. Eggermont, J. J. and Smith, G. (1996) Burst-firing sharpens frequency-tuning in primary auditory cortex, *NeuroReport* **7** 753-757.

12. Scharf, B. (1970) Critical bands, in *Auditory Theory*, ed. J. Tobias (San Diego: Academic Press).

13. Greenwood, D. D. (1990) A cochlear frequency-position function for several species-29 years later. *J. Acoust. Soc. Am.* **87** 2592-2605.

14. Shamma S. A. (1985) Speech processing in the auditory system. II: Lateral inhibition and the central processing of speech evoked activity in the auditory nerve, *J. Acoust. Soc. Am.* **78** 1622-1632.

15. Rhode, W. S and Greenberg, S. (1992) Physiology of the cochlear nuclei, in *The Mammalian Auditory Pathway: Neurophysiology,* ed. A.N. Popper and R. R. Fay (Springer, New York) pp. 94-152.

16. Johnson, D. H. (1980) The relationship between spike rate and synchrony in responses of auditory-nerve fibers to single tones, *J. Acoust. Soc, Am.* **68** 1115-1122.

SIGNAL PROCESSING MODELS FOR THE AUDITORY PERIPHERY

R. KUMARESAN[†], A. RAO[†], M. SANDERSON[‡], A. SIMMONS[‡]

[‡] *Department of Neuroscience, Brown University,*
Providence, RI-02912

[†] *Department of Electrical Engineering, University of Rhode Island,*
Kingston, RI-02881

Our presentation at this conference consisted of two parts. In the first part we argued that nonlinear signal processing in the auditory periphery may be viewed in terms of analytic signals, especially minimum and maximum phase signals. We pointed out that if the information content in the phase and envelope of the signal are equivalent then one may retain only the phase thereby effectively achieving nonlinear compression. This may be viewed as a form of cepstral processing. The second part of the presentation was concerned with modeling the response of the auditory nerve fibers of the bullfrog *Rana catesbeiana* using multiple sinusoidal stimuli. Assuming an integrate-to-threshold model for the neural spike generation process at the haircell-nerve synapse, we present an algorithm for reconstructing the haircell receptor potential given the neural spike train timing.

1 Part I: Auditory Nonlinearity

The ratio of the intensities of the loudest to the softest sounds that the cochlea can handle without permanent damage ranges by ten orders of magnitude or 100 dB. To deal with such a large dynamic range the cochlea is known to process signals using a non-linear signal processing scheme. This can be surmised from the distortion products it produces when two or more tones are simultaneously applied to the ear. However the precise form of this nonlinearity is still unknown. Its form and function, if discovered, will shed light on early sound processing mechanisms of the auditory system and pave the way for improved machine-based acoustic signal processing schemes. Based on current knowledge of cochlear mechanics we propose a signal processing model for the filtering performed by the cochlea. Analytic signals, particularly minimum phase/maximum phase signals are used as tools to model the signal processing function of the cochlea. Based on properties of such signals we argue that the cochlear filtering may be modeled as a form of adaptive filtering in which one attempts to minimize the difference between the envelope of a signal and its instantaneous frequency. Due to space constraints only rudiments of the model are discussed here.

Research supported by NIH grant NS28565 and by AFOSR contract F49620-93-I-0026.

1.1 Key Features of the Nonlinearity:

In this section we outline the essential features of the cochlear nonlinearity which help motivate our signal representation model. Firstly, the function of the mechanical nonlinearity residing in the cochlea is to compress the large dynamic range of the input stimulus into a range suitable for the inner haircells. Consequently, the input-output function for basilar membrane motion becomes highly compressive at moderate to high sound pressure levels. However this dynamic range compression must be achieved with minimal distortion. A key question is what kind of signal representation would afford such a range compression and yet not significantly distort or misrepresent the stimulus signal? Secondly, it is well known that the auditory filters have an asymmetrical shape. That is, the roll-off rate of the filters determined by REVCOR analysis is much higher on the high-frequency side compared to the gentler roll-off on the low frequency side. Finally it has been recognized for a long time that the excitation pattern on the basilar membrane shifts its location when the intensity of the stimulus is increased. This would suggest that the signal intensity and (tonotopic) frequency must be related in the way the signal is represented at the output of the cochlea.

1.2 Signal Representation Model

A complex-valued signal, $s(t) = \phi(t) \pm j\hat{\phi}(t)$ is said to be analytic, if its Fourier transform $S(\omega)$ is one sided; *hat* denotes Hilbert transform. The so called minimum/maximum phase signals which are of the form $e^{\phi(t)\pm j\hat{\phi}(t)}$ are special cases of analytic signals. In this case the log of the envelope and phase are Hilbert pairs. $e^{j\omega_1 t}e^{\phi(t)\pm j\hat{\phi}(t)}$ are frequency translated versions of the minimum/maximum phase signals, the real part of which are $e^{\phi(t)}cos(\omega_1 t \pm \hat{\phi}(t))$. The spectrum of this real signal is essentially confined to one side of the frequency ω_1 depending on the $\pm$ sign. Recall the sharp high frequency cutoff of the cochlear filters. Thus $e^{\phi(t)}cos(\omega_1 t - \hat{\phi}(t))$ could represent the output of a cochlear filter[6]. Since its envelope and phase essentially contain the same information it is sufficient to retain only $cos(\omega_1 t - \hat{\phi}(t))$ thereby achieving 'compression'. In practice an adaptive filter which minimizes the difference between the envelope and phase derivative/instantaneous frequency of its output appears to be a suitable cochlear filter model. Model details will be given elsewhere.

2   Part II: Auditory Nerve Fiber Modeling:

In this part of the paper we present an algorithm for modeling the spike train observed at an auditory nerve fiber. An early model of the auditory periphery, known as the "sandwich model", is shown in Figure 1. Recently, a number of researchers have tried to characterize the auditory periphery of the bullfrog based on this model using Gaussian noise [5] and sinusoidal stimuli [2]. The sandwich model of the auditory nerve consists of a cascade of four elements: 1) the linear time-invariant band-pass filter, $H_1(f)$, which represents the middle ear and hair cell-tectorial membrane dynamics, 2) the static nonlinearity that models the process of hair cell transduction, 3) the low-pass filter, $H_2(f)$, which represents the membrane capacitance and conductance of the hair cells, 4) and a spike generator which supposedly converts the haircell receptor potential $g(t)$, into a train of action potentials. In this paper we propose an algorithm to reconstruct the haircell receptor potential waveform, $g(t)$, given the neural spike train data. In contrast to earlier approaches [4] our approach invokes an explicit model for the spike generator and uses sinusoidal stimuli.

2.1   *Integrate-to-Threshold Model Fitting (ITMF) of Spike Train data*

We invoke an "Integrate-to-Threshold" (IT) model [3] for spike generation at the haircell-synapse, i.e., a model for conversion of $g(t)$ into the spike train $p(t)$. As per this model, an integrator integrates $g(t)$ and compares it to a constant positive threshold value A and initiates a spike if $g(t)$ obeys the equation $\int_{\tau_{k-1}}^{T_k} g(t)dt = A$. The integrator is then reset to zero and the process repeats. The basic premise of our model is that the spikes carry information in the interspike intervals and not just in the spike rate, especially at high stimulus intensities and for sinusoidal stimuli. The pulse position modulation (PPM) [3] implied by our spike generator is ideally suited for this representation. The dc voltage induced by the asymmetric rectifying nonlinearity in the sandwich (when integrated and reset) serves as the underlying 'carrier' for the PPM. Once the receptor potential $g(t)$ is reconstructed, it along with the stimulus $x(t)$ may be used, at least in principle, to identify the filters $H_1(f)$ and $H_2(f)$ and the non-linearity. This is one of our future goals.

2.2   *The ITMF Algorithm:*

We now develop an algorithm to reconstruct the waveform corresponding to the haircell's receptor potential, $g(t)$ given the neural spike train data. Let $x(t)$ represent the input stimulus to the frog's ear consisting of L sinewaves $x(t) = \sum_{l=1}^{L} \lambda_l \cos(2\pi\gamma_l t + \beta_l)$, where λ_l, γ_l and β_l refer to the amplitude, frequency and the phase of the l-th sinusoid. Further, let $p(t) = \sum_{k=1}^{N} \delta(t - \tau_k)$, denote the recorded spike-train data corresponding to the stimulus $x(t)$, where τ_k, $(k = 1, 2, .., N)$ represent the times of occurrences of the spikes. We assume that the filter-rectifier-filter sandwich depicted in Figure 1 is time-invariant. Since the stimulus is composed of sinusoids, which is then subjected to a rectification process, $g(t)$, will consist of intermodulation products which have been lowpass filtered $(H_2(f))$ by the haircell membrane. Hence, $g(t)$ may be modeled as $g(t) = g_{dc} + \sum_{l=1}^{M} g_l \cos(2\pi f_l t + \phi_l)$. The frequencies of these sinusoids, f_l, are a function of the frequencies in the stimulus. For example, if the input stimulus is made up of three sinewaves at frequencies γ_1 , γ_2 and γ_3, then $g(t)$ will be composed sinusoids with frequencies $l\gamma_1 \pm m\gamma_2 \pm n\gamma_3$ Hz for all integers l, m and n[1]. However, only a few of them will have significant amplitudes, due to the low-pass characteristics of the haircell membrane. In addition $g(t)$ will have a significant positive dc component g_{dc}, due to the asymmetry in the haircell rectifying nonlinearity.

Now assume that the number of τ_k values or spikes, N, is much greater than $2M + 1$. Since the spike generation and the data collection process are inherently noisy we expect that the equation $\int_{\tau_{k-1}}^{\tau_k} g(t)dt = A.$ will be only approximately satisfied. Keeping this in mind, if we substitute for $g(t)$ from Eq. 2.2 into the equation $\int_{\tau_{k-1}}^{\tau_k} g(t)dt \approx A$, for each τ_k we have in matrix notation,

$$
\begin{bmatrix}
\Delta\tau_1 & c_{11} & s_{11} & \cdots & s_{M1} \\
\Delta\tau_2 & c_{12} & s_{12} & \cdots & s_{M2} \\
\vdots & \vdots & \vdots & \vdots & \\
\Delta\tau_{(N-1)} & c_{1(N-1)} & s_{1(N-1)} & \cdots & s_{M(N-1)}
\end{bmatrix}
\begin{bmatrix}
g_{dc} \\
g_{c1} \\
g_{s1} \\
\vdots \\
g_{sM}
\end{bmatrix}
=
\begin{bmatrix}
A \\
A \\
\vdots \\
A
\end{bmatrix}
+
\begin{bmatrix}
\epsilon_1 \\
\epsilon_2 \\
\vdots \\
\epsilon_{(N-1)}
\end{bmatrix}, \quad (1)
$$

where $c_{lk} = \int_{\tau_{k-1}}^{\tau_k} \cos(2\pi f_l t)dt$, $s_{lk} = \int_{\tau_{k-1}}^{\tau_k} \sin(2\pi f_l t)dt$, $\Delta\tau_k = \int_{\tau_{k-1}}^{\tau_k} dt$, and $g_{cl} = g_l \cos(\phi_l)$ and $g_{sl} = -g_l \sin(\phi_l)$; ϵ_k account for the random errors which are assumed independent. Let the matrix and vector on the left of Eq 1 be called $\mathbf{X}$ and $\mathbf{a}$ respectively, and the vector on the right, ϵ. Then Eq. 1 may be rewritten as $\mathbf{X}\,\mathbf{a} = \mathbf{A1} + \epsilon$; $\mathbf{1}$ denotes an $(N - 1) \times 1$ vector of all ones. Notice that the matrix $\mathbf{X}$ is entirely known. Setting the threshold, A, to be unity, we estimate the vector of unknown amplitudes, phases and the dc (relative to the threshold) by minimizing the sum of squared error, $\epsilon^T \epsilon$ ($\mathbf{T}$ stands for matrix transpose); this is same as minimizing the squared-norm, $||\mathbf{1} - \mathbf{X}\,\mathbf{a}||_2^2$, and is a standard least-squares problem. Once $\mathbf{a}$ is determined, using the amplitudes and phases in $\mathbf{a}$, the waveform of $g(t)$ (as in Eq. 2.2) is reconstructed, within a scale factor. We now describe model fitting results for

194

synthetically generated $g(t)$ and recorded spike trains.

2.3 Modeling Results

First, the spike-generator model was used to generate a synthetic spike-train data. Its input's, $g(t)$'s, integral is plotted in Fig. 2, along with the waveform resulting from resetting $g_1(t)$ when it reaches the threshold, A. Observe that for a fixed threshold, this model behaves like a PPM [3] with the integral of $g(t)$'s dc providing an implicit PPM carrier. Using our ITMF procedure, we reconstructed an estimate of $g(t)$ (within a scale factor), plotted in Fig. 3 along with the true $g(t)$; they match exactly. In Fig. 3 we have displayed as dots both the original (upper row) and the resynthesized (lower row) spike timings.

Next, we considered a real stimulus, $x(t)$, consisting of tones of frequencies $\approx$ 200 Hz, 250 Hz and 261 Hz with respective amplitudes of -6 dB, 0 dB and -7 dB; they had zero phases. In Fig. 4 we have displayed the raster plot for this stimulus obtained from a fiber with a BF of 127 Hz. In general we observed (see Fig. 5) that, although low frequency AP fibers (BFs $100-500$ Hz) phase-locked to $x(t)$'s envelope, they also showed phase-locking to the stimulus' frequencies. Mid AP and BP fibers, however, exhibited strongest phase-locking to the envelope (see Fig. 6). Using the recorded spike-timings from experiments (30 presentations of $x(t)$ for the BF 127 Hz fiber), $g(t)$ was estimated (for each presentation) using the ITMF procedure and later time-averaged; its ac portion is displayed (solid line) in Fig. 7 along with the ac portion of $x(t)$'s envelope's (dashed-dotted line). The results of another example are shown in Fig. 8. Using our procedure we found that, in general, the averaged receptor potentials resemble the stimulus' envelope.

References

1. Bennett, W.R. (1933) New results in the calculation of modulation products. *Bell System Technical Journal* **12** 228-243.
2. Simmons, A.M. and Shen, Y. and Sanderson, M. (1996) Neural and computational basis for periodicity extraction in frog peripheral auditory system. *Auditory Neuroscience* **2** 109-133.
3. Zeevi, Y.Y. and Bruckstein, A.M (1979) Analysis of "Integrate-to-Threshold" neural coding schemes. *Biological Cybernetics* **34** 63-79.
4. Rieke, F. (1992) Physical Principles Underlying Sensory Processing and Computation. *PhD thesis* University of California at Berkeley.
5. van Dijk, P., Wit, H.P., Segenhout, J.M. and Tubis, A. (1994) Wiener kernei analysis of inner ear function in the American bullfrog. *J. Acoust. Soc. Am.* **95** 904-919.
6. Kumaresan, R and Rao, A. (1995) Minimum/Maximum Phase Decomposition of Signals Inspired By The Auditory Periphery. Proc. of the 29-th IEEE Asilomar Conf. on Signals, Systems and Computers, CA.

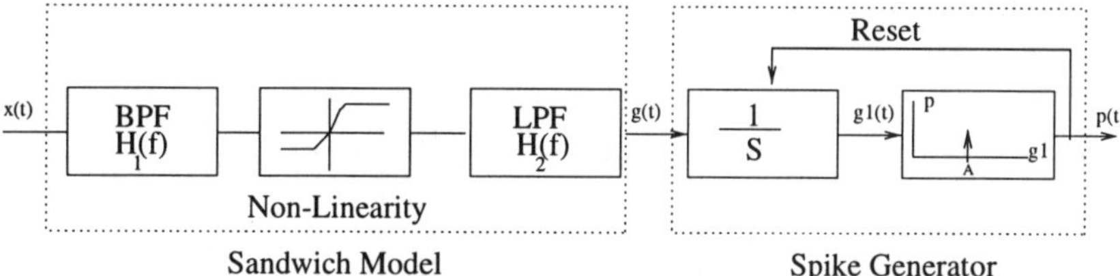

Fig. 1: Sandwich model and the Integrate-to-Threshold spike generator. The output of the filter-rectifier-filter sandwich is the receptor potential, $g(t)$, which then forms the input to the spike generator. A spike is generated at τ_k if $\int_{\tau_{k-1}}^{\tau_k} g(t)dt = A$.

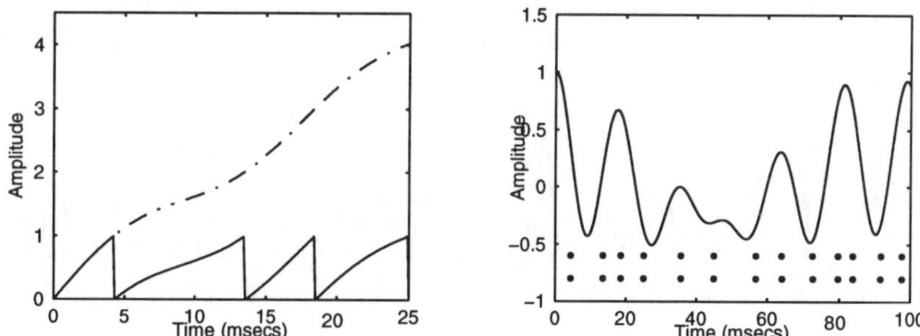

Fig. 2: The integral of a synthetic receptor potential, $\int_0^t g(\tau))d\tau$, is plotted as a dashed-dotted line. Whenever $g_1(t)$ reaches a fixed threshold, A, a spike is generated and $g_1(t)$ is reset to zero; the resulting $g_1(t)$ is shown by a solid line. **Fig.** 3: We have overlaid plots of the original and reconstructed $g_{ac}(t)$; they match exactly. When the reconstructed $g(t)$ was fed to the spike-generator model along with the estimated threshold-value, the spike-train obtained matched the original; both are plotted as dots, lower row and upper row dots respectively.

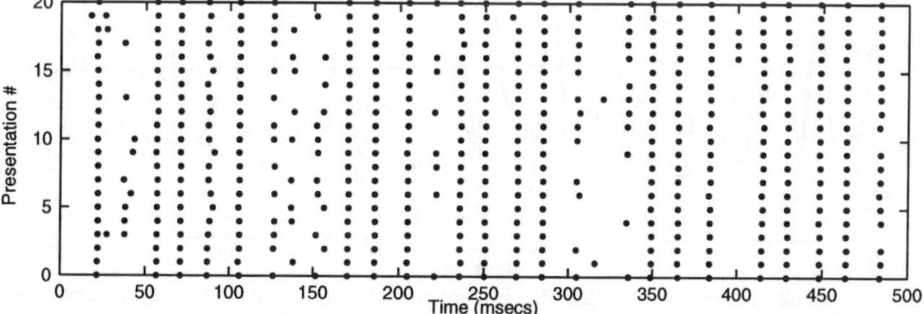

Fig. 4 The recorded spike locations for 20 different presentations of the same stimulus, $x(t)$. The fiber BF was 127 Hz; $x(t)$ had frequencies of $\approx$ 150 Hz, 200 Hz and 261 Hz with amplitudes −6 dB, 0 dB and −7 dB and zero-phases respectively.

196

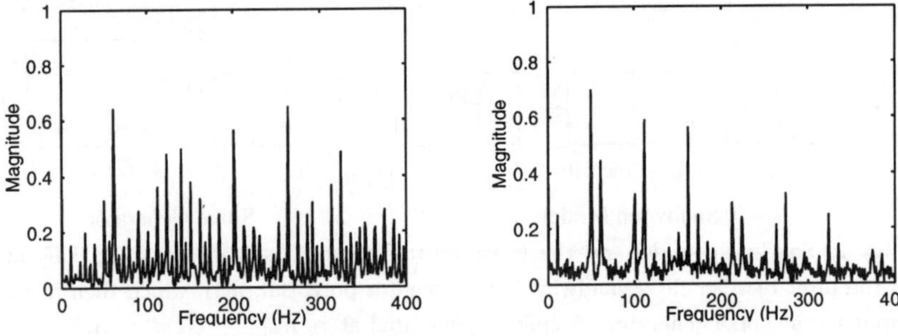

Fig. 5: DFT of the PSTH for the example considered in Fig. 4. In **Fig.** 6 we have displayed the PSTH's DFT for a BP fiber (BF 1240 Hz); $x(t)$ had frequencies $\approx$ 1350 Hz, 1400 Hz, and 1461 Hz; amplitudes and phases were the same (see Fig. 4).

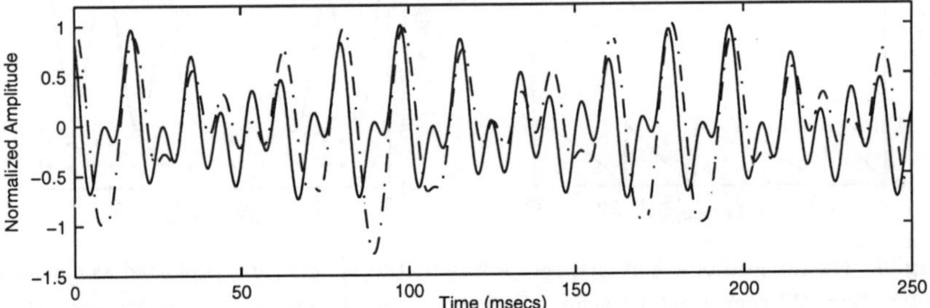

Fig. 7: For the example considered in Fig. 4 (BF 127 Hz), the reconstructed ac receptor potential, $g_{ac}(t)$, is shown by a solid line; ac portion of $x(t)$'s envelope (magnitude of its analytic version) is displayed as a dashed-dotted line. The ITMF algorithm was fed with frequencies 11 Hz, 50 Hz, 61 Hz and 111 Hz.

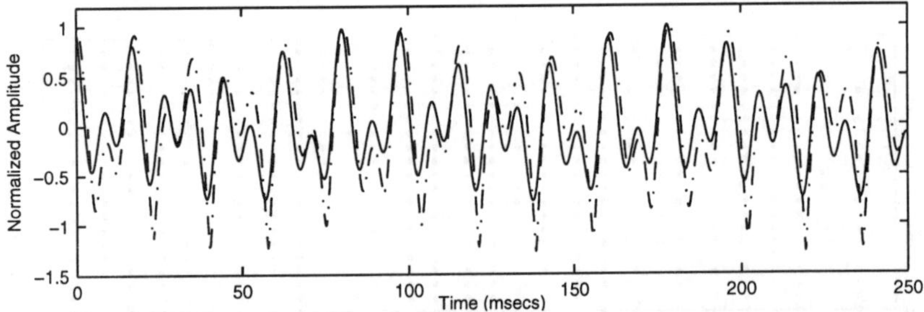

Fig. 8: Another example (BF 122 Hz) is considered. $x(t)$ had same frequencies (150, 200 and 261 Hz); amplitudes were -7, -6, and 0 dB respectively.

ESTIMATING SCALING EXPONENTS IN AUDITORY-NERVE SPIKE TRAINS USING FRACTAL MODELS INCORPORATING REFRACTORINESS

S.B. LOWEN

Department of Electrical and Computer Engineering
44 Cummington Street
Boston University, Boston, MA 02215
lowen@bu.edu

M.C. TEICH

Department of Electrical and Computer Engineering
Department of Biomedical Engineering
44 Cummington Street
Boston University, Boston, MA 02215
teich@bu.edu

Fractal stochastic point processes (FSPPs) provide good mathematical models for long-term correlations present in auditory-nerve fibers in a number of species. Simulations and analytical results for FSPPs concur with experimental data over long times. Refractoriness-modified Poisson point processes, in contrast, model only the short-term characteristics of these data. FSPPs incorporating refractoriness yield superior results over all time scales, and analytical results for the statistics of this model agree closely with both computer simulations and auditory data. Furthermore, these processes provide a superior method for estimating the fractal exponent α, which parametrizes the long-term correlation found in these recordings.

1 Introduction

Certain random phenomena are well described by essentially identical events occurring at discrete times. One example is the registration of action potentials recorded by an electrode near an auditory-nerve fiber [3,16,17]. A (one-dimensional) stochastic point process is a mathematical construction which represents these events as random points on a line. Such a process may be called fractal when a number of the relevant statistics exhibit scaling with related scaling exponents, indicating that the represented phenomenon contains clusters of points over a relatively large set of time scales [11,5,6,7].

The power spectral density (PSD) and the Allan factor (AF) are two statistics which reveal this clustering [7,9,1]. The PSD $S(\omega)$ for a point process, as for continuous-time processes, provides a measure of how power is concentrated as a function of the angular frequency ω. The Allan factor $A(T)$, is defined as the ratio of the Allan variance of the event count in a specified time window

"

T to twice the mean count. The Allan variance, in turn, is the variance of the *difference* between the numbers of counts in adjacent windows of duration T. For an FSPP, over a large range of times and frequencies, it can be shown that [7,9,1]

$$
\begin{aligned}
\text{PSD:} \quad & S(\omega)/\lambda & \approx & \quad 1 + (\omega/\omega_0)^{-\alpha} \\
\text{AF:} \quad & A(T) & \approx & \quad 1 + (T/T_0)^{\alpha},
\end{aligned}
\tag{1}
$$

with λ the average rate of the process, $\alpha > 0$ the fractal exponent, ω_0 a cutoff frequency, T_0 a cutoff time, and $\omega_0^{\alpha} T_0^{\alpha} = (2 - 2^{\alpha}) \cos(\pi\alpha/2)\Gamma(\alpha+2)$ [9,10]. Thus in this mathematical formalism, the fractal exponent α can assume values in excess of unity, as sometimes occurs in auditory recordings [9].

The homogeneous Poisson point process (HPP) is perhaps the simplest stochastic point process, being fully characterized by a single constant quantity, its rate. It is not fractal, but serves as a building block for other point processes which can be. With the inclusion of refractoriness (dead- and sick-time effects), the refractoriness-modified Poisson point process (RM-P) [14,12,15] proves successful in modeling auditory-nerve spike trains over short time scales. With fixed and exponentially distributed [20] random refractoriness together [15], the RM-P predicts an interevent-interval histogram (IIH) of the form

$$
p(t) = \begin{cases} \lambda(1 - \lambda r)^{-1} \left\{ \exp[-\lambda(t - f)] - \exp[-(t - f)/r] \right\} & \text{for } t > f \\ 0 & \text{for } t \leq f. \end{cases}
\tag{2}
$$

where λ is the original rate of events (before refractory effects), f is the portion of the refractory period that is fixed, and r is the mean of the random component.

However, the accurate modeling of the self-similar or fractal behavior observed in sensory-system neural spike trains over long times requires a fractal stochastic point process [16,13,17,4,18,2,9]. A number of FSPP models have been developed [7]; we focus on a particular process, the fractal-Gaussian-noise-driven Poisson process (FGNDP) [7]. The FGNDP is important because Gaussian processes are ubiquitous, well understood, and are completely described by their means and autocovariance functions. Thus only three parameters (including the rate) are required to specify an FGNDP, since, like all FSPPs, it follows Eq. 1. The FGNDP describes the firing patterns of primary auditory afferents quite well over long time scales (several hundred milliseconds and larger) [17], although it does not accurately model neural activity over short time scales. Therefore procedures for estimating the fractal exponent α based on a simple FSPP formalism that ignores refractoriness, such as a least-squares fit to the logarithm of Eq. 1, necessarily yield biased results. The parameter α plays a crucial role in characterizing the auditory-nerve fiber recordings, since this single quantity describes the long-term correlations present in such recordings, and the singularity near zero frequency in the PSD [9].

2 Models Incorporating Refractoriness and Fractal Behavior

Incorporating refractory effects into the fractal behavior of the FGNDP yields the refractoriness-modified version (RM-FGNDP), a new model which does indeed mimic auditory-nerve behavior over all time and frequency scales [8]. Figure 1 shows the AF obtained from a recording of an auditory-nerve fiber under spontaneous conditions (solid curve), and from a single simulation of the RM-FGNDP process (dashed curve). All recordings used in this paper were obtained from one cat auditory afferent fiberhe cat, with a spontaneous rate of 75 spikes/sec, and a characteristic frequency (CF) of 3926 Hz. (Data collection and minimal subsequent processing methods are described in Ref. 9 and references therein.) The two curves agree within the limits imposed by fluctuations inherent in a finite data length; agreement also obtains for other statistics such as the IIH, not shown. Evidently, simulations of the RM-FGNDP process mimic auditory-nerve-fiber data well. Simulations of non-fractal models, in contrast, exhibit AF curves which never exceed unity, and thus are not suitable as models of auditory-nerve firing behavior. Conversely, simulations of

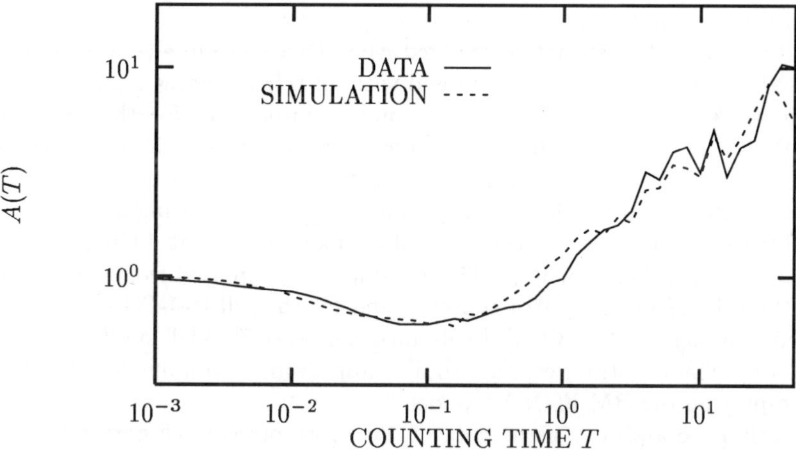

Figure 1: Doubly logarithmic plot of the Allan factor (AF) for auditory-nerve-fiber data recorded under spontaneous conditions (solid curve), and for a simulation of the RM-FGNDP process with parameters chosen to fit the data (dashed curve).

non-refractory models exhibit AF curves which never dip below unity, while those of the data always do.

Fortuitously, for the parameter ranges employed in modeling these spike trains, the effects of the fractal fluctuations are minimal over the time scales where refractoriness dominates, and vice versa; thus these two effects may be decoupled in the modeling procedure. In particular, the IIH plots for the full RM-FGNDP theory, the non-fractal RM-P models, and the data all resemble each other closely.

The AF and PSD for the RM-FGNDP, in contrast, do differ appreciably from those of both the (non-fractal) RM-P and (non-refractory) FGNDP models. We have developed new analytical formulas for these quantities in the presence of generalized refractoriness (including both fixed and exponentially distributed random components) [10], and provide two key results below. For steady-state (equilibrium) counting [12], and for $T \gg f, r$, the AF assumes the form, over all counting times:

$$A(T) \approx \frac{6a^2 + 4a^3 + a^4 + \lambda^2 r^2 (6 - \lambda^2 r^2) - 4\lambda^3 r^3 (1 + \lambda f)}{4(1 + a)^3 \lambda T} + (1 + a)^3 (T/T_0)^\alpha,$$

(3)

with $a \equiv \lambda(f + r)$ [10]; the PSD assumes the form

$$S(\omega) \approx \lambda \left[\frac{1 + \lambda^2 r^2}{(1 + a)^3} + (\omega/\omega_0)^{-\alpha} \right]$$

(4)

for equilibrium counting in the range $\omega \ll 1/f, 1/r$ [10].

Figure 2 provides estimated averaged Allan Factors from a typical simulated FGNDP with $\alpha = 0.5$, both with and without refractoriness (solid curves). Also shown are fits from Eq. 1 for the upper curve, and for the full RM-FGNDP (Eq. 3) model for the lower curve (dashed curves). Both theoretical results match their respective simulations extremely well, particularly at the longer counting times which prove most important in estimating α.

Table I shows the results from a number of simulations at different design values of the fractal exponent α. These results are estimated from the simple FGNDP model of Eq. 1 (fourth column), and for the full RM-FGNDP model with refractoriness of Eq. 3 (third column). The RM-FGNDP model yields a much more reliable estimate of α. Similar improvement obtains for the PSD when employing the RM-FGNDP model [10].

Returning to auditory-nerve data, in Fig. 3 we present AF curves for two stimulus levels: spontaneous firing (no stimulus) as shown in Fig. 1, and +40 db:re threshold at CF. Also shown are the predictions of Eq. 3, obtained from a least-squares fit of the logarithm of the AFs. For the upper and lower experimental data curves, the estimated fractal exponents of these firing patterns

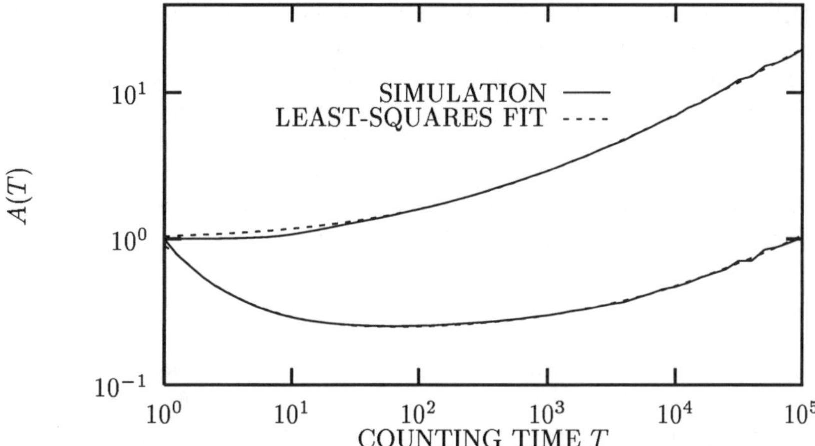

Figure 2: Doubly logarithmic plot of the averaged Allan factor (AF) for simulations of the RM-FGNDP process, with $\lambda = 1$, $\alpha = 0.5$, and $N = 100$ simulations. Upper curves: $f = r = 0$ for simulation (solid curve) and fit from Eq. 1 (dashed curve). Lower curves: $f = r = 1$ for simulation (solid curve) and fit from Eq. 3 (dashed curve).

are $\alpha = 0.71$ and $\alpha = 1.5$, respectively. These are indeed substantially larger than the values $\alpha = 0.48$ $\alpha = 0.96$ obtained without taking refractoriness into account [9]. Within limits imposed by a finite data size, predictions of the RM-

SIMULATION		ESTIMATION	
Fractal Exp.	Refract.	Eq. 3 Bias	Eq. 1 Bias
$\alpha = 0.5$	none	-0.002	-0.046
$\alpha = 0.5$	$f = r = 1$	+0.016	-0.156
$\alpha = 1.0$	none	-0.012	-0.027
$\alpha = 1.0$	$f = r = 1$	-0.015	-0.058
$\alpha = 1.5$	none	-0.019	-0.035
$\alpha = 1.5$	$f = r = 1$	-0.027	-0.090

Table 1: Bias in estimates of the fractal exponent α obtained from the averaged Allan factor (AF) for simulations of the RM-FGNDP process. For all table entries, $\lambda = 1$ and $N = 100$ simulations. Results are reported for three values of α (0.5, 1.0, and 1.5), both with ($f = r = 1$) and without ($f = r = 0$) refractoriness. Bias is calculated by a least-squares fit of the logarithm of the averaged simulated AF plots to the logarithm of Eq. 3, for ten values of the counting time T per decade in the range $10^3 \leq T \leq 10^5$ (left bias column); and to Eq. 1 in the range $10^4 \leq T \leq 10^5$ (right column).

FGNDP model closely follow the AF for the experimental data over all time scales. The PSD predicted by the RM-FGNDP model also accords with that of the data over all frequency scales, as do all other statistics examined to date.

Finally, a similar process, based on a gamma renewal process instead of a Poisson substrate, appears to provide an excellent fit to data collected from neurons in the visual system of the cat, using these same statistics[19]. Thus theoretical results obtained for this process will likely provide a superior method for estimating the fractal exponent of these neurons.

3 Conclusion

Over all time scales, analytical predictions of the refractoriness-modified fractal-Gaussian-noise-driven Poisson point process model, with fixed and stochastic refractory periods together, match statistics of experimental data collected from cat auditory-nerve fibers, and of computer simulations of this process. This model therefore provides the best method known to date for estimating the fractal exponent α of neural recordings.

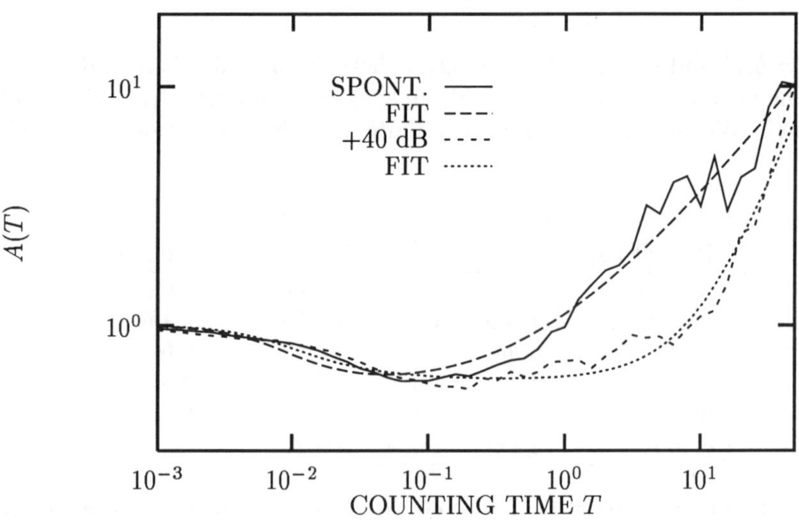

Figure 3: Doubly logarithmic plot of the Allan factor (AF) plot for auditory data (unit L-19, with CF = 3926 Hz, threshold = 19.3 dB SPL, and spontaneous firing rate = 75 spikes/sec.). Upper curves: spontaneous firing conditions (solid curve) and analytical fit from Eq. 3 (long-dashed curve). Lower curves: stimulus applied at CF at +40 dB:re threshold (short-dashed curve) and analytical fit from Eq. 3 (dotted curve).

Acknowledgments

Supported by the Whitaker Foundation under Grant No. CU01455801 and by the Office of Naval Research under Grant No. N00014-92-J-1251.

References

1. Feurstein, M. *et al.*, in preparation.
2. Kelly, O.E. *et al.* (1996) Fractal noise strength in auditory-nerve fiber recordings. *J. Acoust. Soc. Am.* **99** 2210-2220.
3. Kiang, N.Y-S. *et al.* (1965) *Discharge Patterns of Single Fibers in the Cat's Auditory Nerve,* Res. Monogr. No. 35 (MIT, Cambridge, MA).
4. Kumar, A.R. and Johnson, D.H. (1993) Analyzing and modeling fractal intensity point processes. *J. Acoust. Soc. Am.* **93** 3365.
5. Lowen, S.B. and Teich, M.C. (1991) Doubly stochastic Poisson point process driven by fractal shot noise. *Phys. Rev.* A **43** 4192–4215.
6. Lowen, S.B. and Teich, M.C. (1993) Fractal renewal processes generate $1/f$ noise. *Phys. Rev.* E **47** 992–1001.
7. Lowen, S.B. and Teich, M.C. (1995) Estimation and simulation of fractal stochastic point processes. *Fractals* **3** 183–210.
8. Lowen, S.B. and Teich, M.C. (1996) Refractoriness-modified fractal stochastic point processes for modeling sensory-system spike trains. in *Computational Neuroscience,* ed J.M. Bower (Academic, New York), pp. 447-452.
9. Lowen, S.B. and Teich, M.C. (1996) The periodogram and Allan variance reveal fractal exponents greater than unity in auditory-nerve spike trains. *J. Acoust. Soc. Am.* **99** 3585–3591.
10. Lowen, S.B. (1996), Refractoriness-modified Doubly Stochastic Poisson Point Process. *CTR Technical Report* **449-96-15** (Columbia Univ., New York).
11. B.B. Mandelbrot (1983) *The Fractal Geometry of Nature* (Freeman, New York).
12. Müller, J.W. (1974) Some formulae for a dead-time-distorted Poisson process. *Nucl. Inst. Meth.* **117** 401–404.
13. Powers, N.L. and Salvi, R.J. (1992) Comparison of discharge rate fluctuations in the auditory nerve of chickens and chinchillas. in *Abstracts of the Fifteenth Midwinter Research Meeting of the Association for Research in Otolaryngology,* ed D.J. Lim (Association for Research in Otolaryngology, Des Moines, IA), Abstract 292, p. 101.

14. Ricciardi, L.M. and Esposito, F. (1966) On some distribution functions for non-linear switching elements with finite dead time. *Kybernetik* **3** 148–152.
15. Teich, M.C. *et al.* (1978) Refractoriness in the maintained discharge of the cat's retinal ganglion cell. *J. Opt. Soc. Am.* **68** 386–402.
16. Teich, M.C. (1989) Fractal character of the auditory neural spike train. *IEEE Trans. Biomed. Eng.* **36** 150–160.
17. Teich, M.C. (1992) Fractal neuronal firing patterns. in *Single Neuron Computation*, ed. T. McKenna *et al.* (Academic, Boston), pp. 589–625.
18. Teich, M.C. and Lowen, S.B. (1994) *IEEE Eng. Med. Biol. Mag.* **13** 197–202.
19. Teich, M.C. *et al.* (1996) Fractal character of the neural spike train in the visual system of the cat. *J. Opt. Soc. Am.* **A** in press.
20. Young, E.D. and Barta, P.E. (1986) Rate responses of auditory nerve fibers to tones in noise near masked threshold. *J. Acoust. Soc. Am.* **79** 426–442.

ALL-POLE MODELS OF AUDITORY FILTERING

R.F. LYON

Apple Computer, Inc., One Infinite Loop
Cupertino, CA 94022 USA
lyon@apple.com

The all-pole gammatone filter (APGF), which we derive by discarding the zeros from the popular gammatone filter (GTF), and the related all-pole filter cascade (APFC) provide models of auditory filtering with simple parameterization and useful properties. Compared to the GTF, these all-pole models offer fewer parameters, a more controlled behavior of the tuning-curve tail, and an easier way to model level-dependent gain, bandwidth, asymmetry, and center-frequency (CF) shift. The order-N APGF is the Nth power of a filter with one complex-conjugate pair of poles; the GTF has this same set of poles, but, in addition, has spurious zeros on the real axis that complicate its description and behavior. Since the APGF is the Nth power of a simple pole-pair filter, many of its properties—such as gain, bandwidth, delay, and dispersion—are easy to compute as analytic functions of the parameters, which may be tied to sound level or to output power level. Good approximate and empirical results extend these functions to the APFC, which is an efficient tapped filter-cascade structure that has a mathematical link to an underlying traveling-wave structure via the Liouville–Green (or WKB) approximation. Fixing the all-pole filter's tail gain, rather than fixing the peak gain, as we vary parameters with sound level, allows us to construct more realistic models of how the auditory system behaves across levels, emphasizing approximate linearity at low frequencies; variation in the damping parameter of the poles can then be interpreted in terms of automatic gain control near CF. The APGF and APFC represent two steps from the popular GTF toward more flexible, realistic, physically grounded, and efficiently implemented models of auditory filtering.

1 Models of Auditory Filtering

Models of auditory filtering are useful tools for understanding, describing, and emulating experiments in auditory mechanics, auditory physiology, and auditory psychophysics. Linear time-invariant lumped-parameter models (rational transfer functions) form a useful class of filters on which to build, even when we are modeling nonlinear and time-varying properties of the auditory system. The gammatone filter (GTF) is a simple and easily parameterized member of this class that has been used in models of mechanics, psychophysics, and physiology. By contrast, the rounded exponential (roex) filters that are often used in such models are not members of this class, since there is no known phase response that makes the transfer function into a rational function (ratio of polynomials) in the Laplace transform domain; roex filters therefore cannot be implemented as circuits.

In this paper, we consider a further restriction to the class of easily parameterized *all-pole* filter models. We show that the GTF has zeros (i.e., the numerator in its rational transfer function is not a scalar, but rather is a polynomial, whose roots are the zero locations), and that by removing them we arrive at the all-pole gammatone filter (APGF), which has improved properties for auditory modeling.

The GTF and APGF of order N have N coincident poles at a complex-conjugate pair of locations in the Laplace transform's s plane. Relaxing this constraint of coincident poles, we consider filters whose poles are in differing locations, and particularly filterbanks made up of cascades of two-pole filters with progressively varying pole locations—the all-pole filter cascade (APFC). These filters are closely related to wave-propagation models of the underlying cochlear mechanics, and form a bridge between cochlear-mechanics models and the auditory-filter models used in psychophysics and physiology.

Filters with zeros are still of interest, as well, but zeros need to be considered carefully as targeted modifications of all-pole filters, rather than to be accepted as ill-behaved interference effects—as they are in the GTF.

2   Gammatone Filters With and Without Zeros

The GTF and the APGF are closely related auditory-filter models, sharing a complex conjugate pair of order-N poles. The GTF also has N zeros on the real axis in the s plane, inherited from its defining impulse response via the Laplace transform. We define the APGF is defined by discarding those zeros, making it an all-pole filter.

We describe the APGF in terms of its Laplace transform $H(s)$. For conciseness, let the s-plane pole positions be given by the complex number p and its conjugate p^*. Then the APGF is given by:

$$H_{AP}(s) = \frac{K}{[(s-p)(s-p^*)]^N} \tag{1}$$

where K is a constant that we will normally adjusted to give unity gain at DC: $H(0) = 1$. In terms of the Cartesian parameterization of complex pole position $p = -b + i\omega_r$ (as typically used with the GTF), the APGF becomes

$$H_{AP}(s) = \frac{b^2 + \omega_r^2}{[(s+b)^2 + \omega_r^2]^N} \tag{2}$$

The GTF impulse response $g(t) = t^{N-1}\exp(-bt)\cos(\omega_r t + \phi)$—a gamma distribution times a tone—transforms to a rational transfer function with the same poles as the APGF, but with a complicated numerator with N real roots:

$$H_{GT}(s) = \frac{e^{i\phi}[s+b+i\omega_r]^N + e^{-i\phi}[s+b-i\omega_r]^N}{[(s+b)^2 + \omega_r^2]^N} \tag{3}$$

The roots of the numerator—the zeros of the GTF—fall on the real axis in the s plane, at locations that depend on all the parameters. By varying the phase or bandwidth parameters, we can make a zero fall exactly at $s = 0$, so the tail gain can go to zero for particular parameter values.

The differentiated APGF (DAPGF) also has the same poles, and one zero at DC (a numerator factor of s, or differentiator); thus, it is closely related to both the APGF and the GTF:

$$H_D(s) = \frac{Ks}{[(s+b)^2 + \omega_r^2]^N} \tag{4}$$

On a continuum between the APGF and the DAPGF is the one-zero gammatone filter (OZGF), in which the generalized numerator $K(s + \omega_z)$ has *one zero* anywhere on the real axis. We can convert a GTF of any phase to an OZGF by discarding all but one of its zeros.

The GTF and DAPGF, in the form of Laplace transform transfer functions of order $N = 3$, were first used by Flanagan to model basilar membrane motion.[1] Slaney analyzed the GTF and APGF Laplace transforms, including the zeros of the GTF.[2]

Figure 1 shows typical GTF, APGF, and DAPGF transfer functions; Figure 2 shows the corresponding impulse responses. Note that the GTF tail gain depends on the phase parameter (in a complicated interaction with the bandwidth and order parameters), whereas the tails of the APGF and DAPGF are fixed, independent of any other parameters.

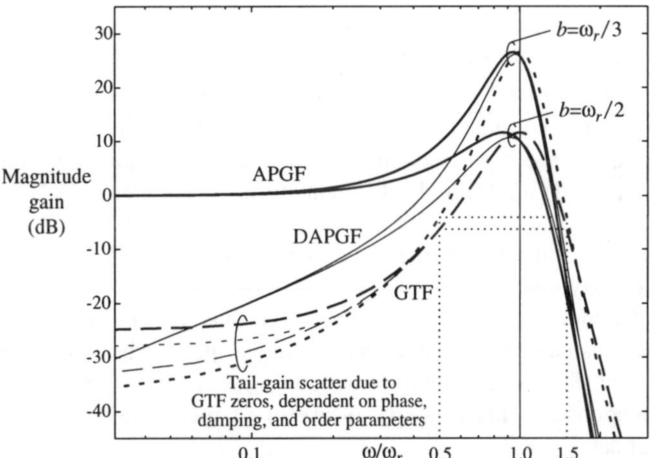

Figure 1: Comparison of GTF, APGF, and DAPGF transfer functions ($N = 6$) for two different values of the real part of the pole location. Dotted lines show the symmetry of the GTF at $f = 1 \pm 0.5$. Each GTF is shown with two phases (0 and $\pi/2$, heavy and light dashed lines, respectively). Notice that the ordering of gain near the peak is not maintained in the tail. The variation in the GTF tail is not accounted for by the usual phase-independent symmetric GTF approximation.

Since the APGF is just the Nth power of the well-studied two-pole filter, its properties—e. g., bandwidth, center frequency (CF), delay, and dispersion—are easy to express analytically. A useful alternative parameterization is that of Q and natural frequency of pole position (QNF parameterization), with $\omega_n^2 = \omega_r^2 + b^2$ and $Q = b/(2\omega_n)$, in which variation of the nondimensional Q or damping factor $1/(2Q)$ models a physical change of damping.

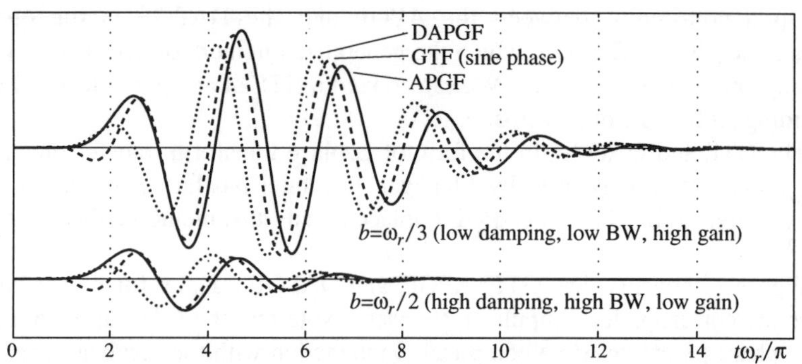

Figure 2: Impulse responses of the APGF, DAPGF, and sine-phase GTF from Figure 1. Note that the GTF's zero crossings are equally spaced in time, while those of the APGF and DAPGF are stretched out in the early cycles.

The magnitude of the GTF transfer function is almost exactly symmetric about a CF of ω_r. In contrast, the APGF and DAPGF are asymmetric (more in line with auditory reality) and have a CF somewhat below ω_r. At low frequencies, the APGF gain is nearly constant (near unity), so we say that it has a *flat* low-frequency tail. The gain of the high-frequency tail, by contrast, falls very rapidly with frequency. The DAPGF, due to the differentiator, has zero gain at DC and a slope of 6 dB per octave at low frequencies, so we say that it has a *sloping* low-frequency tail. Its passband and high-frequency tail are much like the APGF's, although the DAPGF is less asymmetric.

The APGF and DAPGF variants of the GTF thus have the advantage that their transfer functions can have a parameter-dependent passband gain, to implement a level-dependent nonlinearity, while maintaining a fixed tail gain, or linear low-frequency response. This property is useful in modeling psychophysical and physiological data.

3   Filter Cascades

A cascade filterbank is a natural approximate model, via the Liouville–Green (or WKB) method, of the distributed filtering in a nonuniform wave-propagation medium such as the cochlea.[3] Local complex wavenumber solutions allow us to design filters to match the gain and phase of a small section of the cochlea for forward-propagating waves of any frequency. A cascade of such filters can simultaneously compute the filtered model output at a large number of places, or taps, corresponding to a set of characteristic frequencies in a filterbank.

If each filter in such a cascade filterbank is an all-pole filter, then, at every tap, the composite transfer function from the input through all the stages up to that tap is an all-pole transfer function.

The simplest all-pole filter stage that leads to a pseudoresonant response is a two-pole filter, and the resulting APFC is very closely related to the APGF. The differences are that the poles are not coincident, and that each successive tap response has a higher order. The APFC's transfer functions are not quite as sharp and asymmetric as those of the APGF, due to the pole positions being distributed. Figure 3 compares typical APFC (one tap of a filter cascade) and APGF transfer-function magnitudes.

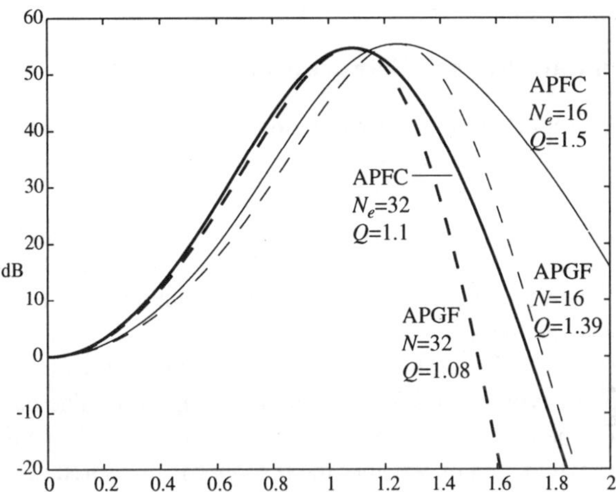

Figure 3: Comparison of APGF and APFC transfer functions. The frequency axis is labeled in units of the tap natural frequency, and parameters are noted in term of pole Q. The APFC needs a large number of stages per factor of e frequency change (N_e) to approximate the APGF shape.

4 Asymmetric Auditory Filters

The APGF is similar in result to Irino's *gammachirp* filter (GCF), which was derived from time–scale optimality but inspired by the need for an asymmetric variant of the GTF.[4] The GCF adds a free parameter to the GTF, controlling how much of a log-time term is added to the phase of the tone:

$$g(t) = t^{N-1} \exp(-bt)\cos(\omega_r t + \phi + c\ln t) \tag{5}$$

The result is a controllable asymmetry that can be zero or of either sign. The APGF, DAPGF, and APFC, on the other hand, have an inherent asymmetry that depends on the pole positions, but have no additional parameters. For auditory filters, the degree of asymmetry seems to be reasonable; we have not done careful fitting yet. Of course, with the extra degree of freedom, the GCF always will be able to provide a closer fit to asymmetry data than can the simpler all-pole models.

The log-time term (with negative c, for the proper sign of asymmetry) corresponds to an instantaneous frequency that starts low and rises hyperbolically to approach the ringing frequency. A similar chirp effect has been pointed out in physiological data,[5] and can also be seen in the instantaneous frequency calculated from an APGF impulse response.

The GCF does not have the linear low-frequency tail, as parameters are varied, that characterizes the all-pole filters—it inherits the GTF's tail sensitivity to parameters (whether the GCF has a rational transfer function is not presently clear, so we cannot claim that it inherits the GTF's zeros).

5 Wide-Dynamic-Range Compression

One of the most important nonlinear functions of the cochlea is its compression of a wide range of sound intensities into a narrower range of cochlear motion intensities at the sensor array, for frequencies near CF (while maintaining near linearity for lower frequencies, and not enough gain to measure at higher frequencies). Studies of cochlear mechanical response since about 1970 have repeatedly demonstrated this frequency-dependent compression in live cochleas, and its absence in dead cochleas.[6]

In live cochleas, the overall input–output intensity curves for frequencies near CF have a slope of typically 0.25 to 0.5 on a log-log plot. The exact slope of this compression nonlinearity depends on the preparation, on the frequency and intensity range to a lesser extent, and on whether the response is measured at a fixed frequency or at the frequency of greatest response, which shifts slightly with level.

Since a wave picks up energy as it travels across a range of places, each little increment of place needs to contribute only a small amount of gain. If the filter cascade model has stages that model small place increments, each filter will need to contribute only a small gain; as the overall gain changes, each filter will have to change only slightly. Similarly, each pole in an APGF will need only a small Q change to effect a large overall gain change.

There are two general forms of compressive nonlinearity that are important to consider, and it is likely that both operate in the real cochlea: instantaneous nonlinear distortion, and feedback parameter variation. For example, the nonlinear model of Kim and associates is actually an APFC with a compressive nonlinearity in each stage;[7] Kim's later suggestions incorporate parameter feedback.[8]

6   Conclusions

Removing the zeros from the popular GTF to make the APGF improves its applicability to auditory modeling in two ways: by decoupling a linear low-frequency tail from the variable-gain peak, and by adding a moderate asymmetry correlated with realistic group-delay dispersion or chirping.

The APFC is an all-pole model, related to, but slightly generalized from, the APGF, that uses noncoincident poles to two advantages: efficient realization of a whole bank of filters in one structure, and an analytic link to underlying wave-propagation models of cochlear filtering.

These all-pole structures provide a natural coupling among gain, bandwidth, and CF shift as we vary one parameter to model a level-dependent nonlinearity in the cochlea.

Acknowledgments

I thank Roy Patterson and Egbert de Boer for encouraging the development of the APGF idea, Carver Mead for helping in the development of the APFC, and Malcolm Slaney for analyzing the gammatone's Laplace transform and zeros.

References

1. Flanagan, J.L. (1960). Models for approximating basilar membrane displacement, *Bell Sys. Tech. J.* **39** 1163–1191.
2. Slaney, M. (1993). An efficient implementation of the Patterson-Holdsworth auditory filter bank, Apple Computer TR #35, Cupertino, CA.
3. Lyon, R.F. and Mead, C.A. (1988) An analog electronic Cochlea, *IEEE Trans. ASSP* **36** 1119–1134.
4. Irino, T. (1996). A 'gammachirp' function as an optimal auditory filter with the Mellin transform, *IEEE ICASSP-96,* Atlanta, 981–984.
5. Møller, A.R. and Nilsson, H.G. (1979) Inner ear impulse response and basilar membrane modelling, *Acustica* **41** 258–262.
6. Rhode, W.S. (1971) Observations of the vibration of the basilar membrane in squirrel monkeys using the Mössbauer technique, *J. Acoust. Soc. Am.* **49** 1218–1231.
7. Kim, D.O., Molnar, C.E., Pfeiffer, R.R. (1973) A system of nonlinear differential equations modeling basilar-membrane motion, *J. Acoust. Soc. Am.* **54** 1517–1529.
8. Kim, D.O. (1986) Active and nonlinear biomechanics and the role of outer-hair-cell subsystem in the mammalian auditory system, *Hear. Res.* **22** 105–114.

CHANGES IN PHASE-LOCKING TO COMPLEX STIMULI PRODUCED BY NOISE-INDUCED HEARING LOSS

E.D. YOUNG, R.L. MILLER, J.C. WONG AND J.R. SCHILLING

*Dept. of Biomedical Engineering and Center for Hearing Sciences, Johns Hopkins Univ.
Baltimore, MD 21205 USA   eyoung@bme.jhu.edu*

Phase-locking of auditory nerve fibers to the vowel /ɛ/ was studied in normal cats and in cats with a noise-induced hearing loss. Fibers in the noise-exposed cats showed elevated thresholds, broadened tuning, and loss of two-tone rate suppression. In normal cats, phase-locking of fibers with best frequencies (BFs) near the second formant showed narrowband responses to components near BF at low levels ($\approx$ 50 dB), synchrony capture by the second formant at intermediate levels ($\approx$70 dB), and broadband responses to harmonics between the first and third formants at high levels ($\approx$ 90 dB). Fibers in exposed animals showed only the broadband response. The results are interpreted in terms of cochlear models.

1 Introduction

Studies of auditory nerve (AN) responses in cochleas damaged by noise or ototoxic antibiotics have been a historically important source of information about the function of inner (IHC) and outer (OHC) hair cells.[2,10,12,19,22] In the AN, OHC damage leads to elevated thresholds and broadened tuning, whereas IHC damage leads to a uniform threshold elevation.[9,11,13] In addition, two-tone rate suppression has been reported to be weakened or abolished in damaged cochleas.[3,22] However, the properties of the damaged cochlea in response to more natural broadband stimuli have been studied only to a limited extent.[4,16] This is unfortunate since these responses can provide useful information about cochlear nonlinearities and can provide guidance in the design of hearing aids.

This paper describes the properties of AN responses to vowel stimuli in cats exposed to acoustic trauma. We show that these responses are similar to responses in the normal (unexposed) cochlea at high sound levels.

2 Methods

Ten cats were used as normal controls and nine cats were exposed to acoustic trauma (110-115 dB SPL free-field noise bands, 50 Hz bandwidth, centered at 2 kHz, for two hours, followed by >44 days recovery). For single unit recording, cats were anesthetized (0.2 mg xylazine and 200 mg ketamine im followed by sodium pentobarbital, $\approx$12 mg/hr iv). Single fibers were recorded in the auditory nerve using standard techniques.

For each fiber, a tuning curve, a measure of two-tone rate suppression, and responses to the vowel /ɛ/, either alone or in the syllable /bɛʃ/, were taken. The vowel was periodic (F0=100 Hz) with formant frequencies F1=500 Hz, F2=1700 Hz, and F3=2500 Hz.

3 Results

Results are shown here for fibers with BFs near F2; these fibers show the phenomena of interest most clearly. A more complete description of the results has been reported elsewhere.[14]

3.1 Tuning curves and two-tone suppression

Figure 1 shows tuning curves of two fibers from normal unexposed cats and two fibers from exposed cats. The normal fibers have low thresholds and tuning within the range normally seen. The exposed fibers have a threshold shift of 50-80 dB in the tip region and somewhat less in the tail region. Fibers with hypersensitive tails and W-shaped tuning curves[13] were not observed with our exposure. The likely nature of the hair cell damage can be inferred from previous studies in cats with similar exposures[11,13]. The threshold elevation in both tip and tail region and the loss of sharp tuning suggest that both IHCs and OHCs were damaged. In addition, relatively few AN fibers with BFs near 2 kHz were encountered in exposed animals, which suggests loss of IHCs leading to loss of response or perhaps degeneration of AN fibers.

Two-tone rate suppression was assessed by presenting excitor tones at BF at a fixed level (10 dB re threshold) simultaneously with suppressor tones at 1.2xBF or at 0.25xBF; the level of the suppressor tone was varied over a 50 dB range.[22] Responses were converted to fractional response (driven rate to the excitor+suppressor divided by driven rate to the excitor alone) and rate suppression was quantified

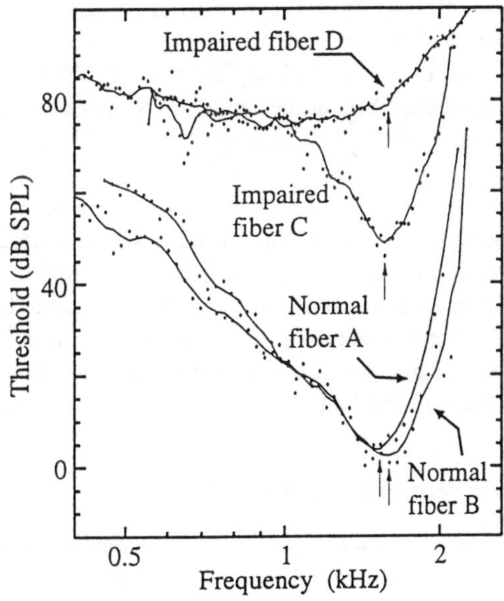

Fig. 1. Tuning curves from normal (A,B) and exposed (C,D) animals. Dots are thresholds and lines are smoothed versions of the dots. Vertical arrows mark the BFs; the exposed fibers' BFs were set at the edge of the steep high-frequency part of the curve.[9]

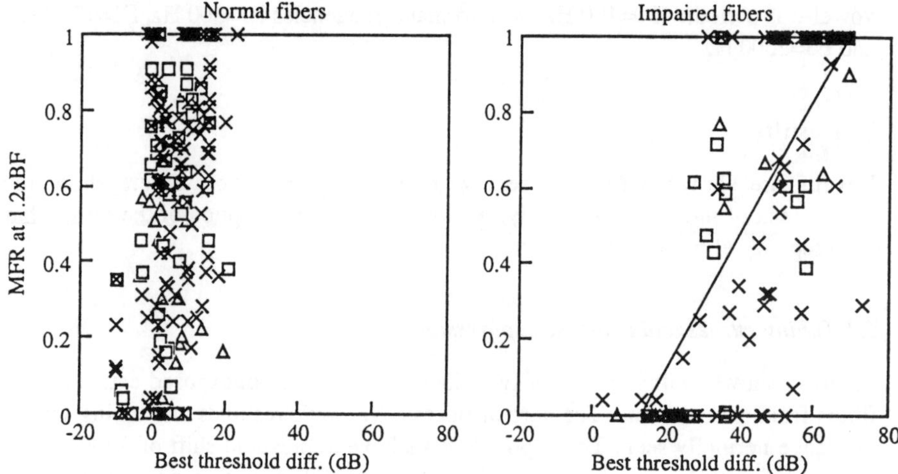

Fig. 2. Plots of MFR versus best threshold difference. Each symbol shows data for one fiber: triangles show low (≤1), squares show medium (>1, ≤18) and Xs show high (>18) spontaneous rate fibers. The suppressor is a tone at 1.2 x BF. Left, data from normal fibers; right, data from exposed fibers.

as the minimum of the fractional response curve (MFR or minimum fractional response). In the absence of suppression, MFR is 1; with complete suppression, MFR is 0.

Results for the above-BF suppressor are shown in Fig. 2, which plots MFR versus best threshold difference; the best threshold difference for each fiber is the shift, relative to the best threshold of Liberman's chamber-reared cats,[8] of the lowest threshold fibers at the same BF as the fiber. In this way, the threshold shift axis is a measure of the local damage to the cochlea; this measure is independent of BF and of variations in threshold related to spontaneous discharge rate. Data are shown in Fig. 2 only for fibers with BFs above 1 kHz because lower BF fibers show reduced rate suppression in normal animals. In the normal population in Fig. 2, the low and medium spontaneous rate fibers almost all show some suppression but many high spontaneous rate fibers show no suppression. In the exposed animals, there is a clear relationship between threshold shift and loss of two-tone rate suppression. The line is a regression line calculated from all the data (R=0.72). Similar results were observed for the below-BF suppressor, except that the effect is weaker (R=0.60).

3.2 Responses to the vowel

Figure 3 shows responses to the vowel at three sound levels for two normal fibers. At the lowest sound level (49 dB SPL), the fibers respond to a cluster of harmonics

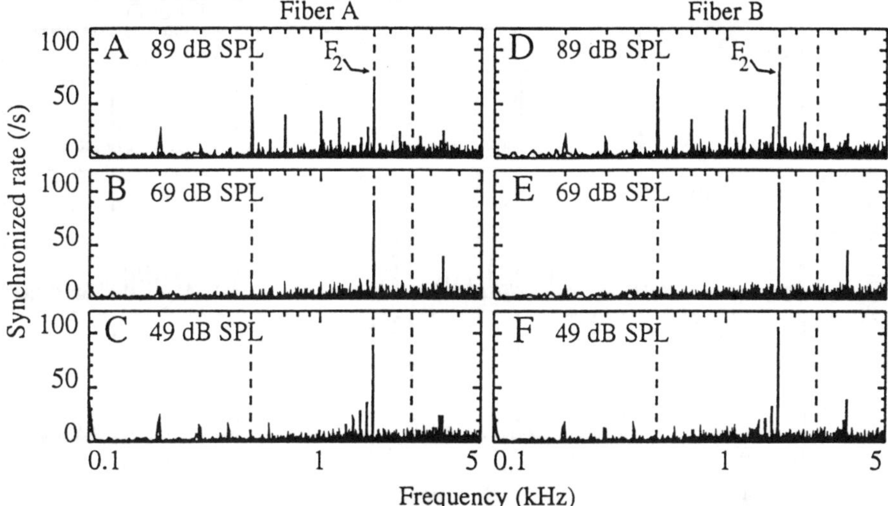

Fig. 3. Responses of fibers in unexposed cats to the vowel; each column shows data for one of the fibers whose tuning curves are shown in Fig. 1. Plots are synchronized rates, equal to the magnitudes of Fourier transforms of PST histograms of responses to the vowel. Dashed lines show the formant frequencies. Both fibers have BFs near the second formant.

near their BFs, which are near F2. The largest response is to F2 (1.7 kHz). Another cluster of response components appears near 3.4 kHz; these are distortion products generated by rectification in the hair-cell/AN fiber synapse.[23] At the intermediate level (69 dB), the fibers' responses are captured by F2, in that phase-locking is observed almost exclusively to F2 and its harmonics; responses to other harmonics are suppressed.

At the highest level (89 dB SPL), synchrony capture disappears and the response becomes quite broadband. Much of the change is due to the appearance of the F1 response. There are rectifier distortion products at the second harmonics of the formants (1 and 3.4 kHz) and at F2-F1 (1.2 kHz). In addition, there are several smaller components that cannot be accounted for by rectifier distortion; these represent a broadband response to many harmonics of the vowel. The broadband response at 89 dB SPL was observed in almost all fibers with BFs near F2 and F3.

The broadband response seen at high levels in normal fibers resembles the phase-locking seen at all levels in noise-damaged cochleas. Figure 4 shows responses to the vowel of two exposed fibers. Fiber C shows a broadband response at all three levels, which includes both F1 and F2, their distortion and intermodulation products, and some extra harmonics of the vowel. Fiber D shows a

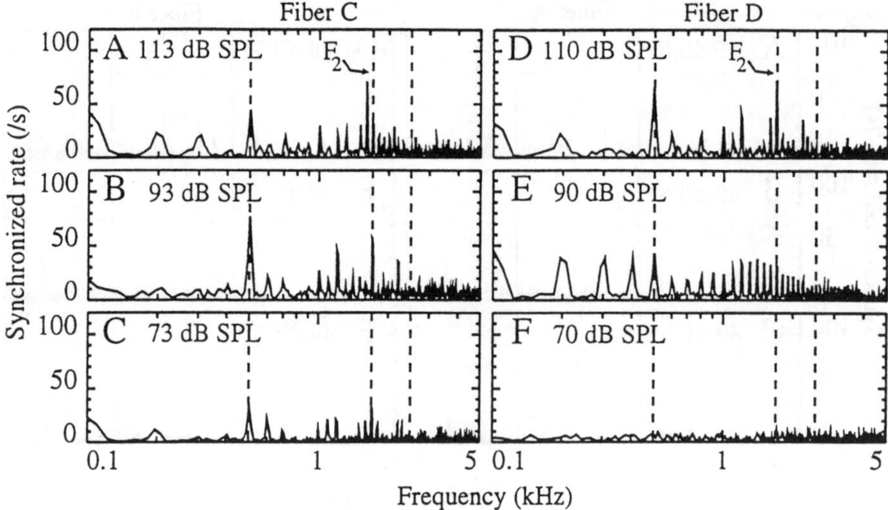

Fig. 4. Synchronized rates of responses of two exposed fibers (tuning curves in Fig. 1) to the vowel. Dashed lines show the formant frequencies of the stimulus.

similar response at the upper two levels, but is below threshold at the lowest level. Synchrony capture by F2 was not observed in exposed animals at any sound level.

4 Discussion

The resemblance between the phase-locking at high levels in normal fibers and the phase-locking at all levels in exposed fibers suggests that a common mechanism is operating in both cases; most likely this is loss of synchrony suppression.[7] The origin of the suppression is unclear, since synchrony suppression can occur through large-signal suppression in a non-linearity, such as the hair-cell/auditory nerve fiber synapse.[5] In a model consisting of a filter, a rectifying compressive nonlinearity, and a point-process spike generator,[1] phase-locking is determined by the filter shape, for a complex stimulus like our vowel. For a narrow filter centered on a formant frequency, phase-locking is observed only to the formant; for a broader filter that passes several harmonics, including two formants, a broad-band phase-locking like Figs. 3A, 3D, and 4 is seen. Thus with this model, the similarity in phase-locking between high levels in normal animals and all levels in exposed animals occurs because the basilar membrane filters are broad in both situations.[11,13,21]

Another possibility is that the responses at high levels in normals and the responses in exposed animals reflect component 2 responses of auditory nerve fibers.[12] However, the transition from component 1 to component 2 in normal animals is accompanied by a 180_ phase shift which is not observed in our data; that is, the phase of the F2 response in Fig. 3 is the same at 69 dB as it is at 89 dB.

We show a reduction in two-tone rate suppression in exposed animals (Fig. 2). It is tempting to speculate that there is a relationship between the loss of two-tone suppression and the loss of synchrony capture in exposed animals. From the discussion above, it is clear that such a relationship cannot be inferred directly from the data as presented. Nevertheless, there is an indirect relationship between the two sets of data. Two-tone synchrony suppression has been demonstrated in BM motion[15,18,20] and is similar to two-tone rate suppression.[20] Suppression at the BM level is thought to occur when the OHC receptor current saturates, so that the gain-enhancing effect of the OHCs is lost.[6,17] In noise-exposed cochleas, the OHCs are destroyed or damaged, which results in broadened tuning and weakening of cochlear suppression. Thus the loss of synchrony capture at high levels in normal animals and the lack of synchrony capture in exposed animals are both caused by loss of OHC function acting, at least in part, through the broadening of the cochlear filter.

Acknowledgments

This research was supported by NIDCD grant DC 00109. Kevin Franck participated in some experiments. Murray Sachs made valuable comments on the manuscript.

References

1. Carney, L.H. (1993) A model for the responses of low-frequency auditory-nerve fibers in cat. *J. Acoust. Soc. Am.* **93** 401-17.

2. Dallos, P. and Harris, D. (1978) Properties of auditory nerve responses in absence of outer hair cells, *J. Neurophysiol.* **41** 365-83.

3. Dallos, P., Harris, D.M., Relkin, E. and Cheatham, M.A. (1980) Two-tone suppression and intermodoulation distortion in the cochlea: Effect of outer hair cell lesions, in *Psychophysical, Physiological and Behavioral Studies in Hearing*, ed. G. van den Brink and F.A. Bilsen (Delft U. Press, Delft) pp. 242-252.

4. Geisler, C.D. (1989) The responses of models of auditory-nerve fibers in a damaged cochlea to speech syllables in noise, *J. Acoust. Soc. Am.* **86** 2192-205.

5. Geisler, C.D. and Greenberg, S. (1986) A two-stage nonlinear cochlear model possesses automatic gain control, *J. Acoust. Soc. Am.* **80** 1359-63.

6. Geisler, C.D., Yates, G.K., Patuzzi, R.B. and Johnstone, B.M. (1990) Saturation of outer hair cell receptor currents causes two-tone suppression, *Hearing Res.* **44** 241-56.

7. Javel, E. (1981) Suppression of auditory nerve responses I: temporal analysis, intensity effects and suppression contours, *J. Acoust. Soc. Am.* **69** 1735-45.

8. Liberman, M.C. (1978) Auditory-nerve response from cats raised in a low-noise chamber, *J. Acoust. Soc. Am.* **63** 442-55.

9. Liberman, M.C. (1984) Single-neuron labeling and chronic cochlear pathology. I. Threshold shift and characteristic-frequency shift, *Hearing Res.* **16** 33-41.

10. Liberman, M.C. and Beil, D.G. (1979) Hair cell condition and auditory nerve response in normal and noise-damaged cochleas, *Acta Otolaryngol.* **88** 161-76.

11. Liberman, M.C. and Dodds, L.W. (1984) Single-neuron labeling and chronic cochlear pathology. III. Stereocilia damage and alterations of threshold tuning curves, *Hearing Res.* **16** 55-74.

12. Liberman, M.C. and Kiang, N.Y. (1984) Single-neuron labeling and chronic cochlear pathology. IV. Stereocilia damage and alterations in rate- and phase-level functions, *Hearing Res.* **16** 75-90.

13. Liberman, M.C. and Mulroy, M.J. (1982) Acute and chronic effects of acoustic trauma: Cochlear pathology and auditory nerve pathophysiology, in *New Perspectives on Noise-Induced Hearing Loss*, ed. R.P. Hamernik, D. Henderson and R. Salvi (Raven Press, New York) pp. 105-135.

14. Miller, R.L., Schilling, J.R., Franck, K.R. and Young, E.D. (1996) Representation of the vowel /eh/ in the auditory nerve of cats with a noise-induced hearing loss. In: *Modeling Sensorineural Hearing Loss*, W. Jesteadt (Ed.), Erlbaum Assoc. (in press, 1996).

15. Nuttall, A.L. and Dolan, D.F. (1993) Two-tone suppression of inner hair cell and basilar membrane responses, *J. Acoust. Soc. Am.* **93** 390-400.

16. Palmer, A.R. and Moorjani, P.A. (1993) Responses to speech signals in the normal and pathological peripheral auditory system, *Prog Brain Res* **97** 107-15.

17. Patuzzi, R.B., Yates, G.K. and Johnstone, B.M. (1989) Outer hair cell receptor current and sensorineural hearing loss, *Hearing Res.* **42** 47-72.

18. Rhode, W.S. (1977) Some observations on two-tone interaction measured with the Mössbauer effect, in *Psychophysics and Physiology of Hearing*, ed. E.F. Evans and J.P. Wilson (Academic, London) pp. 27-41.

19. Robertson, D. and Johnstone, B.M. (1979) Aberrant tonotopic organization in the inner ear damaged by kanamycin, *J. Acoust. Soc. Am.* **66** 466-9.

20. Ruggero, M.A., Robles, L. and Rich, N.C. (1992) Two-tone suppression in the basilar membrane of the cochlea: mechanical basis of auditory-nerve rate suppression, *J. Neurophysiol.* **68** 1087-99.

21. Ruggero, M.A., Robles, L., Rich, N.C., and Recio, A. (1992) Basilar membrane responses to two-tone and broadband stimuli, *Phil. Trans. R. Soc. Lond. B* **336** 307-315.

22. Schmiedt, R.A., Zwislocki, J.J. and Hamernik, R.P. (1980) Effects of hair cell lesions on responses of cochlear nerve fibers. I. Tuning curves, two-tone inhibition, and responses to trapezoidal-wave patterns, *J. Neurophysiol.* **43** 1367-89.

23. Young, E.D. and Sachs, M.B. (1979) Representation of steady-state vowels in the temporal aspects of the discharge patterns of populations of auditory-nerve fibers, *J. Acoust. Soc. Am.* **66** 1381-1403.

TWO COMPONENTS OF ACOUSTIC DISTORTION: DIFFERENTIAL EFFECTS OF CONTRALATERAL SOUND AND ASPIRIN

ANN M. BROWN, HAZEL A. BEVERIDGE

Laboratory of Experimental Psychology, University of Sussex, Brighton BN1 9QG, UK

Acoustic distortion emissions were measured from the ears of human subjects treated with contralateral sound stimulation or aspirin. The responses were elicited by slow sweeps of f_1 frequency with f_2 fixed. Two vectors with differing delays were derived from the emitted distortion. The level of the more delayed component (presumed to be from the distortion product or DP place) was affected by both aspirin and contralateral stimulation, but there was little effect on mean group delay. However, with aspirin, there was a significant change in mean group delay of the overall distortion signal (which was predominantly from the f_2 'place') and a shift downwards in the frequency of the magnitude function. It is suggested that therapeutic doses of aspirin produce a basalward shift of the second frequency map revealed by distortion emissions, reduce cochlear 'amplification', but produce little change in basilar membrane compliance. Contralateral sound causes reduced amplification, but no discernible effect on compliance in either basilar membrane or the 'second' map.

Introduction

Analysis of acoustic distortion products (DPs) generated by low level sound confirms that there are at least two distinct sources contributing to the ear canal sound pressure.[1] The distortion products are generated in the region of stimulus overlap (f_2 place) and propagate to their own place (DP place) on the basilar membrane. The ear canal sound pressure is the vector sum of these two major components which are themselves the vector sum of distributed sources along the cochlear partition. The 'f_2 place' and 'DP place' components are distinguished by their differing mean group delays. Delay from the f_2 place is relatively brief, but delay from the DP place is greater than that for the stimulus frequency emissions (SFEs) evoked by the same frequency range. The latter difference can be attributed to the additional time due to stimulus propagation and distortion generation in the case of propagated DP. Both efferent stimulation and aspirin are thought to affect the putative feedback of energy into the cochlear partition as a result of direct action on basolateral conductance and the hair cell 'motor' respectively.[2,3] In these experiments, we aimed to explore the effect of contralateral sound and aspirin on the acoustic distortion components with differing delays.

Method

The probe contained a Knowles EA 1842 microphone (fully calibrated for sound pressure in an artificial ear) and two Knowles BP 1712 transducers.

Tonal stimuli were generated by two function generators under computer control. A spectral shaper (octave steps, 24 dB/octave slopes) was used to make the swept tone flat across the sweep frequency range. The microphone response was amplified (40 dB) and fed to an EG&G 5210 lock-in amplifier with time constant set to 100 ms. The electrical reference was an artificially generated source of $2f_1-f_2$. Sound levels were measured and adjusted to the required levels in each ear canal.

For the generation of DPs, f_2 was fixed and f_1 was swept in frequency at a rate of 3.2 Hz/s (1.6 Hz/s for $2f_1-f_2$) with f_2/f_1 from 1.41 to 1.01. Stimulus levels were $L_1 = 55$, $L_2 = 40$ dB SPL. The magnitude and phase data collected from the lock-in amplifier were corrected to give magnitude in μV and phase in degrees relative to the reference, after unwrapping at 2π discontinuities. Both traces were smoothed using a 101-point average and the first and last 50 points were excluded from subsequent analysis. The complex conjugates of the raw and smooth waveforms were calculated. The real and imaginary parts of the smoothed waveform were subtracted from the equivalent in the raw waveform. The magnitude and phase of the residual were calculated using the modulus and argument of the resulting complex data. The residual phase was unwrapped at 2π discontinuities. The total and residual magnitude were referenced to the voltage for 0 dB SPL from the system calibration and expressed in dB SPL.

The residual signal detected is referred to as DP residual. The phase slope of f_1 measured in the ear canal was subtracted from the DP phase slope to remove any delay between generation of the 'artificial' DP produced electronically and sound reaching the ear canal. The DP residual phase slope was referenced to the DP, so it is superimposed on the delay already experienced by the major DP component. Where no phase trend could be discerned in the DP or DP residual, the signal was assumed to be noise. The residual delay was usually substantially greater than the overall mean group delay and was assumed to come from the DP place, while the less delayed, major component was assumed to come from the f_2 place (Figure 1).

Subjects, noise administration and aspirin

Broad-band noise at 60 dB SPL rms was delivered to the ears of four subjects (2 M, 2 F). It was generated by a laboratory-made white-noise generator and passed through a spectrum shaper to flatten the ear-canal noise spectrum. This controlled for any frequency-specific effects that could be produced by ear-canal resonances. Noise levels were monitored with a separate microphone in the contralateral ear. Measurements were made without contralateral noise, with noise and then without noise again in the same session.

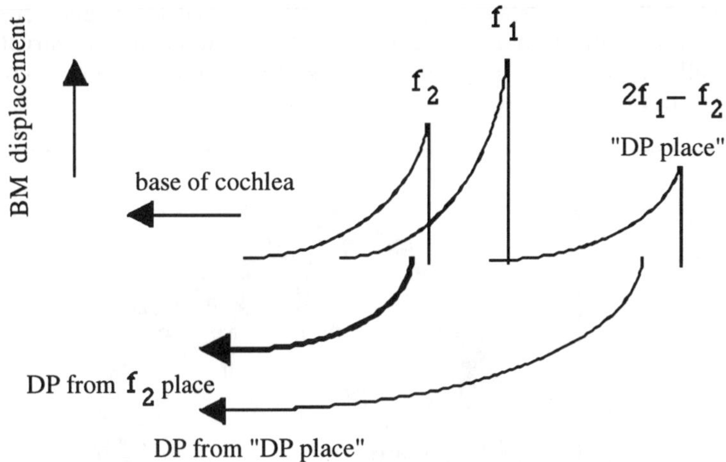

Figure 1: Schematic of the stimuli and distortion product generation and propagation in the cochlea showing origin of two components which sum vectorially to give meatal sound pressure.

Normal hearing male volunteers received three 320 mg capsules of aspirin every six hours for either two or three days. Measurements were made one or more times a week before aspirin was taken, immediately after the course of tablets and then again after a delay of one to two weeks.

Results

Noise

Contralateral broad-band noise was found to affect the amplitude of the emitted distortion product in all subjects with f_2 at 4 kHz without having any pronounced effects on the spectral shape of the amplitude function or on the mean group delay of the acoustic distortion product.[7] The decrease in amplitude under contralateral stimulation (amounting to 1 dB or less) was most pronounced at peaks in the fine structure of the amplitude function. At troughs in the fine structure, the amplitude was either less reduced, not reduced at all or even elevated under contralateral stimulation. There was no change in mean group delay in any of the subjects.

In two of these subjects, distortion level was sufficiently steady across frequency to allow further analysis of the vectors comprising the total distortion signal. An example is shown in Figure 2. This revealed two components with markedly different delays.[1] The results of this analysis indicated that the main effect of the contralateral stimulation was to decrease

222

the level of the more delayed emission: that presumed to emanate from the 'DP place'. This effect could account for the flattening of the fine structure in the overall DP magnitude function and suggests that there is negligible effect on the DP from the f_2 place.

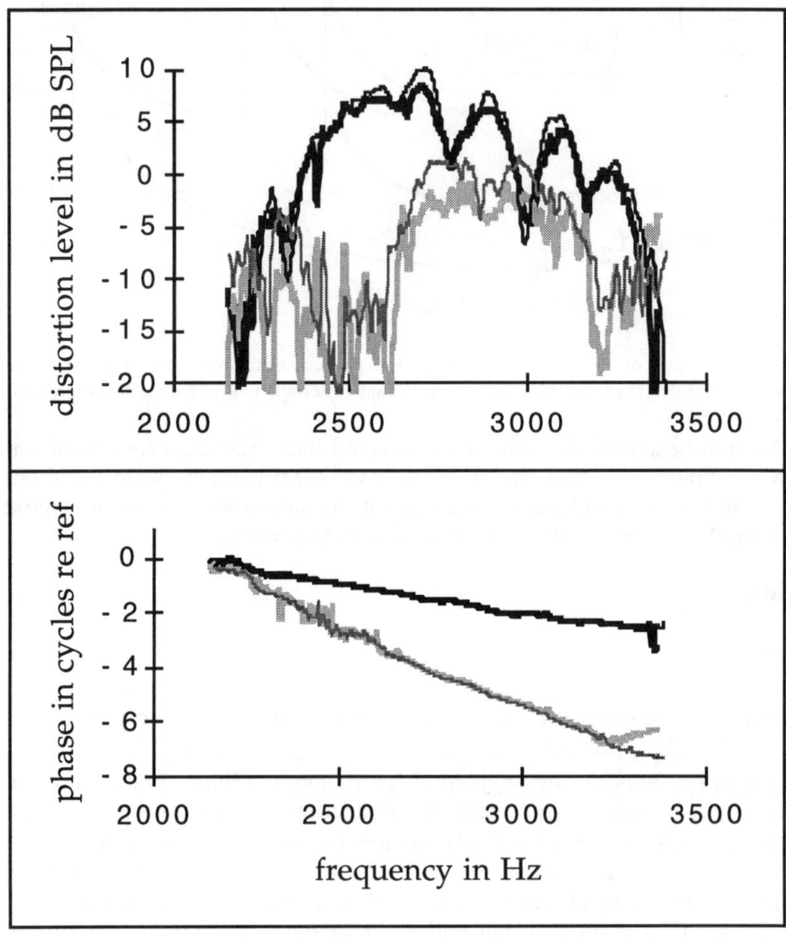

Figure 2: Distortion product magnitude (above) and unwrapped phase (below) for both the major (black lines) and the residual (grey lines) distortion components. Thick lines are data with and thin lines are data without contralateral broad-band noise at 60 dB SPL rms. $f_2 = 4000$ Hz and f_1 swept in frequency. $L_2 = 40$ dB SPL, $L_1 = 55$ dB SPL.

Aspirin

Aspirin was found to decrease distortion level in 5/7 subjects (p < 0.05; paired two-sample t-test, t = 2.04). There was also a significant change in mean group delay in 6/7 subjects (mean reduction 0.42 ms; sd 0.42 ms: p < 0.03; paired two-sample t-test, t = 2.40).

Three subjects had distortion levels which were sufficiently steady across frequency to allow vector analysis as described above. An example is shown in Figure 3. These three showed a depression in level of distortion, a shift in the amplitude function to lower frequencies of between 25 and 100 Hz and a decrease in mean group delay. Vector analysis indicated a differential effect on the two components. Both were decreased in level, but the effect on mean group delay was almost entirely accounted for by the effect on the less delayed component (assumed to be from the f_2 place). The highly delayed 'residual' DP showed negligible change in mean group delay with aspirin. This component was referenced to the overall DP phase, so it represents the round trip delay from the generation site (f_2) to re-emission. Measurement of stimulus frequency emissions in these subjects showed only a very small effect on mean group delay with aspirin.

Discussion

Contralateral sound causes a reduction in re-emission from the DP 'place', suggesting a reduction in amplifier gain alone without any effect on compliance, as evidenced by the lack of change in mean group delay. However, aspirin produces an increase in compliance of the 'filter', causing a downward shift in frequency and a decrease in mean group delay. By contrast, the effect on the DP-characteristic place, as evidenced by the highly delayed, apically-propagated DP component and the SFEs, is simply to reduce feedback without significantly affecting stiffness. Some subjects showed a significant change in level of distortion in the fine structure, without any change in overall level, while in others the total level of distortion was greatly diminished (Figure 3). If the basilar membrane and second filter are modelled as two cochlear maps, as proposed by Allen and Fahey[4] then the results we have seen could be interpreted as a shift basalwards of the second map relative to the first with therapeutic doses of aspirin (Figure 4).

Assuming that the distribution of resonant frequencies of the second map is critical in determining the efficacy of feedback, then the aspirin-induced shift could reduce amplification, thereby elevating thresholds and reducing SFEs. If the phase relationship between the first and second maps is critical in determining frequency selectivity then this, too, will be affected. Comparable doses of aspirin have been shown to impair frequency selectivity by Beveridge and Carlyon.[5] Higher doses of aspirin, as used in experimental animals, appear to cause a shift of the basilar membrane frequency map as well.[6] Such an effect is undetectable with therapeutic doses, as there was a negligible effect on the frequency distribution of SFEs or their mean group delay, or that of the residual DP.

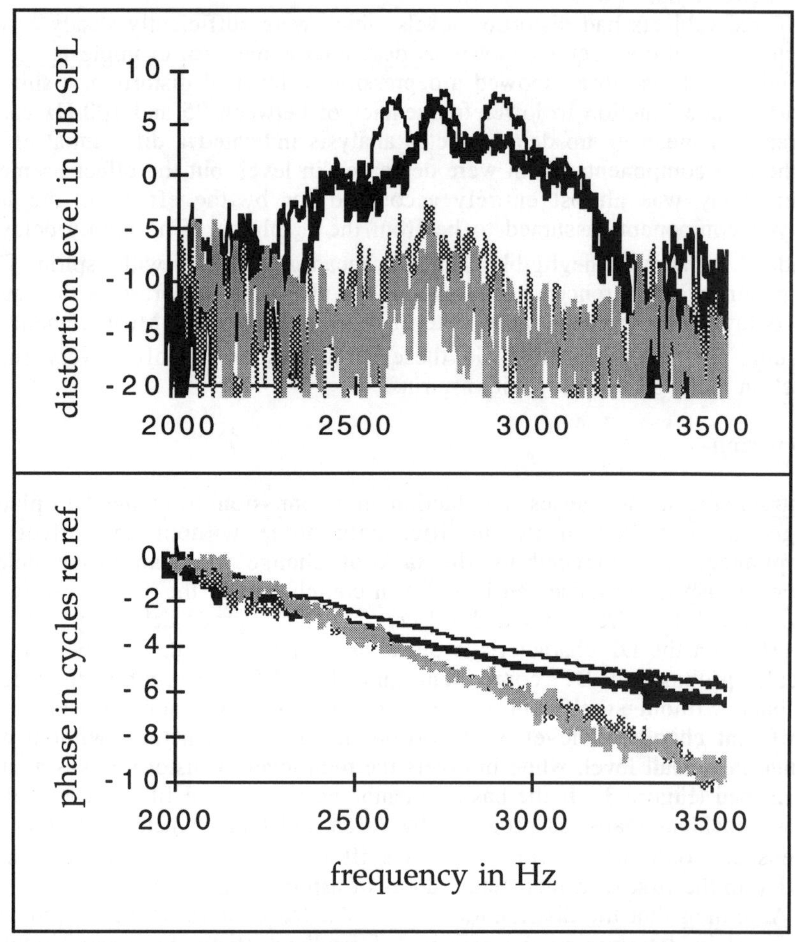

Figure 3: Distortion product magnitude (above) and unwrapped phase (below) for both the major (black lines) and the residual (grey lines) distortion components. Thick lines: with aspirin; thin lines: without aspirin. $f_2 = 4000$ Hz and f_1 swept in frequency. $L_2 = 40$ dB SPL, $L_1 = 55$ dB SPL.

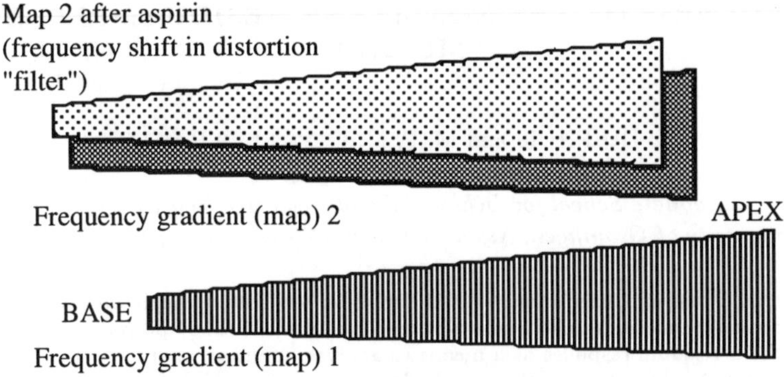

Figure 4: The differential effect of aspirin on two cochlear maps. The first represents that produced by the basilar membrane and any 'active' processes. The second may be attributable to the TM

Acknowledgements

Supported by Wellcome Trust, Hearing Research Trust. Thanks are due to Dr Deirdre M. Williams, Paul Russell and Andrew Stephenson.

References

1. Brown, A.M., Harris, F.P. and Beveridge, H.A. (*J. Acoust. Soc. Am. 100.*, *in press*) Two sources of acoustic distortion products from the human cochlea.
2. Gifford, M.L. and Guinan, J.J. Effects of electrical stimulation of medial olivocochlear neurons on ipsilateral and contralateral cochlear responses. *Hear. Res.* **29**, 179 (1987).
3. Shehata, W.E. *et al.*, Effects of salicylate on shape, electromotility and membrane characteristics of isolated outer hair cells from guinea pig cochlea. *Acta Oto-Laryngolog.* **111**, 707 (1991).
4. Allen, J.B. and Fahey, P.F. A second cochlear-frequency map that correlates distortion product and neural tuning measurements. *J. Acoust. Soc. Am.* **94**, 809 (1993).
5. Beveridge, H.A. and Carlyon, R.P. (accepted *Hear. Res.*) Effects of aspirin on human psychophysical tuning curves in forward and simultaneous masking.
6. Murugasu, E. and Russell, I.J. Salicylate ototoxicity: The effects on basilar membrane displacement, cochlear microphonics and neural responses in the basal turn of the guinea pig cochlea. *Aud. Neuroscience* **1**, 139 (1995).
7. Williams, D.M. and Brown, A.M. (submitted *Hear. Res.*) The effect of contralateral broad-band noise on acoustic distortion products from the human ear.

USEFULNESS OF THE NONLINEAR RESIDUAL RESPONSE METHOD

H. DUIFHUIS and M. P. M. G. VAN DEN RAADT

Department of Biophysics
Graduate School for Behavioral and Cognitive Neurosciences,
University of Groningen, Nijenborgh 4, 9747 AG Groningen, Netherlands

In 1991 Brass and Kemp[1] introduced a method for 'Time-domain observation of otoacoustic emissions during constant tone stimulation'. They proposed the analysis of a residual response as a means to analyze nonlinear characteristics of the inner ear. We have applied their method to analyze properties of nonlinear cochlea models, and conclude that this method provides a sensitive test for amplitude characteristics, but also for phase characteristics of cochlear models. A measurable residual will be a 'fingerprint' of nonlinear, and some (almost) linear, characteristics of the cochlea. Our analysis shows that in addition to amplitude, and (carrier-) phase of the residual, envelope shape is a crucial property. This shape contains the 'delayed' onset of the residual. Typical residual shapes (Brass and Kemp Fig. 6) require significant addition, or phase coherent accumulation, of distortion near the site of generation, which can be in conflict with the notion of a strong phase gradient near the site of maximum excitation. Several quantitative predictions are presented, and implications for cochlear modeling, including the possible role of second filters, are discussed.

1 Introduction

1.1 The nonlinear residual response method

The stimulus paradigm for the nonlinear residual response method is indicated in Table 1. It was developed by Brass and Kemp (1991)[1] as a sensitive tool to measure ear canal responses to an acoustic stimulus in the presence of the same stimulus.[a] The method allows the measurement of relatively weak auditory distortion effects even at the input frequency.

The method requires accurate summation of a continuous background tone and an intermittently presented probe tone. The combination is generated in a sophisticated way, in precisely defined time intervals. Four intervals, of equal duration, are labeled A, B, C, and D. Each interval contains exactly an odd number of half periods of the background tone. Hence, the waveforms of the background tone in consecutive sections differ only by sign (phase shift of π). The probe tone is presented only in intervals C and D, during approximately

---

[a]Meanwhile the term Stimulus Frequency evoked OtoAcoustic Emission, SFOAE, has been generally adopted for the present and related phenomena.

half the interval, with exactly equal shapes (referenced to the onsets of C and D).

The frequency of the background tone, f_b, is subject to the restriction stated above. The frequency of the probe tone, f_p, and the levels of both tones, L_c and L_p, are free.

Table 1: Temporal structure of stimulus $\longrightarrow$ time

A	B	C +probe	D +probe
+background	−background	+background	−background

The residual is obtained by addition and subtraction of the ear canal pressure measured during those four intervals as defined by the rule

$$\text{Residual} = A - B - C + D.$$

Hence its duration is that of a single time segment.

Obviously, the linear residual of the overall stimulus (background tone plus probe tone) is equal to zero. Experimentally however, the residual of the response measured in the ear canal does not cancel completely[1]. Due to the nonlinearity of the system a small component remains.

1.2 Specification of the analysis of the cochlea

For optimal comparison between model results and data we stay close to the stimulus parameters used by Brass and Kemp. One time section was kept at 40 ms. Obviously this limits the maximum spectral resolution to (at best) 25 Hz. Probe tones were shaped with cosine shaped onsets and offsets of 1 ms. Brass and Kemp claim that with this duration of the window no significant high frequency components or other transients are detectable in the residual. Their choice was motivated by the necessity to collect an optimum set of data over a limited period.

The simulations presented in this study have been obtained using a nonlinear one-dimensional cochlea model that is solved in the time domain.[2] The advantage of this model is that nonlinear parameters can be manipulated, in stiffness as well as in damping, that interaction between elements is taken into account, and that time effects (onset and offset transients) are computed properly. The classical Runge-Kutta method was chosen as time integration method with a time step of 2.5 μs [or less].

1.3 Relevant cochlea properties and model parameters

Relevant properties to be considered include:
1. The number of resonators, N, used in the transmission line model.
2. Stiffness and damping profiles over place, $s(x)$ and $d(x)$.
3. Stiffness and damping nonlinearity characteristics.
4. Coupling at ear canal and middle ear.
5. Helicotrema mechanics.

The number of coupled resonators N has been varied between 100 and 3200. In general we used $N = 400$ as a practical choice. The responses for $N = 100$ differ considerably, for $N = 200$ markedly, and for larger N minor high frequency differences are detectable.[b]

Damping, stiffness, and mass profiles determine a place to frequency map, and a 'traveling wave' velocity profile, or/and phase profile or/and Q (quality factor) profile. Following the general trend we keep the mass per unit area independent of x, but examine overall variation by introduction of a global BM-factor that modifies m, d, and s in such a way that frequency map and Q are unaffected. The effect of Q can be studied 'independently' by manipulation of an additional damping factor.

So far results have been obtained for six different choices of the damping functions $d_{NL}(v)d(x)$ and the stiffness functions $s_{NL}(y)s(x)$ $[v = v(x), y = y(x)]$:
The linear case $d_{NL}(v) = 1$, $s_{NL}(y) = 1$; an exponential damping nonlinearity $d_{NL} = \chi \sinh(\alpha v)/(\alpha v)$, $s_{NL} = 1$ (as proposed earlier[3] $\chi = 1$ and $\alpha = 10^4$ s/m parameters and v in m/s); a nonlinear and active damping or generalized Van der Pol oscillator with the additional negative term $2\gamma/\cosh(\beta v)$ where $\gamma = 1$ and $\beta = 10^6$ s/m; a nonlinearity in the stiffness $(d_{NL} = 1, s_{NL} = 1 + \epsilon_s |y|^p)$; a power law nonlinearity in damping $(d_{NL} = 1 + \epsilon_d v^2, s_{NL} = 1)$; and finally the combination of the last two[4].

It should be obvious that the coupling properties at the ear canal/middle ear side and at the helicotrema play a significant part, both in ear and in model. A simplified middle ear and canal coupler are assumed which cover the basic physical properties[5,6].

The apical coupling is more relevant than is generally acknowledged. It determines how fast the cochlea adapts to transients. Of course all transients contain low-frequency components, and a reaction to these components would require efficient properties at the helicotrema. In a linear approximation an optimum impedance match, to the local characteristic impedance if the gradient is sufficiently small,[c] would prevent reflections.

---

[b] The $N = 3200$-value is in fact not appropriate for a macroscopic one-dimensional model.
[c] Formally the Ricatti equation provides the general solution.[7,8]

2 First Results

2.1 The residual of a linear cochlea model

Several properties were studied for equal parameters for probe and background $(L_b = L_p, \ f_b = f_p)$. In the linear case with $N = 400$ there is a clear low-frequency component in the residue (at approx. 100 Hz). This component remains linearly related to stimulus level. This was checked by measuring the residue in absence of the probe, in which case the residue should vanish. An essential difference exists between our computation, based on a single set of intervals A through D, and the experimental data, which involve continuously repeated stimuli. In the first case the transients are clipped at the end of interval D, in the experiments the transient responses are continuously taken into account. Matthews[5] describes a similar effect obtained with his time domain method.

2.2 Nonlinear damping

As indicated above, we so far studied two possible damping nonlinearities, viz. the power law nonlinearity and the exponential nonlinearity that have been suggested and used in cochlear modeling over the years.

As obvious in Fig. 1, the residual has three main characteristics: an initial transient, a relatively stationary part, and a final transient which continues until the end of the frame. Furthermore, at the start of the time section a much smaller transient is present.

The two large transients in the residue came unexpectedly. Apparently this residue displays a strong contribution from the high-frequency part of the cochlea. That is the part that responds fastest, and because of the spectral sensitivity, provides strong transient responses. The cochlear response near resonance grows more gradually, but in that range the phase gradient is larger and vectorial summation can then lead to a weaker result. This is where phase behavior plays an important role. In the simple, straightforward model cochlea two parameters are available to control the phase behavior: The BM-factor that scales m, d, and s, without changing the frequency map; and the d-term by itself, changing the quality factor and phase. It may be clear that the Q-factor presents two opposite effects: a higher Q implies a greater frequency selectivity, and therefore a slower but stronger response ($\Delta f \times \Delta t$ remains constant). It also implies a faster phase transition at resonance, which will reduce the residual response.

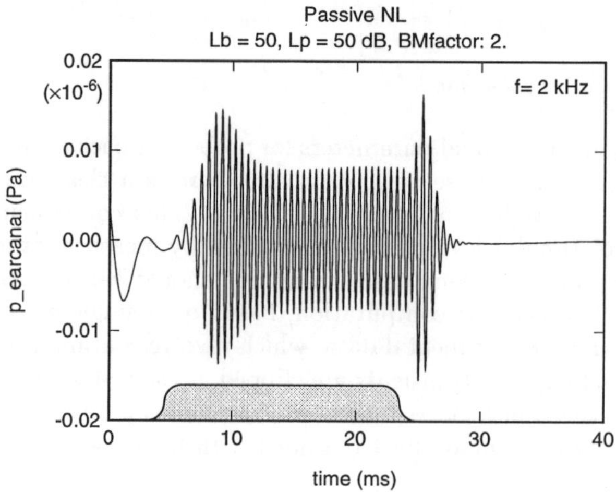

Figure 1: A typical waveform for the nonlinear residual response of the macromechanical time domain model ($f_p = f_b$). The probe duration is indicated at the bottom of the figure.

2.3 Nonlinear stiffness

The question whether the experimentally observed nonlinearity originates in cochlear damping or in cochlear stiffness, or in a combination of both, is still open. On the basis of psychoacoustical as well as neurophysiological data it was concluded about 20 years ago that the most important nonlinear component was an (almost) even nonlinear damping term, supplemented by a weak odd term (generating, e.g., the difference tone) and probably by a weak nonlinear stiffness term.[4,9] Hence the impact of a nonlinear stiffness term was investigated, both separately and in combination with a nonlinear damping function. We choose functions similar to those proposed by Furst & Goldstein.[4] At low levels the discontinuity in the derivative at $y = 0$ [y =partition displacement] can lead to instability in the response. Stiffness nonlinearity does not seem to provide transients above the average continuous response level.

An alternative nonlinear stiffness characteristic, quite different from the one mentioned above is the term associated with the Duffing equation. It gives an odd nonlinear stiffness element, instead of the symmetrical, even element mentioned above. Tentative results indicate that it may produce larger onset 'delays'.

Along this line we started to test the effect of an asymmetric nonlinear stiffness term as assumed to be relevant for hair bundle motion. The primary effect appears to be characterized by overall stiffness reduction, which leads to a basalward shift of the characteristic frequency.

3 Discussion

We started the analysis of stimulus frequency otoacoustic emissions (SFOAEs). The technique, introduced by Kemp and Souter (1988)[10] and expanded by Brass and Kemp[1], was simulated in a transmission-line cochlea model. This nonlinear response residue method has the advantage that temporal measurements are possible at the stimulus frequency.

A nonlinear model cochlea generates a reproducible residual result. A linear cochlea model displays a low-frequency oscillatory response, because the apical part of the cochlea, often beyond the region of resonance, is relatively slow, and it is stimulated by transients in the stimulus. Part of this effect is exaggerated by the use of a too simple middle ear; the appropriate match will reduce high-frequency as well as low-frequency transients.

With a straightforward specification of the acoustic coupler it was possible to predict the levels of the residue. Also global frequency effects and level effects follow the experimental data. In this macroscopic model there is -so far- no apparent need for a second filter.

For the nonlinearities tested, we have not yet been able to mimic every detail of the experimental data. Open questions are the source of strong initial and final transients and for the 'delay' of the residual. As mentioned above, both middle ear properties and cochlear parameters involving the phase characteristics directly affect this result. At least one of those has to be modified to explain the data. The 'delay' caused by the traveling wave is in fact the gradual onset profile of the coupled cochlea elements, and thus formally there is no delay. The time necessary for the residue to reach 50% of the stationary response can be used for a comparison, physically it is determined by the onset properties at the sites where the nonlinearity is prominently present. Likewise, travel time through the fluid back to the ear canal is negligible. Relevant envelope effects are determined by the same onset properties, which incorporates the coupling with all elements in the system.

Acknowledgments

The authors acknowledge the discussions with several colleagues, in particular with P. W. J. van Hengel. The project received support from the Netherlands Organization for Scientific Research (NWO) through the Foundation for Biophysics.

References

1. D. Brass and D. T. Kemp. (1991) Time-domain observation of otoacoustic emissions during constant tone stimulation. *J. Acoust. Soc. Am.* **90** 2415–2427.

2. H. Duifhuis, H. W. Hoogstraten, S. M. van Netten, R. J. Diependaal, and W. Bialek. (1985) Modelling the cochlear partition with coupled van der Pol oscillators. In; J. B. Allen, J. L. Hall, A. E. Hubbard, S. T. Neely, and A. Tubis, editors, *Peripheral Auditory Mechanisms*, pages 290–297, New York. Springer.

3. H. Duifhuis. (1988) Cochlear macromechanics. In; G. M. Edelman, W. E. Gall, and W. M. Cowan, editors, *Auditory Function. Neurobiological basis of hearing*, chapter 6, pages 189–211. A Neurosciences Institute Publication, Wiley, New York.

4. M. Furst and J. L. Goldstein. (1982) A cochlear nonlinear transmission-line model compatible with combination tone psychophysics. *J. Acoust. Soc. Am.* **72** 717–726.

5. J. W. Matthews. (1983) Modeling reverse middle ear transmission of acoustic distortion signals. In; E. de Boer and M. A. Viergever, editors, *Mechanics of Hearing*, Delft U.P., Netherlands.

6. M. P. M. G. van den Raadt and H. Duifhuis. (1993) Different boundary conditions in a one-dimensional time domain cochlea model. In; H. Duifhuis, J. W. Horst, P. van Dijk, and S. M. van Netten, editors, *Biophysics of Hair Cell Sensory Systems*, page 103, World Scientific, Singapore.

7. M. A. Viergever and E. de Boer. (1987) Matching impedance of a nonuniform transmission line: Application to cochlear modeling. *J. Acoust. Soc. Am.* **81** 184–186.

8. Chr. Kaernbach, P. König, and Th. Schillen. (1987) On Ricatti equations describing impedance relations for forward and backward excitation in the one-dimensional cochlea model. *J. Acoust. Soc. Am.* **81** 408–411.

9. J. L. Hall. (1974) Two-tone distortion products in a nonlinear model of the basilar membrane. *J. Acoust. Soc. Am.* **56** 1818–1823.

10. D. T. Kemp and M. Souter. (1988) The dynamics of cochlea pertubations following brief acoustic stimuli and efferent stimulation–otoacoustic and cm data. In; H. Duifhuis, J. W. Horst, and H. P. Wit, editors, *Basic Issues in Hearing*, pages 116–123, Academic, London.

EXCITATION PATTERN SHIFTS: TIME-FREQUENCY EVIDENCE FROM CLICK-EVOKED OTOACOUSTIC EMISSIONS

E.L. LePAGE, N.M. MURRAY, K.TRAN
Hearing Loss Prevention Research
National Acoustic Laboratories, Chatswood, N.S.W., 2067 Australia

M.J. HARRAP
Department of Aerospace and Mechanical Engineering,
Australian Defence Force Academy, Canberra, A.C.T. 2600, Australia

Click-evoked otoacoustic emissions have the advantage of being able to display the temporal dependence of the emission power spectra as 3-dimensional surfaces through the use of the short-time Fourier transform. Such displays have been used to investigate manipulations of human cochlear mechanics, specifically looking for evidence of earlier suggestions that outer hair cell activity produces dynamic remapping of the tonotopy as a primary mechanism. Data were obtained using an Otodynamics ILO88 system. Surface displays of the emissions are quite sensitive to relatively low level manipulations such as pure tone exposures which produce minimal levels of temporary threshold shift (TTS). A pure tone exposure such as 3 kHz, 90 dB SPL, 1 min applied ipsilaterally, producing negligible TTS, still produces significant shifts of frequency in major frequency peaks in the time-frequency plane, predominantly to lower frequency in the subjects tested. Notably, the largest effects upon the spectrum and latency may not be seen for some minutes but the response eventually returns to its original condition.

1 Introduction

The evidence that the cochlea does remap began with the so-called "half-octave shift" exhibited by most parameters (see review, McFadden, 1986) in response to prolonged high level stimulation. One set of more recent mechanical evidence was accompanied by a qualitative model relating OHC motility and mapping (LePage, 1992); the proposed key connecting parameter being tension in the radial fibres of the basilar membrane (LePage, 1990). The evidence for remapping during development is also strong, and it may also be a major response influencing aging, or presbycusis. Such changes may be modelled using slow changes in control parameters such the variation in operating points of the hair cells. As has been observed previously (LePage, 1990, 1992) the modelling of the normal active cochlea has been severely restricted in the past by the implicit assumption concerning the existence of a steady-state, 1:1, unique map between frequency and place. If this restriction were relaxed, even allowing mapping to vary dynamically, a considerable range of new possibilities exist to account for frequency-varying phenomena, particularly those normally protecting the ear from acoustic overload.

In the past, variations in cochlear potentials and neural activity have been largely modelled assuming the mapping remains fixed and that all variations seen are due to local changes. Punctate measurements along the cochlear partition do not provide a truly spatial representation of the activity -- it must be inferred from varying frequency (and be distorted by any history/level-dependent effects). In a

"

linear system this presents no problem; even in a nonlinear system, it depends upon the nature of the nonlinearity. If the nonlinearities were all level-dependent in a way which did not influence the *position or extent* of the travelling wave envelope, the assumption of a unique, 1:1 map is also valid. There is a significant problem, however, if the spatial position of the travelling wave changes as a function of level because many of the assumptions of traditional cochlear models break down. Some possible advantages of having two tuned processes defining two maps have been investigated (Brown and Beveridge, 1996) such that the sharpness of tuning was fixed by the degree of alignment between the two maps -- one fixed, one free to move. The spatial relationship required has been derived from neural data (LePage, 1987) while support for tension variation as the basis supplied by Allen (1966).

However, to sustain the argument that re-mapping occurs dynamically it is necessary to demonstrate unambiguously migration of the spatial extent of the travelling wave, or excitation region, *without requiring a changing of the stimulus or the introduction of an external modulating signal or bias*. The only way of conducting such an experiment is using a wideband stimulus. The "natural" response of the ear is largely obscured by any stimulus in which the response cannot be separated from the stimulus either in time or frequency. These requirements eliminate both white noise and distortion products as the stimulus of choice.

Click-evoked otoacoustic emissions (CEOAE) not only fulfil the key requirements; they also have the advantage of being able to display the temporal dependence of the emission power spectra as 3-dimensional surfaces through the use of the short-time Fourier transform. The most significant disadvantage of the click approach is that it is practically impossible to determine precisely what the energy density is as a function of distance along the cochlear partition. Ideally, the click delivers constant power/Hz which means that per octave (per unit distance along the cochlear partition) the basal end will, relative to the distortion product method, be receiving more energy. Hence the click method tends to weight the active contribution of the basal regions higher than does the DP-method. In practical terms the spectrum of the click is not flat but rolls off from about 5 kHz.

The spectra of CEOAE show much more fine structure than do distortion product otoacoustic emissions (DPOAE) from the same ear (LePage, unpublished results). The notches so characteristic of CEOAE spectra are seldom so deep or sharp with the DPOAEs. This feature may be related to the fact that DPOAE spectra are produced by scanning at a rate somewhat arbitrarily determined by the operator, whereas the "scanning rate" of CEOAE spectra is effectively fixed by the factors controlling the forward and reverse propagation of the travelling wave. That differences exist between the methods is not surprising considering the range of nonlinear activity. CEOAEs also appear very sensitive to acoustic overload. Our hypothesis is that shifting of the excitation pattern is responsible for TTS and that bias in OHC electromechanical operating point is responsible. CEOAEs may be a sensitive indicator of that bias. The rate of recovery from that fatigue may constitute a measure distinguishing ears of differing susceptibility.

The objectives of the study are 1) to obtain time-frequency distributions of the CEOAE responses and observe to what extent systematic frequency and amplitude variations occur, 2) to examine the changes in the distributions with relatively low noise-doses, e.g. a 90 dB tone for short periods.

2 Methods

Click-evoked otoacoustic emissions were obtained using an Otodynamics ILO88 analyser in screening mode, averaging 260 repetitions of the so-called "nonlinear" stimulus click train designed to cancel all linear components of the OAE response. The ear probe was a standard Otodynamics distortion product probe. The first speaker was used for the CEOAE measurement. The preset click stimulus level is 80 dB SPL peak. Array length is 512 samples at a 40ms sample time, while, alternate responses are bandpass filtered (range 1 to 5 kHz) and added into arrays "A" and "B". The period of the stimulus artifact (2.5ms) is zeroed. The total averaging time is approximately 30 s, depending on background noise and the artifact rejection level. Responses are plotted vs time and an FFT is used to determine cross power spectrum between arrays A and B. The FFT of the difference (A-B) is used as an estimate of the noncoherent part of the response (noise).

The ear probe is sealed in the ear canal and remains in place for the entire experiment. In the acoustic challenge experiments, recording was suspended while the second probe speaker was used to deliver the tone. After repeat recordings were obtained, the acoustic load (3kHz, 90dB for a 1 m interval) was applied, after which CEOAE records were taken at 1 m intervals for the next 15 to 20 minutes.

In this series, the time-frequency analysis was continued off line using an Ariel "Cyclops" card using a TMS320C40 processor to compute the short-time FFT of the averaged click-evoked otoacoustic emission. The spectra were created by first dividing the emission signal into a series of consecutive time subintervals using a sliding Blackman window 256 samples in length. Each subinterval andvanced 8 samples yielding 33 subinterval frames of data. The spectrum of each frame was then estimated using an FFT algorithm. These spectra were then arranged in time order to create the time-frequency spectrogram. For all records displayed here the frequency axis displays frequencies from 0 to 6 kHz, the time axis (into the page) from 0 to 10 ms, and the magnitude axis of arbitrary fixed *linear* scale.

3 Results

3.1 Time detail normally seen smeared in the cross power spectrum

For the first pair of records (Figure 1) the subject was selected from a database of 12500 records, to illustrate normal cochlear level-dependent frequency shifts. For the series of experiments examining the effect of loud tone exposure subjects were chosen with high and low level emission strengths. These records are low noise and highly reproducible.

The short-time Fourier transforms are displayed as 3-dimensional surfaces rather than using contour or dot plots (Bray, 1989; Cheng, 1993) because it is essential to see the terrain to appreciate that the successive peaks define a locus representing frequency modulation of isolated segments of activity. For example in Figure 1(a) an otoacoustic emission record is presented with a signal-to-noise ratio of 10 to 15 dB across the frequency band, the short-time Fourier transform shows that the frequency of certain peaks in the response systematically change during the first 10 ms interval time course of the emission, moving to lower frequency by up to half and octave as the response at the peak grows in amplitude. The right ear for the same subject (Fig. 1(b)) shows clearly that the fine structure that we sometimes see in averaged emission spectra is associated with peaks whose frequencies either are strongly dependent on latency, and/or rapid amplitude modulation associated with slight shifts in frequency.

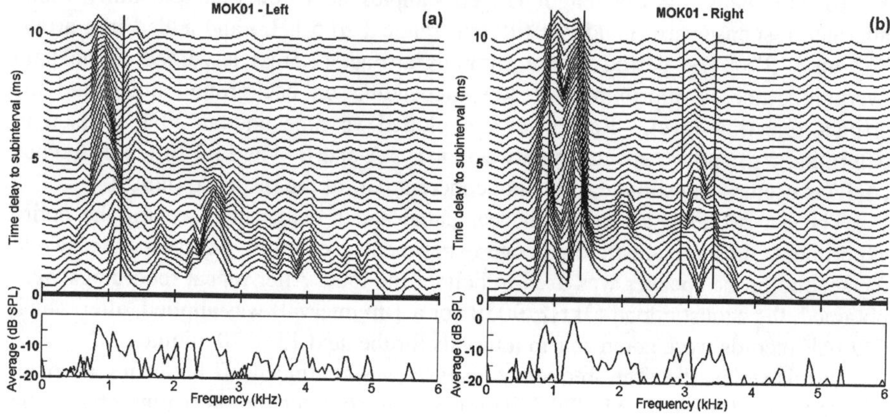

Fig 1: Time-frequency plots for subject with isolated peaks; cross-power and nois spectra below

3.2 *Test of ear regulation - perturbation produced by loud tone.*

As only nine people have been tested this way so far, the results are preliminary. Two data sets are presented here to illustrate the approach. Figure 2 shows results from a female subject with high emission strengths. Fig. 3 shows results from a male with low emission strengths, (due to lack of high frequency emissions), and showing a faster rate of decline (-5 dB/decade) over past five years.

Both families of time-frequency plots for subjects ANM01 and SEJ01 show clearly discernable dynamic changes in response to a tonal exposure of much lower dose than maxima stipulated by Australian Standard AS1269 - Hearing Conservation. It is not clear at this stage how much of the changes are due to noise; however, there is strong evidence of continuities between successive traces.

Pronounced changes were not seen so much above the test frequency of 3 kHz e.g. at 4 kHz, but rather changes were seen at lower frequencies e.g. 1 to 3 kHz.

Low frequency changes were maximal at the time of the maximal change to the overall emission response.

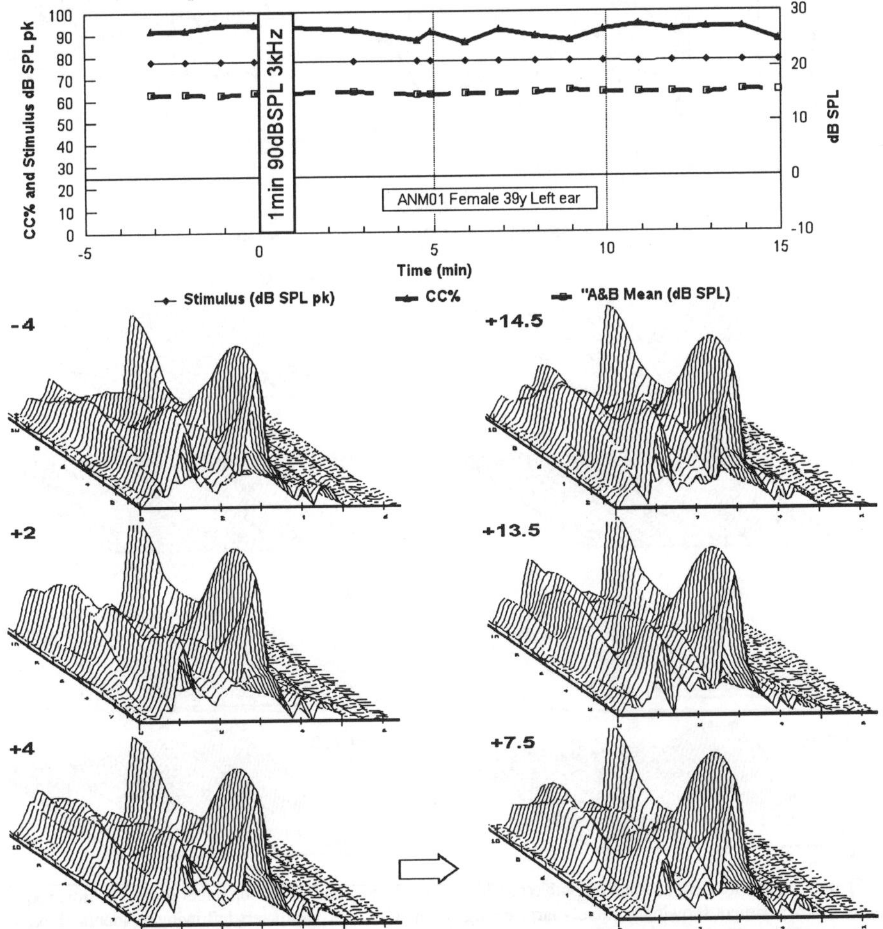

Figure 2: Time-frequency surfaces for subject ANM01 with "tough ear". The top panel shows the time sequence for the experiment showing small change in CEOAE parameters following a 1 minute, 3kHz test tone exposure at 90dB SPL. In this panel the correlation coefficient and stimulus SPL is on the left axis, mean SPL on right. Abcissa is frequency (0 to 6 kHz), time (0 to +10ms) into page, linear magnitude.

4 Discussion

Two classes of responses were represented with the data presented here. The first was examining fine details of the CEOAE response and the second was showing by example that ears differ in terms of how strongly reproducible the emission is following a small acoustic overload. The fact that the frequency of single peaks is clearly seen to bend suggests that the mechanism is exhibiting frequency modulation

238

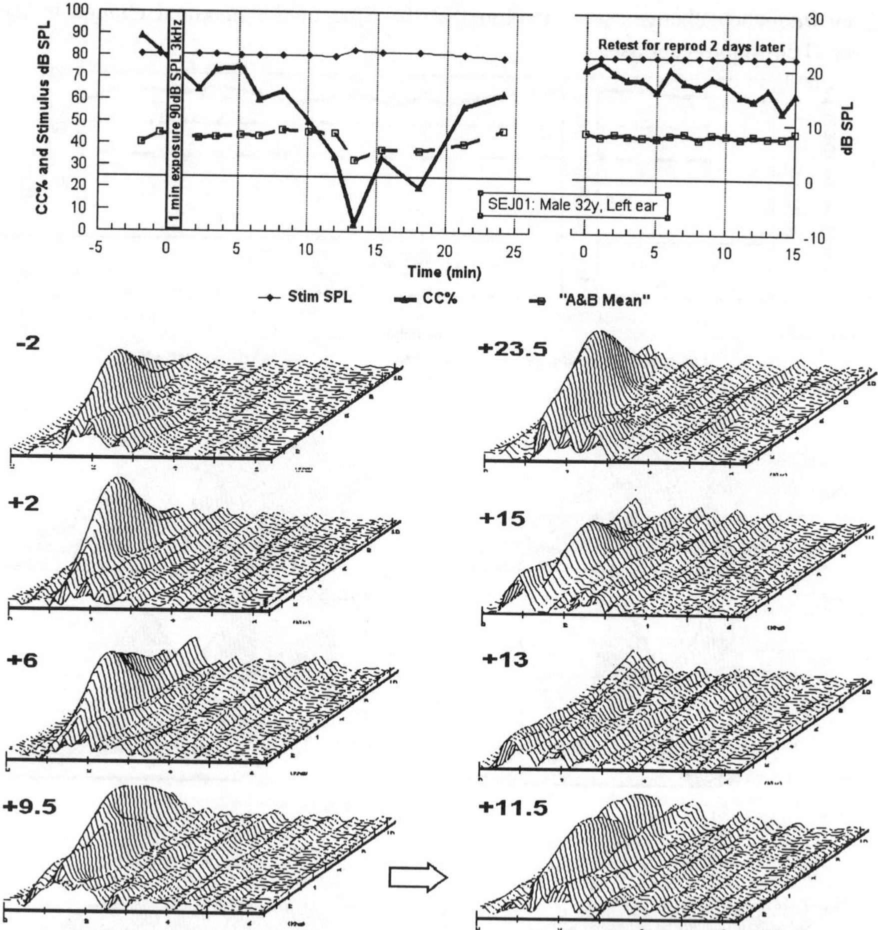

Figure 3. Time-frequency surfaces for subject SEJ01 with a "tender ear". The top panel shows the time sequence for the experiment showing relatively large change in the CEOAE parameters following an identical exposure to ANM01. The largest effect occurs not immediately but some minutes later as seen in the Correlation Coefficient (%) and emission sound level (dB SPL).

over a time course of 5 ms and is associated with higher amplitude components of the response (the cochlear map is preserved at low amplitude locations). We believe this to be the first clear evidence of dynamic mapping effects for a condition of no manipulation, by other tones or bias effects. The frequency modulation seen in figure 1(a) is directly the result of a primary peak at one location having its frequency varied during the course of the local response to the click-evoked travelling wave. Such responses are at least consistent with the hypothesis that a *localised* change has occurred at the site of emission generation and not at some more basal place instantaneously or post-generation.The rapid amplitude modulation occurring at 3.2 kHz (Fig. 1(b)) is responsible for the appearance of sharp notches in the spectrum of the averaged time response. We assert that this variation is a normal part of the dynamic response of the ear to the repetitive click stimulus since it is not the result of any externally applied manipulation. These data are therefore consistent with the notion that OHC force generation is directly modifying the local tonotopy of the cochlea.

In response to the tone, the measures of coherence in the ear of SEJ01 showed a much more dramatic change than those for subject ANM01. The major change in emission strength was not immediate with the cessation of the tone, but delayed for some minutes. Other subjects have shown similar delays. Experiments by Dancer et al. (1992) have shown maximum changes in hearing threshold delayed for anything up to 24 hours after severe exposure. The approach may be useful for characterising susceptibility to hearing loss because, unlike previous experiments on TTS much smaller controlled doses can safely be administered. It would now be extremely useful to refine such a test so that very specific levels of perturbation could incorporate challenge levels which occasion minimal discomfort.

Dynamic mapping may explain why the transition between TTS and PTS is not strongly connected. TTS may be a behavioural indication of a perturbed state of the cochlea leading to a shift in mapping probably in response to an OHC-based control mechanism which manifests itself as a shifted operating point for sound levels over 90dB SPL.

References

1. Allen, J. B., (1996). OHCs shift the excitation pattern via BM tension. In Diversity in Auditory Mechanics, edited by E. Lewis, G. Long, P. Narins, and C. Steele. World Scientific Publishing World Scientific Publishing, Singapore, (this volume).
2. Bray, P. J., (1989). Click evoked otoacoustic emissions and the development of a clinical otoacoustic hearing test instrument. Thesis submitted for the degree of Doctor of Philosophy, University of London.
3. Brown, AM. and Beveridge, HA., (1997). Two components of acoustic distortion: differential effects of aspirin and contralateral sound. In:Diversity in Auditory Mechanics, ed. by E. Lewis, G. Long, P. Narins, and C. Steele. World Scientific Publishing, Berkeley, June 24-28, (this volume).
4. Cheng, J., (1995). Time-frequency analysis of transient evoked otoacoustic emissions via smoothed pseudo Wigner distribution. *Scand-Audiol.* **24** 91-6.
5. Dancer, A. L., Grateau, P., Cabanis, A., Barnabe, G., Cagnin, G., Vaillant, T., and Lafont, D., (1992). Effectiveness of earplugs in high-intensity impulse noise. *J-Acoust-Soc-Am.* **91** 1677-89.
6. LePage, E.L. (1987). A Spatial Template for the Shape of Tuning Curves in the Mammalian Cochlea. *J. Acoust. Soc. Am.* **82** 155-164.

7. LePage, E. L., (1990). Helmholtz revisited: direct mechanical data suggest a physical model for dynamic control of mapping frequency to place along the cochlear partition. In: The Mechanics and Biophysics of Hearing, edited by P. Dallos, C. D. Geisler J. W. Matthews M. A. Ruggero and C. R. Steele. June 25-29, 1990, *Lecture Notes in Biomathematics*, **87** 278-287.

8. LePage, E. L., (1992). Hysteresis in cochlear mechanics and a model for variability in noise-induced hearing loss. In: Noise-Induced Hearing Loss. A. Dancer, D. Henderson R. J. Salvi and R. P. Hamernik, ed(s). Mosby Year Book, St.Louis , 10, 106-115.

9. McFadden, D., (1986). The curious half-octave shift: evidence for a basal-ward migration of the traveling-wave envelope with increasing intensity. In: Basic and Applied Aspects of Noise-Induced Hearing Loss. R. Salvi, D. Henderson R. P. Hamernik and V. Colletti, ed(s). Plenum Press, New York, 295-312.

EFFECTS OF LOOP DIURETICS ON SUPPRESSION TUNING OF DISTORTION-PRODUCT OTOACOUSTIC EMISSIONS IN RABBITS

G.K. MARTIN, B.L. LONSBURY-MARTIN, D. JASSIR, B.B. STAGNER

University of Miami Ear Institute (M805), Box 016960, Miami, FL 33101, USA

gmartin@mednet.med.miami.edu

Suppression tuning of distortion-product otoacoustic emissions (DPOAEs) is often assumed to measure frequency selectivity because the dominant features of suppression-tuning curves (STCs) are similar to the tuning curves of cochlear-nerve fibers. In the present study loop diuretics were used to affect DPOAE generation in order to determine if reversible ototoxicity adversely modified the frequency selectivity of STCs. Contour plots of DPOAE level in the presence of an interference tone were obtained before and after administering diuretics that reversibly reduced or eliminated DPOAEs. Primary-tone pairs were centered at 2.8 or 4 kHz, with $L_1=L_2$ or L_2 lower than L_1. From resulting contour plots, DPOAE level, best-suppressor center frequency, suppressor or tip threshold, and Q_{10dB} measures of tuning were abstracted for several suppression criteria. The major finding was that suppression tuning depended on both primary-tone level and the relative levels of the primaries, with tuning being sharper for lower- than for higher-level equilevel primaries, and sharpest for $L_2<L_1$. Following drug injection, the expected decrease in sharpness of tuning was often not found, and, at times, STCs became sharper than prior to diuretic dosing. These findings imply that STCs and neural-tuning curves may reflect unique cochlear processes.

1 Introduction

Studies of suppression tuning of distortion-product otoacoustic emissions (DPOAEs) in animal models suggest that this measure may provide an index of frequency selectivity. In the bat, Frank and Kossl[2] noted that, as the tuning characteristics of neurons in the ventral cochlear nucleus changed within various specialized frequency regions, DPOAE suppression-tuning curves (STCs) obtained across corresponding frequency extents in other bats demonstrated similar tuning properties. Specifically, in the frequency region between 62 and 72 kHz, which represents a region of specialized thickening of the basilar membrane, the low-frequency tails of both the neural tuning curves (NTCs) and STCs reversed direction. Similarly, in the bobtail lizard,[3] comparisons of the distributions of Q_{10dB} values revealed a close relationship between the NTC and STC measures of frequency selectivity. Together, these observations support the notion that the dominant features of STCs are similar to the tuning characteristics of single cochlear-nerve fibers.

To our knowledge, there have been no direct comparisons between NTCs and STCs recorded from the same animal. One critical problem in making this comparison is determining the parameters under which to obtain STCs, which are elicited by bitonal stimuli, that are comparable to those used to measure NTCs, which are based on single pure-tone stimuli.

The present study was designed to obtain STCs in the same rabbit before and following the performance of experimental manipulations known to reliably alter cochlear-frequency selectivity. Because it is well-established that the administration of ototoxic-loop diuretics, such as ethacrynic acid or furosemide, reduces basilar-membrane[5] and cochlear-nerve fiber[1] tuning, STCs were obtained before and during the recovery of cochlear dysfunction due to diuretic-drug dosing.

2   Methods

Subjects were eight young adult pigmented rabbits. To reduce the confounding effects of the acoustic reflex and potential changes in probe position, $2f_1$-f_2 DPOAEs were obtained from anesthetized animals (ketamine, 50 mg/kg; xylazine, 10 mg/kg). Prior to drug injection, DPOAE measures were determined in response to several primary-tone levels. DPOAE responses included level/frequency functions or DP-grams, i.e., DPOAE level as a function of frequency in response to constant-level primaries, and contour plots, i.e., DPOAE level as a function of systematic changes in the frequency and level of an interference tone (f_{int}). Following acquisition of control measures, rabbits were given an intravenous (IV) injection of either ethacrynic acid (40 mg/kg) or furosemide (100 mg/kg). To observe dynamic changes as the animals recovered from the effects of the diuretic agent, both DPOAE functions were regularly re-measured at ~20-min intervals over the post-drug period that lasted for about 80 mins.

The f_1 and f_2 primary tones were generated by a digital signal-processing (DSP) board in a microcomputer, and presented over ER-2 speakers. Ear-canal sound pressure was measured with an ER-10 microphone, and sampled and synchronously averaged by the DSP board. The f_{int} was digitally added to the f_1 channel.

The primary tones (f_2/f_1=1.25) were centered around the geometric-mean (GM) frequencies of 2.8 or 4 kHz, at L_1=L_2=45, 50, 55, 60, or 65 dB SPL, or with L_2 lower than L_1 by an amount that depended on the level of L_1,[6] ie, L_1,L_2=50,35, 55,45, and 60,55, dB SPL. For each primary-tone pair, the f_{int} was swept in 10 steps/octave, from .25-10 kHz, with the f_{int} level (L_{int}) being systematically increased in 5-dB steps, from 35-85 dB SPL. Data were analyzed as contour plots displaying changes in DPOAE amplitude in the presence of the f_{int} relative to control measures collected in the absence of the f_{int}. Successive contours represented increasing iso-suppression in 3-dB interpolated steps (see Fig 2 below). From these data-point matrices, STCs were abstracted, for suppression criteria of 3, 6, 9, and 12 dB, along with several tuning-curve parameters (i.e., suppressor-center frequency, suppressor threshold, and Q_{10dB}).

3   Results

Suppression tuning was found to depend on both primary-tone level and on the relative levels of the primaries. Specifically, similar to observations established in normal-hearing young humans,[4] tuning was sharper for low-level equilevel ($L_1=L_2$) primaries, and was sharpest with $L_2<L_1$ primaries. Following diuretic administration, the expected decrease in sharpness of tuning was usually not found, even when DPOAE level was reduced at least 5-6 dB, in that, frequently, STCs did not change substantially, or they became even sharper than prior to diuretic dosing. The data of Fig 1 for rabbit #39 compares pre-versus post-furosemide data for the 6-dB suppression criterion using primary-tone levels of $L_1=50$ and $L_2=35$ dB SPL. In this case, which illustrates an example of a minor decrease in tuning, during the post-drug period, the DPOAE amplitude was so drastically reduced, that contour plots could not be obtained until about 40-60 mins following furosemide injection, ie, during the post-3 time interval.

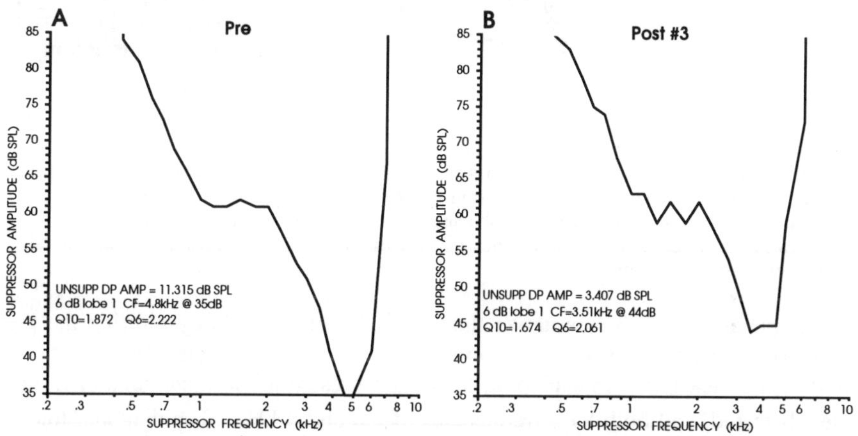

Figure 1: Suppression-tuning curve for R#39 at the 4-kHz GM frequency using a 6-dB suppression criterion during pre- (A) and post-drug (B) intervals. Note the ~8-dB reduction in DPOAE level, the slight reduction in STC tip frequency, the 9-dB increase in suppression threshold, and the slight decrease in the Q_{10dB} value.

In Fig 2, for the animal of Fig 1, the pre/post contour plots obtained over the identical time intervals are shown. These findings describe the major outcome in more detail in that it is clear that at baseline, DPOAE level was sufficiently robust to establish iso-suppression tuning curves that reflect suppression criteria from 3-27

244

dB, in 3-dB steps (Fig 2A). However, as apparent in Fig 2B, DPOAE level was considerably reduced post-drug administration so that only suppression criteria from 3 to 9 dB could be satisfied. However, despite the loss in the 'depth' of suppression, the tuning-curve shapes remained relatively constant.

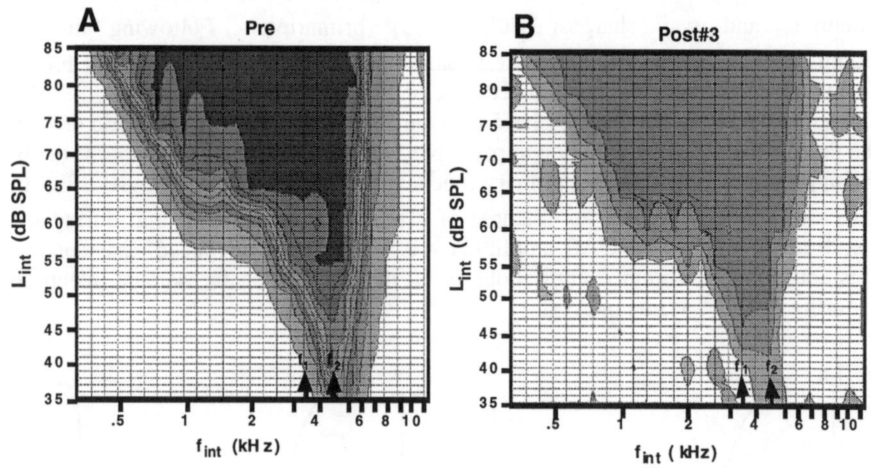

Figure 2: Suppression-contour plots for animal #39 displayed in Fig 1 obtained over the identical time periods--in fact, these data were used to extract the STCs of Fig 1. Note that during the pre- drug period (A) suppression criteria from 3-27 dB were easily obtained as indicated by the increased bands of shading. However, post-drug (B) , the 'depth' of suppression was reduced to 3-9 dB, but the shapes of the iso-suppression tuning curves remained essentially identical.

The panels of Fig 3 summarize the results for all animals by plotting the pre- (abscissa) versus post-drug data points over four recovery intervals for several experimental measures. In each plot, the data represent all combinations of L_1 and L_2 levels tested, and both STC frequencies of 2.8 and 4 kHz. The diagonal line on each plot represents the 'no-change' condition in which pre- and post-drug dosing measures were identical. In each plot, data points falling above the 'no-change' line indicate increases in the response parameter, whereas data plotted below the line reflect decreases in that measure.

In Fig 3A it is clear that immediately post-drug administration (solid circles) DPOAE amplitudes were reduced, on average. However, as recovery continued, emission levels tended to approach baseline amplitudes as evidenced by the closeness of the solid triangle and 'X' data-point symbols to the 'no-change' line. The recovery of DPOAE amplitude with increasing time post-drug injection, was the only temporally ordered effect observed.

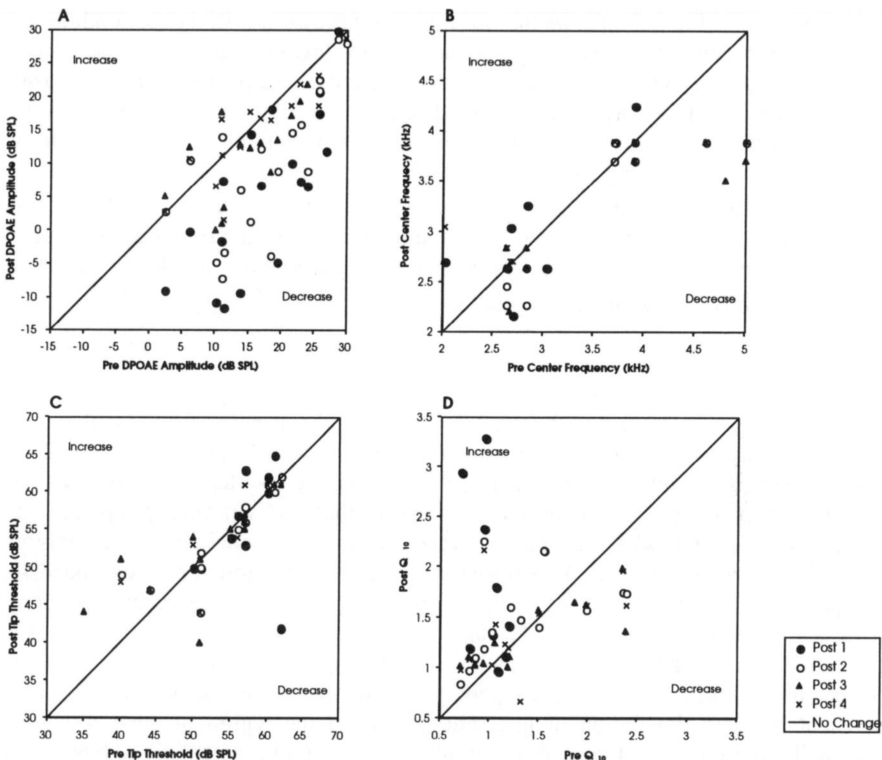

Figure 3: Pre/post-drug comparison plots for all rabbits for all GM frequencies and for all combinations of primary-tone levels. Symbols indicate the approximate measurement times post-injection: post 1=0-20 mins (solid circles); post 2=21-40 mins (open circles); post 3=41-60 mins (solid triangles); post 4=61-80 mins (X'es). A: Changes in DPOAE levels; B: changes in the STC tip frequency; C: changes in STC tip or suppression threshold; D: changes in Q_{10dB} tuning.

Although several lower-frequency outliers are evident in Fig 3B, which plots the pre/post-center or best-suppressor frequency, it is clear that, for the 2.8-kHz GM frequency, whereas the baseline data are centered around 2.8 kHz, tip frequencies are distributed more widely from about 2.3-3.4 kHz during the post-drug period. In contrast, at the GM of 4 kHz, some data points show little diuretic-induced change in that they are centered about the GM frequency during both pre- and post-drug measurements. However, other data reflect a lowering of the best-suppression frequencies during the post-drug interval from about 4.5-5 kHz to ~3.5-4 kHz. It is interesting that the former data set, showing few pre/post changes in STC-tip frequency, represent primarily DPOAEs elicited with equilevel primaries, whereas the latter data evidencing decreases in the tip frequencies of the STC reflect DPOAEs measured with primary tones offset in level.

The data of Fig 3C indicate that for higher suppression criteria, ie, conditions in which suppression thresholds are also necessarily higher, minimal changes occur between the pre- and post-drug injection periods. However, for the lower-suppression criteria, on average, diuretic dosing produced about a 10-dB increase in the threshold of suppression. Finally, although a few examples of decreases in the Q_{10dB} measure of tuning are apparent in Fig 3D, particularly for STCs having the higher pre-drug values, in general, frequency selectivity tended either not to change substantially, or to increase following the administration of the diuretics as reflected by the tendency for Q_{10dB} values to be distributed around the 'no change' line or to increase slightly following drug injection.

4 Discussion

These findings imply that although STCs exhibit the general features of neural-tuning curves, they may not directly measure cochlear-frequency selectivity as evidenced at the level of the basilar membrane or single cochlear-nerve fibers. This interpretation is not too unexpected considering that STCs probably represent the suppression of DPOAE generation processes that are elicited by a two-tone complex. It would, in fact, be surprising if this measure equaled or exceeded the frequency selectivity observed for single-tone tuning. The present findings are more consistent with the notion that STC shape originates primarily from the properties of the interference tone. In this formulation, the shape of the STC arises from this tone's interference with emission generation, which would be minimal or non-existent basal to the region of generation, peak in the region of generation, and gradually diminish as the interfering tone moves more apically. Thus, when pathological factors influence DPOAE generation, such as during the reversible episodes of ototoxicity performed here, as long as the DPOAE is generated, i.e., measurable, the amount of suppression may diminish, but the overall shape of the STC will remain similar to that recorded during the control period. However, if the region of DPOAE generation is dramatically reduced, it could be predicted that the STC would become sharper as observed at times in the present study.

Acknowledgments

The work was supported by the Public Health Service (DC00613, ES03500), and funds from the University of Miami Chandler Chair.

References

1. Evans, E.F. and Klinke, R. (1982) The effects of intracochlear and systemic furosemide on the properties of single cochlear nerve fibres in the cat, *J. Physiol. (Lond.)* **331** 409-428.
2. Frank, G. and Kossl, M. (1995) The shape of $2f_1$-f_2 suppression tuning curves reflects basilar membrane specialization in the mustached bat, *Pteronotus parnellii Hear. Res.* **83** 151-160.
3. Koppl, C. and Manley, G.A. (1993) Distortion-product otoacoustic emissions in the bobtail lizard. II: Suppression tuning characteristics, *J. Acoust. Soc. Am.* **93** 2834-2844.
4. Lecusay, R.A., Fletcher, C.A., Lonsbury-Martin, B.L., Stagner, B.B., Waxman, G.M., and Martin, G.K. (1996) Otoacoustic emissions in normal-hearing humans: Musicians vs non-musicians, *Abstr. Assoc. Res. Otolaryngol.* **19** 25.
5. Ruggero, M.A. and Rich, N.C. (1991) Furosemide alters organ of Corti mechanics: Evidence for feedback of outer hair cells upon the basilar membrane, *J. Neurosci.* **11** 1057-1067.
6. Whitehead, M.L., Stagner, B.B., McCoy, M.J., Lonsbury-Martin, B.L., and Martin, G.K. (1995) Dependence of distortion-product otoacoustic emissions on primary levels in normal and impaired ears. II. Asymmetry in L_1,L_2 space, *J. Acoust. Soc. Am.* **97** 2359-2377.

CHANGES IN COCHLEAR AMPLIFIER MECHANICS DURING DEVELOPMENT

D. M. MILLS, E.W. RUBEL

Virginia Merrill Bloedel Hearing Research Center
University of Washington, Seattle, WA 98195-7923, USA
e-mail:dmmills@u.washington.edu

Development of properties of the cochlear amplifier has been investigated using distortion product emission measurements before and after furosemide injection in 75 Mongolian gerbils, age 14 to 28 days. The base cutoff frequency, marked by the frequency at which the cochlear amplifier gain drops abruptly to zero, increased from below 20 kHz at 14 days to about 56 kHz at maturity. A transformation from frequency to place for the cochlea at different ages was derived from these data. For the transformed cochlear amplifier gain, the basal slope, or rate of increase with distance from the the base, was found to increase steadily during development, so that the length of the active amplification zone decreased from 1.2 mm to 0.7 mm over the period studied. A similar decrease in the length of this zone in the mid base regions could account for the observed decrease, from 18 to 28 days old, in the total cochlear amplifier gain at mid frequencies.

1 Introduction

Development of cochlear function has been studied extensively in gerbils,[1] including recent distortion product emission measurements which extended the frequency range above 50 kHz.[2] For all frequencies above 2 kHz, the cochlear amplifier was found to be essentially mature near the onset of hearing, but hearing function was apparently limited by the passive response of the cochlea. That is, there was evident a sharp falloff in absolute emission amplitude and in cochlear amplifier gain above a certain frequency, and this cutoff frequency increased steadily with age. The sharp falloff was attributed to the passive mechanics of the cochlear base, which necessarily has a finite frequency above which waves cannot propagate along the basilar membrane.[3, 4] This report extends the previous study[2] with a detailed examination of the development of emission characteristics around the base cutoff frequency.

2 Methods

The material presented here is based on distortion product emission studies of a total of 75 gerbils aged 14 days after birth (dab) to adult. Animal preparation, equipment and procedures were as previously reported.[2] For all animals, after baseline measurements were completed, furosemide was administered intraperitoneally to determine the "passive" emission response. The increase in stimulus level, A_c, required to reach the same emission level for the passive response as for the normal value, at low stimulus levels, was taken as an indication of the cochlear amplifier gain.[2] For the first group of gerbils (34 total) measurements were made at octave intervals from 1 to 32 kHz, with parameters optimized to obtain estimates of the cochlear amplifier gain. The measurements on the second group of 41 animals included gain measurements at 1/12 octave intervals around the base cutoff frequency, before and after furosemide administration.

3 Results

3.1 Variation of cochlear amplifier gain with frequency and age

The calculated variation of the gain, A_c, associated with the cochlear amplifier is summarized in Fig. 1 for stimulus frequencies 4 kHz and higher for the two groups. Development of the endocochlear potential (EP) is also shown.[5]

For both groups, the results at midfrequencies (4-16 kHz) agree very well. Near the onset of hearing, the cochlear amplifier gains were near adult values, except at 16 kHz. As the EP increased sharply from 15 to 20 dab, the gains increased at all frequencies. From dab 21 on, with the EP stabilized to its adult values, the gains then decreased, reaching adult values by about 28 dab. The adult values were found to be remarkably constant across frequency, considering the wide variation observed during development. At higher frequencies (20-32 kHz) for both groups the gain of the cochlear amplifier was near zero at the onset of hearing, but attained adult values by about 20 dab. The only difference between the results for the two groups was for 32 kHz, where there was an apparent overshoot for the first group but not the second.

3.2 Variation in base cutoff frequency with age

In the second group of 41 animals, gains were determined at 1/12 octave intervals near the base cutoff frequency for each animal. Typical individual results are presented in Fig. 2A.
For all animals, above some characteristic frequency there was a sharp dropoff in gain, reaching zero in 0.4 to 1 octave. The frequency at which the gain was extrapolated to zero was designated the base cutoff frequency, f_b. Preceding the sharp decline, there was either a plateau where the gain was approximately constant, or there was a relative maximum. In all cases, the plateau edge, or peak frequency, f_p, could be defined as shown. The gain at the plateau edge or peak frequency was designated A_p, as illustrated. Fig. 2B presents the development of the mean values of the frequencies, f_b and f_p.

The mean base cutoff frequency was below 20 kHz at the onset of hearing, but rose rapidly to reach about 40 kHz by 17-18 dab. After this age, it rose more slowly, reaching adult values by about 21 dab. The peak frequency tended to be about a half octave below the base cutoff frequency over most of the developmental period.

250

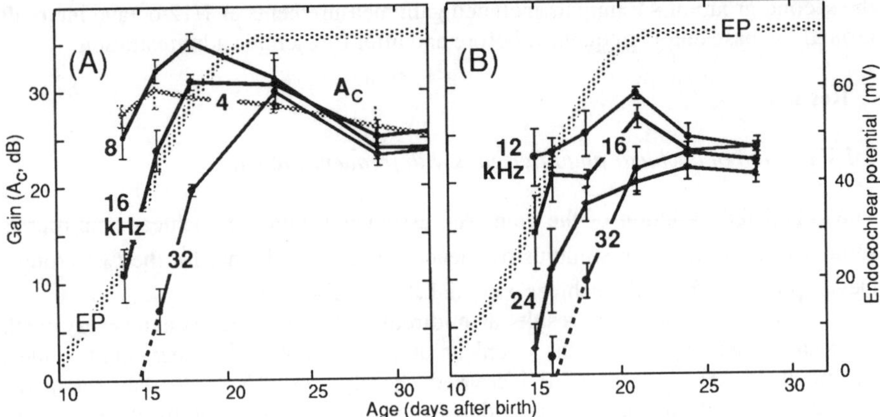

Fig. 1. The mean gain (A_c, left axis) plotted versus the age of the gerbil. The parameter is the stimulus frequency in kHz. Bars indicate standard error of the mean. **(A)** Results for the first group (with 34 gerbils total) using stimulus levels L_1 ten dB higher than L_2. Only frequencies at 4 kHz and above are shown. **(B)** Results for the second group (41 total gerbils) with equal level stimuli. Only frequencies from 12 kHz up were measured in this group.

In general, then, the highest frequency for which the cochlear amplifier gain was near adult values was about a half octave below the frequency at which the gain became zero. The separation between these two frequencies increased to about 0.7 octave during the period 18 to 21 dab, and for adult animals it decreased to about 0.4 octave.

3.3 Frequency-place transformation

The information in Fig. 2B may be used to derive a transformation from frequency to physical distance along the cochlear duct, under suitable assumptions. The essential assumption is that the observed sharp falloff in cochlear amplifier gain with frequency is primarily due to the effects of a finite base cutoff frequency. That is, while there are likely some minor changes in the active amplification processes during development, the development of the active response in the base is assumed to be primarily limited by the development of the passive response of the cochlea.[2,3]

At a given age, the frequency (f_b) at which the cochlear amplifier gain goes to zero is therefore the frequency associated with the location of the extreme basal end of the cochlea ($z=0$). That is, the "characteristic frequency" (CF) at $z=0$ is f_b by definition. As the stimulus frequency decreases below f_b, an actual peak occurs apically of $z=0$ because there is then "room" for amplification to occur at that frequency.[3]   When the stimulus frequency has decreased to f_p, the cochlear response peak has reached near normal or normal values, typically 20-40 dB above the zero gain condition. Note that the distance between the locations associated with f_b and f_p is the distance over which the active amplification must occur at the frequency f_p.

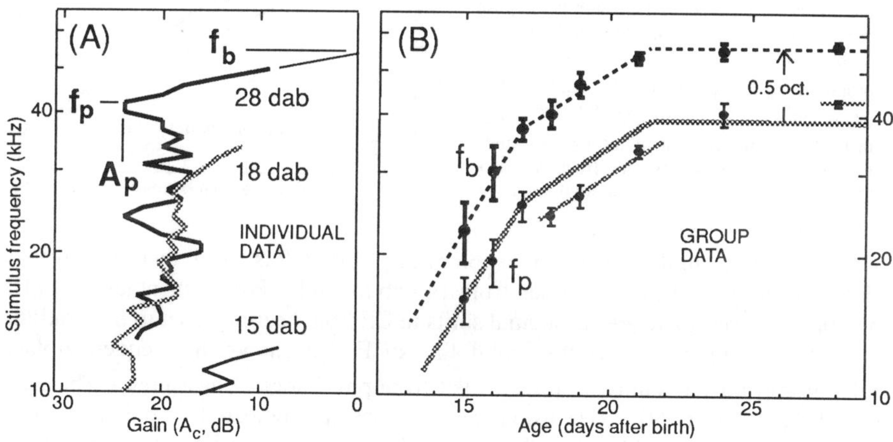

Fig. 2. (A) Individual responses at three different ages from the second group of animals, used to determine the variation of base cutoff frequency with age.   The vertical axis gives the stimulus frequency in kHz and the horizontal the calculated gain, A_c, in dB.   The figure illustrates the determination of the frequency at the leading edge or peak, f_p; the gain, A_p, at the frequency f_p; and the frequency, f_b, at which the extrapolated gain goes to zero. (Animals 95-2105, 2124, 2130). **(B)** The mean values for the derived base cutoff frequencies plotted versus gerbil age. The two parallel lines are shown for comparison, and are 0.5 octaves apart. The upper line is the relationship used in Fig. 3 to obtain the frequency-place transformation. This line indicates the frequency of the extreme basal end of the cochlea, above which the cochlear amplifier gain is zero. In contrast, at a given age the lower curve denotes the highest frequency which obtains normal or near normal amplification from the cochlear amplifier.

Two more simple assumptions are required to convert the results in Fig. 2B to a frequency (CF) to place (z) transform. The first is that, at some distance from the apex, there is no change in CF location with development following hearing onset. This view is supported by results which show no measurable change in CF with development for gerbils at frequencies of 2 kHz and lower.[6] The second assumption required is that between the base and the fixed location, characteristic frequencies are located approximately logarithmically, with equal spacing per octave, as is known for adult gerbils.[7]

For illustrative purposes, we assume that the place for a CF of one kHz is fixed, at the location $z = z_1$ as noted. The resulting frequency-place transform, with age as a parameter, is shown in Fig. 3.

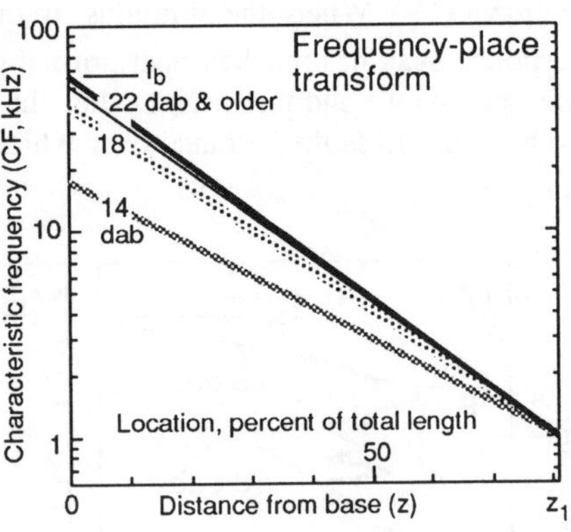

Fig. 3. The derived frequency-place transform for three different ages. For a given frequency on the left, the maximum response is located at a place on the cochlea denoted on the horizontal axis. It is arbitrarily assumed that the 1 kHz place is fixed at the location $z = z_1$. The frequency f_b from Fig. 2B then determines the intercept on the left axis, which is the base ($z=0$). For comparison, the thin solid line next to the adult data on this plot represents the proposed relationship[7] for the adult gerbil, where CF in kHz $= 0.4 * 10^{(0.021 * d)}$. The distance d is the percent of the total distance from the *apex* and is 19% for a frequency of 1 kHz, i.e., z_1 equals 81% of the total length of the cochlea.

Note that, although the cochlear location of the 1 kHz CF is fixed, there is still very little shift at the 2-4 kHz locations from 14 dab to adult. For frequencies of 8 kHz and up, however, there are substantial shifts in CF from hearing onset to maturation.

For comparison, the thin solid line in Fig. 3 shows the frequency-place relationship for the adult gerbil estimated from physiological measures.[7] The base cutoff frequency is 50.3 kHz using this relationship, compared to our adult base cutoff frequency of 56 kHz (Fig. 2B and 3). This is excellent agreement considering the entirely different methods of obtaining these two estimates.

3.4 Variation of cochlear amplifier gain with distance

The frequency response data in Fig. 1A has been transformed by the relationships summarized in Fig. 3, to obtain a determination of the development of cochlear amplifier gain as a function of position along the cochlear duct (Fig. 4).

The most striking result in comparing the gain versus frequency results with those for gain versus distance involves the slope of the gain function near the base. When seen in the frequency domain, the slope appears to change with development in an inverted "U" shaped response. Consider Fig. 2B. At the youngest ages, there was about a half octave separation between the frequencies, f_b and f_p, associated with the zero gain and relative maximum gain respectively. At 18 to 21 dab, however, this separation increased to 0.7 octave. As mature function was attained, the separation decreased back to a half octave and became even smaller for the adult animal. These changes in the mean values were also reflected in the individual examples shown in Fig. 2A. A curvilinear response was also seen in the mean data when the slope itself (i.e., in dB/octave) of the high frequency falloff was plotted (not shown). However, when the data is transformed to the distance scale, this curvilinear response disappears. It does so due to the sharp increase in f_b from 14 to 18 dab associated with a substantial compression of the frequency scale.

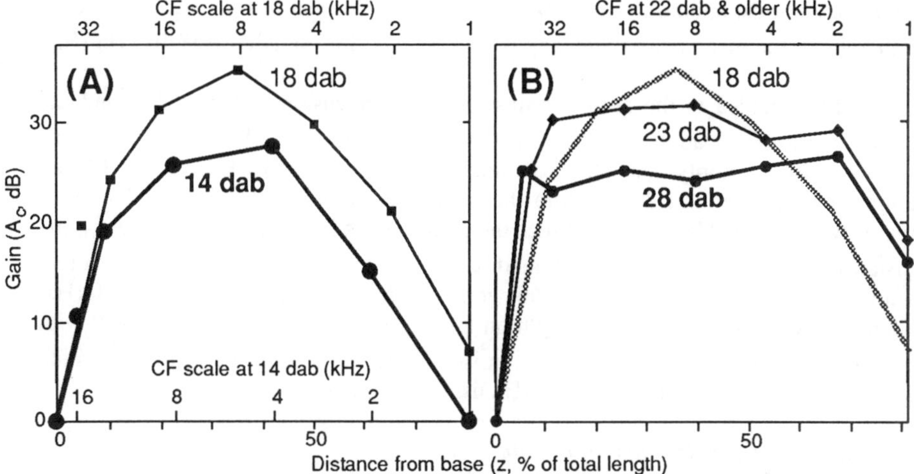

Fig. 4. The cochlear amplifier gain figure, A_C, presented as a function of place along the basilar membrane. Most points were obtained by transforming the data in Fig. 1A using Fig. 3. For responses within about a half octave of the base, however, the more precise data from the second group of animals were used for the gain values. In addition to the mean f_p values shown in Fig. 3, the figure includes the corresponding mean A_p values estimated for the second group:19 dB at 14 dab, 24 dB at 18 dab, and 25 dB for 19 dab and up. At the top of Fig. 4A is given the CF scale at 18 dab, at the bottom of this panel the CF scale for 14 dab, and at the top of Fig. 4B is the adult CF scale. As in Fig. 3, the percentage scale given on the lower axis is obtained from the proposed frequency-place relationship for adult gerbils.[7]

Expressed as a function of the distance along the cochlear duct, the gain at all positions increased from 14 dab to 18 dab. This was also the period of a substantial increase in EP (Fig. 1). At 18 dab, the mid frequency regions of the cochlea amplified the most strongly. The sharply peaked gain seen at 18 dab, however, was transformed by adulthood into a gain which was remarkably flat as a function of position along the BM. For most of the length of the cochlea, except for the extremes, this was accomplished by a reduction in the gain of the cochlear amplifier from its maximum values at 18-23 dab.

4 Discussion

4.1 Changes in length of the active amplification zone

At 14 dab, the cochlear amplifier gain rises sharply at the base, going from zero to normal gain levels in about 10% of the total cochlear length (Fig. 4).The slope of the amplification increases slowly but steadily as the animal ages, so that by maturity this distance has decreased to 6% of the total length. This distance may be taken as equal to the length of the active amplification zone[8] for the stimulus frequency corresponding to the peak frequency, f_p, defined in Fig. 2A. For the 14 dab animal, the mean peak frequency is 13 kHz, and for the adult it is 40 kHz (Fig. 2B).

The cochlea in the gerbil attains its adult dimensions by 10 dab,[9] and the mean length of the adult gerbil cochlea is about 12 mm.[10] With this length, the results in Fig. 4 imply that the active amplification zone at 13 kHz in the 14 dab animal extends about 1.2 mm from the base, but extends only about 0.7 mm by maturity, for a 40 kHz stimulus. Since the gain flattens for frequencies below f_p, the distance of 0.7 mm can be assumed to be the entire distance of the active amplification zone in the normal adult gerbil at the stimulus frequency of 40 kHz. This is only about 0.4 octave in length on the CF scale. This result agrees well with an active zone determination based on noise lesions in the adult guinea pig,[8] which gives 0.8 mm at frequencies near 15 kHz using comparable definitions.

4.2 Changes in cochlear amplifier gain

As measured by emissions, from the age of 14 dab the gain of the cochlear amplifier increases for the mid frequencies, 4 to 16 kHz. These gains reach a maximum value sometime between 18 and 21 dab (Fig. 1). The gain then decreases at mid frequencies, declining (depending on the measure and frequency) about 5-10 dB. This decline is largely accomplished by 24 dab, only 3-6 days after the peak occurs, and is complete by 28 dab. The maximum gain occurs about the same time that the EP reaches mature levels. It is parsimonius to suppose that the sharp increase in gain is driven by the substantial rise in the EP from 14 dab to 20 dab. Subsequently, the length of the active amplification zone at the base apparently decreases (Fig. 2B), and the gain at mid frequencies is reduced (Fig. 4). Taken alone, the decrease in gain could be due to a reduction in gain per unit distance in the relevant frequency range. However, it is parsimonious to assume that the gain per unit length along the cochlea remains constant over this time period, but that the length of the active amplification zone at mid frequencies is reduced, as it is at the basal end.

As an example, consider the 8 kHz region. Suppose at 18 dab the length of the active amplification zone is 1 mm and there is a total gain of 35 dB. If the amplification rate stays the same (i.e., 35 dB/mm), but the length of the active amplification zone is decreased to 0.7 mm, the total gain will decrease to 25 dB, which is the amount observed. It appears that the developmental variation in the cochlear amplifier gain noted previously[2,3] may be accomplished by a shortening of the active amplification zone.

Acknowledgments

Support was provided by research grant NIH DC 00395.

References

1. Ryan A.F. and Woolf, N.K. (1992) Development of the lower auditory system in the gerbil. In: *Development of Auditory and Vestibular Systems II.* ed. Romand ,Elsevier. pp 243-271.
2. Mills, D.M. and Rubel, E.W. (1996) Development of the cochlear amplifier. *J. Acoust. Soc. Am.* **100** 428-441.
3. Mills, D.M., Norton, S.J. and Rubel, E.W. (1994) Development of active and passive mechanics in the mammalian cochlea. *Auditory Neurosci.* **1** 77-99.
4. Puria, S. and Allen, J.B. (1991) A parametric study of cochlear input impedance. *J. Acoust. Soc. Am.* **89** 287-309.
5. Woolf, N. K., Ryan, A.F., and Harris, J.P. (1986) Development of mammalian endocochlear potential: normal ontogeny and effects of anoxia. *Am. J. Physiol.* **250** R493-R498.
6. Arjmand, E., Harris, D. and Dallos, P. (1988) Developmental changes in frequency mapping of the gerbil cochlea: Comparison of two cochlear locations. *Hear. Res.* **32** 93-96.
7. Tarnowski, B.I., Schmiedt, R.A., Hellstrom, L.I., Lee, F.S. and Adams. J.C. (1991) Age-related changes on cochleas of mongolian gerbils. *Hear. Res.* **54** 123-134.
8. Cody, A.R. (1992) Acoustic lesions in the mammalian cochlea: Implications for the spatial distribution of the "active process". *Hear. Res.* **62** 166-172.
9. Harris, D.M, Rotche, R. and Freedom, T. (1990) Postnatal growth of cochlear spiral in mongolian gerbil. *Hear. Res.* **50** 1-6.
10. Schmiedt, R.A. and Zwislocki, J.J.. (1977) Comparison of sound-transmission and cochlear-microphonic characteristics in Mongolian gerbil and guinea pig. *J. Acoust. Soc. Amer.* *61* 133-149.

THE ORIGIN OF OTOACOUSTIC EMISSIONS ELICITED BY ELECTRICAL STIMULATION OF THE COCHLEA

A. L. NUTTALL

Kresge Hearing Research Institute, The University of Michigan Medical School
1301 East Ann Street
Ann Arbor, MI 48109-0506
email: nuttall@umich.edu

T. REN

Kresge Hearing Research Institute, The University of Michigan Medical School
1301 East Ann Street, Ann Arbor, MI 48109-0506
Department of Otolaryngology, Xian Medical University, The People's Republic of China
email: renty@umich.edu

E. DE BOER

Academic Medical Center, Meibergdreef 9
1105 AZ, Amsterdam, The Netherlands
email: E.deBoer@amc.uva.nl

We have shown that electric stimulation of the normal cochlea (e.g., at the round window) causes traveling waves on the basilar membrane.[1] In the current study a two-frequency electric stimulus (f1 and f2) is used to produce an ear canal measured acoustic signal that consists of at least three frequency components, f1, f2, and 2f1-f2. We test the hypothesis that the distortion product (DP) otoacoustic emission at 2f1-f2 originates from the tonotopic location near f2, while the primary otoacoustic emissions originate from the basal turn where the electric stimulus is applied. An acoustic suppressor tone, near f2 in frequency, suppressed f2 as well as the 2f1-f2 DP measured as mechanical components on the basilar membrane at the f2 location. The otoacoustic emission 2f1-f2 DP was suppressed but the f2 (and f1) electrically evoked emissions were not significantly decreased. These results are consistent with the concept that traveling waves are produced as intracochlear outer hair cell-generated acoustic pressure in the potential field of the electric stimulus.

1   Introduction

Otoacoustic emissions are observed in the ear canal of an animal when electric current is applied to the cochlea.[2,3] These emissions are thought to result from intracochlear acoustic pressure produced by the electrically induced motility of outer hair cells (OHCs); and the intracochlear pressure also induces basilar membrane (BM) traveling waves.[1] Otoacoustic emissions resulting from electric current injected into the scala media of apical turn areas of the cochlea have a 'long' delay representing the reverse propagation time of the BM from the topographic location of stimulation.[4,5] These emissions are relatively narrow frequency-band responses where the band is tonotopically consistent with the location of the cochlea being stimulated. In contrast, current applied to the base of the cochlea (e.g., from an electrode on the round window) gives a broad frequency-band otoacoustic emission that has little or no delay other than that which can be attributed to the propagation of the otoacoustic emission from the eardrum to the receiver microphone.[3]

Whereas the origin of the emissions from apical turn stimulation is intuitively consistent with a cochlear location of OHCs tuned to lower frequencies, and having a correspondingly long traveling wave delay, the emissions caused by basal turn stimulation may be different. Basal turn emissions could potentially arise either from the locally stimulated place or from a reflection of traveling wave energy from the characteristic frequency location for the particular stimulus.

2　Methods

2.1　Animals and surgery

The pigmented guinea pigs used in this study were housed in American Association for Accreditation of Laboratory Animal Care-approved facilities. Experimental protocols were approved by the University of Michigan Committee on Use and Care of Animals. After preanesthesia with sodium pentobarbital (30 mg/kg i.p.), anesthesia was induced by an injection of 30 mg/kg of ketamine and 5 mg/kg i.m. of xylazine. Anesthesia was maintained by alternating doses of 30 mg/kg ketamine and 5 mg/kg of xylazine every hour. Redosing with 30 mg/kg of sodium pentobarbital was done every 4 hours. After the animal's head was firmly fixed in a headholder which is electrically isolated from the operating table, a tracheotomy was performed and a ventilation tube inserted into the trachea to insure free breathing. Rectal temperature was maintained at $38 \pm 1°C$.

The bulla was exposed and opened through a ventral approach and the middle ear muscles were cut. A platinum-iridium electrode was positioned against the round window. An Ag-AgCl ground electrode was placed in the soft tissues of the neck, posterior to the bulla.

2.2　Extracochlear stimulation and measurement of EEOAE and BM velocity

Two sinusoidal signals having frequencies f1 and f2 were generated by different oscillators and linearly mixed. This complex signal was delivered to the round window electrode by a constant current stimulator, and level was controlled by an attenuator. A 1 kΩ resistor was connected in series at the return end of the stimulating circuit. Voltage across the resistor was read with an FFT spectrum analyzer (Model SR760, Stanford Research System, Inc., Sunnyvale, CA) and the current through the circuit was calculated. A microphone (Etymotic Research ER-10B, Elk Grove Village, IL) was acoustically coupled to the external ear canal through a plastic speculum. The output signal from the microphone was measured with the FFT analyzer. The possible electrical interference from cross-talk of the electrical stimulus to the microhpone was checked and found to be negligible.

A trigger signal for coherent FFT averaging was derived from the outputs of the oscillators. Amplitudes of electrically evoked otoacoustic emissions (EEOAEs) at frequencies of f1, f2, and 2f1-f2 (the cubic distortion product [DP]) were read from the FFT analyzer.

To measure BM motion, a small hole was made in the bony cochlear wall over the scala tympani of the first turn. Gold-coated glass microbeads (10-30μm diameter) were placed on the scala tympani surface of the BM. A laser Doppler velocimeter (Polytec Corp. OFV 1102), coupled through a compound microscope, measured the velocity of these beads. Velocity signals were analyzed with the FFT analyzer.

2.3 Model

An operational model of an EEOAE from the base of the cochlea is given in Figure 1A. This shows the simple condition where the cochlea is stimulated by a single-frequency (f1) electric current applied at the round window. Figure 1A illustrates current stimulating a restricted area of the basal turn and generating acoustic energy that propagates in both directions. The forward wave behaves just as a normal acoustic traveling wave, by passing through the hypothetical region of the cochlear amplifier (CA) and stopping at the f1 best frequency (BF) location (x1). A left pointing line represents the reflected wave that propagates back to the stapes and emerges as a stimulus frequency otoacoustic emission. Thus, two reverse propagating waves may theoretically arrive at the stapes. The question this study seeks to answer is, which one will dominate?

Figure 1B shows a two-frequency stimulus model. In this illustration, we make the assumption that the locally stimulated OHCs will produce a multi-component reverse wave consisting of f1a, f2a, but no distortion products. There are now two forward propagating acoustic waves which each have reflections (f1b, f2b) from the BF locations (x1 and x2). Additionally, DPs are produced in the region of the CA for f1 and f2,[6] which leads to forward and reverse waves at the DP frequencies (we will measure only the 2f1-f2 intermodulation distortion product). The forward wave behaves as an acoustic traveling wave, passes through another region of cochlear amplification (not shown) and stops in the BF region for the cubic DP (xDP). The forward moving DP would also generate another reverse reflected wave which is not shown in the figure.

The black bar in Figure 1B illustrates the BM location of an externally-applied acoustic suppressor tone. We compare the effect of this suppressor on EEOAEs and BM velocity responses.

3 Results

The experimental protocol was conducted on three guinea pigs with equivalent results in each. Figure 2 shows the result of stimulation of the cochlea with 'low frequency' electrical signals. We define these as low frequencies because 5 kHz is near the low frequency cut-off of the EEOAE

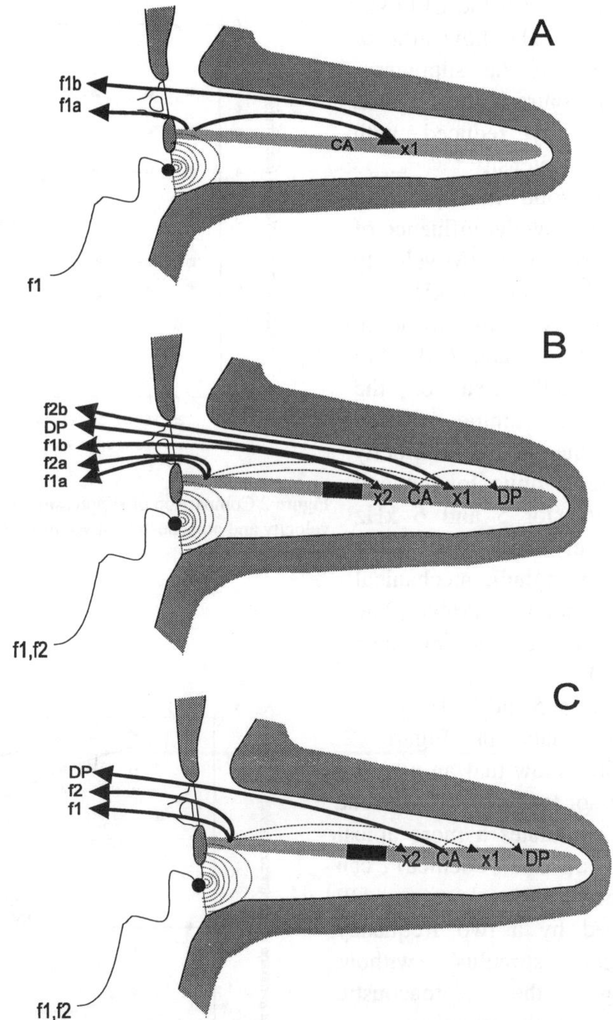

Figure 1 Model of the production of electrically evoked otoacoustic emissions.

transfer function when current is applied to the round window.[3] A current level of 1.2 mA peak-to-peak for the mixed signal of 5 and 6 kHz was delivered to the round window. The f1 (5 kHz) current level was 6 dB stronger than f2. This current produced EEOAEs of approximately 28 and 23 dB SPL, respectively, in the guinea pig ear canal. The cubic DP at 4 kHz was approximately -3 dB SPL. The 7 kHz masker was stepped through an intensity series from 25 to 75 dB SPL. The dotted line curves from the EEOAEs at 5 and 6 kHz show little or no effect of the suppressor tone. In contrast, the DP was systematically reduced with suppressor intensity.

The solid line plots in Figure 2 show the influence of the suppressor on BM velocity recorded at the 18 kHz BF location. At this location, stimuli at 5, 6, and 7 kHz are in the 'tail' area of the mechanical tuning curve. Thus, the local velocity response is quite low, 4 and 2.4 μm/s (for 5 and 6 kHz respectively), for these low frequency stimuli; mechanical DP was not measurable. The suppressor did not influence the BM

responses at 5 and 6 kHz.

The data in Figure 2, therefore, show that an acoustic suppressor tone at 7 kHz (a tone which stimulates a more apical region of the cochlea) can influence the level of the DP produced by a two frequency electrical stimulus without altering the otoacoustic emissions of the primaries.

Figure 3 shows the result obtained when the electric stimulus frequencies were changed to 15 and 18 kHz. These frequencies were chosen to place the f2 stimulus at the BF site of the BM observation.

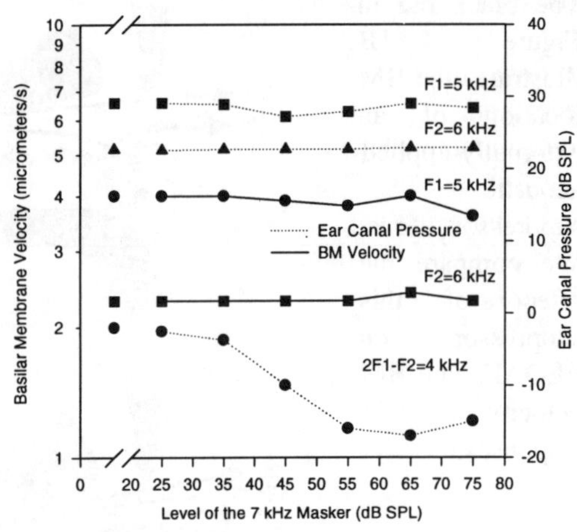

Figure 2 Comparison of suppression of electrically evoked BM velocity and otoacoustic emissions (GP 2368) for 'low frequency stimuli'.

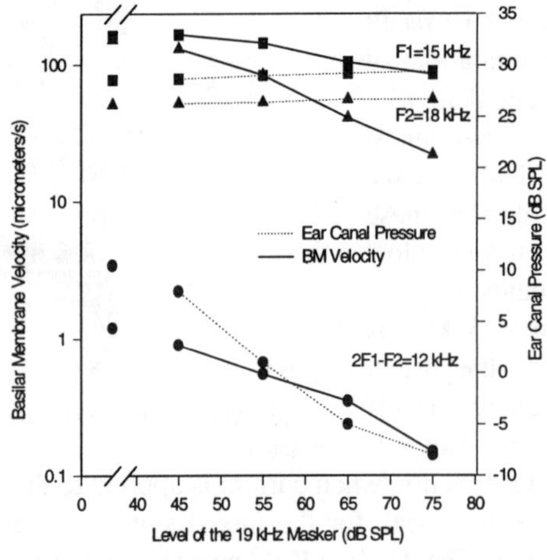

Figure 3 Comparison of suppression of electrically evoked BM velocity and oacoustic emissions (GP 2368) for 'high frequency stimuli'.

The intensity conditions of this test are the same in Figure 2. The dotted curves show that, once again, there was no significant suppression of the EEOAEs that were being recorded for 15 and 18 kHz when the masker acoustic tone of 19 kHz was raised in level from 40 to 75 dB SPL. The cubic DP emission at 12 kHz was suppressed just as for the low frequency case.

BM velocity responses, given by the solid lines, show that the mechanical DP was suppressed with a similar suppression function as the otoacoustic emission DP. This occurs because the BM responses to f1 and f2 are systematically suppressed by the 19 kHz stimulus.

4 Discussion

Ren and Nuttall[3] report a new model for the study of electromotility in the intact cochlea. Alternating current stimulation of the round window gave wide frequency-band otoacoustic emissions. These are thought to result from acoustic energy produced by the OHCs in the base of the cochlea near the stimulation electrode. Nuttall and Ren[1] show that traveling waves result from the acoustic energy produced by basal turn electric stimulation. A traveling wave would occur on the BM which would be amplified by the cochlear amplifier (for a particular frequency) and all related otoacoustic emission phenomena would follow. Therefore, it is not certain that the otoacoustic emissions from electrical stimulation are primary or secondary events.

The results of Figures 2 and 3 showing that the cubic DP emission could be suppressed without a change in the emissions at the stimulus frequencies strongly indicates that the DP is dependent on physiological processes that are separate from the agent producing the EEOAEs at the primary frequencies.[a] Figure 1C presents the model that we propose to account for the data. The suppressor tone, at the black band, would cause two tone suppression of either or both of the propagated acoustic waves, resulting from the electrical stimulation (x1, x2). A BM velocity response measured at those locations would show velocity suppression. The BM velocity response and the cubic DP otoacoustic emission of the mechanical DP, at xDP, would also be suppressed exactly as expected from an acoustic tone suppression experiment. There is, however, no suppression of the EEOAEs, indicating that the

---

[a] If the basal turn hypothesis for the origin of the EEOAEs at the stimulus frequencies is correct, then the fact that the DP can be nearly totally suppressed implies that little or no cubic distortion arises from the local mechanical process (reverse transduction) of the electrically stimulated OHCs, i.e., the reverse transduction is approximately linear. This result is more fully explored by Ren[7]).

origin of these EEOAEs is not a reflection of traveling wave energy at the BF location as a type of stimulus frequency otoacoustic emission.

Acknowledgments

Supported by research grants P01 DC0078 and DC00141 from the National Institute for Deafness and Other Communication Disorders, National Institutes of Health, and SLW 01.011 from NWO, The Netherlands.

References
1. Nuttall, A.L. and Ren,T. (1996) Electromotile hearing: Evidence from basilar membrane motion and otoacoustic emissions. *Hearing Res.* **93** 170-171.
2. Hubbard, A.E., Mountain, D.C. (1983) Alternating current delivered into the scala media alters sound pressure at the eardrum. *Science* **222** 510-512.
3. Ren,T. and Nuttall, A.L. (1996) Extracochlear electrically-evoked otoacoustic emissions: A model for in vivo assessment of outer hail cell electromotility. *Hearing Res.* **92** 178-183.
4. Nakajima, H.H., Olson, E., Mountain, D.C. and Hubbard, A.E. (1994) Electrically evoked otoacoustic emissions from the apical turn of the gerbil cochlea. *J.Acoust. Soc. Am.* **96** 786-795.
5. Xue, S., Mountain,D.C. and Hubbard, A.E. (1995) Electrically evoked basilar membrane motion. *J.Acoust, Soc. Am.* **97** 3030-3041.
6. Kemp, D.T., Brass, D.N., and Souter, M. (1991) Observations on simutaneous SFOAF and DPOAE generation and suppression. In: Lecture Notes in Biomathematics, ed. P. Dallos, C.D. Geisler, J.W. Matthews, M.A. Roggero and C.R. Steele. (Springer Verlag, Berlin) pp 202-209.
7. Ren,T. (1996) Acoustic modulation of electrically evoked distortion product otoacoustic emissions in gerbil cochlea. *Neurosci. Letrs.* **207** 1-4.

WHAT CAN WE LEARN FROM COCHLEAR GROUP DELAYS?

V.F.PRIJS, J-B.J.C. MASUREL, M.B. VERBRUGGEN, E.M.B. DUDOK VAN HEEL

ENT department, University Hospital Leiden
POBox 9600, 2300 RC Leiden, The Netherlands
prys@rullf2.LeidenUniv.nl

Cochlear group delays were determined through distortion product otoacoustic emission (DPOAE) phase gradients. With primary frequencies f_1 and f_2 ($f_1 < f_2$) the group delay of the $2f_1$-f_2 DPOAE was measured using an f_1 sweep and fixed f_2. In order to test effects of changes in cochlear filter two different aspects were investigated. DPOAE delays were analysed in 14 Ménière ears using hearing loss and in 15 normal ears using stimulus level as variables. In the abnormal ears delays were measured at different f_2 values keeping primary levels at L_1=65 and L_2=55 dB SPL. In the normal ears group delays were measured at f_2= 4kHz while primary level was varied. Moreover, the level experiments were simulated with a nonlinear locally active cochlea model from Kanis and de Boer[1,2]. In Ménière patients we find a small significant trend of smaller delays with higher f_2 thresholds revealing a small effect of loss of filter quality on DPOAE delays. In the normal group for higher stimulus level the delay monotonically decreases until L_1=75 dB SPL that again can be attributed to a loss of filter quality. However, the simulated delay only decreases for a narrow stimulus level range (55–75 dB SPL). Furthermore, simulated group delays are substantially lower compared to measured group delays. The discrepancy between model and measurements suggests that the compressive form of the nonlinearity is not correct and that the filter quality in the model is not high enough.

1   Introduction

Determination of group delay from distortion otoacoustic emissions (DPOAEs) is performed by keeping one of the primaries constant while the other is varied. In a simple description DPOAE group delay is half the mechanical group delay at the place of distortion product (DP) generation. This idea is supported by the results of Kimberley et al.[3] and our own results that show a comparable delay-f_2 relation for delays estimated from CAPs and the halved DPOAE delays. We are interested in to what extend other properties of DPOAE delays agree with those measured with CAPs and how these can be related to changes in the cochlear filter.

In this study we tested the relation of DPOAE cochlear delay and filter quality under two conditions. Firstly filter quality was supposed to be decreased as a result of cochlear deterioration in Ménière ears. Eggermont[4] described a decrease in cochlear delay as measured from derived CAPs in a group of Ménière patients. Secondly filter quality was decreased by increase of primary level. In order to interpret the level dependence in relation to cochlear mechanics, we simulated the DPOAE delays by a cochlear model that well reproduces nonlinear cochlear mechanic properties as level dependence, DP production and two-tone suppression: the model of Kanis and de Boer[1,2].

264

2   Methods

2.1   Experimental setup

DPOAEs were measured using a system comprising a PC, a plug-in digital signal processing board (Ariel DSP 16+), a DPOAE probe (Etymotic ER 10C) containing a low noise microphone and two earphones, a microphone amplifier and customized software. The customized software is a modification of the program CUBDISF1, written by Dr. Jont Allen, Bell Labs. The modifications concern (1) the inclusion of phase data to the output file, and (2) improvement of the noise rejection procedures.

Group delay values are calculated by the slope of a straight line fitted through the unwrapped DPOAE phase-frequency curves. These curves are obtained by recording the phase shifts between the primaries and the $2f_1-f_2$ DPOAE for different values of the f_1 frequency, while f_2 is fixed.

2.1.1 Tested ears

In 14 Ménière ears DPOAE delays were determined for 9 different f_2 values. In the abnormal ears delays were measured at 9 different f_2 values (0.5, 0.7, 1, 1.4, 2, 2.8, 4, 5.6 and 8 kHz) keeping primary levels at L_1=65 and L_2=55 dB SPL. We investigated the relation of the DPOAE delays and hearing loss at f_2.

The influence of stimulus level on DPOAE group delay was determined in a group of 9 normally hearing subjects aged between 18 and 25. All 15 investigated ears had pure-tone thresholds better than 10 dB HL. The delays were measured with f_2 fixed at 4 kHz and for wide range of primary levels; L_1 varied between 20 and maximal 90 dB SPL in steps of 5 dB, L_2=L_1-10 dB SPL.

2.2 Model simulations

The active nonlinear model of Kanis and de Boer[1] is a long wave model where the additive pressure of the outer hair cells (OHCS) is implemented as a negative impedance. The saturation of the OHC pressure is described by a hyperbolic tangent. With this model the level simulations were performed using the same stimuli as in the measurements and the DP phase was determined at the place of the stapes.

3. Results

3.1 Ménière ears

As a result of threshold restriction that is imposed by the possibility of measuring DPOAEs only in 10 of the 14 Ménière ears a reliable group delay could be determined. This subgroup had average hearing loss of 28 dB over 0.5, 1, 2, 4 and 8 kHz with a minimum at 2 kHz. Individual delay values rarely were significantly different from normal, but when we separated a high threshold subgroup (n=5; threshold $\geq$ 28 dB HL) their average value was smaller than normal (Fig. 1).

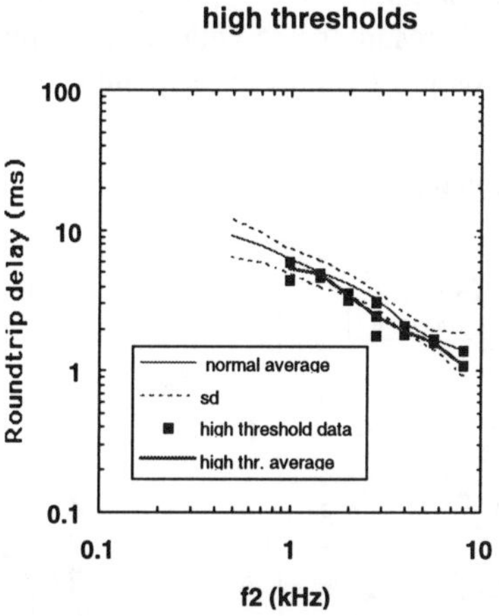

high thresholds

Figure 1: DPOAE- or roundtrip delay is plotted in relation to f_2 for a subgroup with high tone thresholds: average 39 dB HL. As reference normal average with standard deviation for a normal group of 41 ears is presented.

In order to investigate a dependence of group delay on hearing loss multiple regression was performed on the following relation:

$$\log(D(f_2; \theta(f_2))) = a_0 + a_1.\log(f_2) + a_2.\theta(f_2) \tag{1}$$

with $D(f_2; \theta(f_2))$ is DPOAE delay measured at f_2 and $\theta(f_2)$ is audiometric threshold at f_2.

For the 10 Ménière patients a_2 was significantly different from 0 (p=0.0002) having a value of -0.0056 with standard deviation 0.0013 (a_0=0.86 and a_1=-0.64).

3.2. Level variation: model and experiment

3.2.1 General properties of the model in normal ears

The model simulations reflect the common features of the two following experimental results.

a. The phase shift between primaries and DP at the stapes, computed for a number of f_2/f_1 ratios show a linear relation with DP frequency (Fig. 2) as well as a steeper slope for a fixed f_1 than for a fixed f_2[5]. Since in our experiments we restricted to the fixed f_2 paradigm all other simulations were done for a fixed f_2 and sweeping f_1 only.

b. The relation of simulated DP group delay with f_2 can be described as a power function of f_2. This result agrees with experimental data[1] albeit that for most f_2 the model delays are shorter than the experimental ones (Fig. 3).

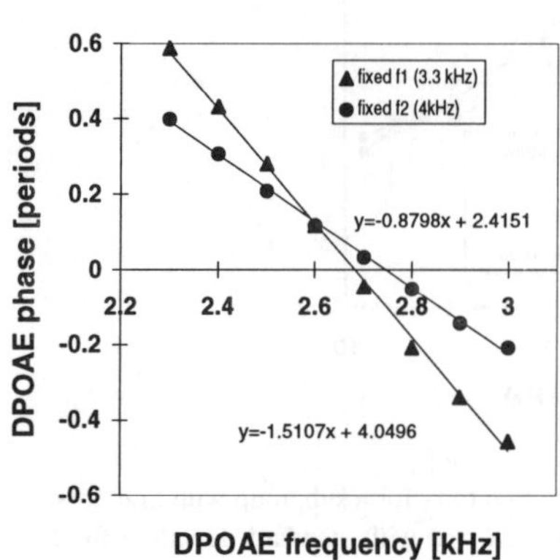

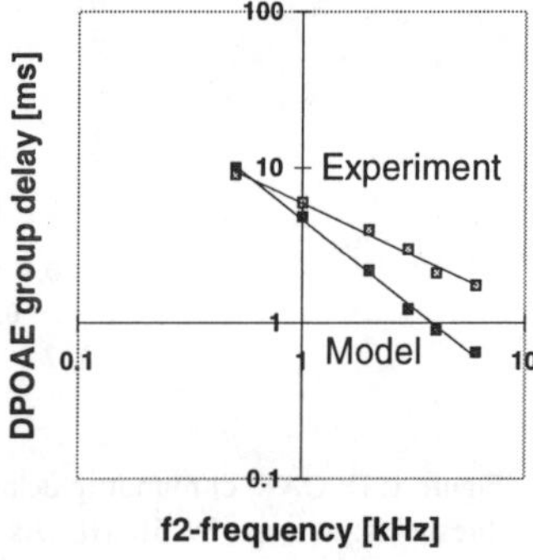

Figure 2: Simulation results: DPOAE phase at the stapes versus DPOAE frequency for both the f_1 and f_2 fixed paradigms. Primary levels are L_1=65 and L_2=55 dB SPL

Figure 3: DPOAE group delay versus f_2 for experiment and model. Both simulation and measurement show a power relation. Experimental data are averages from a group of 41 normal ears (see Fig. 1)

3.2.2 DPOAE group delay as a function of stimulus level: experiment and model

Most of the 15 normal ears showed regular DPOAE phase frequency relations at L_1=65 dB SPL that sometimes deteriorated for lower primary levels. In one of the ears a strong spontaneous otoacoustic emission (SOAE) was present that interfered with the DPOAE. In several ears (6 out of 15) a flattening of phase-frequency curves at the high frequency side for high stimulus levels was recorded (Fig. 4). Clearly for lower stimulus levels the curves are steeper resulting in larger group delays (Fig. 5).

Clearly the simulated DPOAE phase frequency curves are less steep than the experimental ones (Fig. 4). At the lower frequency side the simulated DPOAE phase frequency curves coincide for all levels (Fig. 4, left panel). Most phase-frequency curves exhibit a flattening on the high frequency side. The DPOAE frequency for which this flattening starts is smaller for higher primary levels. These properties result in smaller delays than those measured in the ear canal and in a restricted level region for which the delay decreases with primary level (Fig. 5).

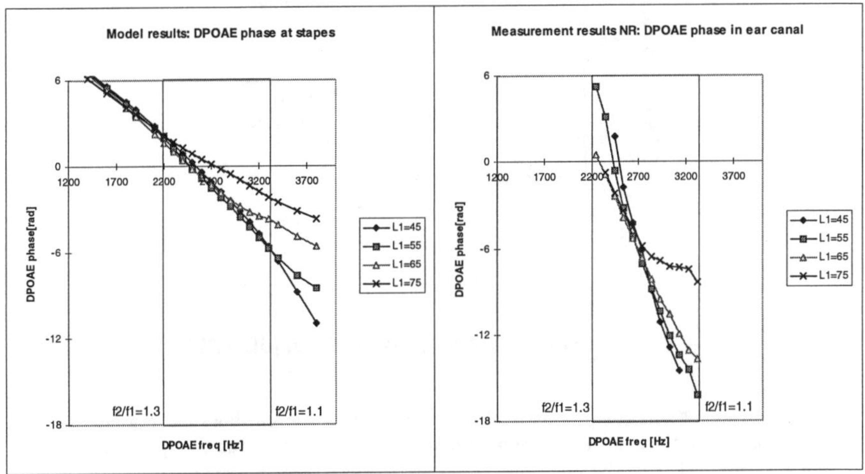

Figure 4: DPOAE phase frequency curves for different primary levels. Left: model simulations. Right: measurement results in one ear.

4. Discussion

4.1. Ménière ears

The multiple regression of the relation of DPOAE group delay with DPOAE frequency and audiometric threshold at f_2 shows a power law relation with frequency and a small but significant decrease of delay with threshold. The power function for phase-frequency relation is not different from normal (Eqn. (1), power is a_1=-0.64; normal power is -0.67).

The average decrease of DPOAE group delay was much smaller than that for the derived CAPs[4] for a comparable group of patients. Eggermont described the decrease to a reduced filter quality and probably the DPOAE results are caused by the same mechanism. Here the simplification of the DPOAE group delay being twice the cochlear delay shows its shortcomings: one would expect an effect that is twice that of the derived CAPs but it is much smaller.

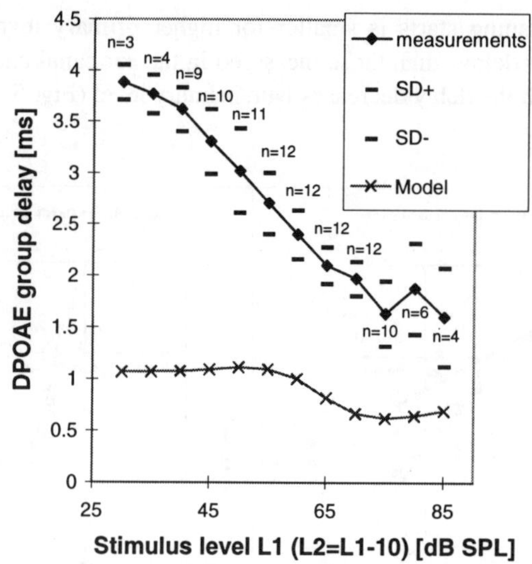

Figure 5: The DPOAE group delay is plotted versus primary levels, both for measurement results and for model simulations. The measurement results are plotted as averages and given with standard deviation. The simulation results are obtained from the same frequency range as for the measurements (see border in Fig. 4).

4.2. Level variation: model and experiment

4.2.1 General properties of the model in normal ears

The Kanis-de Boer model properly reproduces the experimental difference in fixed f_1 and fixed f_2 paradigm[5]. In the simplified description of the DPOAE group delay these differences can be ascribed to differences in cochlear group delay for f_2 and f_1 at the place of DP generation. Such differences are found in measurements of basilar membrane movements[6].

Both the measurements and the simulations show a power law relation between DPOAE group delay and frequency, but the power is smaller for the simulations (Fig 3). Therefore the simulated delays are smaller than the experimental ones for f_2 values above 500 Hz. Probably one of the model parameters has to be recalibrated in a way that the filter quality should increase.

4.2.2 Level dependence

The irregularities in DPOAE found for small levels are possibly due to interactions with chaotic processes near threshold[7]. Since in the Kanis de Boer model these are not incorporated such results lie outside the scope of this study.

The measurements results show a clear decrease in DPOAE group delay for higher stimulus levels. This dependence is thought to be effected by the decrease in quality of the cochlear filter. Although the model simulations show decrease of frequency selectivity for higher stimulus levels,[1] the simulated phase frequency curves do not show a clear slope dependence on level. In this aspect the difference between measurement and simulation is so large that probably essential features of cochlear mechanics are not well incorporated in the model.

The flattening at the high frequency side of the DPOAE phase frequency curves can be the result of two-tone suppression as the frequency where it starts to flatten coincides with the maximum in the DPOAE amplitude frequency curve.

Acknowledgments

We thank Luc-Johan Kanis for the use of his model software.

References

1. Kanis, L. J. and de Boer, E. (1993) Self-suppression in a locally active nonlinear model of the cochlea: a quasi-linear approach, *J. Acoust. Soc. Am.* **96** 3199–3206.
2. Kanis, L. J. (1995) Frequency dependence of acoustic distortion products in a locally active model of the cochlea. In *Cohlear nonlinearity* (Ph.D. Thesis, Amsterdam) 57–70.
3. Kimberley, B. P., Brown, D. K. and Eggermont, J. J. (1993) Measuring human cochlear traveling wave delay using distortion product emission phase responses, *J. Acoust. Soc. Am* **94** 1343–1350.
4. Eggermont, J. J. (1979) Narrow-band AP latencies in normal and recruiting human ears, *J. Acoust. Soc. Am.* **65** 463–470.
5. O'Mahoney, C. F. and Kemp, D. T. (1995) Distortion product otoacoustic emission delay measurement in human ears, *J. Acoust. Soc. Am* **97** 3721–3735.
6. Ruggero, M. A., Rich, N. C., and Recio, A. (1992) Basilar membrane responses to clicks. In *Auditory physiology and perception* ed. Y. Cazals, L. Demany and K. Horner (Pergamon Press, Oxford) 85–92.
7. Keefe, D. H., Burns, E. M., Ling, R., Laden, B. (1990) Chaotic dynamics of oto-acoustic emissions. In *The mechanics and biophysics of hearing* ed. S. Levin et al. (Springer, Berlin) 194–201.

EFFECTS OF SIGNAL DURATION ON THRESHOLD MICROSTRUCTURE IN EARS WITH SPONTANEOUS OTOACOUSTIC EMISSIONS

J. SMURZYNSKI, R. PROBST

*Department of Otorhinolaryngology, University of Basel, Kantonsspital Basel,
Petersgraben 4, CH- 4031 Basel, Switzerland
smurzynski@ubaclu.unibas.ch*

The purpose of the study was to determine the effect of signal duration on psychoacoustic threshold microstructure in the vicinity of spontaneous otoacoustic emissions (SOAEs). Seven normal-hearing subjects who exhibited strong but isolated SOAEs in the 1–3 kHz region were tested using an adaptive 2IFC procedure. Pure-tone signals with a total duration (T) of either 20, 40, 80, 160, or 320 ms were presented monaurally. The frequency of the signal was selected at either ±30, ±20, ±10, ±5, or 0 Hz relative to the SOAE frequency determined before each test using a spectrum analyzer. It was found that in almost all cases, the threshold microstructure associated with SOAEs disappeared for T=20 ms. The slope of the temporal integration function was steeper at the SOAE frequency, with 14.4 dB/decade of duration, than at 30 Hz below or above the SOAE frequency, where the slope was 10.7 dB/decade and 9.0 dB/decade, respectively.

1 Introduction

Microstructure of the threshold of audibility has been associated with spontaneous otoacoustic emissions (SOAEs).[1–3] Spontaneous OAEs occur in the vicinity of threshold minima. There are also threshold minima that are not associated with measurable SOAEs, but that are correlated with strong responses in evoked otoacoustic emissions (EOAEs). Therefore, it has been suggested that all threshold minima are associated with the presence of SOAEs and/or EOAEs.[4]

A study of Cohen[5] examined the influence of signal duration on detection thresholds using pure tones corresponding to peaks and valleys of the audiogram. The results showed that the threshold microstructure diminished as signal duration was shortened. Therefore, the temporal integration function was steeper for frequencies having low thresholds than for frequencies having high thresholds. In that study, however, dip frequencies were not correlated specifically with SOAEs and the temporal integration functions were measured at peaks and valleys separated by approximately 50 Hz.

The purpose of the present study was to determine the effect of signal duration on psychoacoustic threshold microstructure in the vicinity of SOAEs, i.e., within a frequency range of ±30 Hz relative to the SOAE frequency using 5-Hz or 10-Hz frequency steps.

2   Methods

2.1   Apparatus and Stimuli

Pure-tone stimuli were generated digitally and controlled by a Tucker-Davis system linked to a Pentium computer via a fiber optic interface. Signals were delivered to a tested ear through an ER-2 insert earphone. The other ear of a subject, who was seated comfortably in a sound-treated room, was occluded by a foam plug. Signals were gated with a 5-ms cosine-squared rise/fall time. The total duration (the time interval between the beginning and the end of the stimulus) was either 20, 40, 80, 160, or 320 ms, which corresponded to the energy-based duration (t) of 10.3, 30.3, 70.3, 150.3, or 310.3 ms, respectively.[6]

Spontaneous OAEs were measured using an ER10A microphone with no stimulation applied. The microphone output was amplified by 20 dB, high-pass filtered with a cut-off frequency of 400 Hz, and led to a Dynamic Signal Analyzer (Hewlett-Packard 3561A). A spectrum with a span of 200 Hz was based on the average of 10 FFTs of the microphone signal. A high-level SOAE was defined as any narrowband signal that exceeded the noise floor by ^{3}10 dB and was present in two consecutive average spectra of the signal from the ear under test. The frequency of the SOAE was determined using the cursor on the display.

2.2   Subjects

Seven normal-hearing subjects (four men and three women ranging in age from 27 to 42 years) participated. All had SOAEs that were previously documented to be at least 10 dB above the noise floor of the instrumentation. One ear and one SOAE for each subject were targeted for testing. The selection criterion required that: (1) the level of the target SOAE be at least 10 dB above the noise floor in the vicinity of its frequency; (2) no other SOAEs exceeding the noise floor by ^{3}3 dB be detectable in the frequency range of ±200 Hz relative to the target SOAE; (3) the spectrum of synchronized SOAEs[7] show just one peak corresponding to the target SOAE   ±200 Hz. The frequencies and the levels (in dB SPL) of these SOAEs averaged over multiple test sessions were: Subject MB: 1060 Hz, −1 dB; Subject AS: 1165 Hz, +10 dB; Subject JS: 1405 Hz, +4 dB; Subject KH: 1550 Hz, +10 dB; Subject BM: 2235 Hz, −2 dB; Subject KU: 2270 Hz, +1 dB; Subject MI: 2880 Hz, −9 dB.

2.3   Procedure

An adaptive, two-down/one-up 2IFC procedure with feedback was used. Observation intervals, indicated by illuminating the appropriate lights of a response box, corresponded to the total signal duration, which was kept constant within a test session. The observation intervals were separated by 300 ms. A run began with a signal level of approximately 20 dB above the estimated threshold value. The initial step size was 5 dB, and was reduced to 2 dB following the third reversal. The experiment was run in sets of four or five blocks of 60 trials per block. The first four reversals of each block were discarded and the remainder used to obtain an estimate of sensitivity. Blocks were discarded if the standard deviation of the reversals was greater than 3.5 dB.

Prior to running each set, the frequency of the target SOAE (with the accuracy of 1 Hz) was determined using a HP3561A analyzer as described above, to monitor drifts in the SOAE frequency.[8] The frequency of the signal being used within one block of the 2IFC test was randomly selected at either ±30, ±20, ±10, ±5, or 0 Hz relative to the SOAE frequency. The measurement of the SOAE frequency was repeated after each set of threshold tests was completed, and the signal frequency was adjusted if necessary. Each threshold reported is the mean of the estimates from at least three runs for each of the five signal duration values and each of the nine frequency shifts. Order of presentation was randomized across subjects.

3 Results

Figure 1 illustrates an example of threshold microstructure obtained for different values of t from Subject KU. For the longest duration used in the experiment (t=310 ms), a local dip in the threshold curve was observed at the signal frequency corresponding to the SOAE frequency. The depth of this minimum was approximately 7 dB for a ±5-Hz frequency shift relative to the SOAE frequency and approximately 10 dB for a ±30-Hz shift. The dip broadened and the depth decreased with decreasing signal duration. For t=10 ms, the microstructure disappeared. Similar results were obtained for all seven ears with a slightly different behavior of the microstructure obtained for Subject MI. Namely, the dip of the threshold curve did not disappear for t=10 ms and there was an increase of sensitivity in the ±10 Hz range relative to the SOAE frequency with the depth of approximately 4 dB.

Figure 2 illustrates examples of threshold shifts relative to threshold at 310 ms as a function of signal duration for Subject KU. Two signal frequencies are displayed: −30 Hz relative to the SOAE frequency and at SOAE frequency itself. The temporal integration function resulting when the signal frequency corresponded to the SOAE frequency was steeper than when the signal frequency was shifted by 30 Hz. Linear regression analysis showed that a single straight line appeared to fit the temporal integration data quite well. For Æf=−30 Hz, the slope of the regression line was 10.8 dB/decade of duration with the correlation coefficient r=0.998. For the SOAE frequency (Æf=0 Hz), the slope was 15.2 dB/decade with r=0.986. The correlation coefficients were greater than 0.96 for all testing conditions and all seven subjects. Therefore, the values corresponding to the slopes of the temporal integration functions at each frequency shift were averaged over subjects. The results are shown in Figure 3. The mean slope of the temporal integration function was steeper at the SOAE frequency with 14.4 dB/decade than at 30 Hz below or above the SOAE frequency where the slope was 10.7 dB/decade and 9.0 dB/decade, respectively.

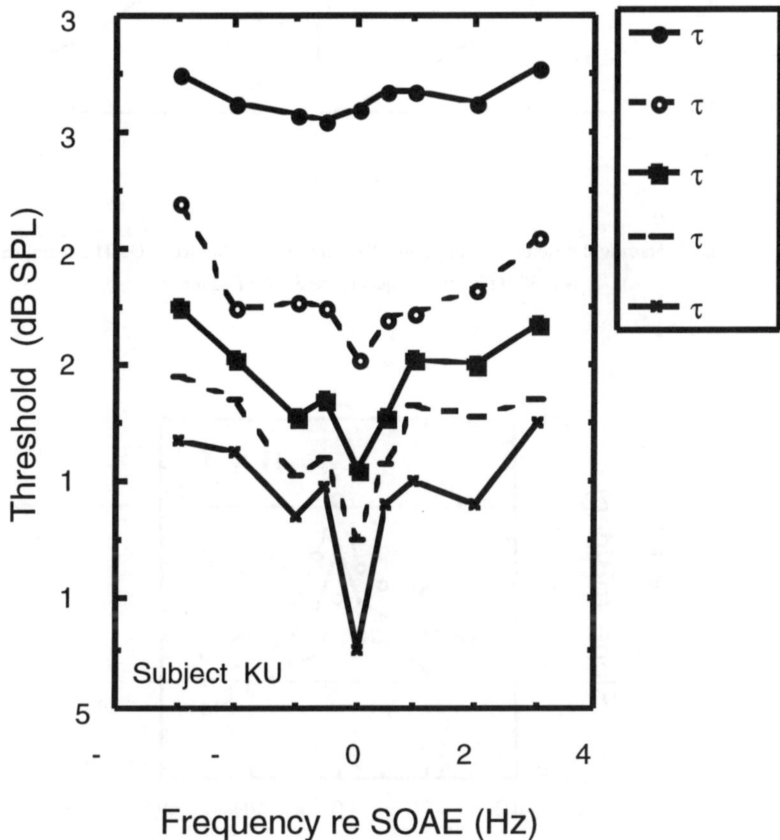

Figure 1: Detection threshold as a function of frequency shift relative to the SOAE frequency (approximately 2270 Hz) for Subject KU. Energy-based signal duration (t) in ms is the parameter.

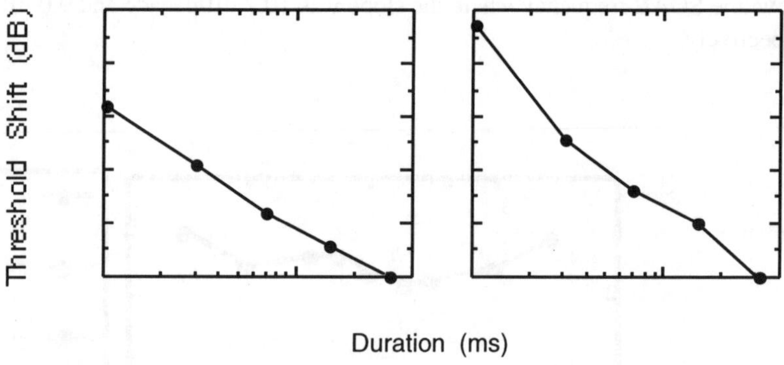

Figure 2: Threshold difference in dB, normalized re: 310 ms. Subject KU. The signal frequency was 30 Hz below or equal to the SOAE frequency.

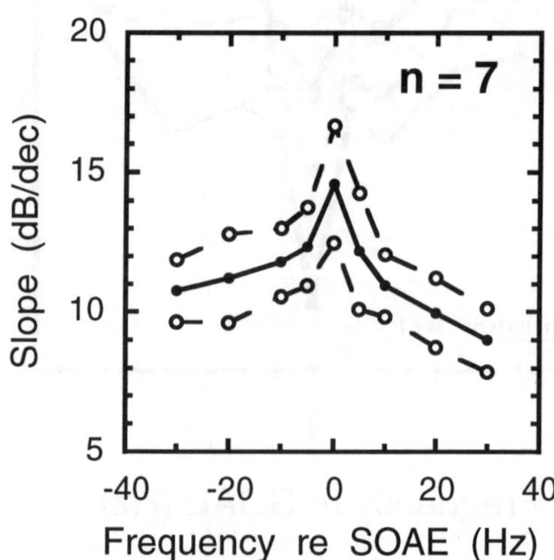

Figure 3: Slope of the temporal integration functions versus the signal frequency relative to the SOAE frequencies. The solid line with filled circles corresponds to the mean, and the dashed lines with open circles correspond to the ±SD from the mean, for 7 ears.

4 Discussion

All seven ears exhibited a clear dip of the threshold microstructure at the frequency of SOAE for the longest duration test signal, which is consistent with previous studies.[1-4] A spontaneous emission may either beat with or be entrained by external tones close in frequency to the SOAE. The ability to detect beating between an SOAE and a test signal depends on the level and duration of the external stimulus, as well as on the frequency separation between the two signals. Some of our subjects reported a perception of roughness for longer duration test signals. That sensation seemed to disappear for stimuli with shorter durations. The signals very close in frequency to the SOAE were often perceived as "tone-like" if the signal duration was relatively long. It seems that the clues that might be available to the subjects for longer duration signals, which results in a dip of the microstructure, are not useful for short signals resulting in a relatively flat threshold microstructure.

Our data, exhibiting a slope of the temporal integration function at the SOAE frequency of 14.4±2.1 dB/decade, are consistent with a study of Cohen[5] who reported a slope for valley frequencies of 12.3 dB/decade. Florentine et al.[9] showed that normal listeners' thresholds decreased by about 8 dB/decade of duration, which is similar to our findings at 30 Hz below or above the SOAE frequency (10.7±1.1 dB/decade and 9.0±1.1 dB/decade, respectively). It has been reported that slope for the peak frequencies of the threshold microstructure is considerably more gradual (5.6 dB/decade).[5] The steeper slope of the temporal integration function at the dip rather than at peak frequencies of the threshold microstructure could possibly be due to energy spread for short signals. The width of the energy spread to frequency bands adjacent to the signal frequency is inversely related to signal duration. The energy splatter will differentially affect detection threshold when the signal frequency is closer to or further from a dip of the threshold microstructure. For signal frequencies shifted relative to a dip frequency, as the bandwidth widens for shorter duration signals, the energy spreads toward the dip frequency. Its detection threshold is lower than that of the signal frequency, which might result in an improvement of detection and a decrease in the depth of the microstructure. Thus, the amount of energy that is available to the auditory system for integration over time depends on auditory sensitivity, which is changing with even relatively small frequency shifts.

Drifts in the frequency and amplitude of SOAEs during an experimental session were noted, similarly to previous reports.[8] The frequency and amplitude changes were typically complete within the first 20–30 minutes of the session when, in almost all cases, the SOAEs decreased in frequency by up to 7 Hz and the level increased by up to 6 dB. These changes were smaller than those observed between recording sessions. Deviations in the frequencies of SOAEs between all test sessions were up to 17 Hz, whereas SOAE levels varied by up to 10 dB. For the longer duration signals used in the present study, the dip frequency of a threshold microstructure was related to its corresponding SOAE frequency and drifted together with it rather than remaining at a fixed frequency.

The processes responsible for threshold microstructure influence many psychophysical measures taken at low stimulus levels, which leads to large intersubject variability. Most psychoacoustical experiments are performed using a limited number of fixed frequencies. Therefore, the ability of a subject to perform a task might depend on the frequency separation between a test signal and a local minimum of the pure-tone threshold. Such data are not available to investigators routinely, although this could be a significant factor in accounting for variability in psychoacoustic testing.

Acknowledgments

This study was supported by a grant from Swiss National Foundation (project Nr. 3200-042241.94/1).

References

1. Long, G.R. (1984) The microstructure of quiet and masked thresholds, *Hear. Res.* **15** 73–87.
2. Long, G.R. and Tubis, A. (1988) Investigations into the nature of the association between threshold microstructure and otoacoustic emissions, *Hear. Res.* **36** 125–138.
3. Long, G.R. and Tubis, A. (1988) Modification of spontaneous and evoked otoacoustic emissions and associated psychoacoustic microstructure by aspirin consumption, *J. Acoust. Soc. Am.* **84** 1343–1353.
4. Zwicker, E. and Schloth, E. (1984) Interrelation of different oto-acoustic emissions, *J. Acoust. Soc. Am.* **75** 1148–1154.
5. Cohen, M.F. (1982) Detection threshold microstructure and its effect on temporal integration data, *J. Acoust. Soc. Am.* **71** 405–409.
6. Gerken, G.M., Bhat, V.K.H. and Hutchison-Clutter, M. (1990) Auditory temporal integration and the power function model, *J. Acoust. Soc. Am.* **88** 767–778.
7. Prieve, B.A. and Falter, S.R. (1995) CEOAEs and SSOAEs in adults with increased age, *Ear Hear.* **16** 521–528.
8. Whitehead, M.L. (1991) Slow variations of the amplitude and frequency of spontaneous otoacoustic emissions, *Hear. Res.* **53** 269–280.
9. Florentine, M., Fastl, H. and Buus, S. (1988) Temporal integration in normal hearing, cochlear impairment, and impairment simulated by masking, *J. Acoust. Soc. Am.* **84** 195–203.

SUPPRESSION AND SYNCHRONIZATION OF OTOACOUSTIC EMISSIONS USING COMPLEX TONES

S. UPPENKAMP, J. NEUMANN, B. KOLLMEIER

Fachbereich Physik, AG Medizinische Physik, University of Oldenburg
D-26111 Oldenburg, Germany
e-mail: stefan@medi.physik.uni-oldenburg.de

Experiments on the interaction of otoacoustic emissions with additionally presented sinusoids and tone complexes have been performed. OAE are recorded in a transient emission paradigm, using clicks, tonebursts and chirplets for stimulation, as well as in a simultaneous emission paradigm using single tones and sweep signals. The components of additional tone complexes are constructed as odd harmonics of half of the stimulus repetition rate. By averaging in the time domain, this results in a complete cancellation of the suppressor signal as well as those parts of the emission which are in phase with it. By changing the averaging paradigm from summation to difference of consecutive single sweeps, a separation of synchronization and "true suppression" is possible. The underlying mechanism is investigated by variation of the spectral shape of stimulus and suppressor signal. Results may be interpreted as responses from a series of coupled oscillators driven by two separate forces. The comparison of OAE tuning and psychoacoustical critical bandwidth provides evidence that basically the same underlying mechanism is tested, that is, the interaction of adjacent places along the cochlear partition.

1 Introduction

Each type of otoacoustic emissions is influenced by additional sound. This has been studied extensively by several authors by presenting sinusoids during the recording of transiently evoked emissions (TEOAE)[1-5], spontaneous emissions (SOAE)[6-8], as well as for distortion product emissions (DPOAE)[9]. This influence is critically dependent on the spectral distance of emission and external sound and gives some information about the tuning properties of the emission generation, which reflects the peripheral preprocessing of sound along the cochlear partition. The observed reduction of emission level may be interpreted in terms of "true suppression", denoting a suppression of emission generation, which results in less acoustic energy emitted by the ear. This appears to be the most obvious explanation, especially for the effect of contralateral noise on the level of evoked emissions[10] (which reflects the efferent control of cochlear micromechanics). However, several observations with spontaneous emissions, such as phase locking in certain stimulus conditions[8] as well as the regular spacing of adjacent emissions[11,12], suggest an interpretation of suppression at least partially in terms of synchronization of a self-sustained or driven oscillator to an additional external force. This interpretation pertains to processes to some extent at a "lower" level and reflects the importance of mechanical coupling of adjacent regions along the cochlear partition.

Within this study, several experiments investigating the influence of additional tones on evoked otoacoustic emissions from normal hearing human subjects are presented. First, the underlying stimulus paradigm will be discussed under the question of synchronization and suppression. Then the influence of widening the suppressor spectrum from a single frequency to a complex of tones will be discussed. In the last part, the potential connection of OAE tuning to psychoacoustical critical bandwidth (CBW) is shown within a notched-noise paradigm [13,14] using identical tone complexes with a spectral notch of varying bandwidth as a suppressor or masker signal, respectively.

2 Methods

An insert ear probe ER-10C is used for the recording of SOAE and TEOAE. The microphone output is connected to a low-noise amplifier SR 560 and then converted to digital using 16 bit A/D converters on a signal processing board (Ariel DSP-32C) in a personal computer. All stimuli are generated digitally and presented to the subjects via 16 bit D/A converters and a computer controlled amplifier. The DSP is used for on-line analysis and signal-conditioning of the recorded emissions, including artefact rejection, FFT, and averaging.

For the recording of TEOAE, two types of stimuli are used. Narrowband stimulation is performed by Gaussian-shaped tone-pulses at a relative bandwidth $\Delta f/f_0$ of 0.17, with carrier f_0 chosen as frequency of a SOAE or near the most dominant peak of the click-evoked emission spectrum [5]. A wider frequency range may be stimulated using chirplets of 3 ms length. They allow a free selection of the signal spectrum by increasing the instantaneous frequency according to the desired spectral shape [15]. Stimuli are presented at a sampling rate of 22.05 kHz and a repetition rate of 10.8 Hz or 21.5 Hz, respectively.

For recording of stimulus frequency emissions (SFOAE) sweep signals of 93 ms and 372 ms length with increasing instantaneous frequency are presented repeatedly. As with TEOAE, averaging in the time domain is performed to improve the signal-to-noise ratio. The presence of SFOAE results in a strongly frequency dependent impedance of the auditory system. A more or less regular pattern in the recorded ear canal signal is visible at low stimulus levels [10]. To extract the nonlinear part due to emissions from the linear part of the passive transfer functions dominated by speaker, auditory canal, middle ear, and microphone, the difference of results at higher and lower stimulus levels is calculated (with the appropriate scaling of the high level results [11]).

All suppressor signals are constructed as single sinusoids or complexes of tones, each individual component of which is an odd harmonic of half of the stimulus repetition rate. This results in a phase difference of π for two consecutive single stimulus intervals and thus the suppressor cancels during the averaging in the time domain. The start phase of each component was chosen randomly to obtain a flat envelope of the suppressor signal.

3   Results and Discussion

3.1   Suppression vs. synchronization

To test the hypothesis of synchronization, the influence of a single tone on a narrowband evoked emission was investigated in more detail with four normal hearing subjects. One example is shown in Fig. 1 for a subject emitting a weak SOAE at 1.04 kHz. A tone pulse with carrier frequency near the spontaneous emission was selected as stimulus. A continuous tone at a nearby frequency was used as suppressor signal. Fig. 1a shows the resulting OAE for a stimulus level of 25 dB HL at different levels of the additional sinusoid. As expected, the level and temporal extent of the TEOAE decreases with increasing suppressor level. The slope of level reduction is about -0.5 dB/dB in this subject. Similar results hold for all subjects emitting SOAE, with a maximum slope of about -1 dB/dB in case of strong SOAE. Generally, the observable effect was small in subjects without SOAE, with a slope of about -0.2 dB/dB. This corresponds to the broader synchronization tuning curves observable in subjects without spontaneous emissions[5].

To distinguish between suppression and synchronization, the difference of each two consecutive single sweeps was calculated during averaging, without any other change of stimulus conditions. The resulting response should consist of three parts: the continuous tone, the SFOAE evoked by this tone, and that part of the TEOAE that is synchronized to the continuous tone. Since the phase relation between primary stimulus and emission is unknown, an off-line extraction of the nonlinear part of the response is performed by calculating the difference of two recordings at different levels of the continuous tone (see sec. 2). The resulting simultaneous emission is shown in Figs. 1b and c. The tone pulse causes a dip in the SFOAE in the same order of magnitude as the tone-pulse evoked OAE shown in Fig. 1a. This dip increases in depth and temporal extent with increasing level of the tone pulse at fixed level of the continuous tone (b) as well as with decreasing level of the continuous tone at fixed tone-pulse level (c). These results may be interpreted under the assumption of a single oscillator as source of the emission driven by two concurrent forces: tone pulse as well as continuous tone may be viewed either as stimulus or suppressor. The total

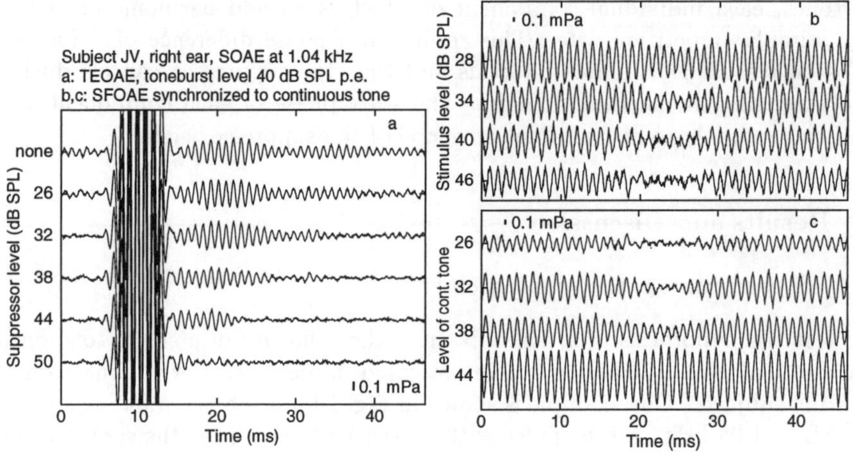

Figure 1: Influence of single tone on toneburst evoked OAE, see text for details.

energy of the emission divides up into one component constituing the TEOAE and a second component constituing the SFOAE, but in total remains constant. Consequently the observed suppression effect in this stimulus paradigm should be considered in terms of synchronization.

3.2 Influence of tone-complex suppressors on TEOAE and SFOAE

With the background from the previous section, the applied stimuli have been extended to a broader frequency range to look at the coupling of a series of emission sources. One example for the results is given in Fig. 2 for a normal hearing subject with several SOAE within a frequency range of 0.5 to 3.0 kHz in both ears at comparatively high levels. TEOAE were recorded using a chirplet with frequencies from 1.25 to 2.5 kHz. The top trace of Fig. 2a shows that the spontaneous emissions are synchronized by the transient stimulus, leading to a continuous response over the whole interstimulus interval of 90 ms (only the first 50 ms are shown here). The presentation of an additional tone complex results in a decrease of synchronization to the chirp, similar to the effect shown before for single tones. First, the frequencies in the complex were selected at a fixed spacing of 1.2 Bark down to 0.1 Bark on the scale of critical bands. Two examples are given in the next two traces of Fig. 2a. The observable effect is dependent on the frequency content of the complex. However, a systematic change with the spectral distance of the single components was not

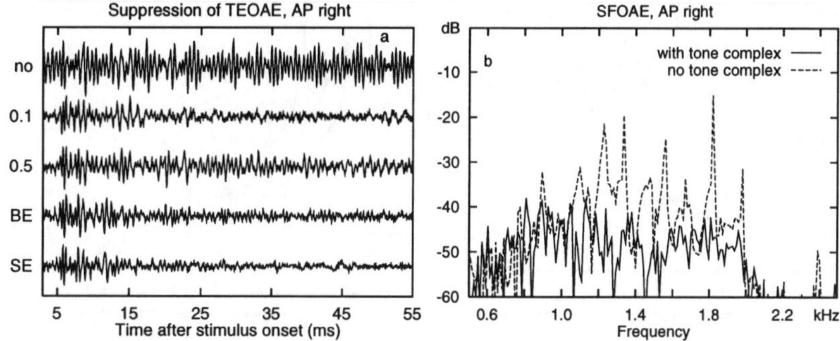

Figure 2: Suppression of TEOAE and SFOAE for a subject with various high-level SOAE using different tone complexes. 0.1, 0.5: 10 resp. 2 components per critical band, BE: components half-way between, and SE: at SOAE frequencies. In (b) complex SE was used.

observable. The largest effect was obtained with a complex containing components at or near the SOAE frequencies. This is demonstrated in the bottom trace of Fig. 2a (SE). Using the SOAE frequencies results in a decrease of the initial evoked response and a complete cancellation in the second half of the interstimulus interval. Selecting frequencies half-way between two particular emissions decreases the initial response as well (BE). However, the response is still partially synchronized to the chirp at 50 ms after onset.

Fig. 2b shows the influence of an additional tone complex on the SFOAE from this ear. The stimulus was a 92 ms-sweep with increasing instantaneous frequency. Restricting the growth of frequency to approximately one octave (1–2 kHz in this case) results in a comparatively slow change with time. The spontaneous emissions are then detectable as SFOAE as well. This is shown by the dotted line. The additional presentation of a tone complex consisting of components at the SOAE frequencies again results in a nearly complete cancellation of the SFOAE (full line). This is in good agreement with the conception of a series of coupled oscillators as emission sources, each of them synchronized to one of the additionally presented sinusoids.

3.3 CBW and synchronization of evoked emissions

Tonebursts as described before were used as test stimuli in a notched-noise masking experiment [13] as well as for narrowband stimulation of otoacoustic emissions. The masker and suppressor signal was generated as tone complex with odd harmonics of half of the stimulus repetition rate $f_r = 10.8$ Hz at a regular spacing of 10 lines per critical band and random start phase for each

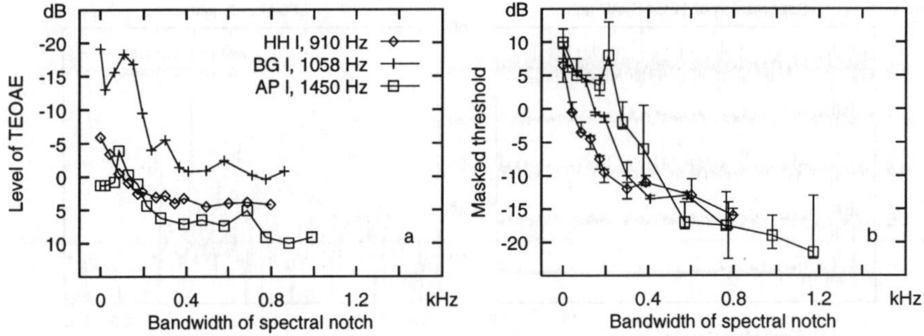

Figure 3: Influence of tone complex with spectral notch on TEOAE and masked threshold for three normal hearing subjects. Center frequencies of complex and toneburst were selected at SOAE frequencies shown in (a). Stimulus level in (a) 20 dB SPL, suppressor level 40 dB SPL, level in (b) is relative p.e. to the masker at 30 dB HL. Note the reversed ordinate in (a).

harmonic. This results in a "noise-like" signal with a periodicity of 93 ms. The masker without spectral notch had a bandwidth of two octaves, centered at the emission frequency. A spectral notch was introduced by omitting components in the center. To keep signal power constant, additional components were added at the lower and upper edge of the complex.

Results of toneburst-evoked OAE and masked thresholds are given in Fig. 3 for three subjects. Narrowband TEOAE (a) are influenced by the tone complex. As expected, the level reduction is maximal using a complex without any spectral notch. The OAE level increases by widening the notch. However, additional minima within a width of 40 Hz up to 300 Hz are visible, that is, within the expected width of one critical band. OAE level is nearly unaffected for wider notches. As for OAE suppression, the threshold (b) is maximal for a masker without spectral notch and decreases by expanding the width. However, even at a bandwidth clearly greater then the expected CBW, a further decrease in threshold is visible. This reflects the very short duration of the stimuli used in this study. Nevertheless, the decreases of masking and OAE suppression with increasing notch width show a similar shape for several subjects (cf. subject BG) even in absolute range. Bandwidth estimates determined from the results of both experiments coincided quite well for subjects with SOAE. This suggests that spectral masking may at least partially be connected to the tuning of OAE generation, as has already shown before for DPOAE [14]. However, the estimate from OAE data was too large even for normal hearing subjects without SOAE. This shows that several additional processes are involved in spectral masking as well as in OAE experiments.

4 Conclusion

The vulnerability effect of an additional sinusoid or tone complex on emission fine structure may be interpreted in terms of synchronization. This is in agreement with the idea of a series of coupled oscillators as source of otoacoustic emissions. OAE tuning as well as basic measures of auditory perception seem to be affected by the interaction of adjacent places along the cochlea in a similar way. However, the "critical bandwidth" measured with OAE experiments can not be used as a predictor of the psychoacoustically measured CBW.

Acknowledgments

Supported by Deutsche Forschungsgemeinschaft DFG Ko 942/11-1.

References

1. Kemp, D.T. (1979) Evidence of mechanical non-linearity and frequency selective wave amplification in the cochlea, *Arch. Otorhinolaryngol.* **224** 37-45.
2. Wit, H.P. and Ritsma, R.J. (1980) Evoked acoustical responses from the human ear: some experimental results, *Hear. Res.* **2** 253-261.
3. Wilson, J.P. (1980) Evidence for a cochlear origin for acoustic re- emissions, threshold fine-structure and tonal tinnitus, *Hear. Res.* **2** 233-252.
4. Sutton, G.J. (1985) Suppression effects in the spectrum of evoked otoacoustic emissions, *Acustica* **58** 57-63.
5. Uppenkamp, S. and Kollmeier, B. (1994) Narrowband stimulation and synchronization of otoacoustic emissions, *Hear. Res.* **78** 210-220.
6. Schloth, E. and Zwicker, E. (1983) Mechanical and acoustical influences on spontaneous oto-acoustic emissions, *Hear. Res.* **11** 285-293.
7. Rabinowitz, W.M. and Widin G.P. (1984) Interaction of spontaneous otoacoustic emissions and external sounds, *J. Acoust. Soc. Am.* **76** 1713-1720.
8. Long, G.R., Tubis, A. and Jones, K.L. (1991) Modeling synchronisation and suppression of spontaneous otoacoustic emissions using Van der Pol oscillators: effects of aspirin administration, *J. Acoust. Soc. Am.* **89** 1201-1212.
9. Kummer, P., Janssen, T. and Arnold, W. (1995) Suppression tuning characteristics of the 2f1-f2 distortion-product otoacoustic emission in humans, *J. Acoust. Soc. Am.* **98** 197-210.
10. Long, G.R., Talmadge, C.L. and Shaffer, L. (1994) The effect of contralateral stimulation on synchronous evoked otoacoustic emissions, *J. Acoust. Soc. Am.* **95** 2844.
11. Zwicker, E. and Schloth, E. (1984) Interrelation of different otoacoustic emissions, *J. Acoust. Soc. Am.* **75** 1148-1154.
12. van Hengel, P.W.J. (1995) Spatial periodicity in the cochlea caused by interaction of spontaneous emissions, in *Advances in Hearing Research - 10th International Symposium on Hearing*, ed. G.A. Manley, G.M. Klump, C. Koeppl, H. Fastl, H. Oeckinghaus (World Scientific, Singapore) pp. 116-124.
13. Patterson, R.D. (1976) Auditory filter shape derived with noise stimulation, *J. Acoust. Soc. Am.* **59** 640-654.
14. Brown, A.M., Gaskill, S.A., Carlyon, R.P. and Williams, D.M. (1993) Acoustic distortion as a measure of frequency selectivity: relation to psychophysical equivalent rectangular bandwidth, *J. Acoust. Soc. Am.* **93** 3291-3297.
15. Neumann, J., Uppenkamp, S. and Kollmeier, B. (1994) Chirp evoked otoacoustic emissions, *Hear. Res.* **79** 17-25.

SIMULTANEOUS MEASUREMENT OF DPOAEs AND BASILAR MEMBRANE VIBRATION BY ACOUSTIC PROBE AND LASER DOPPLER VELOCIMETER

H.WADA, Y.HONNMA

Department of Mechanical Engineering, Tohoku University, Sendai 980-77, Japan

S.TAKAHASHI, T.TAKASAKA

Department of Otolaryngology, Tohoku University School of Medicine, Sendai 980-77, Japan

K.OHYAMA

Department of Otolaryngology, Tohoku Ro-sai Hospital, Sendai 981, Japan

Otoacoustic emissions (OAEs) are believed to be a byproduct of the cochlear amplification, and this amplification is estimated to be caused by the increased basilar membrane (BM) vibration achieved by an active electro-mechanical involvement of outer hair cells. However, the relationship between OAEs and BM vibration has not been clarified. Therefore, in this study, simultaneous measurement of distortion-product OAEs (DPOAEs) and BM vibration was carried out by a commercially available DPOAE measuring system and our own made BM vibration measurement system coupling between a laser Doppler velocimeter (LDV) and a compound microscope.

1 Introduction

Generation mechanism of OAEs is believed as follows: When stimulation is given to the external auditory meatus by a probe earphone, BM vibration is amplified by an active electro-mechanical involvement of outer hair cells[1], this vibration is propagated to the oval window in a retrograde fashion[2], and this signal is detected by a probe microphone. However, the relationship between OAEs and BM vibration has not been clarified.

Many methods have been used to measure BM vibration, e.g. the Mössbauer technique[3], the use of capacitive probe[4], laser homodyne interferometry[5] and laser heterodyne interferometry[6]. Recently, a new method for the measurement of BM vibration using a LDV coupled to a compound microscope and dropping reflective glass microbeads on the BM was developed[7,8]. The advantages of this method are its linearity, wide dynamic and frequency ranges.

In this study, simultaneous measurement of DPOAEs and BM vibration was carried out by a commercially available DPOAE measuring system and our own made BM vibration measurement system coupling between a LDV and a compound microscope, and an attempt was made to clarify the relationship between DPOAEs and BM vibration.

2 Materials and Methods

2.1 Animal Preparation

Healthy albino guinea pigs (250-400g) were anesthetized. Then, they were tracheotomized and artificially ventilated with room air after intramuscular injection of a muscle relaxant. The cochlea was exposed through the ventral approach. Head down position was taken for better access to the BM through a hole 0.5mm in diameter which was opened at the scala tympani of the basal turn. A small quantity of microbeads sucked by the micropipette were dispensed into the cochlea and fell onto the BM. During the cochlear manipulations and measurement, the end-tidal CO_2 concentration and body temperature were kept to be 5% and $38^\circ C$, respectively.

2.2 Measurement System

A laser beam generated by the LDV was reflected at the target, *i.e.* the microbead on the BM. In order to increase reflections of the laser beam, the microbeads (Bright Hyoshiki Reflective Industrial Corp.) of 20 μm in diameter, 9 ng in weight and refractive index 2.2 were applied.

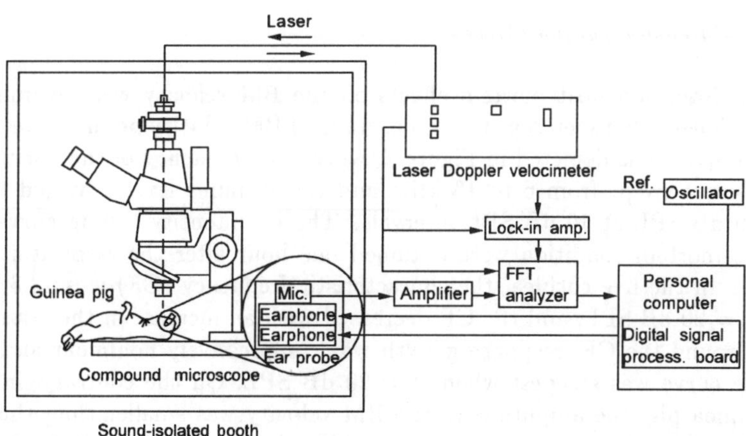

Figure 1: Block diagram of simultaneous measurement system of DPOAEs and BM velocity.

Figure 1 shows a block diagram of the measurement system of DPOAEs and BM velocity. DPOAEs were measured by the CUB^eDIS system (Ver.3.00-C). Two earphones (ER-2, Etymotic Research) and one microphone (ER-10, Etymotic Research) were installed in a ear probe. The measurement system of the BM velocity consisted of a custom made compound microscope (Nikon), a LDV (LV1100, Onosokki), an oscillator (NF-1940, NF Electronic Instruments), a look-in amplifier (5610B, NF Electronic Instruments) and a FFT analyzer (CF-360, Onosokki). Two primary sinusoidal waves at frequencies f_1 and f_2 were generated from the two earphones of the probe, and both the acoustic signals measured by the probe microphone and the BM velocity detected by the LDV were analyzed by the FFT analyzer. Moreover, reference signals of frequency $2f_1 - f_2$ were fed to the lock-in amplifier from the oscillator, and $2f_1 - f_2$ component of the BM velocity obtained by the lock-in amplifier was analyzed by the FFT analyzer. The system was controlled by a personal computer(IBM AT clone). For the purpose of assessing the condition of the cochlea, compound action potentials (CAP) were recorded before measuring the BM velocity. In this study, an attempt was made to measure BM velocity of nearly 130 guinea pigs. However, due to the difficulty of the experiment, good results were obtained from only 10 guinea pigs.

3 Results

3.1 Iso-Intensity Tuning Curve

Stimulus level and post mortem effects on the BM velocity were examined. The relationship between sensitivity, i.e. units of BM velocity per unit pressure versus frequency is depicted in Figure 2, where the frequency of the harmonic stimulus was swept from 6 to 16 kHz, and the stimulus level P varied from 20 to 60 dB SPL at 10 dB SPL intervals. The iso-intensity tuning curves of the post mortem condition were obtained one hour after the respirator was stopped. In the live cochlea, the characteristic frequency (CF) was 13.3 kHz when P = 20 dB SPL, and the CF decreased with an increase in the stimulus level. Around the CF, response growth was compressively nonlinear and the response curve was steepest when P = 20 dB SPL. On the contrary, in the dead guinea pig, the amplitude of the BM velocity was smaller than that of the alive guinea pig in the case of the same stimulus level, and the BM velocity was not obtainable when $P < 30$ dB SPL. Furthermore, the stimulus effect on the CF was not observed, and response growth was linear; in other words, sensitivity was independent of stimulus level.

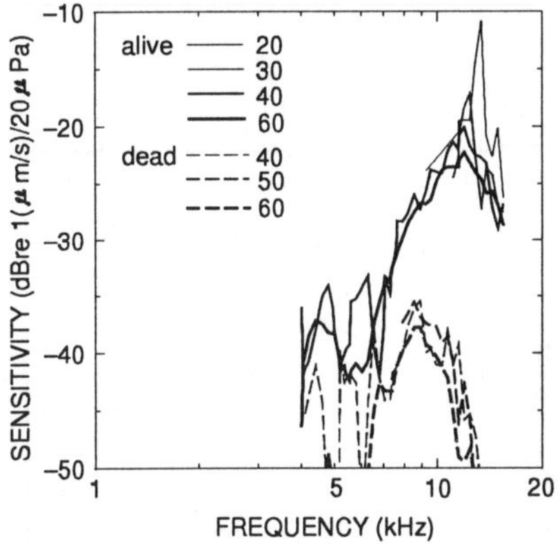

Figure 2: Sensitivity of BM velocity responses to harmonic stimulation. Vertical unit is velocity per unit pressure. The parameter is sound pressure level (dB SPL). Curves of the post mortem condition were obtained one hour after the respirator was stopped.

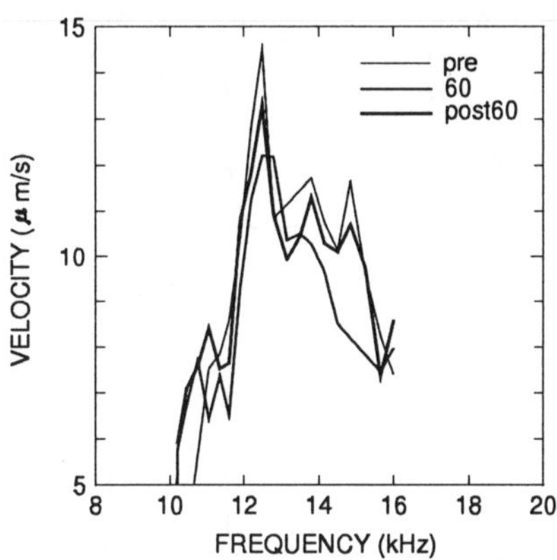

Figure 3: Effect of hypoxia on BM velocity. Pre, before hypoxia; 60, 60 s after the beginning of hypoxia; post 60, 60 s after the end of hypoxia. Hypoxia was given by 2 min intermission of artificial respiration. Stimulus level was 40 dB SPL.

3.2 Hypoxic Effect on BM Velocity

Hypoxic effect on the BM velocity was examined by 2 min intermission of artificial respirator. The results before, during and after the hypoxic episode are shown in Figure 3, where the stimulus frequency was swept from 9 to 16 kHz, and the stimulus level was 40 dB SPL. The amplitude of the BM velocity 60 s after the respirator was stopped was smaller than that before the hypoxic episode almost over the measured frequency region, and the difference was large when the stimulus frequency was larger than the CF. The amplitude of the BM velocity 60 s after the end of hypoxia was almost recovered. However, the amplitude was a little smaller than that before the hypoxia episode.

3.3 Simultaneous Measurement of DPOAEs and BM Velocity

Simultaneous measurement of DPOAEs and BM velocity was carried out, where the stimulus levels of the primaries were 75 and 65 dB SPL, respectively, and their frequency ratio f_2/f_1 was 1.25. Figures 4(a) and (b) show the acoustic signal and BM velocity on a spectrogram, respectively, where

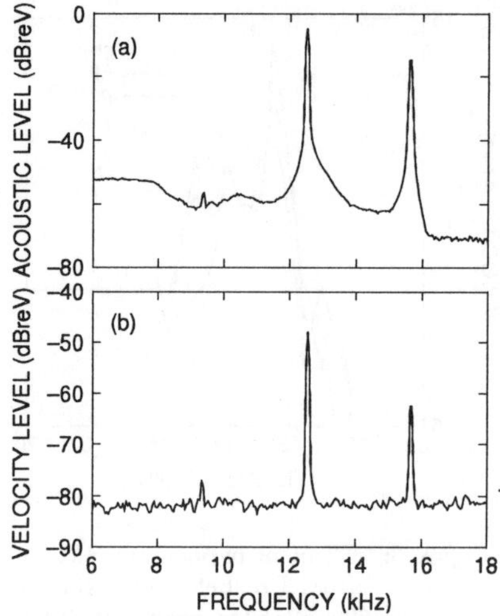

Figure 4: Spectrogram. (a) Acoustic signal. (b) BM velocity. Stimulus levels P_1 and P_2 of the primaries were 75 and 65 dB SPL, respectively, $f_1 = 12.55$ kHz, $f_2 = 15.70$ kHz and $2f_1 - f_2 = 9.40$ kHz.

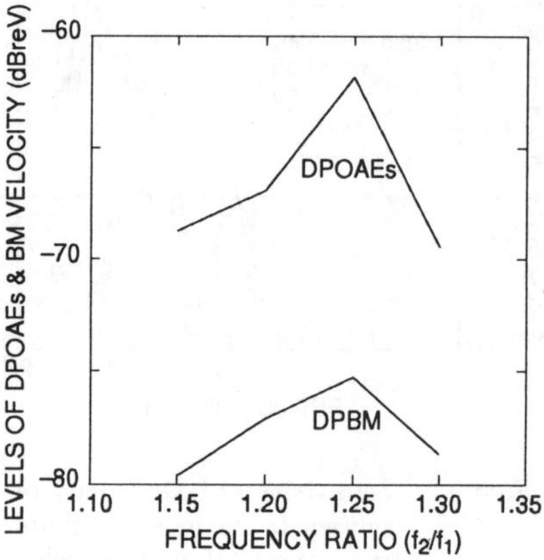

Figure 5: Levels of DPOAEs and BM velocity at $2f_1 - f_2 = 9.40$ kHz (DPBM) versus primary frequency ratio f_2/f_1. $P_1 = 70$ dB SPL, $P_2 = 60$ dB SPL, $2f_1 - f_2 = 9.40$ kHz, $f_2/f_1 = 1.10, 1.15, 1.20, 1.25$ and 1.30.

$f_1 = 12.55$ kHz, $f_2 = 15.70$ kHz and $2f_1 - f_2 = 9.40$ kHz. The reason why such primaries were applied was that the CF where the BM velocity was measured was 9.40 kHz. Clear peaks can be seen at f = 9.40 kHz in both Figures 4(a) and (b). Figure 5 depicts the relationship between the level of DPOAEs at $2f_1 - f_2 = 9.40$ kHz and the primary frequency ratio f_2/f_1 and that between the BM velocity at $2f_1 - f_2 = 9.40$ kHz and f_2/f_1, where $P_1 = 70$ dB SPL, $P_2 = 60$ dB SPL, and $f_2/f_1 = 1.10, 1.15, 1.20, 1.25$ and 1.30. Although the increase and decrease rates of the level of DPOAEs were larger than those of the BM velocity at $2f_1 - f_2$, both the levels of DPOAEs and BM velocity at $2f_1 - f_2$ were largest when $f_2/f_1 = 1.25$.

4 Discussion

One of the advantages of our system would be a size of the cylindrical shaped sensor head, which is 10 mm in diameter and 26 mm in length. Owing to this compact sensor head, installation of the sensor head in the compound microscope was an easy task, and it was comfortable to handle the system during the experiment. Moreover, in spite of the small sensor head, a sensitivity of this system was high, and BM velocity was measurable down to P = 20 dB SPL in a live cochlea and P = 40 dB SPL in a dead guinea pig.

In order to measure relatively low CF (9-12 kHz) compared with 18 kHz of reference 7 and 34 kHz of reference 9, head down position was taken in our experiment. The iso-intensity tuning curves shown in Figures 2 were not so steep around the CF as those of references 7 and 8 . This would be caused by a large angle between the optical axis and the direction of the BM vibration due to head down position. Another disadvantage of the head down position

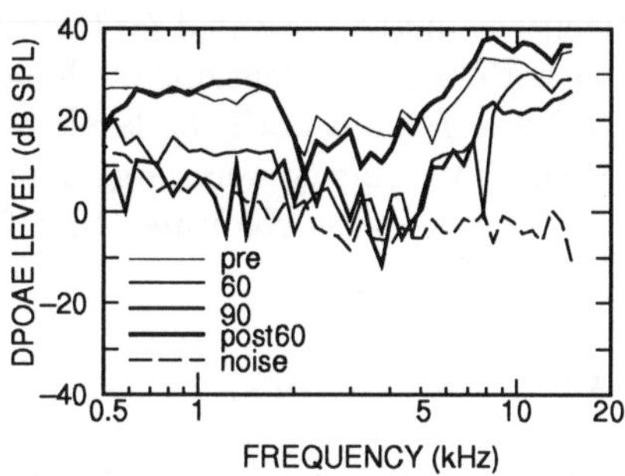

Figure 6: Effect of hypoxia on DPOAEs. Pre, before hypoxia; 60, 60 s after the beginning of hypoxia; 90, 90 s after the beginning of hypoxia; post 60, 60 s after the end of hypoxia; noise, noise level of the measurement system. Hypoxia was given by 2 min intermission of artificial respirator. Stimulus levels of primaries were 70 and 60 dB SPL, and their frequency ratio f_2/f_1 was 1.25.

was that a good condition of the animals did not last for a long time.

Hypoxic effect on DPOAEs will be shown in Figure 6, although this result and those shown in Figure 3 were not obtained simultaneously. Intermission of artificial respirator was 2 min, the stimulus levels of the primaries were 70 and 60 dB SPL, respectively, their frequency ratio f_2/f_1 was 1.25, and the primary frequency f_2 was swept from 16 to 0.5 kHz. The level of DPOAEs decreased over the measured frequency region 60 s after the respirator was stopped, and the level decreased to the noise level in the lower frequency region 90 s after the beginning of hypoxia. The level was recovered over the measured frequency region 60 s after the end of hypoxia. When the amplitude of the BM velocity decreased due to hypoxia, those of DPOAEs and SOAEs[10] also decreased. If the hypoxic condition continued, the level of DPOAEs decreased to the noise level, and SOAEs disappeared[10]. After the end of hypoxia, the amplitude of the BM velocity and DPOAEs was almost recovered, and SOAEs reappeared[10].

Although measurement of cubic distortion of BM velocity by a LDV has already been reported[11], simultaneous measurement of DPOAEs and BM velocity would be presented for the first time in this paper. Clear peaks were seen on both the spectrograms of the acoustic and BM velocity measurement at f $= 2f_1 - f_2$, and both the levels of DPOAEs and cubic distortion component of the BM velocity were largest when $f_2/f_1 = 1.25$.

These results confirmed that OAEs reflected sensitively the dynamic behavior of BM.

Acknowledgments

This work was supported by the Ministry of Education of Japan under Scientific Research Grant (04557074), The Murata Science Foundation (921154) and The Kurata Research Grant (530).

References

1. J.F. Ashmore (1991) *Annu. Rev. Physiol.* **53** 465.
2. H. Wada, K. Ohyama, S. Noguchi and T. Takasaka (1993) In: *Biophysics of hair cell sensory systems*, ed. H. Duifhuis, J.W. Horst, P. van Dijk and S.M. van Netten (World Scientific, Singapore).
3. B.M. Johnstone and A.J.F. Boyle (1967) *Science* **158** 389.
4. J.P. Wilson and B.M. Johnstone (1975) *J. Acoust. Soc. Am.* **57** 705.
5. S.M. Khanna and D.G.B. Leonard (1986) *Hear. Res.* **23** 55.
6. S.M. Khanna, A. Flock and M. Ulfendahl (1989) *Acta Otolaryngol. Suppl.* **467** 151.
7. A.L. Nuttall and D.F. Dolan (1996) *J. Acoust. Soc. Am.* **99** 1556.
8. M.A. Ruggero and N.C. Rich (1991) *Hear. Res.* **51** 215.
9. N.P. Cooper and W.S. Rhode (1992) *Hear. Res.* **63** 163.
10. K. Ohyama, H. Wada, T. Kobayashi and T. Takasaka (1991) *Hear. Res.* **56** 111.
11. A.L. Nuttall, D.P. Dolan and G.Avinash (1990) In: *The Mechanics and Biophysics of Hearing*, ed. P. Dallos, C.D. Geisler, J.W. Mattews, M.A. Ruggero and C.R. Steele (Springer Verlag).

ON COCHLEAR CROSS-CORRELATION FUNCTIONS: CONNECTING NONLINEARITY AND 'ACTIVITY'

E. DE BOER

Rm D2-226, Academic Medical Center, Meibergdreef 9
1105 AZ, Amsterdam, The Netherlands
email: e.deboer@amc.uva.nl

A. L. NUTTALL

Kresge Hearing Research Institute, 1301 E. Ann Street
Ann Arbor, MI 48109-0506, USA
email: nuttall@umich.edu

Experiments were carried out to measure the mechanical response of the basilar membrane (BM) in the basal turn of the guinea-pig cochlea. The stimuli were noise signals that are wide-band with respect to the bandwidth of the measured location on the BM. In this case the input-output cross-correlation function (ccf) can be interpreted in terms of a linearized model of the cochlea[3]. The data from the experiments have been subjected to the 'inverse' analysis in order to find the degree of cochlear 'activity'. This was found to decrease monotonically with increasing stimulus level which effect can be attributed to outer-hair-cell (OHC) compression.

Introduction

That the character of the mechanical impulse response of the cochlea varies with click strength[11] can most easily be explained in terms of a time-varying degree of nonlinearity. In the case of stimulation by stationary wide-band noise a more precise and quantitative explanation is possible by invoking the EQ-NL theorem which refers the measured input-output cross-correlation function (ccf) to that of a linear cochlear model (see section 3 for details). We have stimulated the cochlea with noise signals of which the frequency spectrum encompasses the pass-band of the BM location studied and computed the ccf.[5] With help of the 'inverse solution method'[1,2] we have tried to find out how variations of cochlear 'activity' can be attributed to signal compression occurring in outer hair cells (OHCs).

1   Experimental method

Movements of the basilar membrane (BM) in the basal turn of the cochlea of anaesthetized guinea pigs were measured by focusing the beam of a laser Doppler vibrometer onto a glass bead placed on the BM.[9] Signal generation and data acquisition were done with our own integrated programming system.[5] The stimulus signal was a pseudo-random noise sequence of 4096 data sampled periodically and repetitively (at a rate of 208 k samples per second) thus making for a *continuous* signal. The noise signals were at least one octave wide, and centered at the best frequency (BF) of the BM location studied. Response components outside the main passband, 5-22 kHz, were reduced in magnitude. The cross-correlation function (ccf), i.e., the 'indirect impulse response',[5] was determined by averaging over more than 1000 noise periods. The ccf determined for the BM was *always* corrected for the stapes response.

2 Results I - cross-correlation functions and their interpretation

At a very low stimulus level, the cochlea functions linearly, hence the indirect impulse response (measured with wide-band noise) should be indistinguishable from the directly measured impulse response.[10] Figure 1 shows, in the left panel, (a), the waveform of the cross-correlation function (ccf), for a very low level of stimulation, over a time interval of 2.0 msec. Stimulus intensity is labeled by way of the *attenuation* with respect to the over-all peak level of 100 dB SPL at the ear drum. The best frequency (BF) of the cochlear location studied is 16.6 kHz. The same figure shows in the second panel, (b), the (normalized) frequency spectrum of this ccf on a logarithmic frequency axis. Figure 2 shows, in the same format, results for a considerably stronger stimulus signal, from the same animal. We observe big differences in waveform and spectrum, which are entirely comparable with other findings in experiments on the direct impulse response.[11,5]

Consider now a *cochlear model* that is linear as far as the fluid and the structure of the organ of Corti are concerned, and that contains outer hair cells (OHCs) functioning to *enhance* frequency selectivity. These OHCs are assumed to be nonlinear (compressive no-memory) transducers, and they are the *only* nonlinear elements in the model. The input to the OHCs is a filtered form of the BM velocity (which is in our − generalized − type of model not necessarily taken from only one location), and the OHCs are assumed to produce a pressure (similarly: not necessarily acting at one location) that aids in moving the BM. This model is of a class that includes 'classical' locally active models such as the Neely-Kim model[8] as well as the more recently published feed-forward models of Steele et al.[12] and Geisler and Sang[6] and related models[7]. With low stimulus levels the OHCs give rise to a very frequency-selective response. With stronger stimuli the OHCs tend to become saturated and contribute less to frequency selectivity.

For this type of *nonlinear* model the EQ-NL theorem[3] states that *the input-output ccf for the nonlinear model, determined with a wide-band input signal, is equal to the ccf for a <u>linear</u> comparison model that has exactly the same structure but in which all the OHCs are linear and operate with a reduced efficiency (γ). The main argument in the proof of this theorem is that at the input to the (nonlinear) OHC transducers a composite noise signal is present (with a near-Gaussian distribution)

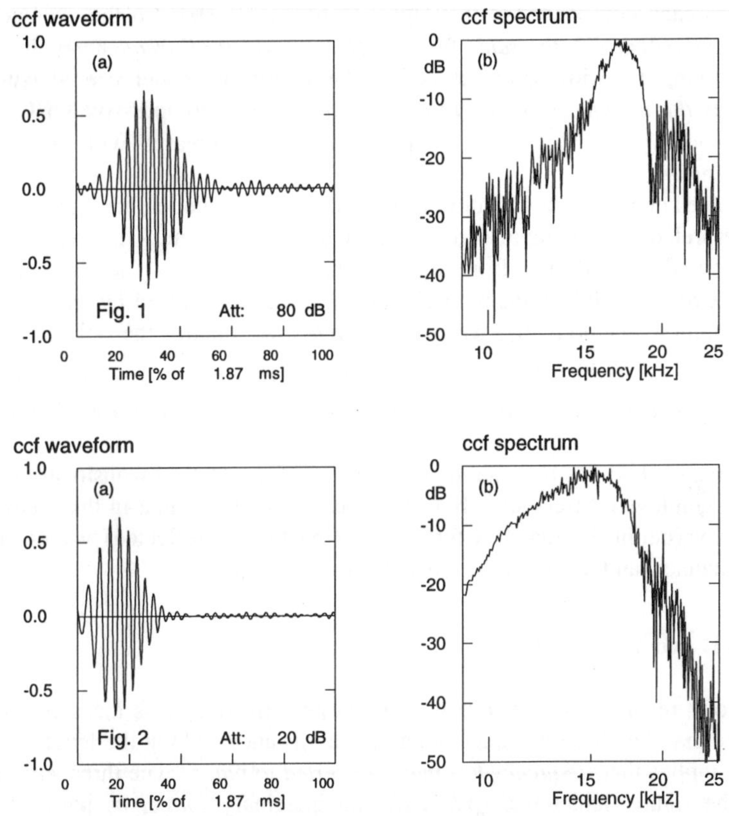

Figure 1 (top). Input-output cross-correlation function (ccf) at a low level of stimulation (attenuation 80 dB). Left panel (a): waveform of ccf, shown on an arbitrary amplitude scale. Right panel (b): spectrum of ccf, shown on a 50-dB scale and normalized with its peak at 0 dB. Frequency scale is logarithmic. Experiment: 0621.

Figure 2 (bottom). Input-output cross-correlation function at a 60 dB higher level of stimulation (attenuation 20 dB), measured in the same animal. Layout as in Fig. 1.

which causes each component of that signal to be *compressed* (in the average) to exactly the same degree – *the same for all OHCs and for all frequencies*. In view of this theorem, the wide-band ccf across the nonlinear model can always be interpreted as *the impulse response of a linear model*. For compressive OHCs, the OHC efficiency (γ) of the linear comparison model decreases with increasing stimulus intensity.

If the cochlea operates like the aforementioned nonlinear model, the measured ccf can be interpreted as the impulse response of a linear system. This leads to the question: how do we derive from that impulse response the 'activity' or the efficiency (γ) of the OHCs in the model? This measure we can find by applying the 'inverse' solution method, by which procedure we obtain the *effective BM impedance* $Z_{\mathrm{BM}}^{\mathrm{eff}}(x)$ (which is a function of cochlear location x) from *the observed response (ccf)*. The inverse solution technique has many problems and subtleties, see for details de Boer.[1,2]

The inverse method has been applied to our data, for a three-dimensional model. The method employed differs slightly from the earlier one[1,2] in that in this study we have used a variation that handles forward and backward (reflected) waves in an equivalent manner[4] and is more robust than the earlier method.

3 Results II - cochlear 'activity'

Figure 3 shows results from the inverse solution performed on ccfs measured in an animal. Note that the abscissa depicts longitudinal distance x along the length of the model, this implies that *frequency has been converted to place*.[2] The three solid-line curves in the figure depict real (*panel a*) and imaginary (*panel b*) parts of the effective BM impedance $Z_{\mathrm{BM}}^{\mathrm{eff}}(x)$ as recovered by the inverse procedure, for three stimulus levels. In order of increasing line thickness they have been measured for increasing levels of stimulation (80, 40 and 10 dB of attenuation). For reasons of clarity, plotting of the impedance is done in a nonlinear way, see the figure legend. The scale for the real part is centered at zero, and that of the imaginary part at the upper border. The dashed line in the *left* panel shows the magnitude of the response (actually, the spectrum of the ccf), also converted to the x-domain; it is drawn only for the weakest stimulus condition (largest attenuation). The dashed curve in the *right* panel shows the corresponding 'resynthesized response', i.e., the response computed from the same model with the impedance $Z_{\mathrm{BM}}^{\mathrm{eff}}(x)$ inserted.[2] All curves are only drawn in the peak region, in other regions they are corrupted by spurious components and internal reflections. From Fig. 3-(a) it is observed that in the region where the response rises the most rapidly, the real part of the impedance $Z_{\mathrm{BM}}^{\mathrm{eff}}(x)$

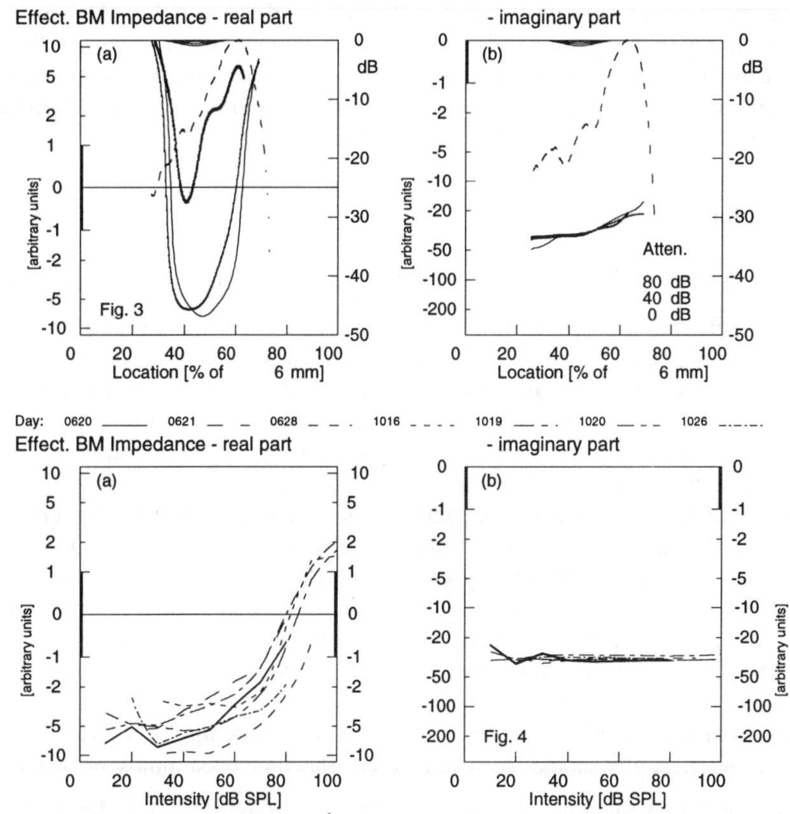

Figure 3 (top). Effective BM impedance, the number 1 on the ordinate corresponds to 100 cgs units (g cm^{-2} sec^{-1}). Values between -1 and +1 are depicted linearly (see thick vertical bands), other values are compressed logarithmically (see scales). Bands along upper edge indicate range of averaging (to be used for Fig. 4). Panel (a): real part; panel (b): imaginary part. Scale for dashed lines (see text for explanation) is on the right. The model used for the inverse solution model is three-dimensional, the width of the BM is assumed to be 0.3 of the width of the channel ($\varepsilon = 0.3$). Experiment: 1019. Three stimulation levels, in order of increasing line thickness: attenuation: 80, 40 and 0 dB.

Figure 4 (bottom). Average value of the effective BM impedance as a function of stimulus level. Ordinate scale as in Fig. 3. Averaging was done over 1.65 mm to the left of the response peak at the lowest level, see bands along upper edge of Fig. 3. Panel (a): real part; panel (b): imaginary part. Seven curves, for experiments: 0620, 0621, 0628, 1016, 1019, 1020 and 1026.

is negative. This feature signifies that *in this region* of the model the OHCs *deliver* acoustic energy to the wave, *in all other regions* they only *dissipate* energy. We also see that the negative excursion of the real part diminishes with increasing stimulus level. In terms of the model, this reduction of 'activity' can be attributed to *compression* occurring in the OHCs with stronger stimuli.

4 Variation of 'activity'

Figure 4 shows how the 'activity' in a region of the x domain varies with stimulus intensity. Each point of a curve signifies the effective BM impedance $Z_{\text{BM}}^{\text{eff}}(x)$ averaged over a small fixed region of the x-domain to the left of the peak of the response (see legend). The impedance is plotted on the same nonlinear ordinate scale as is used in Fig. 3. The seven curves in the figure show results of experiments in seven animals; they are distinguished by line type. We observe that with increasing stimulus level the real part (*left panel*) generally becomes more positive, and eventually crosses the zero line, whereas the imaginary part (*right panel*) varies only little. The deviations due to nonlinearity start in the range from 40 to 60 dB (SPL), and the real part eventually crosses the zero line between 70 and 90 dB (SPL). As said earlier, we can attribute these variations to compression in the OHCs. Incidentally, the real part of the BM impedance is always found to be positive in a 'dead' cochlea, or a dead animal, the negative part lining up neatly with that shown in Fig. 4.

If the nonlinear model of section 3 describes the functioning of the real cochlea, the OHC efficiency γ should be a monotonic function of stimulus intensity. We mainly observe variations in the real part of $Z_{\text{BM}}^{\text{eff}}(x)$, and these follow approximately the same trend in all of our results. The variations in the imaginary part are too small to relate them to those in the real part. We may conclude that these findings (at least) do not contradict the predictions of the EQ-NL theorem.

In our results the real part varies much more, in a relative sense, than the imaginary part. This may indicate that the effective BM impedance $Z_{\text{BM}}^{\text{eff}}(x)$, if we would interpret this as a transformation from velocity to pressure at the *same* location, corresponds to a *non-causal* impulse response. In this connection, it should be remembered that in the very general type of model we are considering the OHCs do not necessarily have to contribute to the effective BM impedance at the same place as where they receive their input. In fact, in the aforementioned feed-forward models[6,12] they receive their input from a more basal location. Therefore, the restrictions applying to a driving-point impedance do not necessarily apply to the effective BM impedance in these cochlear models.

Acknowledgments

This work has been supported by grants from NIH, USA (nr NIDCD-DC-00141) and NWO, The Netherlands (nr SLW 01.011).

References

1. Boer, E. de (1995a) The "inverse problem" solved for a three-dimensional model of the cochlea. I. Analysis, *J. Acoust. Soc. Am.* **98** 896-903.
2. Boer, E. de (1995b) The "inverse problem" solved for a three-dimensional model of the cochlea. II. Application to experimental data sets, *J. Acoust. Soc. Am.* **98** 904-910.
3. Boer, E. de (19-a) Connecting frequency selectivity and nonlinearity for models of the cochlea, *Audit. Neurosci* (in press).
4. Boer, E. de (19-b) A method for forward and inverse solutions of a 3-dimensional model of the cochlea, *J. Acoust. Soc. Am.* (submitted for publication).
5. Boer, E. de and Nuttall, A.L. (19--) The mechanical waveform of the basilar membrane. I. Frequency modulations ("glides") in impulse responses and cross-correlation functions, J. Acoust. Soc. Am. (submitted for publication).
6. Geisler, C.D. and Sang, C. (1995) A cochlear model using feed-forward outer-hair-cell forces, *Hear. Res.* **86** 132-146.
7. Hubbard, A.E. (1993) A traveling wave-amplifier model of the cochlea, Science 259 68-71.
8. Neely, S.T. and Kim, D.O. (1986) A model for active elements in cochlear biomechanics, *J. Acoust. Soc. Am.* **79** 1472-1480.
9. Nuttall, A.L. and Dolan, D.F. (1996) Steady-state sinusoidal velocity responses of the basilar membrane in guinea pig,. *J. Acoust. Soc. Am.* (in press)
10. Papoulis, A. (1985) *Signal Analysis* (McGraw-Hill, Singapore, London), Eq. 9-40, p. 306.
11. Ruggero, M.A., Rich, N.C. and Recio, A. (1992) Basilar membrane responses to clicks, in *Auditory physiology and perception,* ed. Y. Cazals, L. Demany and K. Horner (Pergamon, London) 85-91.
12. Steele, C.R., Baker, G., Tolomeo, J. and Zetes, D. (1993) Electro-mechanical models of the outer hair cell, in *Biophysics of Hair-Cell Sensory Systems*, ed. H. Duifhuis, J.W. Horst, P. van Dijk and S.M. van Netten (World Scientific, Singapore) 207-214.

MID-BAND SENSITIVITY NOTCHES IN APICAL COCHLEAR MECHANICS

N.P. COOPER

Department of Neurophysiology, 275 Medical Sciences Building, 1300 University Avenue
Madison, WI 53706, USA
cooper@neurophys.wisc.edu

The apical cochlea's mechanical responses to both transient (click) and steady-state (tone-pip) acoustic stimulation are used as evidence that two modes of vibration can exist in the cochlea, at least under some experimental conditions. One of these modes is associated with the 'slow' travelling wave of classical studies, and dominates the responses evoked by the low-frequency components of a stimulus [components which fall near or below the location's most sensitive, or best frequency (BF)]. The other mode is associated with a much faster travelling wave, and dominates the responses evoked by the high-frequency (>BF) components of a stimulus. It is this latter mode which gives rise to the high-frequency plateau regions of the location's amplitude and phase transfer functions. Due to their different speeds of propagation, the two modes of response can often be separated (in the time domain) at the apex of the cochlea, such that the properties of each mode can be studied more or less independently[4]. The present report shows how the two modes of vibration might interact in the frequency domain to produce mid-band sensitivity notches of the type observed in several recent studies of the apical cochlea[1-3]. It also shows how the fast mode of response is attenuated when the experimental conditions approximate those occurring in the apical cochlea's natural (i.e. hydraulically sealed) state.

1 Introduction

Several recent reports[1-3] have noted the presence of a sharp notch in the apical cochlea's mechanical tuning characteristics. Some of these reports[1-2] suggest that the notch occurs slightly above the most sensitive or 'best' frequency (BF) for a particular location, while others[3] suggest that it is associated with a tectorial membrane resonance ~0.5 octaves below the BF. In the present report, the possible origins of these 'mid-band' sensitivity notches are investigated through further experimental studies.

2 Methods

The *in vivo* (and occasionally *post-mortem*) tuning characteristics of the apical cochlea were studied in two species (deeply anaesthetised guinea-pigs and chinchillas), using both transient (100µs clicks) and steady-state (30-40ms tone-pips) acoustic stimuli. Responses were recorded from various sites (including both basilar and tectorial membranes) using a displacement sensitive laser interferometer. In order to access these sites, the bulla was opened widely, a small hole was made through the bony wall of the scala vestibuli, and a small tear was made in Reissner's membrane. Small beads (gold coated polystyrene, 25µm diameter) were then introduced into the scala media to reflect the laser beam from the normally transparent structures of interest. The opening into the cochlea was covered with an optically flat cover glass, but no attempt was made to seal the preparation fully (in most experiments). Control responses were measured from the ossicles of the middle ear in each animal. Further details of the surgical approaches, the sound-generation and response recording techniques are given elsewhere[2,4].

3   Results

3.1   *Notches reflect interference between fast and slow response components*

Two pairs of transfer functions relating the vibrations of the apical turn's tectorial membrane to those of the ossicles in the middle ear are shown in Fig. 1. Each pair includes one function which was derived using tonal stimuli (circles in Figs. 1A/C and D/F) and one which was derived using clicks (solid lines). The data in the left column of the figure were recorded from a guinea-pig (GP178), while those in the right column were recorded from a chinchilla (CH23). There are two distinct sensitivity notches in the guinea-pig data (one at ~600Hz, one at ~1kHz; see arrows in Fig. 1A), both of which occur on the high-frequency side of the transfer function's most sensitive, or best frequency (BF≅400Hz). In contrast, there is only one notch in the chinchilla data [see arrow at ~800Hz in Fig. 1D; the BF for this preparation, as estimated from the more reliable (and lower SPL) tone data, was ~500Hz].

The correspondence between the two sets of transfer functions in each species is reasonably good. The correspondence is particularly close with respect to the response phases (solid lines and circles in Figs. 1C/F). The frequency-dependence of both sets of phase characteristics can be modelled reasonably well by two straight line segments (not illustrated in the figure): the first of these would cover the frequency range below ~800Hz, where the observed phases vary rapidly with frequency; and the second would cover the frequency range above ~800Hz, where the phase is almost independent of frequency. The time domain correlates of these two (hypothetical) straight line segments (namely one set of components with a large group delay, and one with almost zero group delay) are clearly visible in the waveforms shown in the insets of Figs. 1C/F; each click response has both a 'fast' and a 'slow' component. It may not be possible to separate these two components entirely in the time domain, but it is possible to separate them to a large extent; and when this is done (for example by considering only those responses which occur either before or after the vertical dashed lines in the insets of Figs. 1C/F), considerable insight can be gained.

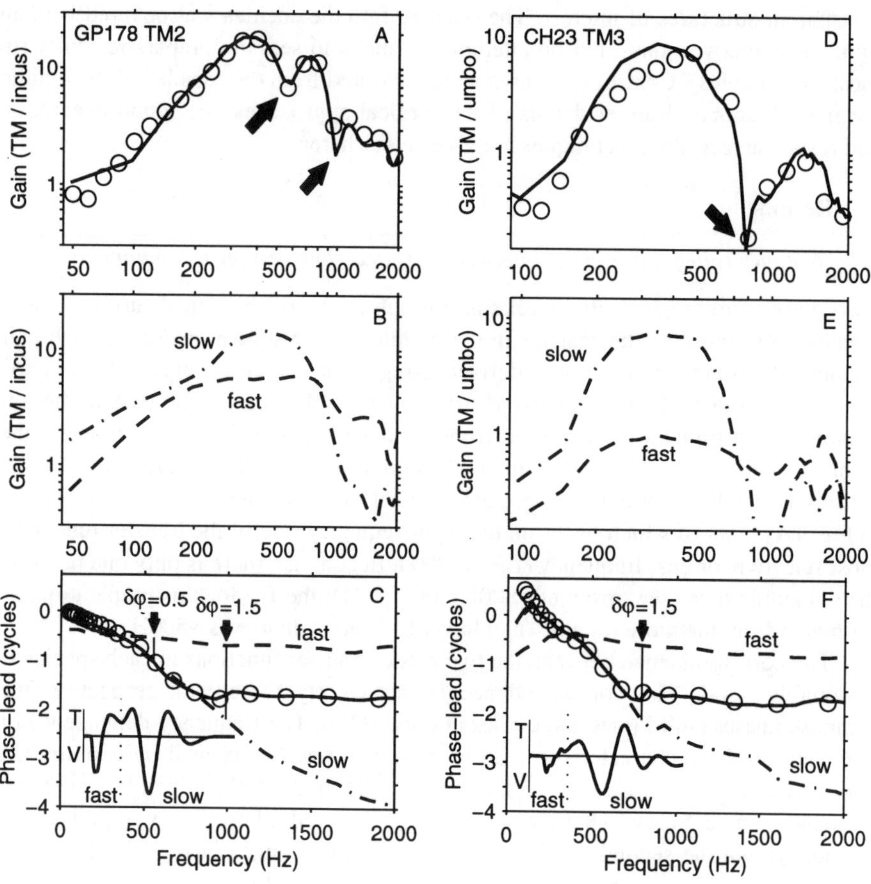

Figure 1: Apical turn transfer functions (TM / incus, TM / umbo) for steady-state (tone-pip; circles) and transient (click; lines) acoustic stimuli. (A) and (D) compare tone-pip and click response amplitudes in the frequency domain. Time domain responses to the clicks are shown in the insets of (C) and (F) [vertical bars indicate ±50nm, horizontal bars 0-7.5ms peri-stimulus time, and scala tympani (S$\underline{T}$) is upwards]. These time domain responses can conveniently be separated into two parts, labelled as fast and slow, by dividing at the vertical dashed lines. The amplitude transfer functions for the two response components then appear as shown in (B) and (E), while the phase transfer functions are as shown in (C) and (F). Solid lines/circles in (C) and (F) show phases corresponding to the amplitude data in (A) and (D). TM vibrations towards ST are shown with respect to 'inwards' motions of the ossicles (as observed during condensation at the eardrum).

The middle row of panels in Fig. 1 shows individual transfer functions for the two components of the click response waveforms (labelled fast and slow in the insets of Figs. 1C/F). Each of these transfer functions was derived following Fourier transformation of a rectangularly windowed subset of the time-domain responses. In contrast to the transfer functions derived using the entire time-domain responses (solid lines in Figs. 1A/D), each of the 'component' transforms has a relatively smooth amplitude spectrum (i.e. there are no obvious notches below ~1kHz in Figs. 1B/E). It should be noted that the amplitude spectrum for the fast response components approaches that for the slow components much more closely in the guinea-pig than it does in the chinchilla. It is also noteworthy that the fast components become larger than the slow ones at frequencies above ~800Hz in both species. Not surprisingly, the phase transfer functions for each of the two response components (dashed and dash-dotted lines in Figs. 1C/F) approximates a single straight line reasonably well [much more closely than the 'combined' phase transfer functions (solid lines) do, for example]. This is particularly true for the guinea-pig data (Fig. 1C), where the fast and slow response components can be separated much more cleanly in the time domain. The most important point of this discussion, however, is that the frequencies at which each of the two combined amplitude spectra (i.e., the transfer functions in Figs. 1A/D) exhibit notches correspond very closely with the frequencies where the two response components occur in anti-phase (i.e. where the dashed and dash-dotted lines in Figs. 1C/F are odd integer multiples of 0.5 cycles apart; see vertical lines in figure). This clearly implies that the notches result from destructive interference between the fast and slow response components.

3.2 *Fast and slow response components differ in many ways*

As the fast and slow response components described above cannot be separated entirely in the time domain, the distinction between them may seem somewhat arbitrary, and their likely physical bases are difficult to interpret. In data described elsewhere, however, the two components are shown to differ from each other in many ways. For example, the fast responses always behave linearly when the intensity of a stimulus is varied, while the slow ones do not[2,4]; the fast responses also appear much more robust than the slow responses, particularly in preparations where the slow responses behave non-linearly[4]; the two response components also have different amplitude and phase profiles across both the radial and longitudinal extents of the cochlear partition[4]; and finally, the fast responses appear particularly sensitive to the hydro-mechanical condition (i.e., the sealed / unsealed nature) of the apical cochlea, while the slow ones do not (see section 3.3).[4] These different behaviours often permit a clearer distinction to be made between the two response components.

3.3   *Fast response components may be artifacts*

One particularly unusual feature of the fast response components is their polarity. In response to the condensation clicks of Fig. 1, for example, the initial movements of the entire apical cochlear partition (not just the tectorial membrane) are directed towards the scala vestibuli. This is counter-intuitive: condensation clicks are known to push the stapes into the cochlea, and to *increase* the pressure in the scala vestibuli. But the observed results suggest that the pressure in the apical turn's scala tympani is greater than that in the scala vestibuli. The only way to reconcile these two observations is to suggest that standing waves exist in the apical turn of the cochlea. These waves might be caused by reflections from the helicotrema, or by reflections from the experimental openings into the scala vestibuli. In the view of the present author, this latter possibility appears somewhat more likely than the former, since the helicotrema is both larger and more closely opposed to the recording site in the chinchilla, while the fast responses are much larger in the guinea-pig (furthermore, comparatively large fast responses are always observed on Reissner's membrane, and this membrane is much closer to the apical opening in both species).

In order to test the hypothesis that the fast response components are associated with standing waves in the immediate vicinity of the scala vestibuli opening, several attempts were made to record the responses from a single location both before and

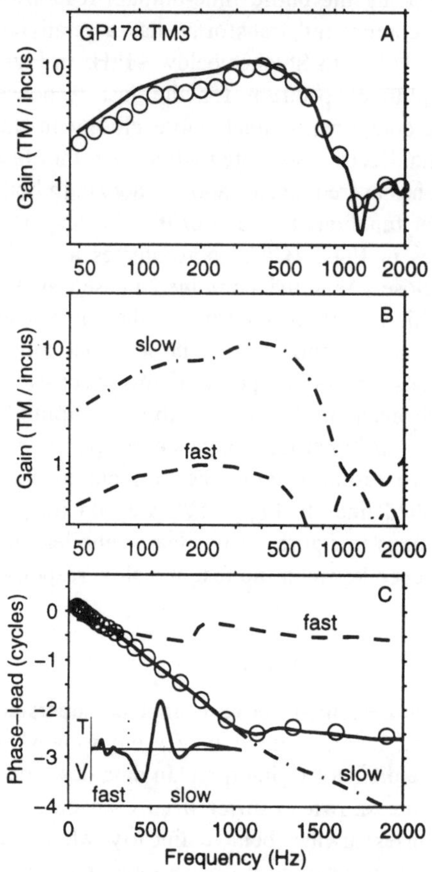

Figure 2: Transfer functions (TM / incus) for steady-state (tone-pip; circles) and transient (click; lines) stimuli under conditions where the opening into the apical cochlea has been sealed using high-vacuum grease. Layout as in Fig. 1. GP178, tones ~ 80dB SPL, clicks ~80dB peak equivalent rarefaction.

after sealing the opening from a hydro-mechanical point of view. The best of the results obtained in these experiments (as judged by the size of the observed effect, and by our confidence that the polystyrene micro-beads had not changed position) are illustrated elsewhere.[4] A somewhat less dramatic example is illustrated in Fig. 2 of the present paper. This shows two transfer functions obtained from the same bead as shown in Figs. 1A-C, under conditions where the experimental cover glass has been sealed onto the shell of the cochlea using a thin layer of high-vacuum grease. This manipulation has two very obvious effects (compare Figs. 1 and 2 A-C; note the switch to rarefaction clicks in Fig. 2): firstly, it decreases the amplitude of the fast response components by a factor of at least five (see Figs. 1/2B, and insets in Figs. 1/2C); and secondly, it either eliminates, or drastically reduces the size (and/or shifts the frequency) of the transfer function notches (see Figs. 1/2A). One other effect of the seal, which is similar to that reported previously[5] *in vitro*, is that it increases the low-frequency sensitivity of the preparation at a rate of ~6dB/octave below ~350Hz. In the example shown in Fig. 2, the peak-to-peak amplitude of the slow response component is ~30% lower than that in Fig. 1, but the low-frequency content of the component is increased. In our best data,[4] the peak-to-peak amplitude of the slow component was almost unchanged, despite the 6dB/octave increase in its low-frequency content.

4   Discussion

This report suggests that the mid-band sensitivity notches which have been observed in several recent studies of the apical cochlea might represent nothing more than (destructive) interactions between two seemingly independent modes of mechanical excitation. One of these modes has many characteristics in common with the 'slow' travelling wave of classical cochlear mechanics,[6] while the other one appears to be associated with a much faster travelling wave - it was introduced here using the concept of standing waves in the apical cochlea, but the pressure waves responsible for the data actually propagate at a finite speed (there is a delay of between 20 and 90µs between the first ossicular responses to a sound and the first apical turn responses). The data of Fig. 2 clearly show that the responses to this second, 'fast' mode of excitation can be reduced considerably by returning the cochlea to a state which approximates that occurring in nature (i.e., by sealing the apical cochlea from a hydro-mechanical point of view). This observation clearly supports the view that the fast components of a response, and all of the response features that can be attributed to them (i.e., the mid-band sensitivity notches, high-frequency amplitude and phase plateaus), might be nothing more than experimental artifacts.

Acknowledgements

Supported by research grant number 5 R01 DC 01910 from the National Institute on Deafness and Other Communication Disorders, National Institutes of Health. The author gratefully acknowledges Profs. W.S. Rhode, C.D. Geisler and E. de Boer for comments on this work.

References

1. Khanna, S.M., Flock, A. and Ulfendahl, M. (1989) Changes in cellular tuning along the radial axis of the cochlea. *Acta Oto-Laryngol.* **suppl. 467**, 163–173.

2. Cooper, N.P. and Rhode, W.S. (1995) Nonlinear mechanics at the apex of the guinea-pig cochlea. *Hear. Res.* **82**, 225–243.

3. Gummer, A. W., Hemmert, W. and Zenner, H.P. (1995) Micromechanics of cellular structures in the mammalian cochlea: Auditory and electrical stimulation, in *Active Hearing,* eds. A. Flock, D. Ottoson and M. Ulfendahl (Pergamon, Great Yarmouth, England) pp. 271–282.

4. Cooper, N.P. and Rhode, W.S. (1996) Fast travelling waves, slow travelling waves, and their interactions in experimental studies of apical cochlear mechanics. *Auditory Neuroscience* **2**, 207-217.

5. Ulfendahl, M., Flock, A. and Khanna, S.M. (1991) Effects of opening and resealing the cochlea on the mechanical response in the isolated temporal bone preparation. *Hear. Res.* **57**, 31-37.

6. von Békésy, G. (1960) *Experiments in Hearing*, McGraw-Hill, New York.

TWO-TONE "LOW-SIDE" SUPPRESSION IN RESPONSES OF BASAL BASILAR MEMBRANE

C.D. GEISLER

Departments of Neurophysiology and of Electrical and Computer Engineering
University of Wisconsin-Madison, Madison, Wisconsin, 53706 USA

A.L. NUTTALL

Kresge Hearing Research Institute, University of Michigan
Ann Arbor, Michigan, 48109 USA

The responses of the basilar membrane (BM) in the basal turn of the guinea-pig cochlea to two-tone stimuli were measured by laser interferometry. One tone was at the characteristic frequency (CF) of the membrane (~17 kHz), the other at a lower frequency (0.2-8 kHz), presented at different intensities. As previously shown, the low-frequency tone suppressed the CF response components. Our principal finding is that, regardless of the degree of suppression, the *sum* of the CF and suppressor displacement amplitudes in the two-tone response was *always* greater than that of the unsuppressed CF response. The suppression of the CF component was both tonic and phasic, synchronized to the suppressor frequency (but only below about 4 kHz). Lower frequency suppressors often produced two phases of suppression (one major and one minor) during each suppressor period. The suppressions are fully accounted for by the "saturating feedback" hypothesis[1].

1 Introduction

Suppression of basilar-membrane response components by a lower-frequency tone ("low-side" suppression) has been demonstrated previously[2-5]. This type of suppression can also be produced by a cochlear-partition model that uses outer-hair-cell feedback forces which "saturate"[6]. To build support for the conclusion that such a model accounts for the physiologically observed suppressions, further comparisons must be made. In particular, the model predicts that the peak height of the two-tone *displacement* will *always* be greater than that of the unsuppressed response, and that the instants within the suppressor tone which produce the maximum amount of suppression will occur when the basilar membrane displacement is maximal into one scala or the other (Figure 6).

We have obtained the requisite physiological data from the basal turn of the guinea-pig cochlea. The results are exactly as predicted by the model, leading us to the conclusion that "saturating feedback" does indeed account for the low-side suppression demonstrated by the basal basilar membrane.

2 Methods

The responses of the basilar membrane in the basal turn of the guinea-pig cochlea were measured with laser interferometry[7]. The stimuli were pairs of tones presented simultaneously for about 20 seconds. One tone, with a frequency near the CF of the location (about 17 kHz), was presented at a constant (weak) intensity. The other tone, harmonically related to the first, was a "low-side" suppressor, with a frequency in the range of 0.2-8 kHz, presented at different intensities. Velocity responses were obtained from small glass beads placed upon the basilar membrane. Signal averaging (1000 segments) was done on 20-ms samples of the responses.

Responses were obtained from 8 different animals. In each animal, only small changes were observed in the compound action potential during surgical preparation, and strong compression was seen in the amplitude-vs-intensity curve taken at CF. In two of those preparations, the CF responses were measured before and after death. In each case, the difference in amplitudes between these two curves (the gain of the "cochlear amplifier") was about 40 dB (Figure 1). Thus, these cochleae were judged to have been in nearly normal condition.

Responses to the two-tone stimuli were formed into period histograms, using the period of the suppressor (or a subharmonic) as the time base. Fourier analysis of the period histograms was used to isolate the high-frequency components (CF plus sidebands) from the low-frequency (suppressor) component. The interferometer measures object *velocity*, so the recorded responses were integrated to obtain BM *displacements* (in nm).

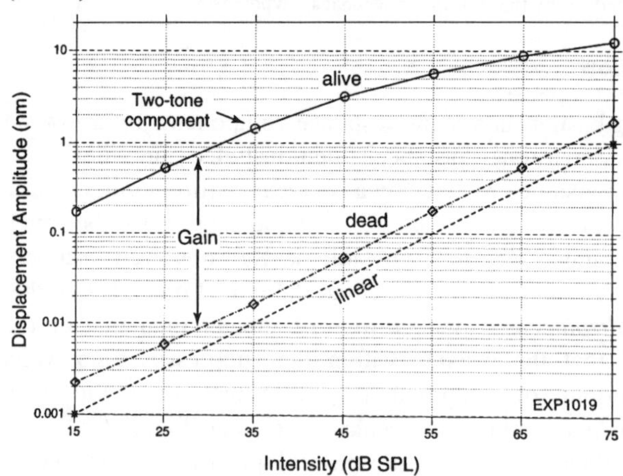

Figure 1: Responses to near-CF tones (17 kHz) before and after death. The level of the near-CF tone used in the two-tone signals is labeled. Typically, it was placed near the onset of amplitude compression (35 dB SPL, in this case).

3 Amplitudes of Responses

The invariant pattern seen in our results is shown in Figure 2, which plots the CF and suppressor-frequency response components elicited by tones of 17 kHz (CF) and 4 kHz presented simultaneously. As seen by others, suppression of the CF component occurred when the suppressor intensity was high enough. Of special interest is the fact that the suppression did not begin until the amplitude of the suppressor reached approximately 3 nm, greater than that of the unsuppressed response (a little over 1 nm). Note that the response component at the suppressor frequency grew linearly over the entire intensity range, as expected.

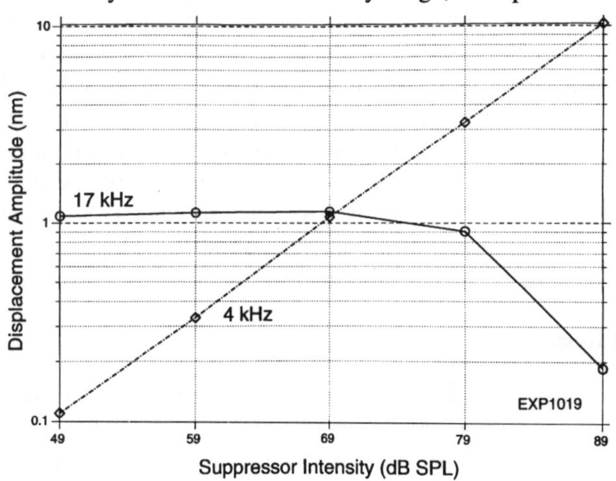

Figure 2: The amplitudes of the CF and suppressor components produced with a 4-kHz suppressor presented at various levels, plotted as functions of suppressor sound level.

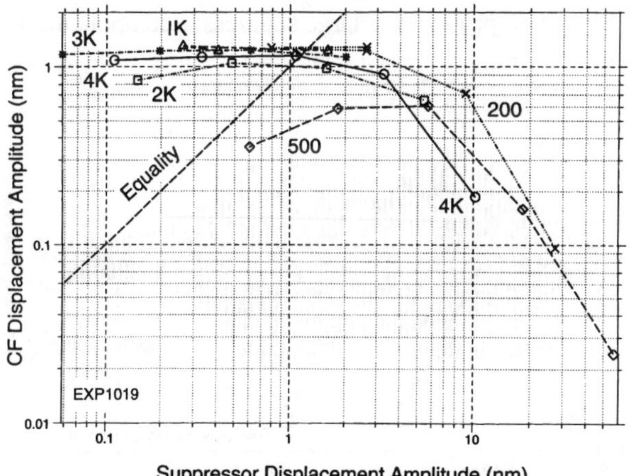

Figure 3: The amplitudes of the CF component produced with suppressors of 6 different frequencies (labeled), presented at various intensities, plotted as functions of suppressor amplitude.

308

In order to compare the suppression patterns obtained with suppressors of other frequencies, these responses have been replotted with suppressor *amplitude* used as the abscissal variable. Thus, the two points in Figure 2 which characterize one two-tone response become one point in Figure 3. The two-tone responses obtained from this same animal with low-side suppressors of 5 other frequencies are also shown.

The pattern of suppression is the same for each suppressor. When the amplitude of the low-frequency component became greater than about 3 nm, suppression of the CF component occurred. This similarity implies that suppressor *displacement*, rather than velocity, determines the magnitude of CF suppression. Moreover, the "equality" line in the figure shows clearly that, in *each* case of suppression, the amplitude of the suppressor component was *always* greater than that of the unsuppressed CF component. Thus, in *all* cases, the *sum* of the two components (approximately the peak value of the two-tone response) was greater than the amplitude of the unsuppressed CF component. This inequality was invariant across all suppressor frequencies in all 8 experimental animals

4 Phases of Responses

The actual waveforms of the suppressor component and the CF-band component (15-17 kHz) obtained with a 200-Hz suppressor are shown in Figure 4, plotted over a complete period of the suppressor. Note that two epochs of suppression occurred, the principle one peaking at about the instant when the basilar membrane was deflected maximally towards scala tympani. The other suppression phase occurred approximately 180° earlier. The suppressor intensity was relatively high in this case (76 dB SPL) and produced a large suppressor component (9.1 nm). With

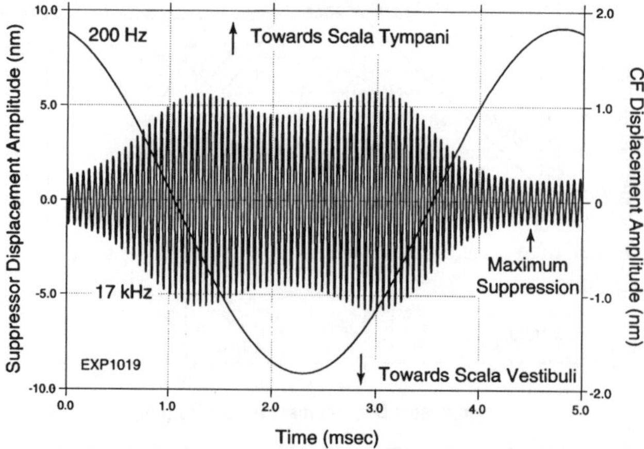

Figure 4 The near-CF band (17±1 kHz) and suppressor component (200 Hz) of the BM's displacement response to a two-tone stimulus. Note the different ordinate scales

lower suppressor intensities, the smaller suppression epoch usually vanished, leaving only the principle one. We observed this same basic pattern (a primary suppression with perhaps a secondary one) in all 4 animals in which we used 200-Hz suppressors. Similar patterns were observed with 500-Hz suppressors in all animals.

The instants of the peaks of all of the primary suppressions produced by 3 of the 4 animals providing useful data with 200-Hz suppressors are shown in Figure 5 (strong harmonic distortion in the 4th animal made its suppression phases ambiguous). As shown, these maximal-suppression instants (individual data points), cluster tightly around the moment of maximum deflection into scala tympani, regardless of suppressor intensity.

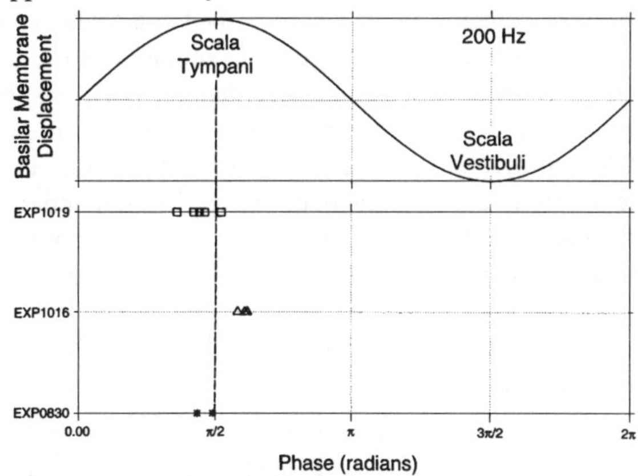

Figure 5: The phases of maximum 17-kHz suppression relative to the phase of the suppressor tone (200 Hz), at different suppressor intensities, for 3 successive experiments.

At higher suppressor frequencies, the instants of maximum suppression were delayed by various small amounts that seemed to vary from animal to animal. Preliminary analysis of these data suggests that the onset of suppression occurred with small idiosyncratic time delays measured in tenths of milliseconds, which (of course) gave larger phase delays as frequency was increased. For suppressor frequencies greater than about 4 kHz, only slight phasic suppression occurred, and that at sub-harmonics of the suppressor frequency.

5   Discussion

When comparable, the responses we have obtained are consistent with almost all previously reported results for low-side BM suppression. In particular, the one-often-two epochs of suppression are very similar to those reported before[2-5], as are the increased amplitudes of displacement peaks for *all* of the responses[5]. Moreover, the phases of our maximum suppression agree with those reported in three of the four relevant reports[2,4,5]; the accuracy of suppression phases reported in the fourth paper[3] has been questioned[5].

In order to test the degree to which the "saturating outer-hair-cell feedback" model can account for our results, we have used an idealization of a measured outer-hair-cell input/output (I/O) curve[8], assuming that it characterizes responses at all stimulus frequencies. As shown in Figure 6, the addition of a low-frequency tone to a CF tone forces the receptor potential further into both of its compressive regions. Thus the voltage waveform in the two-tone case exceeds, at two phases of the suppressor, the output to the CF tone alone (whose envelope is shaded). Since the slope of the I/O curve decreases monotonically at each end, these increased voltage excursions must be more compressed than those of the CF-tone alone. Moreover, since the "rest point" of the input/output curve is asymmetrically placed, the scala-tympani excursions are more highly compressed than the scala-vestibuli deflections. When the suppressor-frequency component is filtered out (it is assumed to have no effect upon the CF amplification process), the receptor potential clearly undergoes two phases of suppression, each corresponding to a BM deflection toward a scala, as in the experimental data (Figure 4). Such a potential would in turn produce a similar pattern of basilar-membrane suppression in a feedback model.

In short, the major characteristics of the basilar-membrane low-side suppression that we report here are qualitatively mimicked by the "saturating feedback" model. Accordingly, we conclude that the model satisfactorily "accounts for" the data.

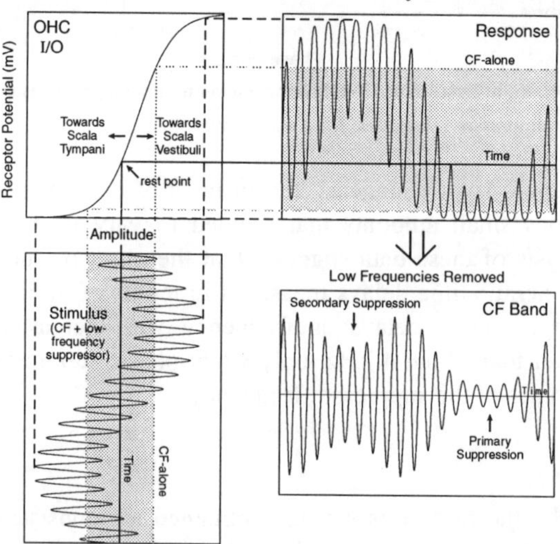

Figure 6: Idealized sketch of an outer hair cell's input/output (I/O) curve, with two-tone input and output waveforms. The envelopes of comparable waveforms evoked by the CF-tone alone are shaded.

By the same token, the model can *not* account for the low-side suppression seen in the responses of low-spontaneous auditory-nerve fibers, for which the peaks of the comparable responses are almost always *less* (sometimes *much* less) in amplitude than the responses to the CF-tone alone[9].

Acknowledgments

This research was supported (in part) by research grant numbers NIDCD-DC00116 and -DC00141 from the National Institute on Deafness and Other Communication Disorders, National Institutes of Health.

References

1. Zwicker, E. (1979) A model describing nonlinearities in hearing by active process with saturation at 40 dB, *Biol. Cybern.* **35** 243-250.
2. Patuzzi, R., Sellick, P.M. and Johnstone, B.M. (1984) The modulation of the sensitivity of the mammalian cochlea by low frequency tones. III. Basilar membrane motion. *Hear. Res.* **13** 19-27.
3. Ruggero, M.A., Robles, L. and Rich, N.C. (1992) Two-tone suppression in the basilar membrane of the cochlea: Mechanical basis of auditory-nerve rate suppression, *J. Neurophys.* **68** 1087-1099.
4. Rhode, W.S. and Cooper, N.P. (1993) Two-tone suppression and distortion production on the basilar membrane in the hook region of cat and guinea pig cochleae, *Hear. Res.* **66** 31-45.
5. Cooper, N.P. (1996) Two-tone suppression in cochlear mechanics, *J. Acoust. Soc. Am.* **99** 3087-3098.
6. Geisler, C.D., Bendre, A. and Liotopoulos, F.K. (1993) Time-domain modeling of a nonlinear, active model of the cochlea, in *Biophysics of Hair Cell Sensory Systems*, eds. H. Duifhuis, J.W. Horst, P. van Dijk and S.M. van Netten (World Scientific, Singapore) pp. 330-337.
7. Nuttall, A.L., Dolan, D.F. and Avinash, G. (1991) Laser Doppler velocimetry of basilar membrane vibration, *Hear. Res.* **51** 203-214.
8. Russell, I.J., Cody, A.R. and Richardson, G.P. (1986) The responses of inner and outer hair cells in the basal turn of the guinea-pig cochlea and in the mouse cochlea grown in vitro, *Hear. Res.* **22** 199-216.
9. Cai, Y. and Geisler, C.D. (in press) Suppression in auditory-nerve fibers of cats using low-side suppressors: II. Effect of spontaneous rates, and III. Model Results, *Hear. Res.*

REISSNER'S MEMBRANE AND THE RETICULAR LAMINA RESPONSE IN THE APICAL TURN OF THE COCHLEA IN A LIVING GUINEA PIG

S.M. KHANNA., L.F. HAO

Columbia University, Department of Otolaryngology and Head and Neck Surgery
630 West 168th Street #11–452
New York, NY 10032
email: smk3@columbia.edu

Vibrations were measured at selected locations on the Reissner's membrane and the reticular lamina in the apical turn of a living guinea pig cochlea, in response to tones applied to the ear canal. The shape of the amplitude and phase response depends on the radial location on the Reissner's membrane and on the specific cochlear structure at the reticular lamina.

1 Introduction

Cooper and Rhode[2] found that in the apical turn of the guinea pig cochleas the tuning at both the tectorial membrane and the basilar membrane were essentially the same as at the Reissner's membrane, concluding that the tuning characteristics of the Reissner's membrane could be used to describe the mechanical behavior of the others. This is in agreement with Békésy's[1] concepts. We have developed a noninvasive technique[4] that allows us to view the organ of Corti and measure the cellular vibrations using its natural reflectivity. We have determined the mechanical responses of the Reissner's membrane and the sensory cells at the reticular lamina and studied their dependence on the radial position.

2 Method

The surgical procedure and the method of access to the guinea pig cochlea is described by Hao and Khanna[3]. Approximately one third of the apical turn was exposed, leaving the modiolus, stria vascularis, and Reissner's membrane (RM) intact. The objective lens of the microscope was optically coupled to the cochlea with a rubber tube filled with tissue culture medium, creating a fluid tight seal. The cochlea was viewed with the slit confocal microscope[5]. A confocal heterodyne interferometer was used for the vibration measurements[6]. The tones were synthesized and the responses were recorded with a DSP system[4].

3 Observations

The normalized tuning curves (meters/microbar) measured at 90dB SPL at four radial locations on the Reissner's membrane are shown in Figure 1: (a) above the inner edge of the Hensen's cells (HC), (b) above the row 3 outer hair cell (OHC), (e) above the inner hair cells (IHC), and (f) above the OSL region. Curve (h) represents

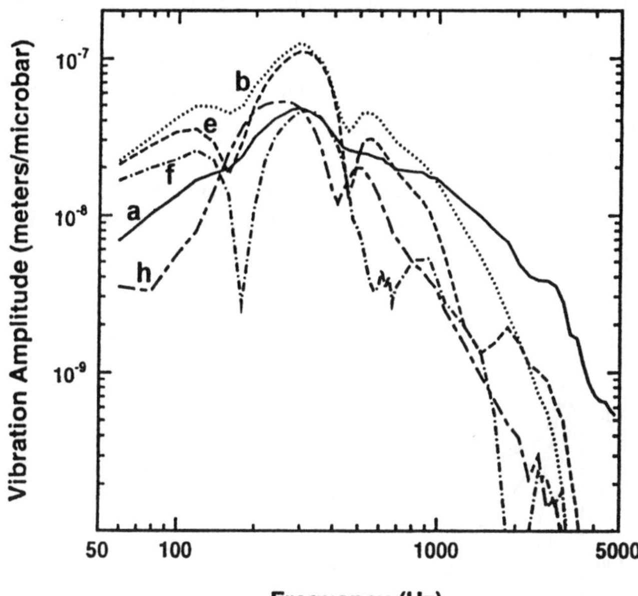

Figure 1: Comparison of normalized vibration amplitude at four radial positions on the Reissner's membrane

the vibration measured at the third row outer hair cell. The four responses are different from each other and from the response of the outer hair cell.

Phase responses measured at the same four radial locations on the RM (a,b,e,f), and at the outer hair cell below (h), are shown in Figure 2. Phase responses measured on the RM (cr) by Cooper and Rhode[2] are included for comparison. The shapes of the phase curves are different at the four radial positions. The phase lag increases as the point of measurement moves from the outside edge of the cochlea toward the modiolus. The first segment of the phase curve, extending from 400 to 600 Hz, has a steep slope, and the other segments (above 600 Hz) have a shallower slope.

Normalized tuning curves obtained at 90 dB SPL are shown in Figure 3 for six radial locations on the reticular lamina: (a) HC at the inner edge, (b) OHC3, (c) OHC2, (d) OHC1, (e) IHC, and (f) edge of OSL. Tuning curves measured at each of these positions are quite similar in shape. The Q_{10} for the tuning curves in this cochlea is 0.98. As we moved from the OSL edge toward the Hensen's cells, the vibration amplitude progressively increased in the CF region by approximately a

314

factor of 12. The ratio of the vibration amplitude measured at the Hensen's cell and the inner hair cell was 7.69. The increase of amplitude in the outer hair cell region (OHC3/OHC1) was 2.15. Similar observations were made in prior temporal bone preparations[4].

Vibration phase plotted on a linear frequency scale is compared in Figure 4 for six radial positions on the reticular lamina: (a) HC at the inner edge, (b) OHC3, (c) OHC 2, (d) OHC1, (e) IHC, and (f) edge of OSL. The curves show a steep portion (−1.65 degrees /Hz) from 100 to about 600 Hz, and a shallower portion (−0.06 degrees /Hz) extending to 3000 Hz. Phase lag increases as we move radially outwards from the OSL to the Hensen's cells. Time delays corresponding to these linear phase shifts are 4.58, and 0.17 msec, respectively.

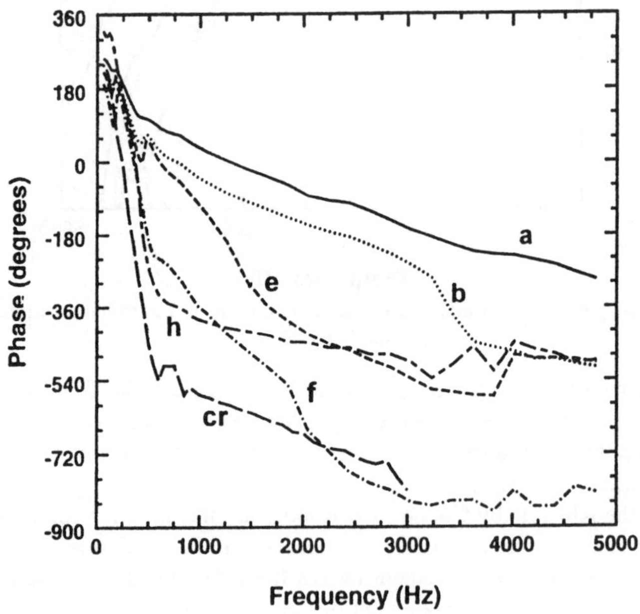

Figure 2: Comparison of phase measured at four radial positions on the Reissner's membrane.

4 Discussion

Measuring techniques that require placing a highly reflective bead to enhance the reflectivity of the structure under study disrupt cochlear integrity. In order to measure deeper structures, such as hair cells, a hole must be made in Reissner's membrane to allow placement of the bead. These manipulations invariably produce trauma and associated changes in the response. Therefore, measurements on different structures are made under inconsistent physiological conditions of the cochlea. Non-invasive measuring techniques, such as ours, allow measurements to be made on all structures under identical physiological conditions, without disrupting the cochlear function.

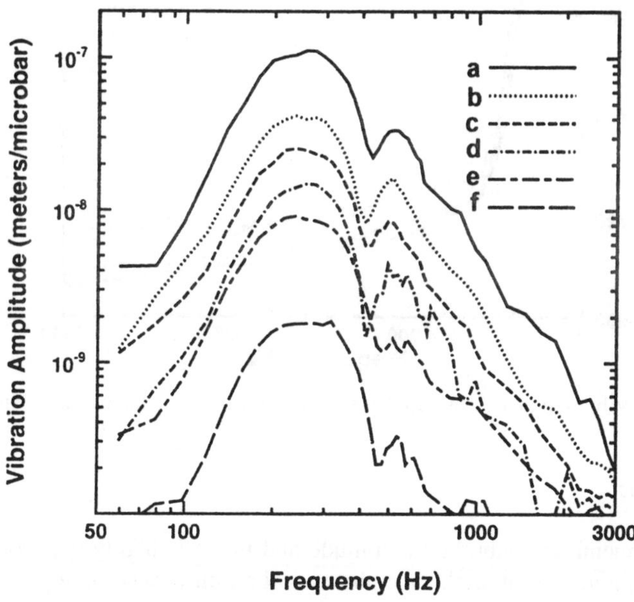

Figure 3: Normalized tuning curves measured at six positions on the reticular lamina.

The experiments presented in this paper show that the shape and magnitude of the tuning curves, and the phase characteristics of the Reissner's membrane, change dramatically with small changes (50 μm) in the radial position. It is clear that Reissner's membrane tuning cannot be described with one curve. It is also shown that the magnitude of the tuning curves obtained at the reticular lamina also change with the radial position. The frequency and phase responses measured at the reticular lamina are different from those measured at the Reissner's membrane. Thus, Reissner's membrane responses cannot be used to represent the reticular lamina responses.

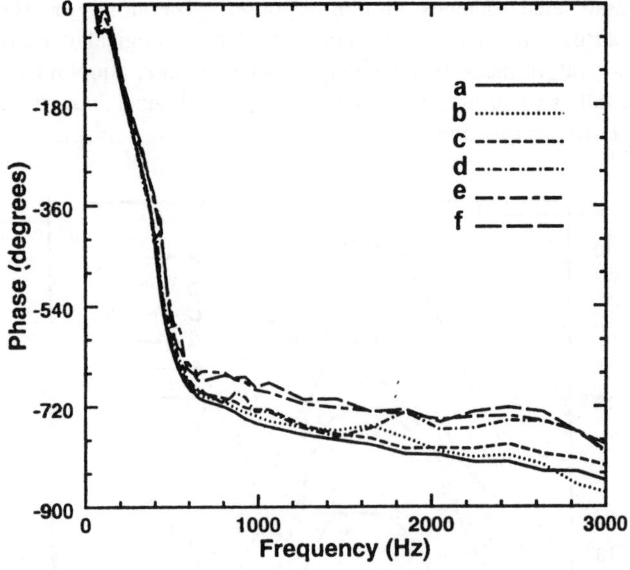

Figure 4: Vibration phase measured at six radial positions on the reticular lamina.

5 Conclusions

1. Reissner's membrane vibration amplitude and phase is highly dependent on the radial position. Reissner's membrane vibrations, accordingly, cannot be described by a single response.
2. The magnitude of the vibration measured at the reticular lamina and the phase delay increases progressively as we move from the osseus spiral lamina radially outward toward the Hensen's cells.
3. Response shapes measured at Reissner's membrane are different from those measured at the sensory cells below. Consequently, measurements made at the Reissner's membrane cannot be used to describe the response of the sensory cells.
4. To fully understand cochlear mechanics, vibrations must be measured at multiple radial locations.

Acknowledgments

Research supported by Emil Capita fund, DRF, and NOHR. We thank G. T. Kaufman, and P. Andreola for their help in preparing the figures.

References

1. Békésy, G. von (1960) In: Wever, E.G. (Ed) *Experiments in Hearing*. New York: McGraw–Hill, p.745.
2. Cooper, N.P. and Rhode, W.S. (1995) Nonlinear mechanics at the apex of the guinea pig cochlea. *Hear.Res.* **82** 225–243.
3. Hao, L. and Khanna, S.M. (1996): Reissner's membrane vibrations in the apical turn of living guinea pig cochlea. (in review).
4. ITER (1989) International Team for Ear Research. *Acta Otolaryngol.(Stockh.) Suppl.* **467** 279.
5. Koester, C.J., Khanna, S.M., Rosskothen, H.D., Tackaberry, R.B., and Ulfendahl, M. (1994) Confocal slit divided-aperture microscope: applications in ear research. *Applied Optics.* **33** 702–708.
6. Willemin, J.F.,Dändliker, R.,and Khanna, S.M. (1988) Heterodyne interferometer for submicroscopic vibration measurements in the inner ear. *J. Acoust Soc. Am.* **83** 787–795.

NONLINEAR MECHANISMS IN THE APICAL TURN OF THE CHINCHILLA COCHLEA.

W. S. RHODE AND N. P. COOPER

Department of Neurophysiology, 275 Medical Sciences Building, 1300 University Avenue
Madison, WI 53706, USA
rhode@neurophys.wisc.edu

Vibration of the organ of Corti has been investigated in the apical region of the chinchilla cochlea using a displacement sensitive laser interferometer with sufficient sensitivity to perform measurements at threshold levels of stimulation. The tectorial membrane in the region of the outer hair cells vibrated with the largest amplitude of any portion of the organ of Corti. The range of frequency and intensity of the nonlinearity is considerably different than has been previously reported for mechanics in the base of the cochlea. The region of nonlinearity consists of all frequencies but a more restricted intensity range than found in the basal region of the cochlea. The region of the nonlinearity also correlates with the occurrence of a *dc* response and two-tone suppression. Comparison with auditory nerve fiber responses indicates that the neural response are largely determined by the mechanics in this region.

1 Introduction

Nonlinear mechanisms in the base of the cochlea likely explain much of the nonlinear behavior in recordings from the auditory nerve.[1,2,3] In contrast, little evidence has been obtained from the apical cochlear region to support the notion that mechanics of the organ of Corti in this region were similar to that of the basal region. This is most probably due to the difficulty of accessing the apex of the cochlea and maintaining a viable preparation in the apical region. We believe that we have now largely succeeded in this goal and can demonstrate both similarities and differences with the mechanics of the basal region of the cochlea.

While numerous attempts have been made to measure the vibration of either Reissner's membrane and/or the various structures of the organ of Corti in the apical cochlea, only one study has revealed nonlinear input/output functions. These were observed in the region of a notch seen in the transfer curves of the motion of Reissner's membrane. The nonlinearity had both compressive and expansive regions and occurred principally at high stimulus levels. It was proposed that the interaction of two vibration modes could explain the observations.[4] The present results support the conventional explanation as formulated for basal cochlear mechanics.

2 Methods

Recordings were made in the apical region of the chinchilla cochlea using a displacement-sensitive laser interferometer[4]. The vibration studied was usually that of the tectorial membrane near the outer hair cells, a region that has been shown to vibrate with the largest amplitude of any structure of the organ of Corti[5]. Full details are given elsewhere.

3 Results

3.1 Nonlinear TM input/output (I/O) functions.

Nonlinear I/O functions for the displacement is a sine qua non for the existence of cochlear mechanical nonlinearity. An I/O function obtained at a location in the cochlea approximately 4 mm from the apex, with a characteristic frequency of 500 Hz is shown in fig. 1. The dotted line illustrates a linear I/O relation. The deviation from linearity is apparent at all of the frequencies tested. Estimations of the contribution due to the cochlear amplifier (CA) range between 6 and 25 dB based on these experiments.

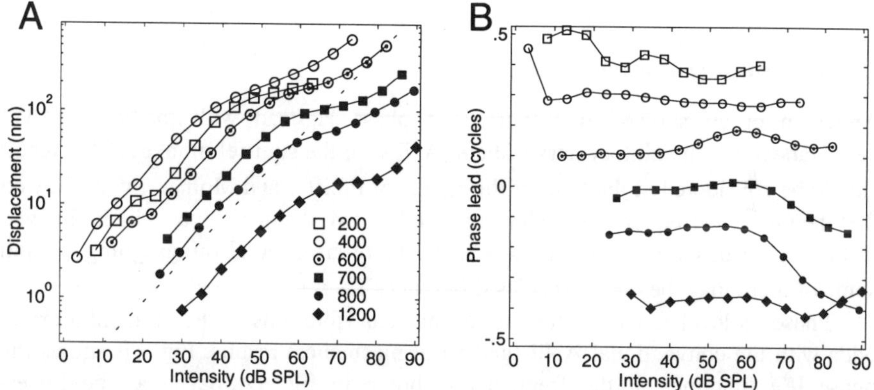

Figure 1: A. A partial set of the I/O functions obtained for CH38 with a linear guide line (dotted line). B. The corresponding phase data. Each curve has been arbitrarily shifted (vertically) so that the data are arranged in frequency.

The I/O functions can be used to construct isointensity curves, as shown in fig. 2. The highest curve (thinnest line) corresponds to 20 dB SPL with additional curves at 6 dB intensity increments and increasing line weights. The higher level

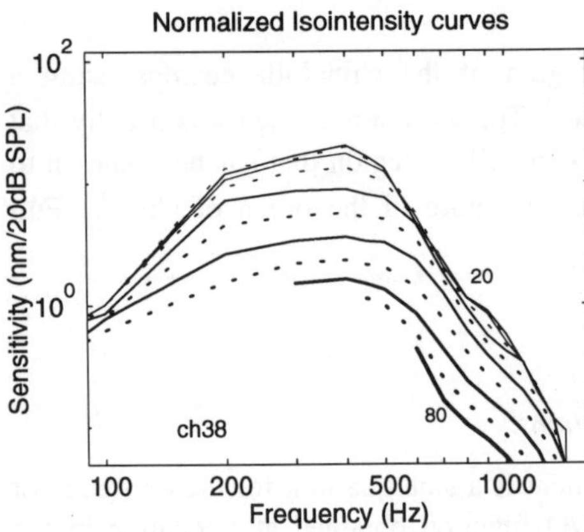

Figure 2. A set of normalized transfer ratios for the tectorial membrane (CH38). In this case the transfer ratios are all normalized to the lowest level shown which is at 20 dB SPL. The increment between the transfer curves is 6 dB. If the vibration was linear then all of the curves would have superimposed exactly. The thickest solid curve corresponds to 80 dB SPL. Solid and dotted lines are alternated for consecutive levels.

(>20 dB SPL) curves are all normalized to the 20 dB SPL level. If the displacements varied linearly all curves would overlie one another. In contrast to the basal region, the nonlinearity extends over a very wide (> 3 octaves) frequency region. The compression is restricted in level to between 35-85 dB SPL in this and other experiments.

3.2 Nonlinear I/0 phase functions.

Anderson et al[6] showed that there is a phase lag/lead with increasing level below/above CF in auditory nerve fibers (ANFs) of the squirrel monkey. This result should be considered in the light of the results of Pfeiffer and Molnar[7], who showed that the phase vs frequency transfer function had two distinct slopes which changed in the region of CF = 1kHz in cat. Clearly there are several things going on and some of them may be due to species differences[8].

Phase vs level functions for the mechanical vibrations in the chinchilla are at odds with the conventional ANF (and basal mechanics) results. Fig. 1B shows the phase I/O functions at the frequencies shown in fig. 1A. Even at the lowest frequency there is a phase change with level. Below CF there is initially a phase lag that increases with level. At CF there is relatively little overall phase change yet at low levels there is an increasing phase lead followed by a lag with increasing level. For frequencies > CF the initial phase change is a small lead followed by a lag at decreasing lower levels as frequency increases. Note the Λ-shaped function of level. There are rapid phase changes as large as 180° in the high frequency region that are not shown here and are associated with an amplitude notch.

3.3 Auditory nerve fiber responses.

In order to compare the mechanical transfer functions to the neural behavior, recordings were made from chinchilla ANFs. ANF behavior is complicated by a number of factors including the variable thresholds, spontaneous rates, and CF related parameter variability. The preparation we used was almost the same as for the mechanical studies so as to minimize differences. The only difference was that we did not open the apex of the cochlea as in the mechanical studies since we believed that this would result in a lower success rate for recording for extended periods.

The phase results are more complicated than can be completely described here. Nevertheless, this indicates that the widely held view of phase vs level has to be modified. We have many examples of different phase vs level behavior and/or changes with level that invert the direction of change with increasing frequency.

Examples of the phase behavior for two units are shown in figure 3. The phase I/O functions have been shifted an arbitrary amount to order them from low to high frequencies in the vertical direction. This highlights the pattern of phase vs level change vs frequency (e.g., fig. 3A). The pattern shown in fig. 3B is quite similar to that found for the TM mechanics (fig. 1B), in particular, it shows a Λ-shaped pattern near CF and an increasing lag for f > CF.

There is a transition around 1kHz in the phase vs level functions. Most fibers with CF > 1 kHz show a lag with increasing level both below and above CF. Some

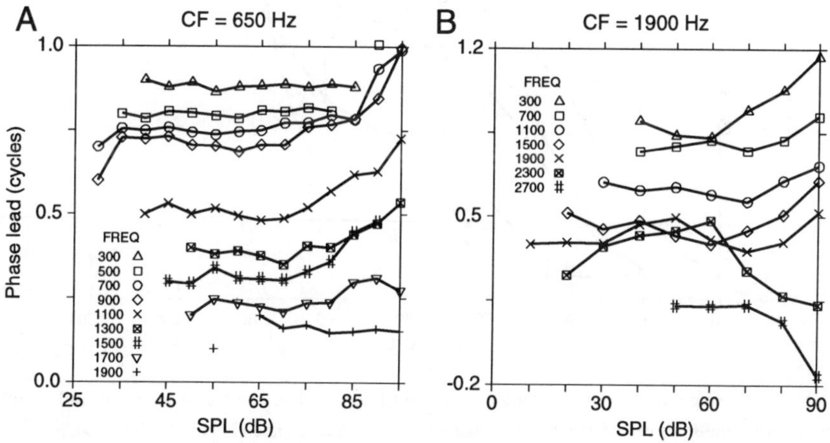

Figure 3. A. A set of I/O phase curves for an auditory nerve fiber with a CF of 650 Hz. B. A set of I/O phase curves for an auditory nerve fiber with a CF of 1900 Hz. Units were recorded from a preparation that was similar to the one used for the mechanics- a wide open middle ear.

units have only a relatively small phase change at CF. However, many I/O phase functions have a V- shaped function (f < CF) and Λ-shaped function above CF as seen in fig. 3B. Occasionally large (~180°) phase changes are observed.

3.4 ANF rate-level functions.

Yates[9] introduced a technique that recovers the basilar membrane displacement I/O functions from ANF rate-level functions. It relies on the fact that the I/O curves in the tail portion of high-CF fibers occur in the linear portion of the mechanical response. Since there are no tails for low-CF ANFs this technique cannot be applied here. However, the general idea allows one to speculate that the region of the rate level functions that have the same slopes at low levels is a linear region. According to the ANF data collected here, the nonlinear region is between 50 and 85dB SPL. The start of this region is indicated by the left most arrows in fig. 4. The right most arrows correspond to a second inflection that we hypothesize as the transition to a high level linear response.   This 50 -80dB SPL nonlinear region agrees with the typical compressive region for TM mechanics.

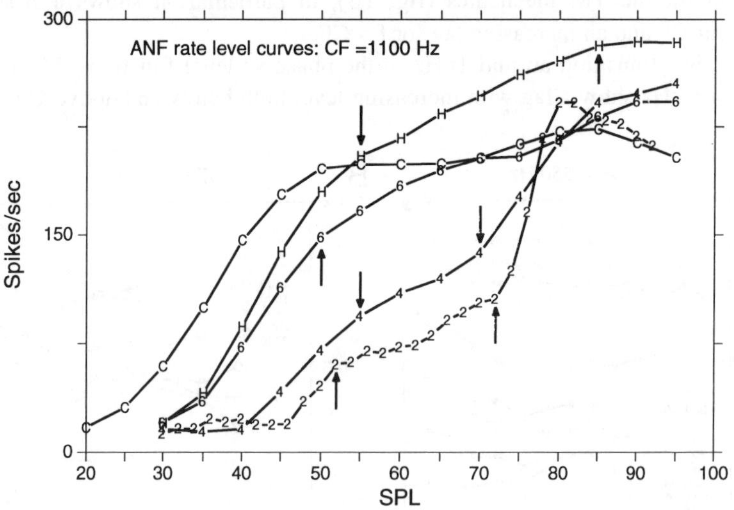

Figure 4. ANF rate level curves for a unit with a BF of 1100Hz. The number symbols indicate the frequency in multiples of 100 Hz. C is the characteristic frequency and H is for 1400 Hz (>CF). The arrows indicate the region hypothesized to be compressive of compression.

3.5 Mechanical tuning curves vs frequency tuning curves (MTCs vs FTCs)

One can derive mechanical isodisplacement curves at a small displacement that are the analog of ANF FTCs. The MTCs for two experiments (solid lines) are shown in fig. 5 along with three FTCs (dashed lines) for ANFs taken with the bulla open as in the mechanical measurements. The FTCs were obtained from response areas obtained with 10dB increments in stimulus level. The FTCs show the same slopes as the MTCs, both above and below CF. The FTCs also have approximately the same bandwidth and minima as the 1nm MTCs. The tips of the FTCs could be as much as 10 dB lower than shown due to the data collection limitations (10dB level increments) and as such maybe closer to the MTCs than shown.

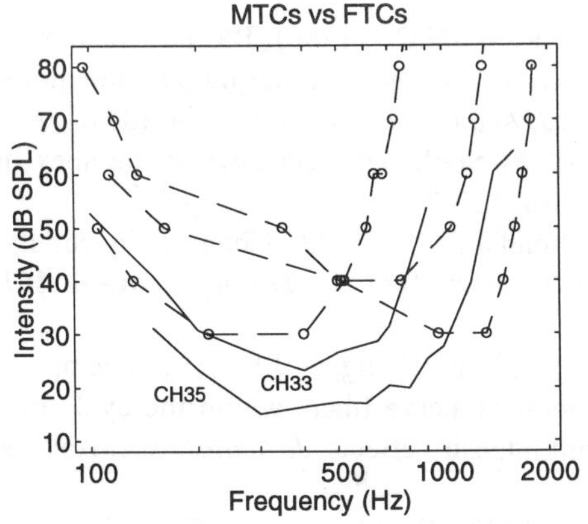

Figure 5. A comparison of the threshold curves for both the mechanics (MTCs at 1nm) and ANF FTCs. The ANFs have several CFs and each was constructed from a 15% isorate curve obtained from response area data. The data were collected with 10dB level increments so that in the threshold could be off as much as 10dB.

4. Discussion

There are both similarities and differences in the mechanics between the basal and apical regions of the cochlea. The nonlinear mechanics of the basal region are no longer in doubt and are quite well understood; the main role of the CA in this region is to provide a large gain in the region of CF. The tip portion of the FTC results from the gain. In the apex there is no tip to the FTCs and there is a gain of as much as 40 dB provided by the middle ear over that in the high frequency region.

Based on both mechanical and ANF studies, it appears that compression operates between 35-85 dB SPL over the entire frequency range in the apical region of the chinchilla cochlea. Other aspects of this study have shown both two-tone suppression[10] and a dc displacement that correlates with the presence of compression. The dc was less than the ac response, with typical values in the 15-30nm range toward scala vestibuli[11], and saturated with increasing levels.

Acknowledgments

Supported by research grant number 5 R01 DC 01910 from the National Institute on Deafness and Other Communication Disorders, National Institutes of Health.

References

1. Rhode, W.S. (1971) Observations of the vibrations of the basilar membrane in squirrel monkey using the Mössbauer effect. *J. Acoust. Soc. Am.* **49**, 1218-1231.

2. Sellick, P.M., Patuzzi, R. and Johnstone, B.M. (1982) measurements of basilar membrane motion in the guinea-pig using the Mössbauer effect. *J. Acoust. Soc. Am.* **72**, 131-141.

3. Robles, L., Ruggero, M.A. and Rich, N.C. (1986) Basilar membrane mechanics at the base of the chinchilla cochlea. I. Input-output fuinctions, tuning curves and response phases. *J. Acoust. Soc. Am.* **80**, 1364-1374.

4. Cooper, N.P. and Rhode, W.S. (1995) Nonlinear mechanics at the apex of the guinea-pig cochlea. *Hear. Res.* **82**, 225–243.

5. Khanna, S.M., Flock, A. and Ulfendahl, M. (1989) Changes in cellular tuning along the radial axis of the cochlea. *Acta Oto-Laryngol.* **suppl. 467**, 163–173.

6. Anderson, D.J., Rose, J.E., Hind, J.E. and Brugge, J.F. (1971) temporal position of discharges in single auditory nerve fibers within the cycle of a sine-wave stimulus: Frequency and intensity effects. *J. Acoust. Soc. Am.* **49**, 1131-1139.

7. Pfeiffer, R.R. and Molnar, C.E. (1970) Cochlear nerve fiber discharge patterns: relationship to the cochlear microphonic. *Science*, **167**, 1614-1616.

8. Dallos, P. (1970) Low-frequency auditory characteristics: Species dependence. *J. Acoust. Soc. Am.* **48**, 489-499.

9. Yates, G.K. (1990) Basilar membrane nonlinearity and its influence on auditory nerve rate-intensity functions. *Hear. Res.* **50**, 145-162.

10. Cooper, N.P. and Rhode, W.S. (1996) Two-tone suppression and two-tone distortion in apical and basal cochlear mechanics. ARO, abstr. #220, p55.

11. Rhode, W.S. and Cooper, N.P. (1996) Nonlinear mechanics in the apical turn of the chinchilla cochlea *in vivo*. Auditory Neurosci.

WIENER-KERNEL ANALYSIS OF BASILAR-MEMBRANE RESPONSES TO WHITE NOISE

A. RECIO, S.S. NARAYAN AND M.A. RUGGERO[+]

The Hugh Knowles Center and [+] Institute for Neuroscience
Northwestern University, Evanston, IL 60208, USA
e-mail: ars@merle.acns.nwu.edu

Basilar-membrane responses to white noise were recorded at the base of the chinchilla cochlea. The noise stimulus and the basilar-membrane responses were cross-correlated to obtain the first- and second-order Wiener kernels. The first-order kernel consists of a relatively undamped oscillation whose period decreases exponentially (time constant = 0.2 ms) until it reaches the inverse of the characteristic frequency (CF). Whereas most kernel oscillations become smaller with increasing stimulus intensity, the initial oscillation remains constant. The second-order Wiener kernel is very small, perhaps entirely artifactual. The first-order kernel suffices to predict fairly accurately the responses to the noise stimulus.

1 Introduction

At the base of the mammalian cochlea, basilar-membrane responses to sound are nonlinear. This nonlinear behavior has been demonstrated using responses to single tones and clicks. Although linear systems are completely described by transfer functions derived from either stimulus (i.e., the responses to arbitrary stimuli can be accurately predicted from the transfer function), this is not the case for nonlinear systems. To study such systems, Norbert Wiener proposed a description consisting of a sum of nonlinear functionals derived from responses to white noise. Lee and Schetzen[1] fleshed out Wiener's proposal by developing the cross-correlation method of kernel estimation.

The first-order Wiener kernel (which is the impulse response when the system is linear) contains the linear part of the system and may contain contributions from odd-order nonlinearities. The second-order Wiener kernel provides information on quadratic and higher-order even nonlinearities. [The impulse response contains information about all nonlinearities.] First-order kernels, introduced to auditory physiology by de Boer[2], have been used to study basilar-membrane vibrations[3-4] and low-CF neurons in the auditory nerve and cochlear nucleus[5-8]. Second-order kernels have been estimated in a few studies of the auditory nerve and cochlear nucleus[6,8-9] and have been useful in obtaining timing information (i.e., group delays at CF) for neurons that do not phase lock to CF stimuli. In the present investigation we extend our previous work on Wiener-kernel analysis in the auditory nerve[9] to basilar-membrane responses in the chinchilla[4].

326

2   Methods

Basilar-membrane vibrations were recorded, using a laser velocimeter, at a site of the chinchilla cochlea located 3.5 mm from the oval window. Laser light was reflected from glass microbeads placed on the basilar membrane. Acoustic stimuli were delivered via a Beyer DT-48 earphone. Stimuli were usually bursts (100 ms on, 300 ms off) of analog Gaussian white noise (General Radio 1381, 15 or 20 kHz bandwidth) presented 512 to 4096 times. The noise level ranged from 5 to 65 dB/√Hz (SPL, re 20 μPa). In a few instances, noise stimuli (< 30 dB/√Hz) were presented continuously for a maximum of 5 min. Wiener kernels were estimated by cross-correlating the basilar-membrane response with the noise stimulus.

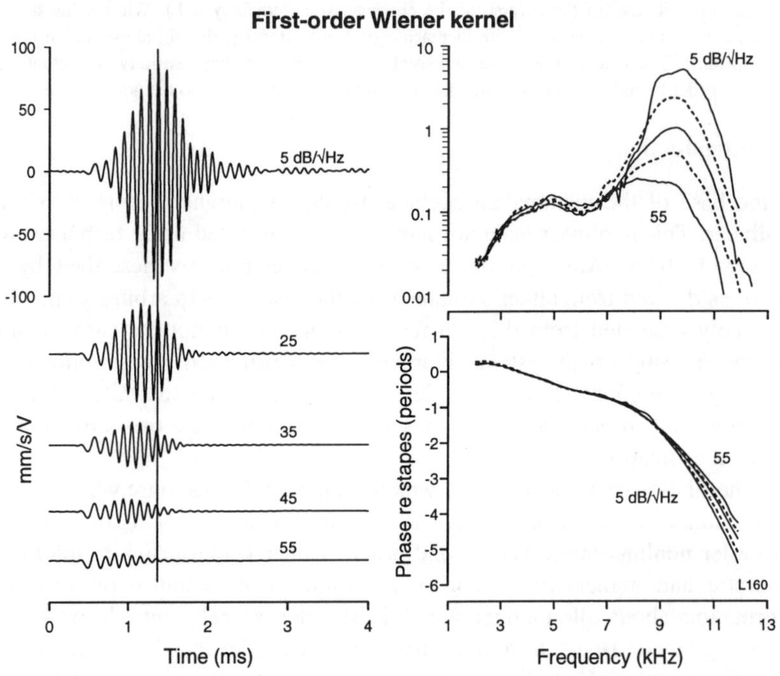

Figure 1: First-order Wiener kernels (left column) obtained for different noise levels and their magnitude and phase spectra (right column). Zero time corresponds to the onset of the electrical noise stimulus.

3   Results

The first-order Wiener kernels (Figure 1, left column), consist of relatively undamped oscillations with period predominantly matching 1/CF (CF measured from responses to tone pips). If the cochlea were a linear system, the kernels obtained at different noise intensities would be identical. In fact, as the noise intensity increases, only the initial period of the oscillation remains constant, whereas later oscillations of the kernels diminish in size and the center of gravity of the responses moves to earlier times (vertical line).

The right column in Figure 1 shows the magnitude and phase spectra of the first-order kernels. Response magnitudes at frequencies near CF (around 9 kHz) decrease with increasing noise intensity but remain constant for frequencies below 7 kHz. Similarly, response phases vary with stimulus intensity at frequencies near CF but do not change below 7 kHz. The phase-vs.-frequency curves have their largest group delays near CF. The phases of high-intensity kernels lead low-intensity ones at frequencies above CF and, to a lesser extent, lag low-intensity ones at frequencies immediately below CF.

3.1 Envelope-Frequency Representation of First-Order Wiener Kernels

The first-order Wiener kernels exhibit frequency modulation: the period of the individual oscillations decreases systematically with time (Figures 1–2). We used the analytic signal representation of the first-order kernel to describe separately its envelope and instantaneous frequency. The magnitude of the analytic signal is the envelope of the waveform and the derivative of its phase approximates the instantaneous frequency (lower left panel in Figure 2). As the intensity increases, the center of gravity of the envelope shifts to lower times (upper right panel in Figure 2). The instantaneous frequency grows exponentially until it reaches a plateau near CF (with a time constant of approximately 0.2 ms). In contrast to the envelope, the instantaneous frequency varies little with stimulus intensity (lower right panel in Figure 2).

3.2 Absence of Minimum-Phase Behavior in Basilar-Membrane Responses

In minimum-phase systems, the amplitude and phase spectra are entirely interdependent and their group delays are smaller (at all frequencies) than those of any other system with the same amplitude spectrum. At the auditory periphery of the chinchilla, middle-ear responses have the minimum-phase property[10]. To determine whether basilar-membrane responses also possess this property, "minimum" phases were computed from the magnitude spectrum of first-order Wiener kernels (modified with arbitrary high-frequency slopes) according to Bode theory[11]. The computed minimum phases, together with the measured amplitude spectrum, were used to synthesize minimum-phase approximations to the first-order kernels.

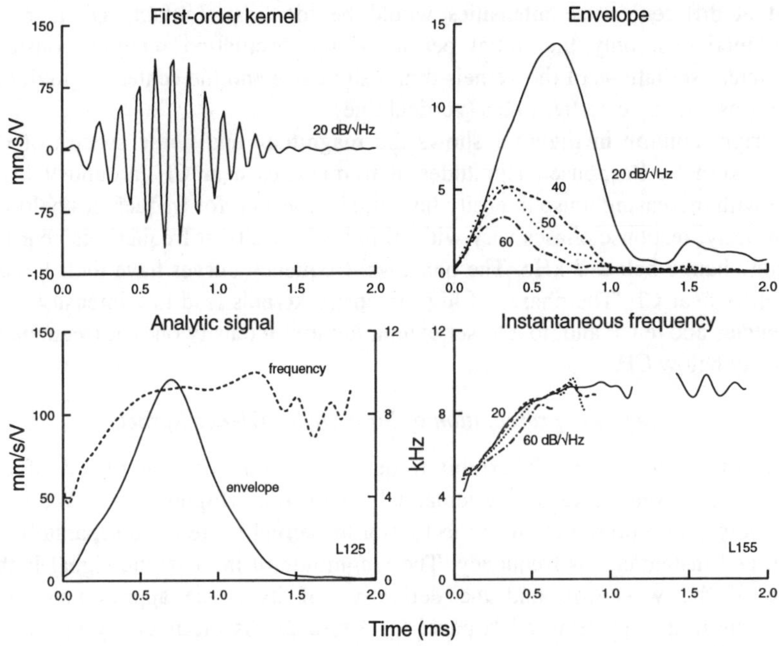

Figure 2: Analysis of first-order kernels into envelope and frequency components. Zero time corresponds to the onset of stapes movement. The right-column responses were measured in a single cochlea (parameter indicates stimulus intensity). Instantaneous-frequency curves are truncated as the envelopes dip below 1 mm/s/V.

Synthetic minimum-phase kernels (not shown) lack the frequency modulation seen in measured kernels, have envelopes that differ from those of the measured kernels and display additional onset "delays." Minimum-phase responses – including those based on spectra terminated with very steep high-frequency slopes (e.g., −180 dB/octave) – have group delays that are smaller near CF than those of the measured kernels. Increasing the terminal slope lengthens these delays but does not improve the match between the measured and synthetic kernels. This result indicates that first-order kernels cannot be modeled as minimum-phase filters and disagrees with literature[12-13] that has likened basilar-membrane responses to minimum-phase systems.

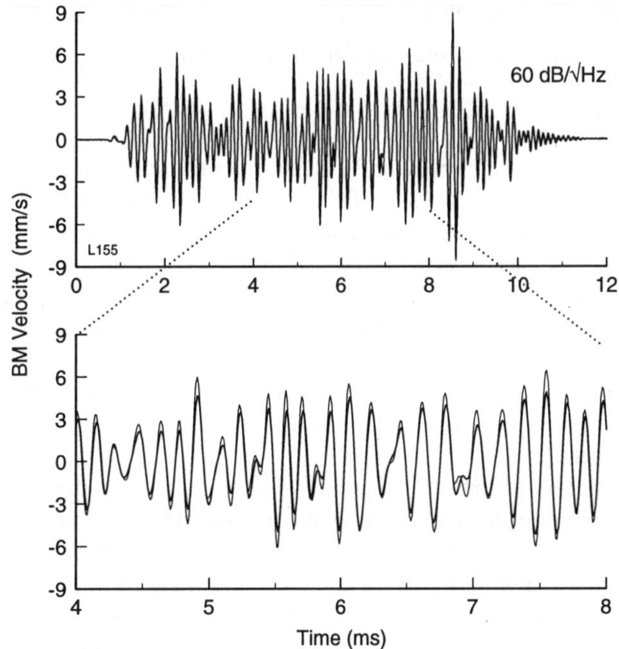

Figure 3: Average basilar-membrane response to multiple presentations of frozen noise (thick line) and prediction based on the first-order kernel (thin line). The duration of the stimulus was 10 ms, presented every 50 ms.

3.3 Predictions Using First-Order Wiener Kernels

To evaluate the predictive power of the first-order kernel, the noise stimulus was filtered in the frequency domain using the corresponding kernel (i.e., measured with the same stimulus intensity) and the filtered signal was compared to the average basilar-membrane response. At 60 dB SPL, the first-order kernel accounted for 90% of the variance of the basilar-membrane response (Figure 3). At lower intensities, 40 and 50 dB SPL, the first-order kernel accounted for 90% and 76% of the variance, respectively.

3.4 Second-Order Wiener Kernels

Second-order kernels (not shown) were small, probably approaching the linearity limits of the laser velocimeter. Their spectra did not exhibit DC or second-order harmonic components but did contain components around $|f_1+f_2| = CF$. These may be artifacts inherent in the cross-correlation in two-dimensions.

4 Discussion

The first-order Wiener kernels of basilar-membrane responses to noise strongly resemble responses to clicks[14]. This resemblance indicates that even-order nonlinearities are absent or very small at the chinchilla basilar membrane (in contrast with their prominence in the auditory nerve[9]). Accordingly, the second-order Wiener kernels are small and the first-order Wiener kernels predict reasonably well the responses to noise (Figure 3). The absence of even-order nonlinearity and the nonlinear growth of the first-order kernels with stimulus intensity jointly imply the existence of a significant odd-order nonlinearity. Such a nonlinearity may be contained in the first-order kernel but may also be demonstrable in third- and higher-order odd kernels.

The onset delay of first-order kernels (Figure 2) and responses to intense clicks (not shown) is no longer than 25–30 μs relative to stapes motion (i.e., even shorter than our previous estimate of 90 μs[14]). This delay at the 3.5–mm site of the chinchilla basilar membrane is substantially shorter than the 300–390 μs measured at the 6–7.8 kHz site of the squirrel monkey cochlea[15], presumably located some 8.3–9.5 mm from the oval window (according to Greenwood's map[16]). The relatively large difference between the delay estimates for chinchilla and squirrel monkey may indicate that the traveling wave slows down considerably in the range between 3.5 and 8.3–9.5 mm or it may reflect a genuine species difference. Alternatively, the short onset delay measured in the chinchilla may result from an artifact[17] that mimics an early and linear basilar-membrane oscillation.

Acknowledgment

Work supported by NIH grants P01-DC-00110-21 and R01-DC-00419-9.

References

1. Lee, Y.W. and Schetzen, M. (1965) Measurement of the Wiener kernels of a nonlinear system by cross-correlation, *Inter. J. Control* **2** 237–254.
2. de Boer, E. (1967) Correlation studies applied to the frequency resolution of the cochlea, *J. Aud. Res.* **7** 209–217.
3. de Boer, E. and Nuttall, A.L. (1995) Frequency modulation in impulse responses and cross-correlation functions of basilar membrane motion in the guinea pig, *ARO Mid-Winter Meeting Abstracts* **18** 187.

4. Recio, A., Narayan, S.S. and Ruggero, M.A. (1996) Wiener-kernel analysis of basilar membrane responses to white noise, *ARO Mid-Winter Meeting Abstracts* **19** 55.

5. Møller, A.R. (1977) Frequency selectivity of single auditory-nerve fibers in response to broadband noise stimuli, *J. Acoust. Soc. Am.* **62** 135–142.

6. Wickesberg, R.E. (1982) Wiener kernel analysis of the response of neurons in the anteroventral cochlear nucleus of the cat, Ph.D. Dissertation, University of Wisconsin.

7. Carney, L.H. and Yin, T.C.T. (1988) Temporal encoding of resonances by low-frequency auditory nerve fibers: single-fiber responses and a population model, *J. Neurophysiol.* **60** 1653–1677.

8. van Dijk, P., Wit, H.P., Segenhout, J.M. and Tubis, A. (1994) Wiener kernel analysis of inner ear function in the American bullfrog, *J. Acoust. Soc. Am.* **95** 904–919.

9. Temchin, A., Recio, A., van Dijk, P. and Ruggero, M.A. (1995) Wiener-kernel analysis of chinchilla auditory-nerve responses to noise, *ARO Mid-Winter Meeting Abstracts* **18** 174.

10. Ruggero, M.A., Rich, N.C., Robles, L. and Shivapuja, B.G. (1990) Middle-ear response in the chinchilla and its relationship to mechanics at the base of the cochlea, *J. Acoust. Soc. Am.* **87** 1612–1629.

11. Thomas, D.E. (1947) Tables of phases associated with a semi-infinite unit slope of attenuation, *Bell Syst. Tech. J.* **26** 870–899.

12. Zweig, G. (1976) Basilar membrane motion, in *Cold Spring Harbor Symposium on Quantitative Biology* (Cold Spring Harbor Laboratory of Quantitative Biology, Cold Spring Harbor), 619–633.

13. Koshigoe, S. and Tubis, A. (1982) Implications of causality, time-translation invariance, linearity, and minimum-phase behavior for basilar-membrane response functions, *J. Acoust. Soc. Am.* **71** 1194–1200.

14. Ruggero, M.A., Rich, N.C. and Recio, A. (1992) Basilar membrane responses to clicks, in *Auditory Physiology and Perception* (Y. Cazals, L. Demany and K. Horner, eds.), Pergamon Press, London, 85–91.

15. Robles, L., Rhode, W.S. and Geisler, C.D. (1976) Transient response of the basilar membrane measured in squirrel monkey using the Mössbauer effect, *J. Acoust. Soc. Am.* **59** 926–939.

16. Greenwood, D.D. (1990) A cochlear frequency-position function for several species – 29 years later, *J. Acoust. Soc. Am.* **87** 2592–2605.

17. Cooper, N.P. and Rhode, W.S. (1996) Fast travelling waves, slow travelling waves and their interactions in experimental studies of apical cochlear mechanics, *Auditory Neuroscience* (in press).

COCHLEAR MECHANICAL NONLINEARITY REFLECTED ON BM VELOCITY I-O FUNCTION SLOPE AND ITS BEHAVIOR AT HIGH SOUND LEVELS

M. ZHANG, D.F. DOLAN, A.L. NUTTALL

Kresge Hearing Research Institute,
The University of Michigan, Ann Arbor, MI 48109-0506

It has been widely reported that cochlear nonlinearity only manifests itself at middle stimulus intensity range. At low (< 40-50 dB SPL) and high (> 80 dB SPL) levels, the basilar membrane (BM) input-output (I-O) functions assume a linear slope. In contrast to this three segment theory, our study found that a normal BM I-O function has a nonlinear shape throughout the entire physiological intensity range. Also we found the possibility that the cochlear amplifier reverses its role from enhancing to suppressing the gross response as stimulus intensity grows beyond a certain level.

The measurements of cochlear BM velocity were made from the guinea pig first cochlear turn (CF 18 kHz) by using a laser Doppler vibrometer (Polytec Corp., OFV 1102) with its laser beam focused on a glass bead placed on the BM. With the help of a lock-in amplifier, we were able to measure the BM responses from -5 dB SPL to 115 dB SPL and found that a normal BM I-O function has a nonlinear shape in entire physiological range (from 5 dB SPL and above). When linearity in BM I-O functions at low intensities is observed, we demonstrate that this results from suppression of cochlear nonlinearity, which probably originates from damage to the cochlear amplifier.

By using loud sound to suppress the nonlinear cochlear mechanics while keeping the linear mechanics intact, we were able to separate the linear BM I-O function from the gross response. We found that in some of our tested animals, that the gross BM I-O function showed a crossing with the linear BM I-O function at very high intensities (generally > 105 dB SPL). Since the cochlear amplifier is probably responsible for the frequency selective nonlinearity in the cochlea, one interpretation for this crossing of I-O function is that the cochlear amplifier reverse its role from enhancing to suppressing the gross cochlear response when intensity grows to a certain level, in the manner of an autoamtic gain control system.

Acknowledgement

This work was supported by NIH NIDCD DC00141.

A NEW APPROACH TO COCHLEAR MECHANICS AND CUBIC DISTORTION TONES BY INTRACOCHLEAR ACOUSTIC PRESSURE MEASUREMENTS IN THE GUINEA PIG.

P. MAGNAN, P. AVAN[*], A. DANCER, R. PROBST[+], J.SMURZYNSKI[+]

French-German Institute of Saint-Louis, PO Box 34
68301 Saint-Louis, France
**Biophysics Laboratory, University of Auvergne, 63001 Clermont-Ferrand, France*
+HNO Klinik, Kantonsspital, 4031 Basel, Switzerland
e-mail : Paul.Avan@u-clermont1.fr

Direct intracochlear measurements of acoustic pressure were carried out in scala vestibuli and tympani of the first and second turn of a guinea pig inner ear with pairs of pure tones as stimuli. The amplitude and phase characteristics of the resulting cubic distortion tone (CDT) were determined both in the cochlea and the external auditory meatus. Comparisons of the amplitude and phase of CDT in the first and second turn allowed to gain information about the way CDT are propagated in the cochlea. Forward and backward travel times appeared to be very short.

1 Context of this research

The fine tuning of a normal cochlea is thought to result from subtle processes combining "passive" hydrodynamics i.e propagation of a pressure wave along the cochlear partition[1] and so-called "active" mechanisms likely involving bidirectional transduction at the level of the motile outer hair cells of the organ of Corti. Two phenomena are typical of a normally tuned cochlea: firstly, basilar membrane movements exhibit a highly nonlinear growth function with the level of a pure-tone stimulus when the location under measurement is tuned to its frequency.[2] Secondly, cochlear responses to pairs of pure tones with neighboring frequencies (f_1 and f_2, with $f_2 > f_1$) contain combination tones that can be recorded in the external ear canal as otoacoustic emissions after backward propagation through the middle ear[3]. The most prominent one in many mammals is called cubic distortion tone (CDT) at frequency $2f_1 - f_2$. Published data[4,5] suggest that CDTs are generated around the place tuned to f_2 where maximum nonlinear interaction exists between the two primary tones; then they should be propagated both in the forward direction, like regular sounds, to the place tuned to $2f_1 - f_2$ where neural responses can be detected, and in the backward direction, through the middle ear. Along these propagation pathways, CDTs are supposed to undergo (i) an amplitude change while traveling through the cochlear amplifier hypothesized by Davis[6] to account for cochlear sensitivity, and (ii) a phase shift depending on travel time.

However, the previous contentions remain largely speculative to-date. A recent experiment[5] failed to reveal any amplitude change of CDT during their cochlear travel that might be attributed to amplification. An alternative interpretation of these results was proposed in the framework of a local cochlear amplifier.[7] Most available evaluations of CDT travel time come from group latency derivations in the external ear canal: when f_1 varies while f_2 and the alleged intracochlear generation site of CDT are kept fixed, the phases of external-ear CDTs exhibit conspicuously large variations suggestive of a long delay -exceeding several cycles- between primary tone interaction and CDT detection at the external auditory meatus. Although such a delay is often interpreted as reflecting the round-trip propagation delay of the classical traveling wave, a large part of it might arise from strictly local cellular filtering processes as well. In the last ten years, outer-hair cell mechanisms have proved to be of prominent importance for normal cochlear function, whereas passive cochlear hydrodynamics alone appeared more and more as relevant to a dead or overstimulated cochlea.

Whatever the interpretation, it is remarkable that most of the direct intracochlear measurements following the pionnier experiment of Rhode,[2] describe the velocity of the cochlear partition[8,9] while little is known about intracochlear pressure,[10,11] so that cochlear impedance cannot be approached except by theoretical models. The goal of the present work was to perform direct intracochlear measurements of acoustic pressure in scala vestibuli and tympani of the first and second turn of a guinea pig cochlea with a pair of pure tones as stimuli. The amplitudes and phases of resulting CDTs were obtained in the first and second turn and in the ear canal so that some characteristics of their intracochlear propagation could be derived.

2   Methods

10 pigmented female guinea pigs weighing from 250-350 g were used for this experiment. They were deeply anesthetized with urethane (1.6 g/kg) and fixed in a holder. The left bulla was widely opened ventrolaterally and an acoustic probe was sealed into the left external ear canal. It was a modified version of the Cubdis system (Allen, Bell Labs, 1990), with a tapered end so as to fit a guinea pig's ear canal. It contained two plastic tubings connected to two earphones (ER2, Etymotic) and a miniature low-noise microphone (ER10B). Pairs of pure-tone stimuli at frequencies f_1 and f_2 were generated by the two-channel Ariel DSP16 board of a PC computer that controlled the whole experiment, and separately sent to the earphones with adjustable sound levels. The microphone recorded the acoustic signal in front of the eardrum, consisting of primary tones together with combination tones produced by the cochlea, including the CDT at $2f_1$-f_2. This signal was preamplified (x100), digitized, time-averaged (1 to 4 s) and stored. The amplitudes and phases of primaries and CDTs were computed using FFT. The built-in calibration procedure of Cubdis was not considered to be valid owing to the modifications of the probe to fit a guinea pig's ear. Actual calibration was made in-

the-ear with the help of a B&K 4180 probe inserted close to the tympanic membrane and stored for further processing.

A CDT measurement session consisted in sweeping f_2 from 1-17 kHz (20 points per octave) while keeping f_2/f_1 equal to 1.35 so that CDT frequency was one octave below f_2. The target levels of primary tones were 60 dB SPL at f_1 and 50 dB SPL at f_2. These levels could not be obtained exactly at all the frequencies of a sweep because it was impossible to bypass the incorrect calibration procedure of Cubdis software, however the actual stimulus levels and phases at the eardrum were computed offline. CDTs were monitored at the very beginning of the experiment, then after every step of the surgical procedure which consisted in carefully drilling calibrated holes (0.15 mm diameter) through the bony wall of scala vestibuli of the first and second turn (SV1 and SV2), and in some animals, in scala tympani of first turn (ST1). The distances of these holes to the oval window were approximately 4 and 10 mm, corresponding to characteristic frequencies of 9-10 kHz and 2-3 kHz.

A calibrated pressure probe containing a miniature piezoresistive transducer (Kulite) was specially designed for this experiment. It was filled with silicon liquid to adapt the transducer impedance to that of cochlear liquids. The tube prolonging its conical hood fitted exactly the holes drilled into the cochlear scalae. During a CDT measurement session, the pressure probe was adapted to one of the holes in the cochlea so that intracochlear pressure was monitored in parallel with ear canal acoustic signal. In the meantime, the other cochlear holes were plugged using conical pieces of appropriate diameter. The output of the probe amplifier was digitized, time-averaged and Fourier-transformed to extract the characteristics of frequency components at f_2, f_1 and $2f_1$-f_2. So, simultaneous measurements of the amplitude and phase of intracochlear and external-ear-canal acoustic pressure were available for primary tones and CDT. Amplitudes and phases of CDT measured in SV1 and SV2, or SV1 and ST1, were compared for identical sound characteristics in the ear canal. Comparisons of intracochlear vs. ear-canal sounds are described in a companion paper[12]. All sound levels were expressed in dB re 20 µPa, referred to as dB SPL in the following.

3 Results

CDT amplitudes in the ear canal never changed by more than 2 dB compared to their initial values, at all frequencies throughout an experiment. The stability of intracochlear measurements was also ascertained by repeated pressure measurements whereas the probe was moved from a hole to another. All CDTs disappeared in less than 5 min after euthanasia at the end of the experiment.

The level of ear-canal CDT (fig.1) was about 20 dB SPL (± 5 dB) and intracochlear CDT levels were 30-32 dB larger in scala vestibuli whatever the frequency.[12] CDT pressure in ST1 (fig.1) was 15-20 dB smaller than in SV1 at all

336

frequencies below 5 kHz and this difference gradually decreased so that CDT pressures were identical in SV1 and ST1 above 8-9 kHz corresponding to the characteristic frequency of the 1st-turn hole place. It can be inferred that the differential pressure due to CDT and exerted at the level of basilar membrane was correctly represented by CDT pressure in SV1 at all frequencies below 8 kHz.

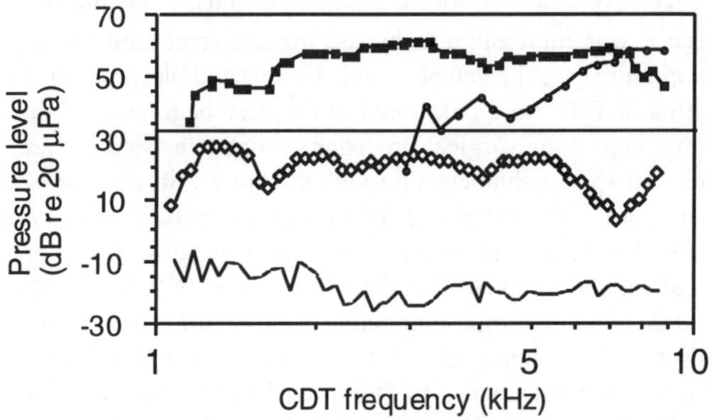

Figure 1: CDT level in SV1 (filled squares), ST1 (open squares) and ear canal (open diamonds). Noise background is given in the ear canal (solid line) and in the intracochlear pressure detection system (dashed line).

The amplitude and phase of CDT pressure in SV1 were plotted with reference to CDT pressure in SV2 at all frequencies between 1.5 and 9 kHz (fig.2). The amplitude curve was quite flat and showed almost no difference between SV1 and SV2 at frequencies below 4 kHz and above 8 kHz. CDT amplitude was larger in SV1 than SV2, by approximately 5 dB, between 5 and 7 kHz. For comparison, the level of primary tone pressure in SV1 systematically exceeded the corresponding level in SV2 by an average of 6 dB between 1.5 and 8 kHz.

The difference between CDT phases in SV1 and SV2 also exhibited a smooth variation from 1.5 to 8 kHz, with little variance. Three intervals could be separated, namely [1.5, 3] kHz, [3, 4] kHz and [4, 8] kHz for CDT frequencies. In the first one, CDT in SV1 presented a phase lag with respect to SV2, which was maximum for lower frequencies (mean 50°, SD 25°) then gradually decreased when CDT frequency got closer to 3 kHz. CDT phase was identical in SV1 and SV2 between 3 and 4 kHz then CDT phase in SV1 increasingly led the corresponding measurement in SV2, so that the phase lead reached 250° (SD 42°) at 8 kHz.

Data interpretation needs to be based upon a few assumptions, namely that CDT are generated close to the place tuned to f_2, and that they are propagated both apically to the place tuned to $2f_1-f_2$, and basally to the middle ear. Sweeping f_2 corresponds to moving the positions of CDT sources and of the place of maximum response to CDT, with respect to the fixed measurement points. It seems possible to separate three typical situations.

-For primary tones around 3 and 2.25 kHz with a CDT at 1.5 kHz, the generation site of CDT is supposed to be close to the hole drilled in SV2. CDT is also measured in SV1 after propagating backward over about 6 mm. Indeed a phase lag is measured and its amount provides an estimation of backward travel time from 2nd to 1st turn i.e. 0.09 ms on average.

-For primary tones around 6 and 4.5 kHz and CDT at 3 kHz, the generation site of CDT is right between the two holes in SV1 and SV2. Thus the phase of CDT measured at both holes is expected to lag that of CDT at its source. The difference between these two measured phases should be close to zero, as depicted on fig.2.

-When primary tone frequencies are about 10 and 7.5 kHz, the CDT at 5 kHz is generated close to the measurement point in SV1. The phase of the CDT measured in SV2 should exhibit a lag due to forward propagation to the place tuned to 5 kHz. Fig.2 shows that this phase lag is close to 50° at 5 kHz: this would correspond to a forward travel time of 0.03 ms.

Discussion

Repeatable measurements of intracochlear pressure were obtained in response to low-level calibrated sounds in the ear canal. CDTs were important to assess in such an experiment for two main reasons. Firstly, there is wide acceptance that CDTs reflect the integrity of the cellular processes which lead both to fine tuning and nonlinear basilar membrane motion. Clinical evidence indicates that there is a systematic correspondence between elevation of hearing threshold at frequency f_2 and decrease of CDT level at $2f_1-f_2$. The remarkable stability of ear-canal CDT throughout the experiments demonstrates that the surgical preparation and the repeated probe positioning manipulations were not detrimental to the so-called "active" cochlear processes. Secondly, in contrast to the primary tones used as stimuli, CDTs are generated on the basilar membrane therefore they provide the unique opportunity to analyze the mechanisms of intracochlear forward and backward propagation of sound, using an energy source that can be displaced along the basilar membrane.

The measured properties of intracochlear pressure at primary and CDT frequencies can be considered as relevant to the issue of basilar membrane stimulation provided a few conditions are met. Firstly, intracochlear pressure has to be independent of transducer depth in the scalae as assumed in long-wave models, and Nedzelnitsky[11] showed that this is valid at least in the cat's first turn. The second point is that differential pressure is the actual value of interest for basilar membrane stimulation. First turn measurements of CDT pressure in scala tympani suggest that pressure in SV1 provide a reasonably good estimation of differential pressure at low frequencies.

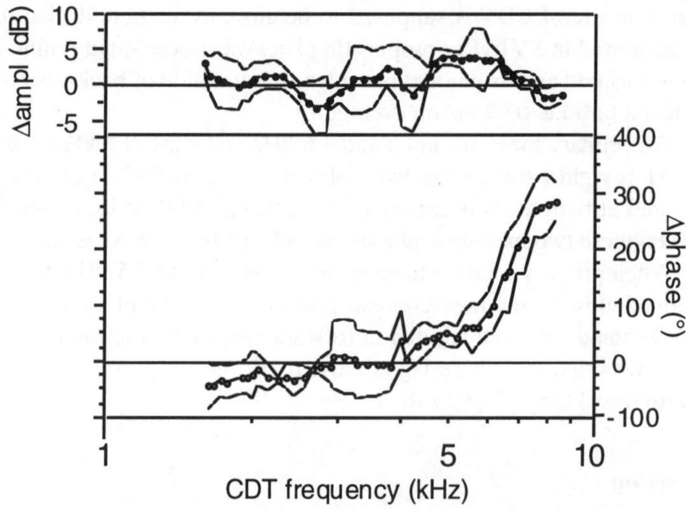

Figure 2: CDT amplitude and phase difference between measurements in SV1 and SV2 (mean, mean ± S.D.): the phase in SV1 exhibits a lag for lower CDT frequencies.

Intracochlear pressure measurements of CDTs as reported here do not allow to draw definitive conclusions about the generating mechanisms of distortion-product otoacoustic emissions: instead of the map of cochlear pressure, its values at only two fixed cochlear locations can be analyzed. Nevertheless, the observed results can be contrasted with a few theoretical models that predict explicitely the amplitudes and phases of CDT.[5,7,13] Allen and Fahey[5] developed a model of transmission line with negative resistance over some regions in order to account for the cochlear amplifier.[6] They argued that if the amplifier gain is larger than unity, CDT pressure wave should be amplified when it propagates over the negative resistance area, when its source and its detection place are on different sides of this area. Experimentally, they failed to measure any gain during such processes. Our data are consistent with their report. Although challenging [5], some locally active cochlear models[7] predict fairly flat CDT pressure patterns along the whole cochlea, for a large range of frequency ratios f_2/f_1, and are consistent with our present data as well. The computational model of Geisler et al,[13] applied to the same ratio f_2/f_1 as here, predicted that the phase of intracochlear CDT be minimum at the vicinity of the place tuned to f_2 and they interpreted this place as the site of energy generation for CDT. Phase varied rapidly during forward and backward propagation. From their fig.5 it can be inferred that the phase difference between CDT pressures at two fixed points in the first vs second turn should vary from lag to lead when CDT frequency increases and be close to zero for intermediate frequencies. However, the predicted phase lags and leads are an order of magnitude larger than those measured on fig.2. The small phase shifts reported here may even be consistent with models of independent resonators instead of traveling wave ones.[14]

In summary, the present results show that intracochlear pressure measurements can be performed without disturbing the fragile tuning mechanisms. No clear evidence of large pressure changes nor phase shifts as expected in a traveling-wave cochlear amplifier model has been obtained. Further measurements will be useful to clarify these fundamental and controversial aspects of cochlear micromechanics and hydrodynamics.

References

1. von Békésy, G. (1960) Experiments in hearing. McGraw Hill, New York .
2. Rhode, W.S. (1971) Observations of the basilar membrane in squirrel monkeys using the Mossbauer technique. *J.Acoust.Soc.Am.* 49, 1218-1231.
3. Kemp, D.T. (1979) Evidence of mechanical nonlinearity and frequency-selective wave amplification in the cochlea. *Arch. Otorhinolaryngol.* 224, 37-45.
4. Robles, L., Ruggero, M.A. and Rich, N.C. (1993) Two tone distortion in the basilar membrane of the cochlea. *Nature* 349, 413-414.
5. Allen, J.B. and Fahey, P.F. (1992) Using acoustic distortion products to measure the cochlear amplifier gain on the basilar membrane. *J.Acoust.Soc.Am.* 92, 178-188.
6. Davis, H. (1983) An active process in cochlear mechanics. *Hear.Res.* 9, 79-90.
7. Kanis, L.J. and de Boer, E. (1993) DP emissions in a locally-active nonlinear model of the cochlea. In: *Biophysics of hair cell sensory systems*, ed. D.Duifhuis . World Scientific Singapore. 304-311.
8. Khanna, S.M. and Leonard,D.G.B. (1982) Basilar membrane tuning in the cat cochlea. *Science* 215, 305-306.
9. Sellick, P.M., Patuzzi ,R. and Johnstone, B.M (1982) Measurement of basilar membrane motion in the guinea pig using the Mossbauer technique. *J.Acoust.Soc.Am.* 72, 131-141.
10. Dancer, A and Franke, R. (1980) Intracochlear sound pressure measurements in guinea pigs. *Hear.Res.* 2, 191-205.
11. Nedzelnitsky, V. (1980) Sound pressures in the basal turn of the cat cochlea. *J.Acoust.Soc.Am.* 68, 1676-1689.
12. Magnan, P., Probst, R., Smurzynski, J., Avan, P. and Dancer , A. (1997) Direct measurement of the inverse transfer function of the guinea pig middle ear. In: Diversity in Auditory Mechanics. World Scientific Singapore,
13. Geisler, C.D., Bendre, A. and Liotopoulos, F.K. (1993) Time-domain modeling of a nonlinear, active model of the cochlea. In: *Biophysics of hair cell sensory systems*, ed. D.Duifhuis (World Scientific Singapore. 330-337.
14. Dancer, A. (1992) An experimental look at cochlear mechanics. *Audiology* 31, 301-312.

CAN THE TRAVELLING WAVE BE CHALLENGED BY DIRECT INTRACOCHLEAR PRESSURE MEASUREMENTS?

A. DANCER

French-German Research Institute of Saint-Louis
68301 Saint-Louis, France
dancer@nucleus.fr

P. AVAN

Laboratoire de Biophysique, Université d'Auvergne
63001 Clermont Ferrand, France
paul.avan@u-clermont1.fr

P. MAGNAN

HNO-Universitätsklinik, Kantonsspital
4031 Basel, Switzerland
magnan@ubaclu.unibas.ch

The intracochlear acoustic pressure was measured from 20 Hz to 20,000 Hz in the 4 turns of scala vestibuli and in the 3 first turns of scala tympani of the guinea pig cochlea. These measurements allowed (i) to re-evaluate the travel time in the cochlea from differential cochlear microphonic data, and (ii) to calculate the differential pressure acting on the cochlear partition in the 3 first turns. At high stimulation levels and for frequencies close to the characteristic frequency of each recording site the phase lag of the cochlear partition displacements is around half-a-cycle (reference: acoustic pressure at the base of scala vestibuli). Therefore, it is concluded that the whole cochlear partition is excited almost simultaneously from base to apex. Consequently, the large phase lags which are observed for frequencies close to the characteristic frequency at low stimulation levels in the active cochlea could arise entirely from active cellular processes which are coupled to cochlear mechanics.

1 Introduction

The displacements of the stapedius footplate inside the oval window produce volume displacements of the perilymph and variations of the acoustic pressure at the base of the scala vestibuli. This signal induces mechanical events in the cochlear fluids and the sensory structures of the organ of Corti.

In 1863, Helmholtz assumed that the transverse fibers of the basilar membrane act as small resonators and that this "bank of resonators" is excited simultaneously. However, it was difficult to imagine isolated resonators inside the cochlea. Their small damping, necessary to provide the frequency selectivity, would not allow the perception of rapid variations of pitch and loudness.

According to later theories, the displacements of the stapes produce a travelling wave (TW) on the basilar membrane (BM) (Wever and Lawrence[1], Bekesy[2]). Bekesy was the first to observe the displacements of the cochlear structures in models[3] and in anatomical specimens[4] at very high levels. Bekesy considered that the TW, sharpened up by lateral inhibition (which constitutes its essential complement), solved the problem of the cochlear frequency selectivity and the speed of the analysis without the need of sharply tuned resonators.

The TW theory was formalized by Zwislocki[5,6]. According to Zwislocki, the one-dimensional long wave model corresponds to a TW which transports the energy along the cochlea and presents a phase lag which can reach a few cycles at the location corresponding to the maximum displacement for a given frequency. Like in a delay line, for each location along the cochlear partition the beginning of the displacement of the cochlear structures (i.e., following an impulse to the stapes) occurs after a given delay which increases exponentially with the distance to the base. This theory was questioned by Wever and Lawrence[1] who stated that "...the basilar membrane responds to this pressure by movements that are practically in phase over the most active region of the membrane". Bekesy admitted some doubts too by publishing with the two preceeding authors[7] a paper in which it is stated that the term "travelling wave" could in fact correspond only to a temporal succession of events not explicitly implying the transfer of the energy by the wave itself.

In fact, the basic TW theory did not explain the cochlear frequency selectivity because the hypothesis of lateral inhibition proposed by Bekesy was invalidated by the recording of the tuning curves of unit nerve fibers[8] and later on by the recording of the tuning curves of the BM itself on cochleas in very good physiological condition[9].

More sophisticated cochlear models were proposed to overcome these difficulties[10]. Significant advance was achievied by taking into account the interactions (resonance coupling) between the stereocilia and the TM[11-13]. Thereby, the shape of the responses approaches the characteristics of the mechanical or neural tuning curves measured on living cochleas.

Nevertheless, descriptions of the cochlear active phenomena (first hypothesized by Gold[14]) demonstrated that two different types of mechanisms coexist inside the cochlea: the ones, passive, correspond to the cochlear hydromechanical phenomena (and the micromechanics of the organ of Corti), the others, active and highly dependent on the condition of the outer hair cells[15], are responsible for the sensitivity and the frequency selectivity of the cochlea.

Nowadays, the one-dimensional long wave model with its accumulating phase lag and its long propagation delay is no more indispensable to explain the cochlear responses at low levels. Lewis et al.[10] stated : "...there is no obvious reason to discard the suggestion that the phase behavior of the mammalian cochlea, which is prime evidence for the travelling wave model being approximately correct, arises entirely from cellular processes which are coupled to cochlear mechanics". Nevertheless, the former interpretation of the TW is used as a leitmotiv to interpret a lot of physiological phenomena which are actually closely related to the active mechanisms: latency of the unit responses, of the compound action potentials (CAP), of the acoustic otoemissions... .

With the help of intracochlear acoustic pressure measurements[17,18], we shall try

342

to answer simple questions: how are the cochlear structures excited by the acoustic stimuli, are they excited all at once (like in the Helmholtz's theory) or is there a finite delay due to a TW, how large is this delay ?

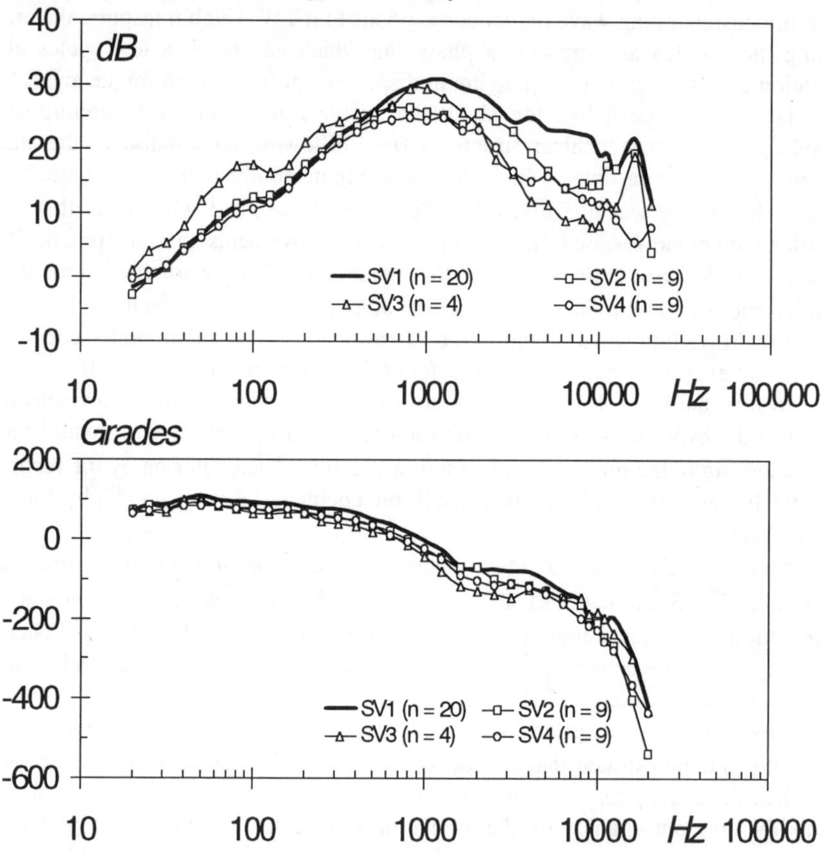

Figure 1: Amplitude and phase of the acoustic pressure in the four turns of scala vestibuli (ref: acoustic pressure in front of the tympanum, bulla open)[18]

2 Travel time

It is possible to evaluate the travel time from the cochlear microphonic potential (CM). When it is recorded by means of differential electrodes in the linear range of its input-output function and at frequencies lower than the characteristic frequency (CF) of the recording site, the CM amplitude is directly proportional to the amplitude of the displacements of the BM located between the electrodes[19]. As the velocity of the TW is independent of the wavelength in the one-dimensional long wave models, the travel time (T) can be computed from the relation: $T = \phi/2\pi f$. According to Dallos and Cheatham[19] T is slightly larger than two periods of CF of the recording site. Now, if we take as a reference the phase of the acoustic pressure at the base of scala vestibuli[18] instead of the phase of the signal in front of the eardrum at the low frequencies[19], we measure a delay of 0.025 ms in the first turn (4 mm from base, CF = 10 kHz), of 0.25 ms in the second turn (9-10 mm from base, CF = 2 kHz), and of 1 ms in the third turn (14-15 mm from base, CF = 0.7 kHz).

These delays correspond only to a fraction of the CF period (and are also much shorter than the values calculated by Zwislocki[20,21]).

CM results are confirmed by various direct measurements of the BM displacements (for a review see Dancer[21]). As an example, Wilson and Johnstone[22] measured the BM displacements in the basal turn of the guinea pig cochlea. In these experiments it is generally agreed[23] that the surgical preparation disrupted the active processes. Then, close to CF the phase lag relative to the input signal to the cochlea is about $\pi/2$[24]. This value is appreciably lower than that found for sharply-tuned responses as recorded by Sellick et al.[9] in cochleas in very good physiological condition, and is in agreement with the response of a simple resonator[25].

Actually, many other results point in the same direction: decrease of the BM phase lag after an acoustic trauma (Patuzzi et al.[26]), CAP and unit fibers latency in normal and noise exposed cochleas (de Boer[27], Salvi et al.[28])...

3 Intracochlear acoustic pressure observations

The intracochlear acoustic pressure was measured in the four turns of scala vestibuli in the guinea pig cochlea (fig. 1). The phase is nearly the same from base to apex: this is a first indication of a simultaneous excitation of the whole cochlear partition. Similar measurements performed in the three first turns of scala tympani (fig. 2) allow to calculate the differential acoustic pressure acting on the cochlear partition in the three first turns. As the phase of the pressure in scala vestibuli is the same from base to apex (fig. 1), the phase of the differential pressure (and of the differential CM) can be represented by taking as a reference that of the input signal to the cochlea (the acoustic pressure at the base of scala vestibuli) (fig. 3). In these conditions, the phase of the differential pressure and of the differential CM recorded on the same cochleas compare well and do not exhibit large phase lag accumulation.

Because of the unavoidable "spatial integration", these measurements cannot be considered as representing the actual micromechanics of an element of the organ of Corti when stimulated close to CF. However, they show that, at least below CF, the form of the curve is similar to a resonance.

4 Conclusion

From these measurements we can conclude that up to CF the hydromechanical phenomenons look relatively simple and close to the Helmholtz's theory in which a bank of resonators more or less damped are excited simultaneously. It is not

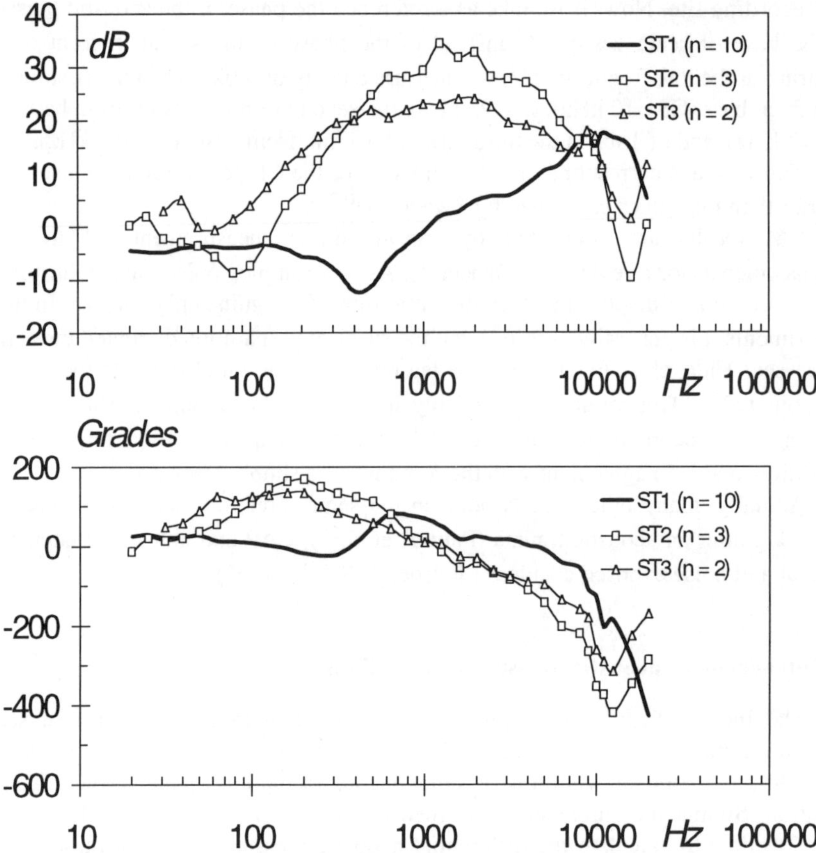

Figure 2: Amplitude and phase of the acoustic pressure in the three first turns of scala tympani (ref: acoustic pressure in front of the tympanum, bulla open)[18]

possible to observe the large phase lags and the long delays which, according to the one-dimensional long wave theory, characterize a travelling wave which transports the energy along the cochlea[5,6]. This conclusion is supported by the recent and more general statement of de Boer and Nuttall[29] "...in a realistic model supporting both long and short waves, the contribution (to the travelling time) due to wave propagation will be small".

The large phase lags measured in cochleas in good physiological condition (especially at CF) depend on the presence of the outer hair cells and are probably due partly to the action of the cellular active processes[30] (phase lags larger than $1/2$ can also originate from passive resonances assuming that several spring-mass systems: cilia, tectorial membrane... are coupled). By stating that "the travel time in

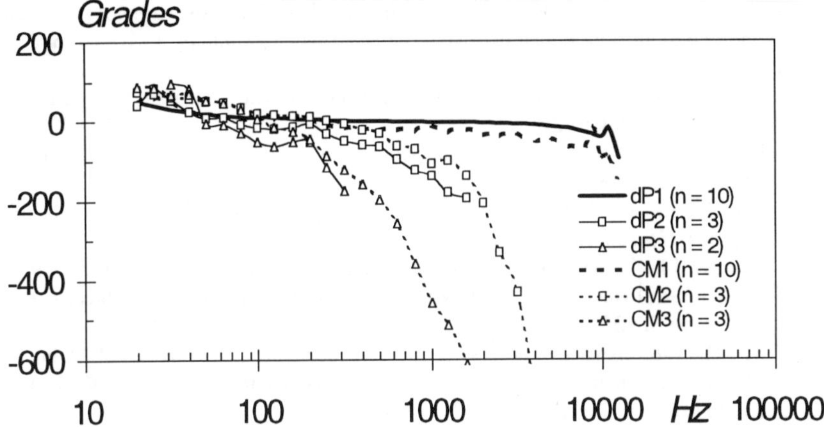

Figure 3: Phase of the differential pressure and of the differential CM in the three first turns of the guinea pig cochlea (ref: acoustic pressure at the base of scala vestibuli)[18]

the real cochlea is small compared to the time due to the resonance build-up" de Boer and Nuttall[29] support this interpretation and come to the same conclusion as put forward by Lewis et al.[10] and Dancer et al.[21,25].

It is now possible to re-examine the interpretation of some cochlear physiological phenomena: i.e., the latency of the neural responses, of the evoked oto-acoustic emissions and distortion products..., according to the actual hydromechanical behaviour of the cochlea.

References

1. Wever, E.G. and Lawrence, M. (1954) Physiological Acoustics, Princeton New Jersey, Princeton University Press, 245–293.
2. Bekesy, G. (1960) Experiments in hearing, Mc Graw-Hill, New York, Toronto and London.
3. Bekesy, G. (1928) Zur Theorie des Hörens; Die Schwingungsform der Basilarmembrane, *Physik Zeits.* **29** 793–810.
4. Bekesy, G. (1942) Über die Schwingungen der Schneckentrennwand beim Präparat und Ohrenmodell, *Akust. Zeits.* **7** 173–186.
5. Zwislocki, J.J. (1946) Über die mechanische Klanganalyse des Ohres, *Experientia* **2** 10–18.
6. Zwislocki, J.J. (1948) Theorie der Schneckenmechanik : qualitative und quantitative Analyse, *Acta Oto-Laryng. Suppl.* **72** 1–76.
7. Wever, E.G., Lawrence, M. and Bekesy, G. (1954) A note on recent developments in auditory theory, *Proc. of the Nat. Acad. of Sc. of USA.***40** 508–512.
8. Kiang, N.Y.S., Watanabe, T., Thomas, E.C. and Clark, L.F. (1965) Discharge patterns of single fibers in the cat's auditory nerve, *Res. Monograph.* **35**, M.I.T. Press, Cambridge, USA

9. Sellick, P.M., Patuzzi, R. and Johnstone, B.M. (1982) Measurement of basilar membrane motion in guinea pig using the Mössbauer technique, *J. Acoust. Soc. Am.* **72** 131–141.

10. Lewis, E.R., Leverenz, E.L. and Bialek, W.S. (1985) The vertebrate inner ear, (CRC Press Inc. Boca Raton) 248 p.

11. Allen, J.B. (1980) Cochlear micromechanics - a physical model of transduction. *J. Acoust. Soc. Am.* **68** 1660.

12. Zwislocki, J.J. and Kletsky, E.J. (1980) Micromechanics in the theory of cochlear mechanics. *Hearing Res.* **2** 505–512.

13. Zwislocki, J.J. (1986) Analysis of cochlear mechanics, *Hearing Res.* **22** 155–169.

14. Gold, T. (1948) Hearing II. The physical basis of the action of the cochlea, *Proc. R. Soc. London B.* **135** 492–498.

15. Davis, H. (1983) An active process in cochlear mechanics, *Hearing Res.* **9** 79–90.

16. Neely, S.T. and Kim, D.O. (1983) An active cochlear model showing sharp tuning and high sensitivity. *Hearing Res.* **9** 123–130.

17. Dancer, A. and Franke, R. (1980) Intracochlear sound pressure measurements in guinea pigs, *Hearing Res.* **2** 191–205.

18. Magnan, P., Dancer, A., Evrard, G., Vassout, P. and Avan, P. (1995) Etude de la propagation et de la dissipation du signal acoustique au niveau de l'oreille interne du cobaye, *French-German Research Institute of Saint-Louis, France,* Rpt. R116/95.

19. Dallos, P. and Cheatham, M. A. (1971) Travel time in the cochlea and its determination from CM data, *J. Acoust. Soc. Am.* **49** 1140–1143.

20. Zwislocki, J.J. (1974) Cochlear waves : interaction between theory and experiments, *J. Acoust. Soc. Am.* **55** 578–583.

21. Dancer, A. (1992) Experimental look at cochlear mechanics, *Audiology.* **31** 301–312.

22. Wilson, J.P. and Johnstone, J.R. (1975) Basilar membrane and middle ear vibration in guinea pig measured by capacitive probe, *J. Acoust. Soc. Am.* **57** 705–723.

23. Wilson, J.P. (1991) Cochlear mechanics, In: Auditory physiology and perception, eds. Y. Cazals, L. Demany and K. Horner, Proceedings of the 9th International Symposium on Hearing, Carcans, June 9-14, 1991.

24. Wilson, J.P. and Evans, E.F. (1983) Some observations on the "passive" mechanics of cat basilar membrane, In: Mechanics of Hearing, eds. W.R. Webster and L.M. Aitkin (Monash Univ. Press). 30–35.

25. Dancer, A. and Franke, R. (1989) Mechanics in a "passive" cochlea: travelling wave or resonance ? *Il Valsalva,* **LXV**, suppl. 1, 1–5.

26. Patuzzi, R., Johnstone, B.M. and Sellick, P.M. (1984) The alteration of the vibration of the basilar membrane produced by loud sound, *Hearing Res.* **13** 99–100.

27. de Boer, E. (1979) Travelling waves and cochlear resonance, *Scand. Audiol.,* **Suppl. 9** 17-33.

28. Salvi, R.J., Henderson, D. and Hamernik, R.P. (1979) Single auditory nerve fiber and action potential latencies in normal and noise treated chinchillas, *Hearing Res.* **1** 237–251.

29. de Boer, E. and Nuttall, A.L. (1996) Cochlear travel time and minimum phase, In: Proceedings of the 19th Midwinter Research Meeting of the *Association for Reasearch in Otolaryngology*, Abstract **228** 57.

30. Mammano, F. and Nobili, R. (1993) Biophysics of the cochlea: linear approximation, *J. Acoust. Soc. Am.* **93** 3320–3332.

THE DESIGN AND PURPOSE OF AN INTRACOCHLEAR PRESSURE SENSOR

E.S. OLSON

Physics Dept., Princeton University, Princeton
NJ 08544, USA

S. BORAWALA

Pharmacology Dept., Rutgers University, Piscataway
NJ 08855, USA

The characteristics of intracochlear pressure are dictated by both the cochlea's basic geometry and the micromechanical properties of the cochlear partition. Measurements of intracochlear pressure made with precise spatial localization with respect to the partition will address compelling questions about cochlear mechanics, and seek to quantify the mechanical impedance of the partition and locate regions of energy gain. We have constructed an intracochlear pressure sensor with the requisite properties for such measurements: a size small enough to access the cochlea without undo trauma, a sensitivity to pressures at the level where nonlinearities are present, and a response to frequencies throughout the auditory range.

1 Motivation for Pressure Measurements

The frequency dependence and spatial variation of intracochlear pressure are shaped by the mechanics of the cochlear partition. Therefore, experimental probes of intracochlear pressure inform our understanding of the partition's properties and action. Our measurements will be made in the base of the gerbil cochlea, where the basilar membrane (bm) is visible through the round window, allowing for precise positioning of the sensor close to the bm. Cross partition pressure will be estimated using measurements of pressure close to the bm in scala tympani, and the pressure in scala vestibuli in the extreme base. In scala tympani, a series of measurements in the vertical direction (perpendicular to the bm) between 20 and 200 μm from the bm will generate a pressure "map" that will be used to estimate the pressure gradient at the bm. This gradient gives fluid motion, and by extension, bm motion. Thus, we will capture nearly simultaneous measures of cross partition pressure and basilar membrane motion. The analysis of these measurements will allow us to estimate (1) the mechanical impedance of the cochlear partition, which is the mathematical embodiment of its micromechanics and (2) the local energy loss or gain of the traveling wave.

2   The Sensor

2.1 *Design*

We have constructed a pressure sensor tailored for intracochlear measurements. The ideal pressure sensor is small enough to not impair cochlear operation, sensitive enough to measure pressures for which cochlear nonlinearity is present, does not load or distort the intracochlear pressure field, and possesses a frequency response which allows for measurements through the characteristic frequency in the gerbil base, approximately 40 kHz[1]. Our sensor, illustrated in Figure 1, has an outer diameter of 167 µm, can reliably measure pressures of 20 mPa[a] (60 dB SPL) with a .02 Hz bandwidth, has a stiffness similar to that of the cochlear partition[2], and has a response which is nearly flat with frequency through at least 45 kHz. These properties are not uniformly ideal but are a substantial improvement over previous intracochlear sensors in size and frequency response. The sensor's sensitivity is similar to that of previous intracochlear sensors (but over a much wider range of frequencies), and because of the substantial pressure gain of inner ear pressure relative to sound pressure[3,4], should be adequate to monitor the cochlea's nonlinear operation. The mechanical impedance of our sensor is comparable to that of previous intracochlear sensors[3], and is calculated as approximately 5×10^{13} Ns/m[5] at 1 kHz. We will perform tests in order to gauge the perturbation of the intracochlear pressure field by the sensor.

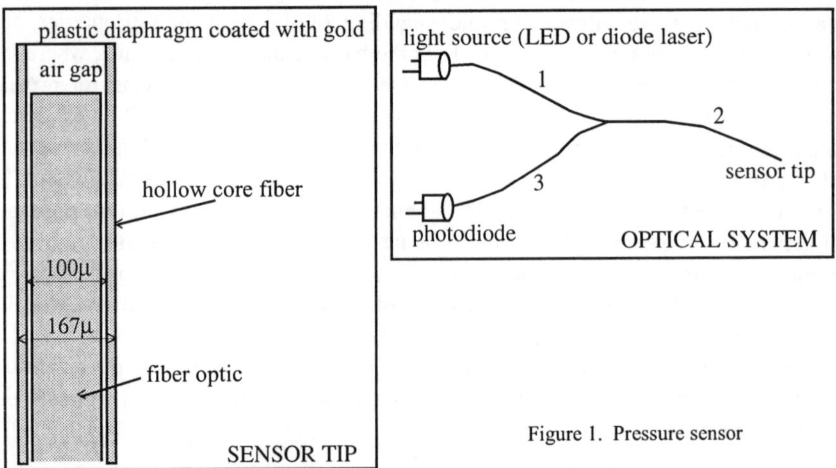

Figure 1. Pressure sensor

The sensor tip is composed of a plastic thin film diaphragm on a glass hollow core fiber (Polymicro Technologies, Phoenix, AZ) with inner and outer diameters of

---

[a] Ongoing improvements may increase this sensitivity

The sensor tip is composed of a plastic thin film diaphragm on a glass hollow core fiber (Polymicro Technologies, Phoenix, AZ) with inner and outer diameters of 100 and 167 µm respectively. The diaphragms have been made of a variety of plastics, but we have concentrated our efforts on polyvinyl formal (formvar) and optical adhesive 60 from Norland (New Brunswick, NJ). The diaphragm has a thin coat of gold evaporated on its outer surface to make it reflective.

The pressure induced flexing of the diaphragm is monitored optically. Arm 1 of a fiber optic coupler (a fiber optic beam splitter, Gould, Millersville, MD) is attached to the light source. This light splits 50:50 into the two output arms of the coupler, only one of which is used. (The second output arm is optically sunk.) The output arm, arm 2, is threaded into the back of the hollow fiber until it is positioned 50-100 µm from the diaphragm. Light reflected back into arm 2 comprises the signal and is detected by the photodetector, attached to arm 3.

The optical technique used to monitor the diaphragm position is an optic lever[5], a position detection scheme which is based on geometric optics, and is specific to fiber optic systems. The amount of light that returns from the reflecting diaphragm to the fiber core depends linearly (over an ample working range) on the deflection of the membrane. The light source is typically an LED, although we have also used a low-noise, low-coherence diode laser (for higher power), and a high coherence diode laser (in which case the system is an interferometer) with improved signal:noise. To date, the LED is the optimal light source for long-term signal stability.

2.2 *Calibration*

The sensor is calibrated absolutely in water[6]. The sensor head is immersed a known distance (0.5 to 2 mm) under the surface of a small vial of water on a piezoelectric shaker, which is vibrated with a known amplitude. This produces a hydrodynamic pressure proportional to the immersion depth, the fluid density, and the acceleration amplitude. In Figure 2a, the shaker amplitude was set to deliver calibration pressures of 60 and 80 dB SPL. The sensor's response is relatively flat through at least 45 kHz[b]. The calibration in water is approximately -37dB V at 80dB SPL.

An independent calibration was performed using the substitution method, in air. Tones of approximately 60 and 80 dB SPL were recorded by a Bruel and Kjær microphone (1/4", type 4135). Then the sensor was substituted for the B&K microphone, and used to record the same tones. The result is shown in Figure 2b. The calibration in air agrees with that in water. In Figure 2c, we plot the phase of the sensor output minus the phase of the output of the B&K microphone.

---

[b] The calibration in Figure 2a is only approximate because the shaker is not well calibrated *itself*, and its motion is not adequately flat at calibration frequencies. A more exacting calibration will be performed shortly using a shaker with a built in accelerometer.

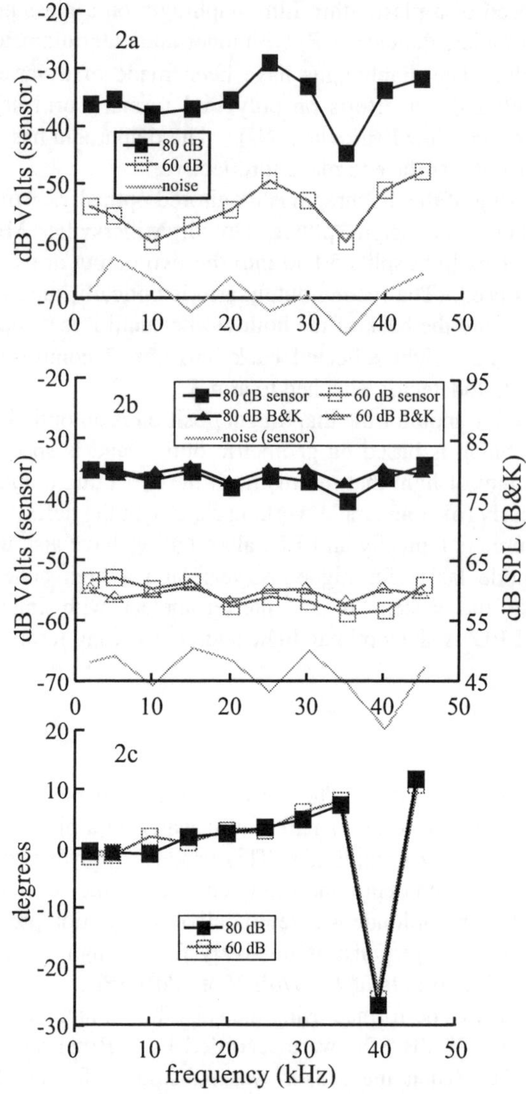

Figure 2. Calibration. (Signal averaging 50 seconds/point. LED light source.)

2a. Absolute calibration in water. (Approximate at this time, see text.)

2b. Substitution calibration in air. Amplitude of sensor output compared to that of Bruel and Kjaer microphone at SPLs of approximately 60 and 80 dB.

2c. Substitution calibration in air. Phase of sensor output - phase of microphone output.

3   Intracochlear Pressure Maps as a Probe of Cochlear Micromechanics

Intracochlear pressure maps will provide a localized probe of cochlear mechanics, a complement to the measurements of partition motion that have become extremely refined in recent years. The following describes a rather coarse strategy for extracting particular quantities from the measurements. Another, more conservative analysis strategy is to use the maps to fuel and test two and three-dimensional cochlear models.

In the following we assume that pressures and motions are in the form $\text{Re}\{Ae^{i\omega t}\}$, where the amplitude A is complex.

3.1 *Cross Partition Pressure*

We would like to know the pressure across the cochlear partition: the difference between the pressure just below the basilar membrane and that just above the partition. We can directly measure the pressure just below the basilar membrane, but cannot measure the pressure just above the partition due to anatomical restrictions. The cross partition pressure will be inferred from a measurement in scala vestibuli well away from the partition, and a measurement in scala tympani close to the partition, as described below.

The pressure in the cochlea is typically thought of as comprising two separate pressures. (See, for example, Lighthill[7].) P is the mean of the pressures in scala vestibuli and scala tympani; it is an acoustical standing wave and is governed by the tube-like geometry of the cochlea, without reference to the partition. p is the deviation from the mean. It describes the cochlear traveling wave, and is governed by the impedance of the cochlear partition. In a system with a symmetric geometry, p is of equal magnitude and opposite sign in the two scalae. Close to the partition, p is expected to have a much more pronounced spatial variation than P, and we will assume that P is approximately uniform in the radial and vertical directions at a particular longitudinal location. In general, pressures measured far from the partition will be assumed to have a relatively gradual spatial variation. The cross partition pressure close to the partition is the quantity we wish to find. The following relationships are approximations that assume a symmetric geometry, and apply only in the extreme base, where the pressure release of the round window zeros the scala tympani pressure far from the partition. Overbars indicate pressures far from the partition which vary gradually in space. The subscript 0 indicates pressures close to the partition. The subscript t indicates pressure in scala tympani, v that in scala vestibuli. p_{cross} is the cross partition pressure.

$$\bar{P_t} = P - \bar{p} = 0$$
$$\bar{P_v} = P + \bar{p} = 2P$$
$$P = \bar{P_v}\Big/2$$
$$P_{t0} = P - p_0$$
$$P_{v0} = P + p_0$$
$$p_{cross} = P_{v0} - P_{t0} = 2p_0$$
$$p_0 = \bar{P_v}\Big/2 - P_{t0}$$
$$p_{cross} = \bar{P_v} - 2P_{t0} \tag{1}$$

3.2 Basilar Membrane Motion

The pressure measured at several closely spaced vertical positions close to the partition will be used to estimate the vertical component of the pressure gradient *at* the partition. The pressure gradient is the fluid force, and produces acceleration of the fluid, convection of velocity gradients (a nonlinear term) and, where viscosity is significant, fluid velocity. Fluid viscosity is expected to produce significant drag only in a boundary layer next to the basilar membrane[8] (within about 20 μm or less at frequencies above 1 kHz). We will work outside this layer. Because the spatial extent of velocity gradients is much greater than the excursions of the partition and fluid the nonlinear convective term is negligible. Therefore, the pressure gradient is approximately proportional to fluid acceleration. Close to the partition the vertical component of fluid acceleration will reflect the acceleration of the basilar membrane, and will provide an estimate of the basilar membrane motion. In the following, P_t is pressure, measured in scala tympani, a is acceleration, z is vertical displacement, ω is angular frequency, and ρ is fluid density. The subscript z indicates the vertical component, 0 indicates close to the basilar membrane, t indicates scala tympani, f indicates fluid, and bm indicates basilar membrane.

$$\nabla P_t = -\rho a \,(\text{linearized description, neglecting viscosity})$$
$$\frac{\partial P_t}{\partial z} = -\rho a_z = \rho z_f \omega^2$$
$$z_{bm} \approx z_{f0} = \left.\frac{\partial P_t}{\partial z}\right|_0 \Big/ \rho\omega^2 \tag{2}$$

3.3 Mechanical Impedance of the Partition

The mechanical impedance of the partition is defined here as the ratio of cross partition pressure to vertical partition velocity.

$$\text{Mechanical impedance} \equiv Z \equiv \frac{P_{cross}}{v_{bm}}$$

$$\text{From (1) and (2):} \quad Z = \frac{\overline{P}_v - 2P_{t0}}{i\left.\dfrac{\partial P_t}{\partial z}\right|_0 \Big/ \rho\omega} \tag{3}$$

3.4 *Energy Gain or Loss*

At frequencies for which the real part of Z is negative, the partition is delivering energy to the traveling wave. The time averaged power absorbed (when positive) or delivered (when negative) by the partition per unit area is found as:

$$\text{Power} = \frac{1}{2}\text{Re}\{p_{cross}v_{bm}^*\} \tag{4}$$

Acknowledgments

A portion of this work was done at Rutgers University in Newark NJ, with funding from the N.S.F. and the Howard Hughes Medical Institute. Current support for this work is from the N.I.H. The authors are grateful for the assistance of Reg Cook, Joe Santos-Sacchi, Marcus Meinhoffer, Dana Anderson and Ed Bonder.

References

1. Xue, S., Mountain , D.C. and Hubbard, A.E. (1995) Electrically evoked basilar membrane motion, *J. Acoust. Soc. Amer.* **97** 3030-3041.
2. Olson, E. and Mountain, D.C. (1991) In vivo measurement of basilar membrane stiffness, *J. Acoust. Soc. Amer.* **89** 1262-1275.
3. Dancer, A. and Franke, R. (1980) Intracochlear sound pressure measurements in guinea pigs , *Hear. Res.* **2** 191-205.
4. Nedzelnitsky, V. (1980) Sound pressures in the basal turn of the cat cochlea, *J. Acoust. Soc. Amer.* **68** 1676-1689.
5. Cook,R. and Hamm,C. (1979) Fiber optic lever displacement transducer, *Appl. Opt.* **18** 3230-3241.
6. Schloss, F. and Strasberg, M. (1962) Hydrophone calibration in a vibrating column of liquid, *J. Acoust. Soc. Amer.* **34** 958-960.
7. Lighthill, J. (1981) Energy flow in the cochlea, *J. Fluid Mech.* **106** 149-213
8. Steele, C. (1974) Behavior of the basilar membrane with pure-tone excitation, *J.Acoust. Soc. Amer.* **55** 148-162.

THE COCHLEA IS AN AUTOMATIC GAIN CONTROL SYSTEM AFTER ALL

J.J. ZWISLOCKI, Y.M. SZYMKO, L.Y. HERTIG

Institute for Sensory Research, Syracuse University
Syracuse, NY 13244, USA
joe_zwislocki@isr.syr.edu

Intracellular alternating potentials of the organ of Corti of Mongolian gerbils, recorded in the frequency and time domains, indicate that the cochlear compressive nonlinearity is due mainly to non-instantaneous automatic gain control. This is so because of relatively small distortion of output waveforms at medium SPLs and time constant asymmetry between the on and off transients.

1 Introduction

We first should introduce some clarifications. "Automatic gain control" (AGC) is used by us according to the classical concept that designates a dynamical process with a finite time constant, usually longer than the period of oscillation of the controlled signal. Accordingly, instantaneous nonlinearity is excluded.

It has been amply established that the mammalian cochlea has nonlinear dynamic characteristics, that is, its gain[1-3] and tonotopic map[4-7] vary with signal amplitude. Apparently, these nonlinearities do not seem to be accompanied by either automatic gain control (AGC) or compatible waveform distortion. AGC would be expected to manifest itself in temporal adaptation, such as is well known in the auditory-nerve fibers[8,9]. However, Russell and Sellick[3] saw no such adaptation in their pioneering recordings of receptor potentials of cochlear inner hair cells (IHCs), and their finding has been confirmed by others[10,11] and extended to the basilar membrane[12].

Diverse models have been proposed to explain the paradoxical relationships. Some of the most prominent ones have been reviewed by deBoer[13]. In all of them, instantaneous nonlinearities seem to be assumed to make the models compatible with Russell and Sellick's[3] finding of no adaptation. In view of strong compression evident in cochlear input-output functions, such nonlinearities must produce extreme waveform distortion, which is not present in the measured waveforms, however. To make the model waveforms and the resulting distortion products compatible with the empirical ones, various filtering schemes are introduced. One of us[14] published preliminary experimental results showing that, at moderate SPLs, wave distortion at the cellular level was too small to be accounted for by empirically determined cochlear filter functions.

The problem could be avoided if AGC with a sufficiently long time constant were present. We describe here experiments showing that, although no adaptive amplitude decay is evident in cochlear responses to tone bursts, their overall temporal amplitude patterns are compatible with the presence of AGC with a time constant on the order of one period of oscillation.

2 Experiments Showing the Presence of AGC

The experiments were performed on 8 Mongolian gerbils aged 10 to 15 weeks and weighing between 65 and 78 g with the help of methods described in the past on several occasions[15].   Receptor potentials of Hensen's cells were recorded intracellularly. It was demonstrated previously[15,16] that the magnitude and phase characteristics of these cells are practically the same as of the OHCs, except for a multiplicative magnitude constant. These cells are much easier to find and to hold than the OHCs.

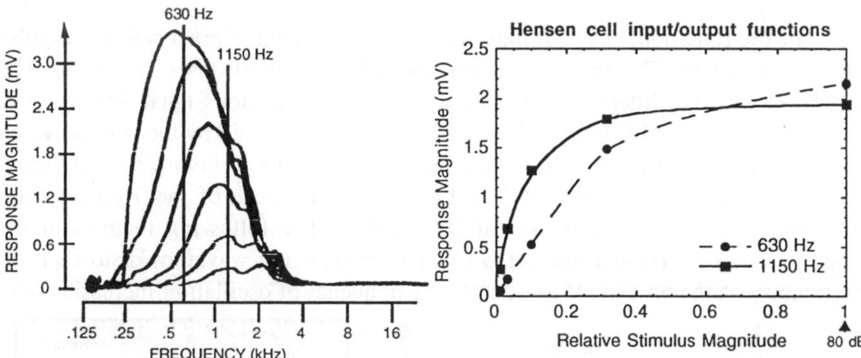

Figure 1: Intensity series of intracellular Hensen's cell transfer functions (40 to 90 dB SPL in 10 dB steps). The vertical lines indicate the frequencies at which intensity- time domain analysis was performed (Gerbil 2/15/96: EP=90 mV; RP=-84 mV).

Figure 2: Input-output functions constructed from he transfer functions of Figure 1.

In the frequency-domain experiments, alternating potentials picked up by the electrodes were amplified and filtered by a lock-in amplifier. Their magnitude as a function of sound frequency was displayed on the screen of a storage oscilloscope, whose horizontal deflection was made proportional to log frequency. The setup allowed us to record intensity series of continuous transfer functions within about a minute — 6 sec per transfer function. Input-output functions could then be constructed from the series at any sound frequency of interest by sectioning the curves vertically. A series of transfer functions obtained on a Hensen's cell of a

356

sensitive cochlea is shown in Figure 1 for SPLs ranging between 40 and 90 dB in 10 dB steps. The small irregularity between 1 and 2 kHz is ascribed to the middle ear. Several features of the curves should be noted for further reference: 1) the routinely observed frequency shift of the response peak from somewhat above 2 kHz downward to .5 kHz at 90 dB, in particular, the shift from about 1.4 kHz at 50 dB to about 0.95 kHz at 70 dB; 2) the peak ratio of about 1/3.25 (approximately -10 dB) between the 70 and 50 dB curves; 3) the amplitude ratios of 1 (0 dB) and 1.5 (3.5 dB) between the location of 630 Hz and its second- and third-harmonic locations of 1.26 and 1.89 kHz and also of 3.8 (11.5 dB) and of 12 (22 dB) between the 1.15 kHz location and its second- and third-harmonic locations at 2.3 and 3.45 kHz, respectively; and 4) a secondary maximum in the vicinity of 2.7 kHz. Input-output functions for the frequencies of 0.63 and 1.15 kHz have been constructed from Figure 1 according to the intersections of the transfer curves with the vertical lines and are plotted in Fig. 2 on linear scales. Note the strong compression extending down to at least 40 dB in both curves but especially in the 1.15 kHz curve.

For the time-domain recordings, the signals consisted of practically rectangular tone bursts 10 to 17 msec in duration repeated at 30 to 80 msec intervals. The responses were not filtered but RMS averaged on a Princeton Signal Averager (50 to 250 repetitions). Examples of responses generated at 70 dB by the cell for which the transfer functions of Figure 1 were obtained are shown in Figure 3. For Figure 3a, the signal frequency was at 1.150 kHz, near the peak of the 70-dB transfer function. For Figure 3b, it was at 0.63 kHz. The following features of the responses are of particular interest to this paper: 1) small waveform distortion; 2) asymmetry of the on and off transients; 3) frequency of oscillation increasing with

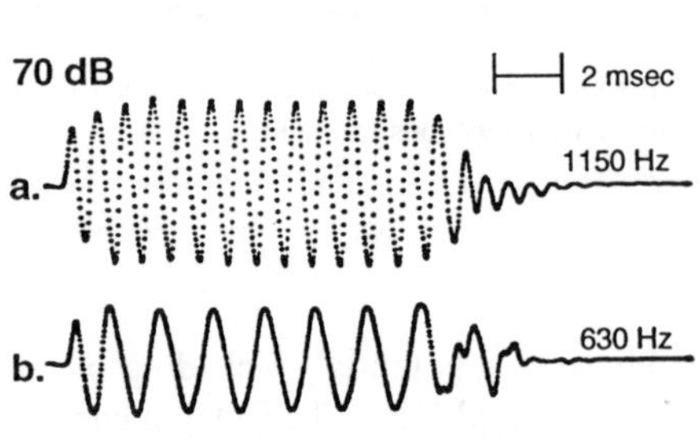

Figure 3: Responses of the cell of Figure 1 to tone bursts.

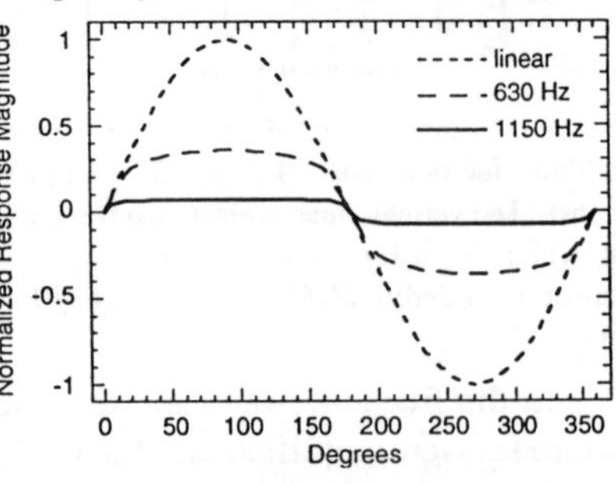

Figure 4: Distorted sinusoids constructed from an undistorted sinusoid using the input-output functions of Figure 2 on the assumption of symmetry with respect to zero ordinate. The symmetry assumption is not entirely realistic but appears reasonable in view of the empirical waveforms of Figure 3.

time in the off transient of Figure 3a; and 4) waveform perturbation in the off transient of Figure 3b. We discuss the significance of these features one by one.

1) The waveform distortion is smaller than predicted from the compressive input-output functions of Figure 2. The predicted waveforms are shown in Figure 4. One could argue that the distortion was reduced by filtering according to the transfer functions of Figure 1. However, we found the filter effect to be too small to account for the practically undistorted 1.15 and 0.63 kHz waveforms of Figure 3. The wave-form discrepancy speaks against an instant nonlinearity.

2) The on/off transient asymmetry seen in particular in Figure 3a is a characteristic of AGC, as is well known in radio and related technologies. It can be shown mathematically that decreasing gain near signal onset decreases the effective time constant of the onset-amplitude buildup. Reciprocally, increasing gain after signal termination prolongs the off transient. Our calculations have yielded an on time constant of 0.373 msec and an off time constant of 1.8 msec, with a ratio of 4.85. Similar relationships have been obtained for other preparations. When a linear-system time constant is calculated from the estimated Q factor of the medium SPL transfer functions of Figure 1, a numerical value of about 0.4 msec is obtained. To further show that a cochlea-like system, but linear and without AGC, produces symmetrical (more accurately, antisymmetrical) on and off transients, we studied them on a hardware model of the cochlea endowed with both basilar-membrane and tectorial-membrane resonance systems. An example of the obtained results is shown in Figure 5. The time-constant symmetry between the on and off amplitude patterns is apparent. The relatively long buildup and decay patterns resulted from a somewhat sharper tuning than is usually encountered in natural cochleas.

3) Comparison of the magnitudes and frequencies of the response peaks in Figure 1 to the corresponding magnitudes and natural frequencies in Figure 3a shows that the magnitudes and the frequencies are coupled. As the peak response in Figure 1 decreased by about 10 dB when the SPL was decreased from 70 to 50 dB, the frequency location of the peak increased from 0.95 to about 1.4 kHz. During the off transient of Figure 3a, the response frequency changed from the frequency of 1.15 kHz of the driving signal at 70 dB to a natural frequency of about 1.45 kHz when the response amplitude decreased by 10 dB. Thus, equal frequencies were coupled to approximately equal peak amplitudes, whether the response was driven or resulted from a natural, free oscillation. Both the gain change and the frequency change seem to depend on a common mechanism. In a preceding study[17], it was shown that the frequency of the response peak is controlled by the active feedback. It seems reasonable to extend this conclusion to the natural, free oscillation in the off transient and, as a consequence, to the AGC.

4) A closer look at the wave-form perturbation in the off transient of Figure 3b

indicates that the perturbation is produced by an oscillation at a natural frequency of the system, the same as measured during the off transient of Figure 3a.

On the basis of the above results, it seems to us reasonable to conclude that the mammalian cochlea is endowed with a non-instantaneous AGC and that the AGC results from the active feedback. The asymmetry of on/off transients clearly evident in basilar-membrane vibration described by Ruggero and Rich[12] is consistent with the existence of AGC.

3 Experiments Indicating a Second Natural Frequency

On the basis of their measurements of basilar-membrane transients produced by clicks, DeBoer and Nuttall (1996) have recently suggested the possibility of a second natural frequency in cochlear oscillatory responses. It is not clear if the second frequency they observed resulted from the dependence of the natural frequency on the response magnitude, as described above, or constituted a separate natural frequency that could result from a second resonance system. Below, we describe

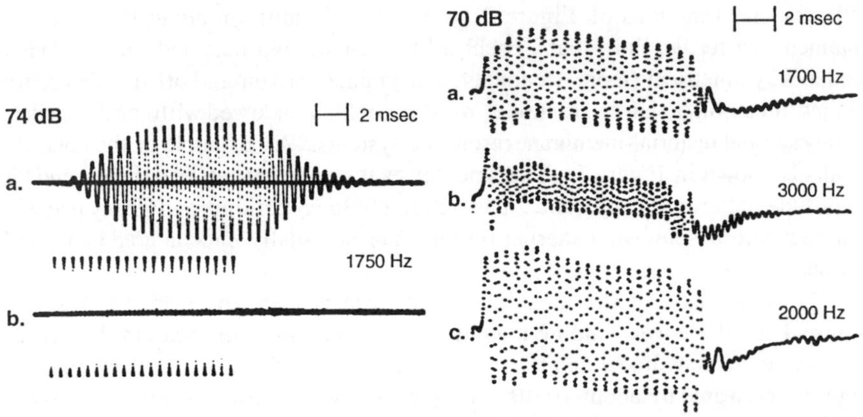

Figure 5: Response of a hardware electrical-network model of the cochlea[20] to the similar tone bursts as used for Figure 4. The bottom trace (b) is the stimulus.

Figure 6: Responses of a Hensen's cell of another gerbil (EP=80 mV; RP=-85 mV), which had similar transfer functions to those of Figure 1, to tone bursts at sound frequencies higher than the frequency of the transfer-function amplitude maximum at 70 dB. The responses at 2000 and 3000 Hz were magnified relative to the response at 1700 Hz.

briefly experiments showing that a second natural frequency does exist.

The experiments were a continuation of the time-domain experiments described above with the difference that higher stimulus frequencies were used. Examples of results obtained on one sensitive cochlea with transfer functions similar to those of

Figure 1 are shown in Figure 6. In all instances the stimulus was at 70 dB SPL. In Figure 6a, the driving sound frequency was at about 1.7 kHz, in Fig. 6b, at about 3.0 kHz and, in Fig. 6c, at about 2.0 kHz. The transient magnitude decayed almost monotonically in both a and b, except for a transition period immediately at the termination of the tone burst in a. However, the transient frequencies differed. In a, where a relatively low stimulus frequency was used, the transient frequency was estimated at 2.4 kHz. In b, on the other hand, where a relatively high stimulus frequency was used, the transient frequency was estimated at 2.8 kHz. A more complicated transient pattern is shown in c. It is associated with an intermediate stimulus frequency. Here, both the amplitude and the frequency seem to be periodically modulated with a modulation frequency of roughly 0.3 kHz. In the first visible wave burst, the frequency has been estimated at roughly 2.7 kHz; in the second, at roughly 2.35 kHz. The two frequencies correspond to the lower and higher transient frequencies of Figures 6a and b, respectively. Because of the very rough frequency estimates and the natural-frequency dependence on the response amplitude, the differences between 2.7 and 2.8 kHz on the one side and between 2.35 and 2.4 kHz on the other cannot be regarded as significant. Since the modulation frequency is roughly equal to the frequency difference between the two transient components of Figure 6c, it is reasonable to conclude that the modulation has resulted from beats between the two components.

The whole transient pattern described above is of the kind that would be expected from two mistuned coupled resonators. In this connection, it should be noted that, in many cochlear transfer functions recorded at the basilar-membrane or hair-cell levels, a secondary maximum can often be discerned. Such a maximum seems to have been first observed by Rhode[1] in basilar-membrane vibration. It was explained by one of us on the assumption of a parallel tectorial-membrane resonance[18,19].

Acknowledgments

We thank A. Wixson and R. Mitchell for technical help. Work supported in part by NIDCD and in part by Syracuse University.

References

1. Rhode, W.S. (1971) Observations of the vibration of the basilar membrane in squirrel monkeys using the Mössbauer technique, *J. Acoust. Soc. Am.* **49** 1218—1231.
2. Sellick, P.M., Patuzzi, R. and Johnstone, B. M. (1982) Measurement of basilar membrane motion in the guinea pig using the Mössbauer technique, *J. Acoust. Soc. Am.* **72** 131—141.
3. Russell, I.J. and Sellick, P.M. (1978) Intracellular studies of hair cells in the mammalian cochlea, *J. Physiol.* **284** 261—290.

4. Rose, J.E., Hind, J.E., Anderson, D.J. and Brugge, J.F. (1971) Some effects of stimulus intensity on response of auditory nerve fibers in the squirrel monkey, *J. Neurophysiol.* **34** 685—699.

5. Møller, A.R.(1978) Frequency selectivity of the peripheral auditory analyzer studied using broad band noise, *Acta. Physiol. Scand.* **104** 24—32.

6. Honrubia, V. and Ward, P.H. (1968) Longitudinal distribution of the cochlear microphonics inside the cochlear duct (guinea pig) *J. Acoust. Soc. Am.* **45** 1443—1450.

7. Zwislocki, J.J. (1991) What is the cochlear place code for pitch? *Acta Otolaryng. (Stockholm)* **111** 256—262.

8. Kiang, N.Y-S. (1965) Discharge Patterns of Single Fibers in the Cat's Auditory Nerve, *MIT Res. Monograph* **35** (MIT Press, Cambridge, Mass.) .

9. Smith, R.L. and Zwislocki, J.J. (1975) Short-term adaptation and incremental responses of single auditory-nerve fibers, *Biol. Cybernetics* **17** 169—182.

10. Goodman, D.A., Smith, R.L. and Chamberlain, S. C. (1982) Intracellular and extracellular responses in the organ of Corti of the gerbil, *Hearing Res.* **7** 161—179.

11. Dallos, P. and Cheatham, M.A. (1989) Cochlear nonlinearities reflected in inner hair cell responses, in *Cochlear Mechanisms*, ed. J.P. Wilson and D.T. Kemp. (Plenum Publishing Corp., London) pp. 197—203.

12. Ruggero, M.A. and Rich, N.C. (1991) Application of commercially-manufactured Doppler-shift laser velocimeter to the measurement of basilar-membrane vibration, *Hearing. Res.* **51** 215—230.

13. deBoer, E. (1993) Some like it active, in *Biophysics of Hair Cell Sensory Systems*, ed. H. Duifhuis, J.W. Horst, P. van Dijk and S.M. van Netten (World Scientific, Singapore) pp. 3—22.

14. Zwislocki, J.J. and Chatterjee, M. (1993) Direct evidence for automatic gain control in the cochlea, *J. Acoust. Soc. Am.* **94** 1811.

15. Zwislocki, J.J., Slepecky, N.B., Cefaratti, L.K. and Smith, R.L. (1992) Ionic coupling among cells in the organ of Corti. *Hearing Res.* **57** 175—194.

16. Oesterle, E. and Dallos, P. (1989) Intracellular recordings from supporting cells in the guinea pig cochlea: AC potentials, *J. Acoust. Soc. Am.* **86** 1013—1032.

17. Zhang, M. and Zwislocki, J.J. (1996) Intensity-dependent peak shift in cochlear transfer functions at the cellular level, its elimination by sound pressure, and its possible underlying mechanisms. Hearing Res. (in press).

18. Zwislocki, J.J. (1980) Five decades of research on cochlear mechanics. *J. Acoust. Soc. Am.* **67** 1679—1685.

19. Zwislocki, J.J. and Kletsky, E.J. (1982) What basilar-membrane tuning says about cochlear micromechanics. *Am. J. Otolaryngol.* **3** 48—52.

20. Zwislocki, J.J. (1983) Cochlear micromechanics- a model and some of its consequences. In: *Mechanisms of hearing*, R.W. Webster and L.M. Aitkin, eds., Monash University Press, Clayton, Victoria, Australia, pp. 21—26.

THE EFFECT OF EFFERENT STIMULATION AND ACETYLCHOLINE PERFUSION ON BASILAR MEMBRANE DISPLACEMENT IN THE BASAL TURN OF THE GUINEA PIG COCHLEA

I.J. RUSSELL, E. MURUGASU

School of Biological Sciences, University of Sussex, Falmer, Brighton, BN1 9QG, U.K.
I.J.RUSSELL@sussex.ac.uk

Electrical stimulation of the olivocochlear bundle (OCB), and intracochlear acetylcholine (ACh) perfusion of scala tympani, reversibly linearized the compressive phase of BM displacement to tone-evoked displacements of the basilar membrane (BM) measured with an interferometer in the basal turn of the guinea pig cochlea. Following OCB stimulation, the tip of the BM isoresponse tuning curve was elevated by up to 24 dB and frequency-shifted downwards by < 0. 5 kHz, while the bandwidth (Q_{10dB}) decreased from a mean of 8.2 to 7. Perfusion of the scala tympani with either Ca^{2+} free artificial perilymph or 100 μM TMB-8 reversibly blocked the ACh-induced suppression of tone-evoked BM displacements whilst the suppression was augmented and prolonged by 10 μM cyclopiazonic acid but irreversibly blocked by 100 μM ryanodine.

1   Introduction

The termination of fibres from the olivo-cochlear bundle (OCB) on outer hair cells (OHCs) has led to speculation that, through the modification of both the electrical and mechanical properties of the OHCs, the OCB controls the gain of electromechanical feedback from the OHCs and, hence, the sensitivity and frequency selectivity of the cochlea. The action of the OCB on the sound-evoked responses of the cochlea is mainly inhibitory. Excitation of the medial component of the OCB attenuates the click-evoked compound action potential, enhances the cochlear microphonic and alters the level of acoustic distortion measured at the external auditory meatus (reviewed by Wiederhold[1]). OCB-mediated inhibition is frequency dependent; suppression of BM displacement[2], IHC receptor potentials[3] and afferent nerve fibre activity[4] is greatest at the peak of the tuning curve. Acetylcholine (ACh) has been implicated as the neurotransmitter of the medial OCB system (reviewed by Eybalin[5]). However, there have been no direct, *in vivo*, measurements of the effects of ACh on tone-evoked BM displacements. In this paper we describe the effects of electrical stimulation of the OCB and ACh perfusion of the scala tympani on tone-evoked BM displacements and how the effects of Ach perfusion are modified by low extracellular Ca^{2+} and agents which interfere with the uptake and release of intracellular Ca^{2+}.

2　Methods

A description of the methods of preparation, experimental techniques and stimulus presentation has been given elsewhere[2,6]. Recordings were made from pigmented guinea pigs (230-320 g) anaesthetised with the neurolept anaesthetic technique (0.06 mg atropine sulphate s.c., 30 mg/kg pentobarbitone i.p., 4 mg/kg droperidol i.m.; 1 mg/kg phenoperidine i.m.). The animals were tracheotomized, artificially respired and core temperatures were maintained at 37°C. The OCB was electrically stimulated at the point where it crosses the fourth ventricle (150 s^{-1} for 80 ms). The scala tympani of the basal turn was perfused with solutions at a rate of 2.5 µl per minute through a fine cannula (< 100 µm diameter) inserted through a small incision in the round window with an outflow through a fenestra in the basal turn. BM displacements were measured through the fenestra in the basal turn using the self-mixing effect of a laser diode[2,6]. This technique is sensitive enough to measure light reflected directly from the 10 µm diameter spot on the BM produced by the focused laser beam. BM displacements were analysed with a two channel lock-in amplifier. Tone burst 100 ms duration, rise time 2ms with onset times delayed 60 ms with respect to the onset of OCB stimulation, were delivered every 200 ms.

3　Results

3.1　Level and frequency dependent OCB suppression of BM displacement

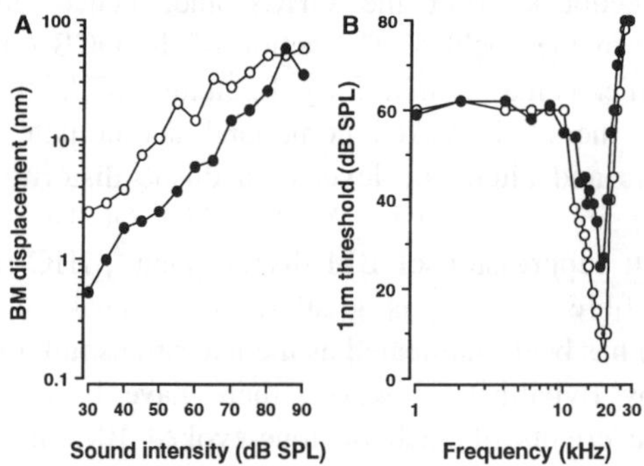

Fig. 1 A) BM displacement as a function of level for an 18 kHz tone close to the CF (17.5 kHz). B) 2nm isothreshold tuning curve. Open symbols: 100 ms tone alone. Closed symbols: 60 ms burst of OCB stimulation preceeds onset of tone by 40 ms. (from Murugasu and Russell[2])

The level and frequency dependent action of OCB stimulation on BM displacement was measured from locations with characteristic frequencies (CFs) between 14.5 kHz and 18 kHz. The effect of OCB stimulation on the displacement of the BM as a function of level (displacement/ level function) was measured at the CF of the measuring site (Fig. 1A) and at frequencies above and below this. OCB stimulation reversibly reduced the dynamic range of the compressive phase by 18.3 dB +- 4.6 dB (mean +- s.d, n = 7). The isoresponse tuning curve plotted before and during OCB stimulation (Fig. 1B) exemplifies the frequency dependency of OCB stimulation on BM displacement. The tip of the tuning curve is elevated but without a change in the sensitivity of the low-frequency tail. The OCB-induced suppression of BM displacement was reversibly blocked following perfusion of the scala tympani with 1μM strychnine in artificial perilymph[6].

3.2 ACh perfusion of the scala tympani mimics OCB action on BM displacement

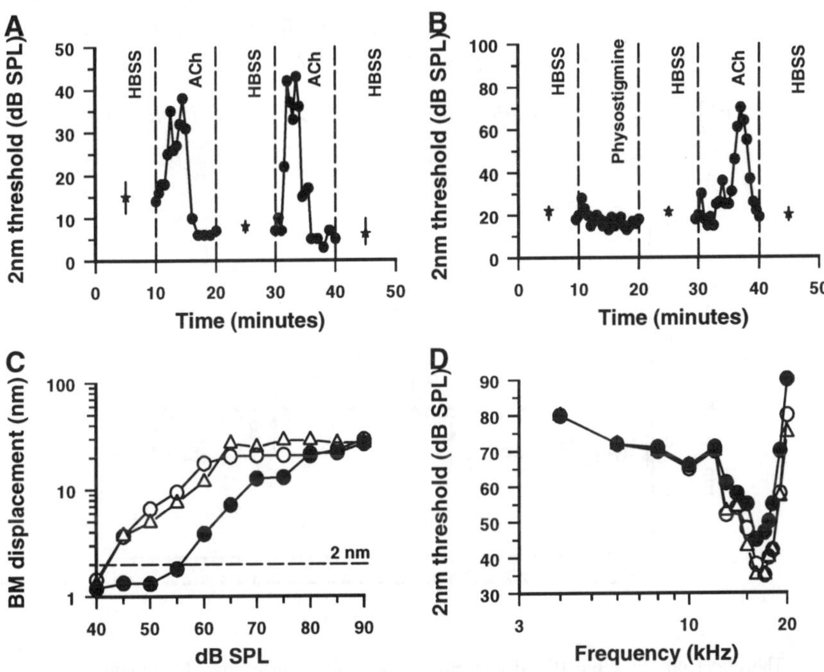

Fig. 2. A) 2 nm BM displacement threshold, at the 15 kHz CF of the measuring point on the BM, as a function of time during continuous perfusion with 100 μM ACh/ 20 μM Phy in HBSS. B) BM displacement threshold remained unchanged by perfusion with 20 μM Phy but was reduced by subsequent perfusion with 100 μM ACh/ 20 μM Phy (ACh). The stars and bars represent the mean ± s.d. threshold from 10 readings measured during HBSS perfusion. C) BM displacement -level functions at 14 kHz (CF 15 kHz) and D) BM 2nm isoresponse tuning curve (CF 18 kHz) measured before (open circle), during (filled circle) and after (open triangle) ACh perfusion of the scala tympani (from Murugasu and Russell[6])

The effect of OCB stimulation was mimicked by perfusing the scala tympani with 100 µM ACh/ 20 µM physostigmine (Phy) which induced a transient 20 -25 dB SPL rise in the 2 nm BM displacement threshold (Fig. 2A, 3C). After 4 - 5 minutes of continuous perfusion, ACh caused a suppression of tone-evoked BM displacements followed by desensitisation which persisted for the 10 min perfusion period. Perfusion with 20 µM Phy alone had no effect on BM displacement but subsequent perfusion with Phy/ ACh transiently reduced BM sensitivity (Fig. 2B). Sensitisation to ACh perfusion was restored after the ACh was washed out with artificial perilymph (HBSS). A displacement-level function at CF is shown in Fig. 2C where, following ACh perfusion, the compressive phase of BM displacement was reversibly linearised with the greatest effect at low to moderate levels. ACh perfusion effected the tuning curve by causing an elevation of the tip (24.2 ± 7.0 dB SPL, n = 21) with greatest suppression on the high-frequency slope of the tip and with either no change in the CF or a shift to lower frequencies of < 0.5 kHz.

3.3 *Extracellular calcium mediates the effect of ACh on BM displacement*

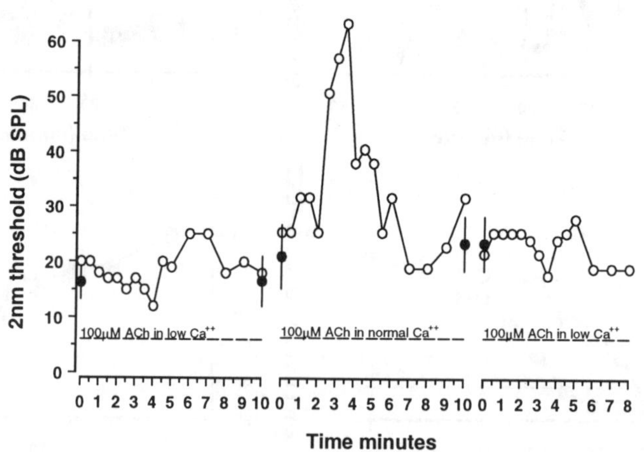

Fig. 3. The effect on the 2 nm BM displacement threshold of successive 10 minute scala tympani perfusions with HBSS (wash), 100 µM ACh in nominally calcium-free HBSS, and ACh in HBSS. Solid symbols represent the means and standard deviations of the threshold measured during the washing periods in 5 minute periods immediately before and after the ACh perfusion (from Murugasu and Russell[6]).

Ca^{2+} is thought to be important for the ACh-mediated regulation of OHC function[7,8]. In experiments reported here, the 2 nm threshold for BM displacement was not altered by perfusion of the scala tympani with the modified HBSS solution, but when the normal HBSS solution was replaced by a nominally Ca^{2+}-free HBSS solution, the suppressive effect of 100 μM ACh/ 20 μM Phy on BM displacement was blocked (Fig. 3). Perfusion of 100 μM ACh/ 20 μM Phy in the presence of low Ca^{2+} did not increase the 2 nm displacement threshold above control. This effect of low Ca^{2+} on ACh perfusion was reversed when the normal-Ca^{2+} HBSS solution was reinstated and 100 mM ACh/ 20 mM Phy again caused elevation of the 2 nm BM displacement threshold.

3.4 Cyclopiazonic acid prolongs the effect of ACh on BM displacement

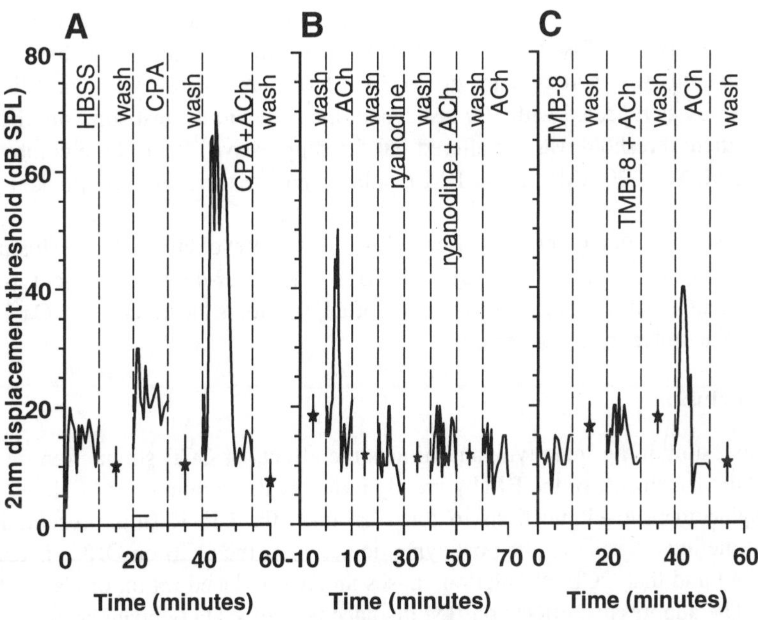

Fig. 4. The effect on the 2 nm BM displacement threshold of successive 10 minute perfusions of the scala tympani with A) HBSS (wash), 100 μM ACh, and ACh together with 10 μM cyclopiazonic acid (CPA). B) HBSS, 100 μM ACh, and ACh together with 100 μM ryanodine. C) HBSS, 100 μM ACh, and ACh together with 100 μM TMB-8. The horizontal lines beneath the CPA traces signify the 10 minute perfusion period. The stars represent the means and standard deviations of ten measurements of the threshold made during the washing periods (from Murugasu and Russell[6]).

Cyclopiazonic acid (CPA) is an inhibitor of the Ca^{2+}-ATPase in the sarcoplasmic/ endoplasmic reticulum which pumps Ca^{2+} back into these intracellular stores[9]. In these experiments, 10 μM CPA was added to the test solution containing 100 μM ACh/ 20 μM Phy. The addition of 10 μM CPA alone did not appear to alter the 2 nm BM displacement threshold, but it enhanced and prolonged the effect of ACh suppression on BM displacement (Fig. 4A). The duration of 4.25 ± 0.82 minutes ACh suppression was increased to between 8 and 10 minutes (n = 4) and the level of the suppression increased from 24.2 ± 7.0 dB to between 42 and 45 dB (n = 4) in the presence of 10 mM CPA.

3.5 *Ryanodine and TMB-8 block the effect of ACh on BM displacement*

At micromolar concentrations, the plant alkaloid, ryanodine, blocks intracellular Ca^{2+} channels which mobilise Ca^{2+} from intracellular stores[10]. When the scala tympani was first perfused with 100 μM ACh/ 20 μM Phy, the 2 nm displacement BM threshold was increased by up to 30 dB SPL for about 4.5 min. When the experiment was repeated with 100 μM ryanodine added to the test solution, the 2 nm displacement threshold was not altered but the suppressive effect of the combination of 100 μM ACh/ 20 μM Phy on BM displacement was irreversibly blocked (Fig. 4B).

Similar, but reversible effects (Fig. 4C) were obtained by perfusing the scala tympani with 100μM TMB-8 [8-(N,N-diethylamino)octyl-3,4,5-trimethoxybenzoate], which has been reported to block the release of Ca^{2+} from intracellular stores in smooth muscle[11].

4 Conclusion

ACh perfusion of the scala tympani mimics the effects of OCB stimulation on tone-evoked displacements of the BM by greatly reducing the compressive nonlinearity of the displacement-level functions to tones around the CF. Results presented here support the hypothesis that the post-synaptic action of the OCB on OHCs is calcium dependent and that OCB stimulation causes an ACh-induced influx of Ca^{2+} into the OHCs. The suppressive effects on BM displacement of scala tympani perfusion with ACh appears to be mediated through Ca^{2+}-induced Ca^{2+} release from intracellular stores and may be similar to the "slow effect" of OCB stimulation[12].

Acknowledgements

We thank James Hartley for designing and constructing electronic equipment. Supported by grants from the Medical Research Council and Hearing Research Trust. E. Murugasu is a recipient of a Lee Kuan Yew Scholarship fund and a Burghard Fellowship from the Royal College of Surgeons.

References

1. Wiederhold, M.L. (1986) Physiology of the olivocochlear system, In: *Neurobiology of Hearing,* ed. R.A. Altschuler et al., (Raven, New York) pp. 349-371.

2. Murugasu, E. and Russell, I.J. (1996). The effect of efferent stimulation on basilar membrane displacement in the basal turn of the guinea pig cochlea, *J. Neurosci.* **16** 325-332.

3. Brown, M.C., Nuttal, A.L. and Masta, R.I. (1983) Intracellular recordings from cochlea inner hair cells: effect of stimulating the crossed olivocochlear efferents, *Science* **222** 69-72.

4. Wiederhold, M.L. and Kiang, N.Y.S (1970) Effects of electric stimulation of the crossed olivocohlear bundle on single auditory-nerve fibres in the cat, *J. Acoust. Soc. Am.* **48** 950-965.

5. Eybalin, M. (1993) Neurotransmitters and neuromodulators of the mammalian cochlea, *Physiol. Rev.* **73** 309-373.

6. Murugasu, E. and Russell, I.J. (1996). The role of calcium on the effects of intracochlear acetylcholine perfusion on basilar membrane displacement in the basal turn of the guinea pig cochlea, *Auditory. Neurosci.* (in press).

7. Housley, G.D. and Ashmore, J.F. (1991) Direct measurement of the action of acetylcholine on isolated outer hair cells of the guinea pig cochlea, *Proc. R. Soc. Lond. B.* **244** 161-167

8. Evans, M. (1996) Acetycholine activates two currents in guinea-pig outer hair cells, *J. Physiol. (Lond)* **491** 563-578.

9. Seidler, N.W., Jona, I., Vegh, M. and Martonosi, A. (1989) Cyclopiazonic acid is a specific inhibitor of calcium-ATPase of sarcoplasmic reticulum, *J. Biol. Chem.* **264** 17816-17823.

10. Tsai, T.D. and Barish, M.E. (1995) Imaging of caffeine-inducible release of intracellular calcium in cultured embryonic mouse telencephalic neurons, *J. Neurobiol.* **27** 252-265.

11. Malagodi, M.and Chiou, C.Y. (1974) Pharmacological evaluation of a new calcium antagonist, 8-(N,N-diethylamino) octyl 3,4,5-trimethoxybenzoate hydrochloride (TMB-8): Studies in smooth muscle, *Eur. J. Pharmacol.* **27** 25-33.

12. Sridhar TS, Liberman MC, Brown MC, Sewell WF (1995) A novel cholinergic "slow effect" of efferent stimulation on cochlear potentials in the guinea pig. *J Neurosci.* **15** 3667-3678.

EFFERENT INHIBITION AS A FUNCTION OF EFFERENT STIMULATION PARAMETERS AND SOUND FREQUENCY: TESTING THE OHC-SHUNT HYPOTHESIS

J.J. GUINAN JR.

Eaton-Peabody Laboratory, Massachusetts Eye and Ear Infirmary,
243 Charles Street, Boston, MA 02114, USA
jjg@epl.meei.harvard.edu

It is widely believed that outer-hair-cell (OHC) fast motility acts to amplify basilar membrane motion. Since OHC fast motility is controlled by the voltage across the OHC membrane, efferent synapses may inhibit by shunting OHC receptor currents thereby reducing receptor voltages and OHC motion. For such a shunt to produce substantial reductions in the receptor voltage, the OHC synaptic conductance must exceed the OHC non-synaptic admittance which increases approximately in proportion to frequency due to the OHC membrane capacitance. This prediction was tested in anesthetized cats by measuring the inhibition produced by stimulation of medial efferents on tone-pip-evoked compound action potentials (CAPs). For a given shock rate, the shock level which produced a criterion CAP reduction increased dramatically with sound frequency for two cats, but on a third cat, it increased only for low shock rates. Thus, most of the data are consistent with the OHC-shunt hypothesis. In addition, the data provide a fundamentally new view of the parametric dependence of efferent inhibition that is not consistent the current view (obtained from experiments using clicks) that the growth of efferent inhibition with increased efferent firing is independent of sound frequency.

1 Introduction

There is considerable evidence that medial efferents inhibit auditory-nerve responses at low sound levels by reducing basilar-membrane motion.[5,14] At low sound levels, the motion of the basilar membrane is thought to be increased by an active process involving fast motility in outer hair cells (OHCs), a process termed the "cochlear amplifier".[2] Medial efferents form large synapses on OHCs that seem ideally situated to modify the action of OHCs, thereby decreasing the gain of the cochlear amplifier and inhibiting auditory-nerve responses.[9]

Perhaps the simplest way that medial efferents might reduce the gain of the cochlear amplifier is by shunting OHC receptor currents. OHC fast motility is controlled by the OHC membrane voltage[19] so that shunting OHC receptor currents would reduce the receptor potentials, the motion response and, ultimately, the gain of the cochlear amplifier. However, at frequencies above the OHC membrane cut-off frequency (which is <1 kHz[10,15]), the OHC ac receptor voltage is limited by the OHC membrane capacitance.[2,19] Thus, for a synaptic shunt to substantially reduce the receptor potential, the synaptic conductance must exceed the OHC non-synaptic admittance. At frequencies well above the OHC cut-off frequency, this admittance is mostly capacitative and increases approximately in proportion to frequency. Thus with the "OHC-shunt hypothesis," the efferent synaptic conductance must exceed a level that increases approximately in proportion to sound frequency.

Described here is a preliminary test of this prediction, with efferent synaptic drive changed by varying the efferent firing rate and the number of efferents which fire (i.e. by changing shock rate and shock level). The inhibition of tone-pip-evoked auditory-nerve compound action potentials (CAPs) was used to assay the efferent effect as a function of sound frequency.

2 Methods

In anesthetized cats, we activated medial efferents by stimulation with a midline electrode[8]. The inhibition of CAPs was measured with tone pips presented continuously at 10/s, and 1 sec bursts of efferent shocks delivered every 5 seconds. Shock timing was chosen so that shock artifacts did not obscure the CAP responses. CAP responses were averaged over 8-16 shock bursts during the one second before the shocks, and during the period of steady-state CAP inhibition (typically the last 0.5 sec of the shock burst). For each sound frequency, tone pips were presented at a sound level selected so that the maximum CAP inhibition was similar (60-90%) across frequency. To minimize the effects of differences in efferent innervation density and absolute efferent inhibition at different frequencies, at each frequency we used an efferent inhibition criterion which was 10% of the maximum efferent inhibition at that frequency. We also used test frequencies which straddled the peak of the efferent innervation density (which reaches a maximum at about 9 kHz [9,12]).

3 Results

Our results are preliminary and from only four cats, three with substantial amounts of data. Fig. 1 shows data from one cat and illustrates CAP inhibition with variation of efferent shock rate, shock level and sound frequency. These data show that the dependence of efferent inhibition on one parameter varied with the settings of the other parameters. For instance, increasing the shock rate reduced the shock level necessary to produce inhibition, i.e. when the efferents are firing at a higher rate, fewer efferents need to be excited to produce inhibition. This tradeoff suggests that the overall efferent drive must exceed some "threshold" level before producing substantial inhibition. Furthermore, the inhibition as a function of shock rate or shock level is a function of sound frequency. As sound frequency was increased, the dynamic ranges of the other variables decreased (Fig. 1, left).

The pattern of efferent inhibition in Fig. 1 is consistent with the prediction of the OHC-shunt hypothesis that the synaptic conductance must exceed a level that increases approximately in proportion to sound frequency. This is illustrated in Fig 1, right, which shows the shock level needed to achieve 10% of the maximum efferent-induced suppression of the CAP at each frequency. These data were obtained by interpolation from the curves at left. Fig. 1, right, shows that at higher sound frequencies, higher shock levels are needed to produce 10% inhibition, as predicted.

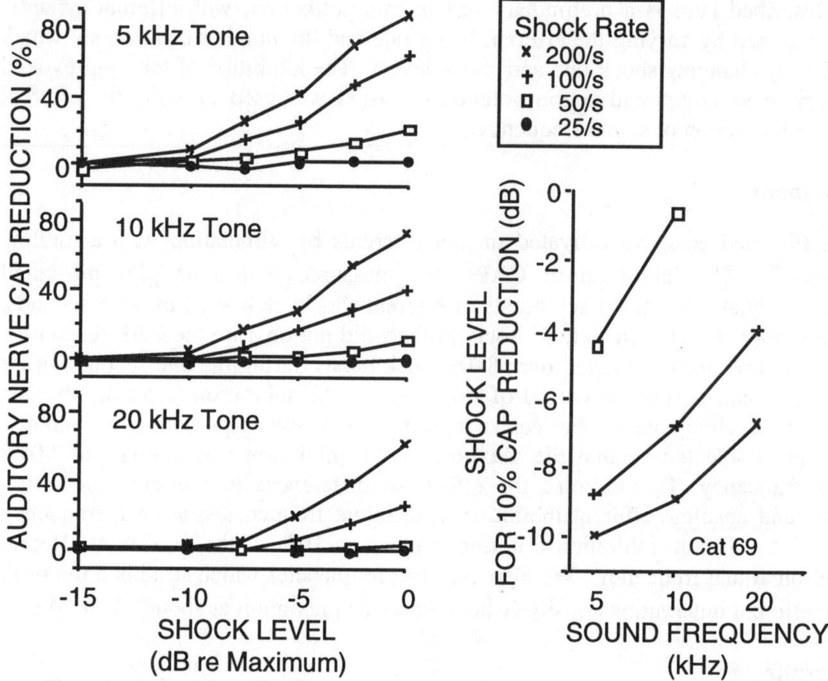

Figure 1: Suppression of auditory-nerve compound action potential (CAP) responses to tone pips as functions of shock level (left abscissa) and shock rate (symbol key in inset). Note that as sound frequency is increased, the effective dynamic ranges of shock rate and shock level contract. Right: The shock levels which produced 10% of the maximum efferent CAP suppression at each frequency. Symbols code different shock rates. Note that the 10% suppression level increases with frequency, as predicted by the shunt theory. The sound levels for the 5, 10 and 20 kHz tone bursts were: 55, 55 and 65 dB SPL.

The shock levels needed to reach the 10% suppression criterion in two other cats are shown in Fig. 2. Cat 78 (Fig. 2, right) shows a pattern similar to that in Fig. 1 with the shock levels for 10% suppression increasing rapidly with frequency over a wide range of frequencies. However, cat 77 (Fig. 2, left) shows this pattern only at the lowest shock rate. At shock rates of 100/s and 200/s, there was almost no change in the shock levels needed to achieve 10% suppression across three octaves of sound frequency. Thus, most, but not all, of our data show a pattern consistent with the predictions of the OHC-shunt hypothesis.

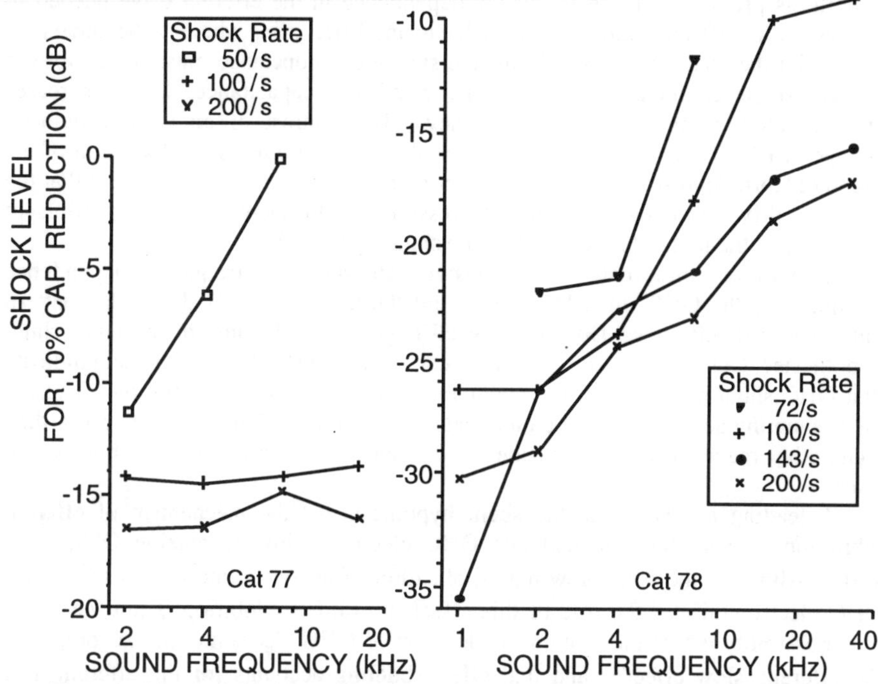

Figure 2: The shock levels which produced 10% of the maximum efferent CAP suppression at each frequency. For cat 77, the sound levels for the 2, 4, 8 and 16 kHz tone bursts were: 45, 46, 43 and 44 dB SPL. For cat 78, the sound levels for the 2, 4, 8, 16 and 32 kHz tone bursts were: 45, 45, 46, 35, 33 and 40 dB SPL.

4 Discussion

4.1 The OHC-shunt hypothesis

There are several hypotheses for how medial-efferents might lower the gain of the cochlear amplifier. (1) The OHC-shunt hypothesis. (2) Efferents modulate OHC electromotility by making OHCs less stiff.[3] (3) Efferents hyperpolarize OHCs and change the voltage-to-motion operating point, thereby producing less OHC motion.[17] (4) Efferents do not change OHC motion but they reduce the coupling of OHC motion back to the basilar membrane (e.g. by distorting the organ of Corti). (5) Efferents reduce OHC receptor potentials by the efferent-induced reduction of endocochlear potential (EP). There is evidence for this last hypothesis, but the EP change accounts for only a small fraction of efferent inhibition at low sound levels.[9,18,20] Medial efferents may also inhibit electrically,[9] but this effect probably has little influence on the cochlear amplifier or responses to low-level sounds.

A major difference between the shunt hypothesis and the others is that the shunt hypothesis predicts a strong frequency dependence in the efferent drive needed to produce a significant reduction of cochlear amplifier gain, whereas the others do not. With the OHC-shunt hypothesis, the synaptic conductance must come close to or exceed the conductance of the OHC membrane capacitance, which increases approximately in proportion to frequency. By contrast, if an efferent-induced change in EP, OHC electromotility, hyperpolarization of OHCs, or distortion of the organ of Corti depresses cochlear amplifier gain, there is no reason to expect that the synaptic drive necessary for this depression would increase in proportion to frequency at the high rate predicted by the shunt hypothesis.

Two of our three cats with extensive data show the frequency dependence predicted by the OHC-shunt hypothesis, but the third cat (#77) shows this pattern only at low shock rates. Does this partial negative result rule out the OHC-shunt hypothesis? Our interpretation is that for cat 77 at high shock rates, the data indicate that OHC shunting is the not the major mechanism of efferent inhibition. Thus, if OHC shunting accounts for the data in cats 69, 78 and in 77 at low shock rates, then some other mechanism must provide the efferent inhibition in cat 77 at high shock rates.

A leading alternative to the shunt hypothesis for the mechanism of efferent inhibition is that efferents modulate OHC electromotility by making OHCs less stiff.[3] Although the data show that application of acetylcholine (ACh) modulates OHC electromotility,[3] the role of this effect in efferent inhibition is not yet clear. One possibility is that the efferent modulation of OHC electromotility accounts for the efferent 'slow effect'[21] and that OHC shunting accounts for the efferent 'fast effect.' Two things favor this interpretation: (1) Only the slow effect appears to provide protection against acoustic trauma.[16] It seems reasonable that an efferent-induced change in OHC stiffness, which is a mechanical change expected to have effects at all sound levels, might affect damage from sounds over 100 dB SPL. In contrast, one would not expect efferent shunting, which acts by reducing the gain of the cochlear amplifier, to do much at sound levels over 100 dB SPL. (2) The slow effect requires tens of seconds to build up, and decays after about 5 minutes,[21] a time course compatible with the artificial application of ACh to OHCs. In contrast, the fast effect builds up in a fraction of a second as does the efferent-induced conductance change (shown by the efferent-induced changes in cochlear microphonic (CM) and endocochlear potential (EP)[8,9]). Thus, efferent modulation of OHC electromotility may produce the 'slow effect,' and existing data on OHC electromotility do not rule out the shunt hypothesis as producing the 'fast effect'.

All considered, do our data prove that the shunt hypothesis produces efferent fast inhibition? Despite some data not conforming, most of the data show a dramatic increase of the shock level that produces a criterion decrease in auditory-nerve CAP. Thus, most of the data are *consistent* with the shunt hypothesis producing fast efferent inhibition. It might be argued that ACh does not produce a large enough change in OHC conductance[1] for the shunt hypothesis to work.

However, the results of ACh application experiments are not conclusive because it is very difficult to artificially deliver an adequate concentration of ACh without accumulating significant desensitization before the peak of the response is reached. The efferent-induced increase CM at high frequencies[11] indicates that efferents do produce a conductance increase in the right range. Furthermore, to inhibit the cochlear amplifier, efferents may not need to significantly reduce OHC receptor potentials; it may be sufficient to change their phase. Changing receptor-potential phase only requires that the synaptic conductance reach a fraction of the resting OHC admittance. The increase in cochlear microphonic and the change in endocochlear potential produced by efferents provide strong evidence that medial efferents do produce a significant change in OHC conductance.[6,8,9,11] Thus, if OHC receptor potentials are important for the cochlear amplifier, then OHC shunting must play some role in efferent inhibition. Note that OHC shunting would affect OHC transmembrane voltage and have a similar frequency dependence whether the OHC transmembrane voltage originated from that OHC's receptor current or from currents external to the OHC.[2] All in all, available evidence is consistent with the view that the OHC transmembrane voltage controls the cochlear amplifier and cochlear sensitivity at low sound levels, and that medial-efferent-induced OHC shunting is an important factor in producing efferent inhibition at low sound levels.

A final question is the source of the results at high shock rates for cat 77 that do not appear to fit with the OHC-shunt hypothesis. If an efferent-induced change in OHC stiffness[3] can be produced fast enough (in a small fraction of a second), it would be a candidate for producing the cat 77 data at high shock rates. Alternately, several, perhaps all, of the possible means by which efferents might lower the gain of the cochlear amplifier (listed earlier) may play a role. It may be that the dominant mechanism depends on the experimental conditions.

4.2 The parametric dependence of efferent inhibition

Whatever the theoretical implications, our data indicate the need for a new conceptualization of the parametric dependence of medial efferent inhibition. Previous studies showed that efferent inhibition of click-evoked CAPs is a function of efferent shock rate with the greatest inhibition at 200-400 shocks/s.[4,6-8] It has generally been assumed that the inhibition versus shock rate function for clicks applies at all sound frequencies. Figs. 1 and 2 show that this assumption is not correct. There are clear differences in the parametric dependence of efferent inhibition across sound frequency. Considering the highest shock level in Fig. 1, for 5 kHz, 50 shocks/s produces 25% as much inhibition as 200 shocks/s, but for 20 kHz, 50 shocks/s produces only 9% as much inhibition as 200 shocks/s (Fig 1, left). Thus, these data provide a fundamentally new view that the dependence of efferent inhibition on efferent firing rate changes with sound frequency and the number of efferents firing.

A trade in effectiveness between the number of efferents which fire and their firing rate is not surprising, but the implications of such a trade have not been described previously. The data suggest that 50% of medial efferents firing at 200/s might produce the same effect as 100% of the efferents firing at 100/s. Preliminary data on the number of medial efferents recorded at the vestibulo-cochlear anastomosis which fire in response to midline shocks suggest that a response proportion of 50% of fibers firing is a realistic estimate for a typical experiment with "good" efferent stimulation.[13] It may be that shock rates as high as 200-400/s are required to produce large (20 dB) inhibitions because only a small fraction of efferents fire in response to shock stimulation. In contrast, binaural sounds, which are thought to evoke activity in all medial efferents,[9] may produce large efferent inhibitions at firing rates in the 100/s range because all medial efferents are firing. These ideas help to resolve the origin of the discrepancy between the rates found optimal with shock-excitation of efferents and the rates actually recorded from efferents.

Acknowledgments

This work was supported by grant 2 RO1-DC00235 from the National Institute on Deafness and other Communications Disorders, National Institutes of Health.

References

1. Ashmore, J.F. (1992) Mammalian hearing and the cellular mechanisms of the cochlear amplifier. in *Sensory Transduction*, eds. D.P. Corey and S.D. Roper (Rockefeller U. Press. New York) pp. 395–412.
2. Dallos, P., and Evans, B.N. (1995) High-frequency motility of outer hair cells and the cochlear amplifier, *Science* **267** 2006–2009.
3. Dallos, P., Sziklai, I., Lin, X., He, Z.Z., and Evans, B.N. (1996) Efferent control of cochlear mechanics: Outer hair cells. in: *Diversity in Auditory Mechanics Symposium.*
4. Desmedt, J.E. (1962) Auditory-evoked potentials from cochlea to cortex as influenced by activation of the efferent olivocochlear bundle, *J. Acoust. Soc. Am.* **34** 1478–1496.
5. Dolan, D.F., and Nuttall, A.L. (1994) Basilar membrane movement evoked by sound is altered by electrical stimulation of the crossed olivocochlear bundle, *Asso. Res. Otolaryngol. Abstr* **17** 89.
6. Fex, J. (1962) Auditory activity in centrifugal and centripetal cochlear fibers in cat, *Acta Physiol. Scand.* **55** 2–68.
7. Galambos, R. (1956) Suppression of auditory activity by stimulation of efferent fibers to the cochlea, *J. Neurophysiol.* **19** 424–437.
8. Gifford, M.L., and Guinan, J.J., Jr. (1987) Effects of electrical stimulation of medial olivocochlear neurons on ipsilateral and contralateral cochlear

responses, *Hearing Res.* **29** 179–194.

9. Guinan, J.J., Jr. (1996) The Physiology of Olivocochlear Efferents. in: *The Cochlea* , eds. P.J. Dallos, A.N. Popper, and R.R. Fay, New York: Springer-Verlag, pp 435–502.

10. Housley, G.D., and Ashmore, J.F. (1992) Ionic currents of outer hair cells isolated from the guinea pig cochlea. *J. Physiol.* **448** 73–98.

11. Kittrell, B.J., and Dalland, J.I. (1969) Frequency dependence of cochlear microphonic augmentation produced by olivo-cochlear bundle stimulation. *Laryngoscope* **79** 228–238.

12. Liberman, M.C., Dodds, L.W., and Pierce, S. (1990) Afferent and efferent innervation of the cat cochlea: quantitative analysis with light and electron microscopy, *J. Comp. Neurol.* **301** 443–460.

13. McCue, M.P., and Guinan, J.J., Jr. (unpublished).

14. Murugasu, E., and Russell, I.J. (1996) The effect of efferent stimulation on basilar membrane displacement in the basal turn of the guinea pig cochlea, *J. Neurosci.* **16** 325–332.

15. Preyer, S., Hemmert, W., Pfister, M., Zenner, H.-P., and Gummer, A.W. (1994) Frequency response of mature guinea-pig outer hair cells to stereociliary displacement, *Hearing Res.* **77** 116–124.

16. Reiter, E.R., and Liberman, M.C. (1995) Efferent-mediated protection from acoustic overexposure: Relation to "slow effects" of olivocochlear stimulation, *J. Neurophysiol.* **73** 506–514.

17. Roddy, J., Hubbard, A.E., Mountain, D.C., and Xue, S. (1994) Effects of electrical biasing on electrically-evoked otoacoustic emissions, *Hearing Res.* **73** 148–154.

18. Ruggero, M.A., and Rich, N.C. (1991) Furosemide alters organ of Corti mechanics: Evidence for feedback of outer hair cells upon the basilar membrane, *J. Neurosci.* **11** 1057–1067.

19. Santos-Sacchi, J., and Dilger, J.P. (1988) Whole cell currents and mechanical responses of isolated outer hair cells, *Hearing Res.* **35** 143–150.

20. Sewell, W.F. (1984) The effects of furosemide on the endocochlear potential and auditory-nerve fiber tuning curves in cats, *Hearing Res.* **14** 305–314.

21. Sridhar, T.S., Liberman, M.C., Brown, M.C., and Sewell, W.F. (1995) A novel cholinergic "slow effect" of olivocochlear stimulation on cochlear potentials in the guinea pig, *J. Neurosci.* **15** 3667–3678.

DOES ACTIVITY IN THE OLIVOCOCHLEAR BUNDLE AFFECT DEVELOPMENT OF THE AUDITORY PERIPHERY?

E.J. WALSH, J. MCGEE
Boys Town National Research Hospital
555 North 30th Street
Omaha, NE 68131 USA
walsh@boystown.org

The role of the olivocochlear bundle (OCB) during development, if any, is unknown. However, on the basis of findings made in experiments designed to address that question, a developmental blueprint implicating the OCB in cochlear development has emerged. In that plan, OCB fibers affiliated with the medial divisions make transient axosomatic contact with inner hair cells throughout much of the first two postnatal weeks of feline life, rhythmically modulating their output and, consequently, the discharge activity of neurons throughout the auditory neuraxis. We hypothesize that the coactivation if inner hair cells by OCB activity and sound stimulation, and the resulting oscillation of sensory signals resulting from that interaction, provides a functional basis for the selective formation of sensory cell-primary afferent synapses underlying the developmental refinement of tonotopy. On the basis of an as yet unknown trigger, medial OCB fibers subsequently "detach" from inner hair cells, establish axosomatic contacts with outer hair cells and, thereby, induce cytodifferentiation related to outer hair cell vitality, "energizing" the cochlear amplifier. This blueprint was derived from the combined results of several experiments generally designed to determine the role of the OCB in feline development. These included both OCB stimulation and lesion paradigms and employed standard extracellular recording techniques to study auditory nerve and cochlear nucleus neuronal responses to sound stimulation.

1. Introduction

Our first insight into the possibility that olivocochlear efferents may regulate cochlear transduction in a novel manner in immature mammals arose in the context of the rhythmic temporal discharge cadence produced by auditory nerve fibers (ANFs) in response to sound.[10] The property of response rhythmicity, the inability of immature auditory neurons to maintain a sustained steady-state response to a long-duration stimulus (>100 ms) and instead to discharge in periodic bursts, is universal in immature auditory neurons, occurring in over 80% of all ANFs and neurons thus far studied.[9-10] An example of responses produced by a rhythmically responding neuron recorded from the cochlear nuclear complex (CN) of a 6-day-old cat compared to one from an adult is shown in Fig. 1.

This response feature has been studied comprehensively, and has been shown to vary with stimulus level, but is independent of stimulus frequency.[10] Specifically, burst frequencies increase in direct proportion to level, increasing by as much as 8 Hz over a neuron's dynamic range. The frequency of bursting ranges between 5 and 15 Hz, with individual bursts lasting approximately 75 ms, although the duration of each burst, but not burst frequency, is highly variable in central neurons. The source of this conspicuous response feature, however, had never been investigated.

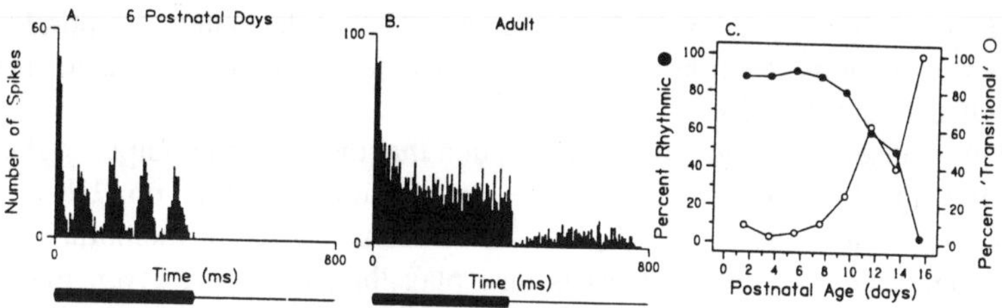

Figure 1: Peristimulus time histograms (PSTHs) obtained from a CN neuron of a 6 postnatal day old kitten (A) and from an adult (B) are shown. In C, the percentage of CN neurons responding rhythmically, and out of those the percentage which displayed rhythmicity at low sensation levels (SLs) and sustained steady-state responses at high SLs ('transitional') are plotted as a function of postnatal age.

In 1988, Walsh and McGee[10] hypothesized that efferents running in the OCB were the source of the rhythmicity, basing that conjecture on several observations, including the finding that the sound-elicited spike trains of individual efferent fibers recorded from adult cats were also rhythmic at relatively low, suprathreshold stimulation levels.[4] In addition, an abundance of anatomical data available at the time suggested that the OCB projections innervate the inner hair cell (IHC) region and not outer hair cells (OHCs) early in functional development (Fig. 2).[6] Moreover, at least a portion of the OCB innervation is directly to IHCs via axosomatic synapses, a circumstance that is essentially unknown in adults except, perhaps, in the apex of the cochlea; i.e., synaptic contacts between IHCs and efferents have not been described in other regions of the adult cochlea.

Spike train bursts dominate the temporal response profile of auditory neurons from birth through the 10th postnatal day (Fig. 1c), corresponding to the time interval that efferent innervation occurs. By the third postnatal week, adultlike

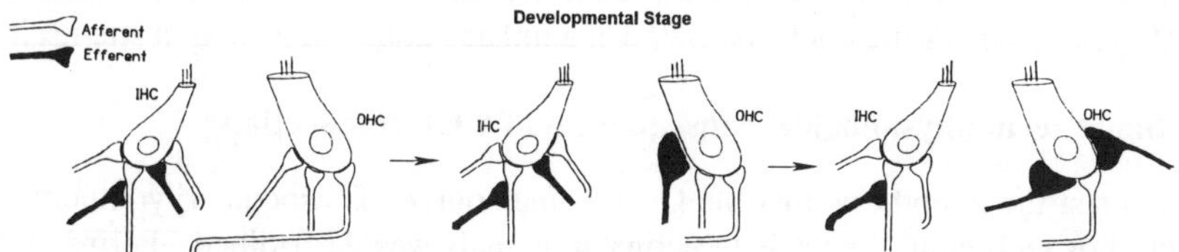

Figure 2: Schematic illustration is shown depicting the developmental sequence of afferent and efferent innervation of IHCs and OHCs. These patterns were generated from descriptions reported by Pujol et al.[6] for the kitten.

sustained steady-state responses are uniformly observed in ANFs and CN neurons that respond tonically. Toward the middle of the second postnatal week, neurons typically enter a transitional stage, during which low level, suprathreshold stimulation produces rhythmic responses, but higher level stimulation results in sustained steady-state temporal firing patterns. Level-dependent temporal response features of auditory neurons at this developmental stage are similar to those from adult OCB fibers (Fig. 3).

These observations led to the proposition that the rhythmic output of the OCB is delivered to the afferent system via axosomatic contacts on IHCs, directly modulating their output. The modulation of primary afferent membrane potentials via axodendritic efferent contacts is also plausible; however, given that the vast

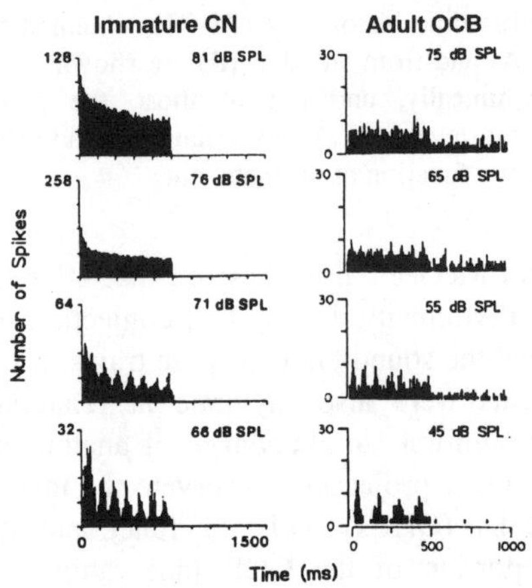

Figure 3: PSTHs obtained at several sound levels are shown for a CN neuron recorded from a 13-day-old kitten (left column) and for an OCB fiber recorded from an adult cat (right column). Tonebursts used to construct PSTHs on the left were 750 ms in duration, whereas those on the right were 500 ms. PSTHs in the left column are adapted from Walsh & McGee[10] and in the right column from Liberman & Brown.[4]

majority of afferent responses are rhythmic early in development and that rhythmic responses never occur among ANFs of adult animals, most of which are innervated via efferent axodendritic contacts, we posit a linkage at the transduction site itself.

2. Short-term physiological consequences of OCB transection

To test the hypothesis that the OCB is the source of response rhythmicity, the effect(s) of sectioning the OCB in perinatal animals was determined. Perinatal cats ranging in age from 5-9 postnatal days of age were anesthetized with sodium pentobarbital and a standard craniectomy into the posterior fossa allowed a portion of the cerebellum to be removed, visualizing both the floor of the fourth ventricle and the auditory nerve/cochlear nuclear complex. Standard extracellular recording techniques were used to record spike activity from ANFs and CN neurons. The temporal firing patterns in response to acoustic stimulation were determined for a sample of neurons, and if all neurons responded rhythmically, an incision, roughly 2 mm deep, was made on the midline of the fourth ventricle floor, extending from its most anterior aspect to beyond the facial genu posteriorly. Following determination of the outcome of the midline cut, an off-midline lesion was made unilaterally along the same longitudinal range, but with the knife angled 45° relative to the brainstem floor at the level of the sulcus limitans. In animals with midline lesions, only crossing fibers of the OCB are interrupted, affecting principally, but not entirely, the fibers from the MOC division. Incisions made sufficiently lateral to the midline, however, interrupt the entire OCB projection to one ear.

Temporal response patterns were altered by midline lesions, however, rhythmicity was only partially affected. A portion of neurons encountered after the transection produced sustained responses, although most units continued to respond rhythmically (Fig. 4). In most rhythmically responding neurons with an intact OCB, the degree of discharge rate modulation in PSTHs approaches 100%. Following midline lesions, there was a notable reduction in the depth of modulation. This result is consistent with the idea that the OCB influence is attenuated, but not eliminated under conditions of partial de-efferentation.

After a brief recording period following a midline lesion, an off-midline lesion designed to transect the entire bundle was attempted. In every case thus far studied, complete interruption of the bundle resulted in the complete loss of rhythmicity (Fig. 5). That is, all neurons encountered following an off-midline lesion, exhibited PSTHs to long-duration tonebursts that were similar to adult responses. Identical results were obtained by producing an off-midline lesion alone. These results support the hypothesis that the OCB causes the bursting spike train observed in immature animals.

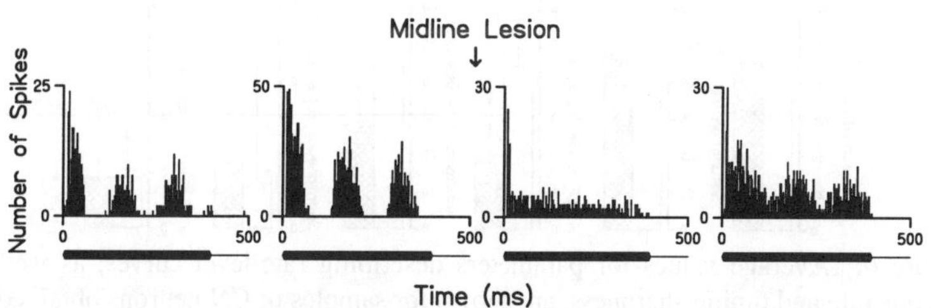

Figure 4: PSTHs taken before and after a midline lesion was made at the floor of the fourth ventricle in a 6-day-old animal are shown. Each panel represents responses from different CN neurons.

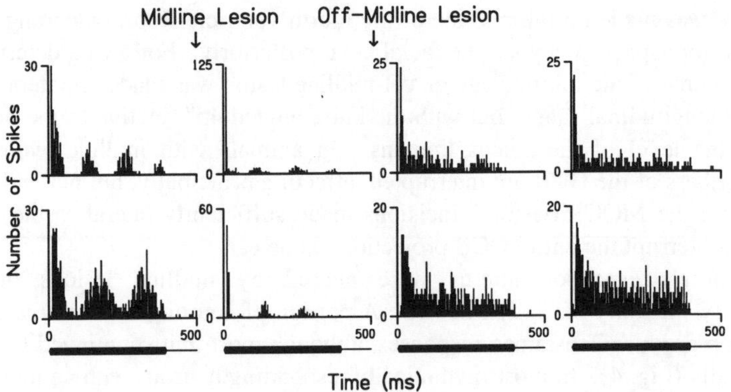

Figure 5: PSTHs from two 6-day-old animals (separate rows) obtained before and after a midline lesion, and following a second lesion made ipsilateral to the recording site ("off-midline") are shown. Each panel represents responses from different CN neurons.

In addition to the abolition of response rhythmicity, the average maximum discharge rate of neurons encountered in the post-lesion period was lower than that of the pre-lesion sample (Fig. 6). Similarly, mean rate-level slope decreased as a consequence of the lesion, whereas average dynamic range did not change. These results suggest that overall excitation within the afferent auditory system was diminished following OCB interruption, a finding that is consistent with a decrease in the excitatory drive onto IHCs and the resulting reduction of their output. Thresholds to acoustic stimuli were typically unchanged, indicating that generalized trauma was not a factor associated with the consequences of brainstem lesions.

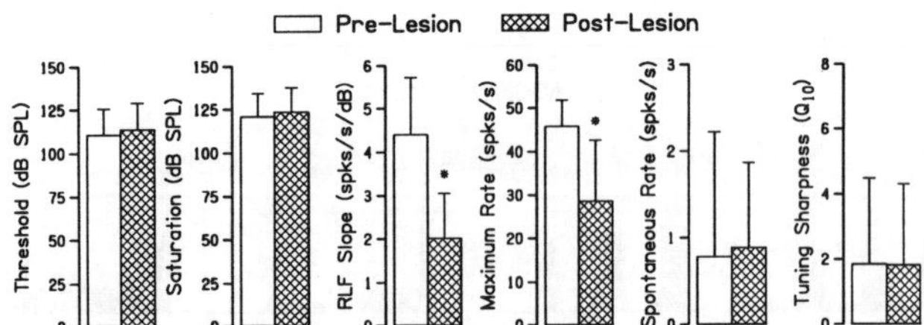

Figure 6: Average values for parameters describing rate-level curves, as well as for spontaneous rate and tuning sharpness, are shown for samples of CN neurons obtained before lesioning and following complete section of the OCB (off-midline incision). Standard deviations are indicated and asterisks identify pre- and post-lesion results which are statistically different based on a student's t-test ($p < 0.001$).

3. Discussion

Based on the results of experiments designed to assess the immediate consequences of OCB transection, it is evident that efferent effects on cochlear output are unique early in the postnatal life of cats. However, the outcome raises the obvious question of whether or not the rhythmic quality of sound driven spike trains are epiphenomenal or play a role in the development of the system or in the processing of information.

We subscribe to the view that OCB generated rhythms are important developmental factors that may set up local cues for synapse refinement in circuits throughout the auditory neuraxis (rhythmic activity is expressed ubiquitously throughout the auditory system). The view is drawn, in part, from similarities between the stimulated bursting of auditory neurons and spontaneous bursting patterns thought to promote synapse refinement in the visual system.[7] We argue that discharge bursts evident in responses of ANFs and central auditory neurons reflect cueing signals as in the eye, and that synapse consolidation, possibly relevant to the refinement of tonotopic frequency-space maps, occur as the cochlea acquires function sequentially along a well characterized developmental gradient that sweeps along its longitudinal axis. In this model, this "wave" of cochlear development substitutes for the waves of spontaneous discharges that are necessary for local synapse refinement in the developing eye.

Supporting evidence for this view includes the observation that supernumerary dendrites have been detected in neonatal animals,[5] and that ANF tuning curves from animals chronically deprived of cochlear efferents since near the time of birth are never as sharply tuned as the most frequency selective fibers found in control animals.

Although not the focus of this report, we have examined the physiology of ANFs in a set of adult animals that were de-efferented as neonates and were reared in the absence of the OCB influence. Only cases with complete or nearly complete loss of tunnel crossing fibers are considered in this review. Surgical and transection procedures followed in chronic de-efferentation studies are detailed in Walsh, McGee & Liberman.[12]

In completely, or nearly completely de-efferented ears, it appears that spontaneous discharge rates are diminished, although the outcomes are highly variable from animal to animal, possibly reflecting variable degrees of interruption of the LOC system, and possibly the uncrossed MOC system. Thresholds at characteristic frequency (CF) are elevated and tuning curves are generally abnormal, occasionally exhibiting hypersensitive tails and low tip-to-tail ratios, and there is a diminished tendency to encounter ANFs in the mid-CF range (Fig. 7). We interpret the abnormalities involving tuning curve tip-to-tail ratios and thresholds as a failure of the OCB system to influence the development of active processes underlying cochlear amplification. In other words, the olivocochlear system appears to play a critical role in the development of the OHC system.

We raise the discussion of experiments on chronically de-efferented animals to address the question, does the interruption of OCB fibers projecting to IHCs affect the refinement of synapses between IHCs and primary afferent dendrites; i.e., eliminating spike train bursts may eliminate dendritic pruning, leaving supernumerary branches in contact with multiple sensory cells. While the anatomical studies that could answer this question directly are underway, results from ANF recordings support the contention. Specifically, when sharpness of

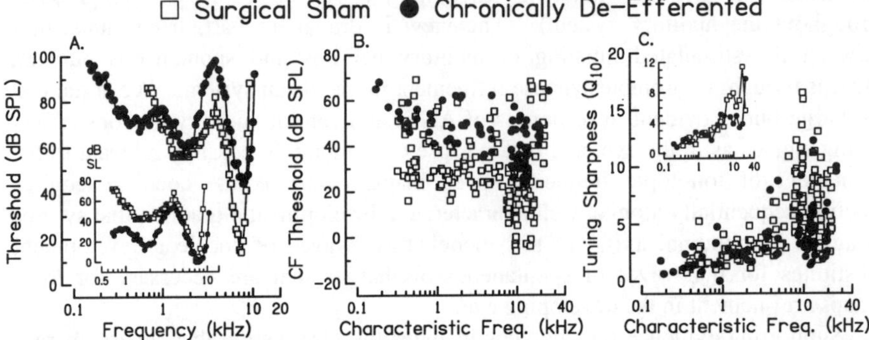

Figure 7: A: An example of a FTC recorded from an ANF from an animal that was chronically de-efferented (off-midline lesion only) during development (surgery was performed at 4 postnatal days [pnd] and recordings conducted at 7.7 postnatal months) is compared to one obtained from a surgical sham (surgery at 14 pnd and recordings at 15 months). In the inset, FTCs are normalized relative to each fiber's CF threshold. CF thresholds (B) and tuning sharpness (C) are plotted as a function of characteristic frequency for an animal that was reared following lesions made at both the midline and laterally at the floor of the fourth ventricle on 3 pnd (recordings made at 6.6 months). Results from a surgical sham are shown for comparison (surgery at 4 pnd and recordings at 12.7 months). Corresponding averages of tuning sharpness, computed every 0.3 octaves, are shown in the inset in C.

tuning is considered, ANFs from chronically-lesioned animals, while not significantly different on average, do not reach the high degrees of tuning observed in ANFs from normal animals or surgical shams (Fig. 7c). This outcome is exactly what one would expect if dendritic fields were not pruned from a span of several IHCs to one, as in the adult; i.e., ANFs connected to multiple IHCs would be less frequency selective, but not dramatically so. However, an alternative possibility requires consideration. If efferents affect the differentiation and or expression of OHC motility, and if cochlear amplification is diminished as a long-term consequence of OCB transection in neonates, ANF frequency-selectivity in lesioned animals may be diminished as well. It is also possible that acoustic trauma is a factor relating to results observed in these studies, but such an explanation is unlikely based on results of chronic de-efferentation in adults.[3] Experiments designed to consider these possibilities are underway.

Thus, we conclude that OCB efferents do indeed play a "critical" role in the development of peripheral auditory function, possibly both at the level of IHCs and OHCs. Furthermore, we suggest that their role at IHCs is the refinement of synapses and at OHCs the development of some aspect of cochlear amplification.

Additional support for the view that the OCB functions uniquely early in development is based on the effects of contralateral acoustic stimulation (CAS) on cochlear output.[2] CAS does not produce obvious changes in cochlear output during the first 7 to 10 postnatal days. These results, combined with the fact that acute de-efferentation in perinatal animals does alter the response properties of auditory neurons to ipsilateral stimulation, suggest that the ipsilaterally driven OCB path is active in neonates, but that input from the contralateral ear, if present, is insufficient to exert additional, detectable effects on cochlear output.

At about the end of the first postnatal week, CAS both suppresses and enhances evoked activity in ANFs, as in adults.However, between 13-23 postnatal days, it appears that CAS induced enhancement of cochlear output is more common than it is in adults. We propose that this phenomenon represents a transitional period, during which MOC fibers switch their physiological allegiance from IHCs to OHCs.

In summary, we propose the following developmental scheme: At birth, MOC fibers invade the cochlea and innervate IHCs through axosomatic contacts. The consequence of normal transduction and rhythmic efferent coactivation of IHC conductances results in a temporally modulated signal (Fig. 8) that is important in generating local cues that are used to refine synapses between IHCs and primary afferent dendrites. This process occurs as a gradient along the length of the cochlea and lasts for approximately two postnatal weeks.

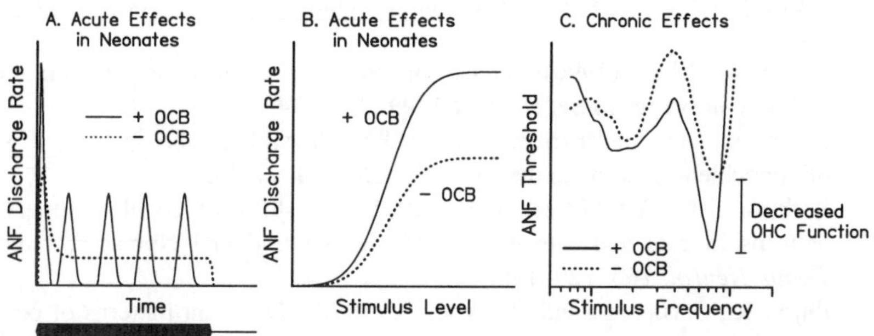

Figure 8: Schematics are shown summarizing the acute effects of complete OCB lesions on responses in neonatal animals (A, B) and the chronic effects of OCB lesions during development (C).

During the next, overlapping developmental stage, as LOC fibers descend to innervate the neuropil of primary afferents[8], MOC fibers shift their physiological actions from IHCs to OHCs. The explicit role of the OCB at this stage of development is unclear. Based on the work of He et al.,[1] OHCs do not require continual OCB contact to develop fast contractility, the motor for active mechanics. However, the OCB may induce OHC differentiation enabling the complete expression of the mechanisms responsible for cochlear amplification, after which its presence may no longer be required.

Acknowledgments

The authors would like to acknowledge the efforts of Ms. J. Lackey, a graduate student, and Dr. S. McFadden, a postdoctoral fellow, both of whom participated in a subset of experiments reported here. We would also like to acknowledge an ongoing collaboration to study the consequence of chronic de-efferentation with Dr. M. C. Liberman, a project to which we allude in this review. We also express deep gratitude to R. Felner, B. Flegas, J. Jenkins, M. Kliment, T. Krivohlavek, J. Lackey, Y. Liu, T. Molloy, L. Song and Y. Zhang for participating in the dedicated, intensive postsurgical care of lesioned animals. Their extraordinary efforts literally made the research on chronically de-efferented animals possible. The effects of acute de-efferentation were reported at the annual meeting of the Society for Neuroscience.[11] This research was supported by grant number 3 P01 DC00215 from NIH-NIDCD.

References

1. He, D.Z.Z., Lin, X., and Dallos, P. (1996) Full expression of outer hair cell motility during ontogeny does not require the influence of innervation, *Assoc. Res. Otolaryngol. Abstr.* **19** 88.
2. Jenkins, J.J., McGee, J. and Walsh, E.J. (1993) Developmental changes of auditory nerve responses to efferent stimulation, *Soc. Neurosci. Abstr.* **23(1)** 34.
3. Liberman, M.C. (1990) Effects of chronic cochlear de-efferentation on auditory-nerve response. *Hear. Res.* **49** 209-224.
4. Liberman, M.C. and Brown, M.C. (1986) Physiology and anatomy of single olivocochlear neurons in the cat, *Hear. Res.* **24** 17-36.
5. Perkins, R.E. and Morest, D.K. (1975) A study of cochlear innervation patterns in cats and rats with the Golgi method and Nomarski optics, *J. Comp. Neurol.* **163** 129–158.
6. Pujol, R., Carlier, E. and Devigne, C. (1978) Different patterns of cochlear innervation during the development of the kitten, *J. Comp. Neurol.* **177** 529–536.

7. Shatz, C.J. (1994) Role for spontaneous neural activity in the patterning of connections between retina and LGN during visual system development, Int. *J. Devl. Neurosci.* **12(6)** 531–546.

8. Simmons, D.D., Manson-Gieseke, L., Hendrix, T.W. and McCarter, S. (1990) Reconstructions of efferent fibers in the postnatal hamster cochlea, *Hear. Res.* **49** 127–140.

9. Walsh, E.J. and McGee, J. (1987) Postnatal development of auditory nerve and cochlear nucleus neuronal responses in kittens, *Hear. Res.* **28** 97–116.

10. Walsh, E.J. and McGee, J. (1988) Rhythmic discharge properties of caudal cochlear nucleus neurons during postnatal development in cats, *Hear. Res.* **36** 233–248.

11. Walsh, E.J., McGee, J. and Lackey, J. (1995) Acute lesions of the olivocochlear bundle eliminate sound-evoked discharge rhythmicity of immature auditory neurons, *Soc. Neurosci. Abstr.* **21(1)** 127.

12. Walsh, E.J., McGee, J. and Liberman, M.C. (1996) The long-term physiological consequences of sectioning the olivocochlear bundle in neonatal cats, (in preparation).

SCALA MEDIA VOLTAGE RESPONSES TO SINUSOIDAL CURRENT STIMULATION

S. XUE

Division of Otolaryngology-HNS, Box 3550
Duke University Medical Center
Durham, NC 27710, USA
sx@dukehrl.mc.duke.edu

Voltage responses to sinusoidal current injection were measured in the second turn scala media (SM) and in the round window (RW) of the gerbil cochlea. Frequency responses of the recording electrode and the amplifier were measured *in situ*, and the results were used to correct the recorded voltage responses. The differential SM-RW voltage response was computed digitally. The results of the experiments, agreeing with classical measurements of cochlear electroanatomy, showed low-frequency input impedance of about 3 kΩ for the second turn SM. The SM-RW voltage response at high frequency, however, was somewhat unexpected. Very little magnitude attenuation and phase lag occurred when the frequency of the injected current went up to 39 kHz. Thus, the one-dimensional cable model used to describe electrical properties of the SM did not fit the data in this study when commonly accepted parameters were used for the model.

1 Introduction

In studies of electrically-evoked otoacoustic emissions and basilar membrane motion, a fundamental question has been, *what voltage responses are evoked by sinusoidal current injected into the scala media (SM) of the cochlea?* These responses determine the electrical input to the outer hair cells, which presumably produce motion through electrical-to-mechanical transduction. With acoustic stimulation to the cochlea, the receptor current of the hair cells, although different from the injected current in scale and distribution, sums up and produces a measurable potential (cochlear microphonic) in the SM.   Dallos and Evans[1] proposed that the extracellular potential generated by the excited hair cells could, in turn, provide the driving force for the high-frequency motility of the outer hair cells. This mechanism is subject to the generation of the SM voltage by the excited hair cells and the coupling between the driving and driven outer hair cells. With either electrical or acoustic stimulation, the voltage responses in the SM are governed by the electrical properties of the scalae, i.e., the electroanatomy of the cochlea.

Since the work of von Békésy[2], a number of studies, both experimental and theoretical, have focused on the cochlear electroanatomy.[3-5] Few classical experimental studies, however, considered the reactive elements of the cochlea and the frequency response of the SM in the high frequency range that interests us today. The purpose of this study is twofold: to measure, directly, the SM voltage responses to sinusoidal current injection in the gerbil cochlea, thereby providing a reference basis for the studies involving current injection into the SM; and to use these measurements, comparing them to the cable model predications, to gain further insight into the cochlear electroanatomy.

2   Methods

Figure 1 shows the experimental setup. Two micropipettes were introduced into the SM at the second turn of the gerbil cochlea. Typical endocochlear potentials measured with the electrodes were between 85 and 90 mV. The distance between the two electrodes varied among experimental animals (0.2–0.8 mm). The electrodes were shielded to a point near the tips. Sinusoidal current (10–20 µA peak) was injected into the SM via the basal electrode, and SM voltage responses were recorded from the other electrode. Electrical pickup between the electrodes was examined by lifting the stimulating electrode just off the cochlear surface while maintaining the driving voltage command (60 V) to the electrode.

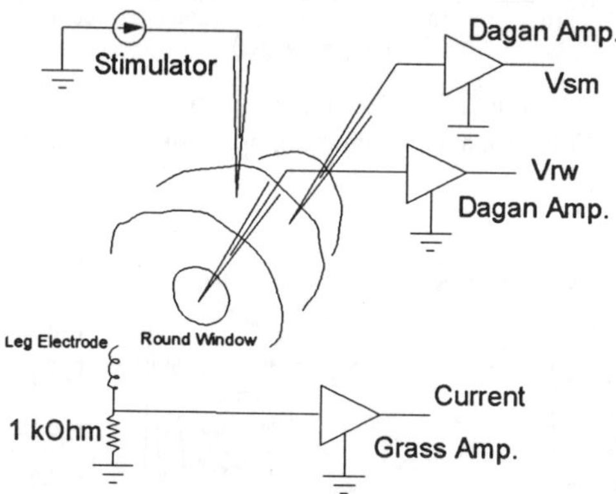

Fig. 1. Experimental Setup. Vsm: scala media voltage; Vrw: round window voltage.

The pickup was found to be very small. The animal was electrically isolated from the recording and stimulating grounds by plastic ear bars and mouth clamp. An *in situ* calibration of the frequency response of the recording electrode and the amplifier was performed. The calibration method was similar to that used by Baden-Kristensen and Weiss.[6] While the stimulating electrode was disconnected, a voltage command signal (1V peak) was applied to the leg electrode. This command voltage and the voltage recorded by the electrode were compared to obtain the frequency-response calibration of the electrode. The recording system with capacitance compensation typically had a cutoff frequency of 20–30 kHz. After the SM voltage measurement, the recording electrode was moved to the round window, and the voltage response in the round window was then measured. The frequency response of the current-monitoring amplifier was also characterized and used to correct the current recording. The recorded voltage responses from the SM and the round window were normalized by the simultaneously sampled current and were corrected according to the frequency response of the electrode. Differential SM-round window (SM-RW) voltage responses were then computed digitally by subtracting the two voltage responses. The data were compared with the predictions of a one-dimensional cable model of the SM[7].

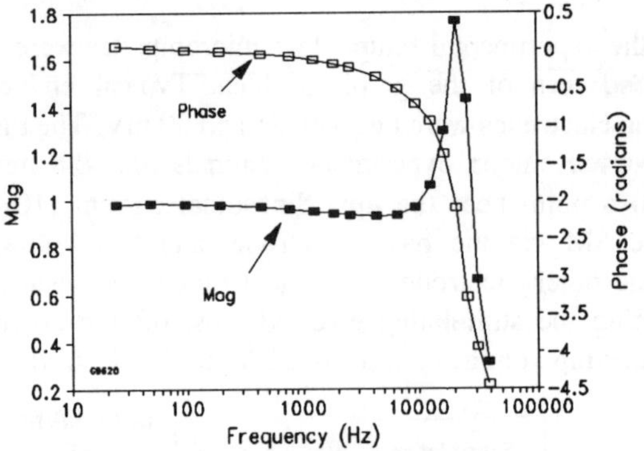

Figure 2: SM electrode frequency response.
Filled squares: magnitude; open squares: phase.

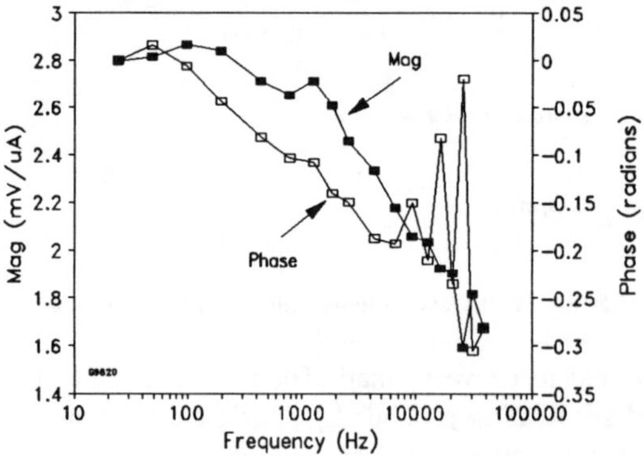

Figure 3: SM-RW differential voltage response.
Filled squares: Magnitude; open squares: phase.

3   Results

Figure 2 shows the frequency-response calibration of the recording electrode in the SM. A similar calibration was also seen when the recording electrode was moved to the round window. Figure 3 shows the SM-RW differential voltage response. In this experiment, the distance between the current injecting electrode and the voltage measuring electrode was 0.7 mm. In all animals examined, the low frequency magnitude response was between 2.5 and 3.5 mV/μA. These values gave an effective SM resistance of about 3–4 kΩ, depending on the assumptions about the space constants of the SM (*see Discussion*). It is evident that the SM voltage evoked at high frequency decreased very little from that at low frequency, and the phase lag was also very small. This is a quite unexpected result since the SM has often been viewed as a simple RC lowpass filter with a cutoff frequency around 1 kHz. At frequencies higher than 10 kHz, the magnitude and phase responses contained more noise, indicating a limitation of the method used to obtain the SM-RW differential voltage response.

4 Discussion

The SM has been modeled as an electrical cable (core-conductor) because of its

$$|V(x, j\omega)| = \frac{r_a I_0 \lambda}{2(1+\omega^2 \tau^2)^{\frac{1}{4}}} \, e^{-\frac{x}{\lambda}\sqrt{\frac{\sqrt{1+\omega^2\tau^2}+1}{2}}}$$

$$\angle V(x, j\omega) = -\frac{x}{\lambda}\sqrt{\frac{\sqrt{1+\omega^2\tau^2}-1}{2}} - \frac{1}{2}\tan^{-1}(\omega\tau)$$

anatomy. The frequency response equations derived from such a model[7] are
where I_0 is the amplitude of the injected current, ω is the angular frequency of the current, x is the distance from the current injection site, λ is the space constant, τ is the time constant, and r_a is the intracellular resistance per unit length of cable.

Using reasonable parameters from the literature, we were unable to make the model fit the data. Because of the small magnitude attenuation and phase lag with increasing frequency, the best fit between the model results and the data would require the use of a very small time constant. Figure 4 shows a result of the model using commonly accepted parameters, compared to the data. It is clear that only in the low frequency region does the model fit the data well.

It is possible that the problem could arise from the data collection, as the experiments were technically quite challenging and prone to many potential pitfalls. In particular, the voltage measurements in the SM and RW were not done simultaneously; therefore any impedance change in an animal's body or in the ground electrode could contribute to the measured differential voltage responses. The problem could also be entirely different, i.e., the cable model may not describe the SM voltage response properties qualitatively under the differential recording scheme used in these experiments. It was assumed that the conductance of the combined scala tympani (ST) and scala vestibuli (SV) was much larger than that of the SM, so that the voltage in the perilymphatic space was more or less uniform and at the electrical ground. This assumption should not be too far off, at least for low frequencies, if we consider some of the classical findings of cochlear electroanatomy[4] where the resistances from the SM to ST and SV were much larger than those connecting the latter two scalae to the blood vessel system within the cochlea (the ground). However, at high frequency when capacitive conductances need to be considered, this assumption may not be valid. Another implied assumption is that the SM voltage responses are linear to levels of injected current when the voltage responses are normalized to current to compute the SM-RW differential response. Because of the voltage-dependent conductances in the hair cells and other nonlinear electrical properties, the linear assumption, when used, may cause significant errors in data, especially when the current level is not stable during the data collection procedures.

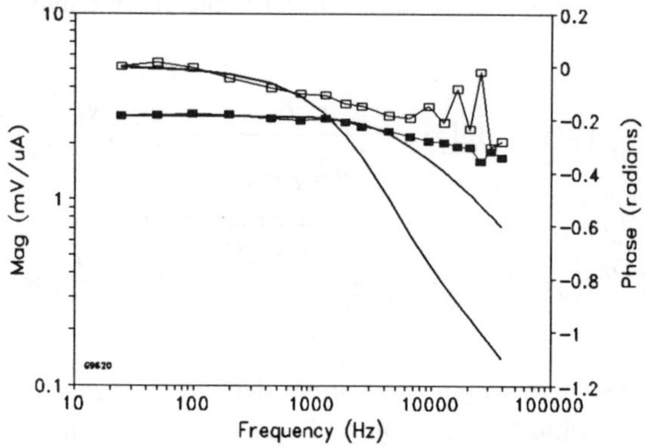

Figure 4: Comparison of the data shown in Figure 3 with the one-dimensional cable model. Filled squares: magnitude; open squares: phase. The model parameters: $\tau = 0.04$ ms, $\lambda = 4.0$ mm, x =0.7 mm (measured), Ra = 1.67 kΩ/mm.

The present study differed from the classical measurements of the electrical properties of the SM in two ways: (1) sinusoidal stimulation was used instead of square pulses; (2) an explicit cable model and its frequency responses were used to fit the data. Do these methods enable better estimation of the space and time constants of the SM space and make it possible to predict the spatial summation of SM potentials? Preliminary results from these experiments do not seem sufficient for these goals. The SM voltage measurement obtained from a single distance from the stimulating electrode yielded good clues to what the time constant of the SM could be, but the model, when fitting such data, was not sensitive to values of the space constant. The best estimate the space constant would be arrived at by measuring SM voltage at more than one distance from the current injection site in the same animal.

Acknowledgments

This work was supported by a grant from The Whitaker Foundation. The author thanks Ann S. Tamariz for editorial assistance.

References

1. Dallos, P. and Evans B.N. (1995) High-Frequency motility of outer hair cells and the cochlear amplifier. *Science* **267** 2006–2009.
2. von Békésy, G. (1951) The coarse pattern of the electrical resistance in the cochlea of the guinea pig (Electroanatomy of the cochlea). *J. Acoust. Soc. Am.* **23** 18–28.
3. Misrahy, G.A., Hildreth, K.M., Shinabarger, E.W. and Gannon, W.J. (1958) Electrical properties of the wall of endolymphatic space of the cochlea (guinea pig). *Am. J. Physiol.* **194** 396–401.
4. Johnstone, B.M, Johnstone, J.R. and Pugsley, L.D. (1966) Membrane resistance in endolymphatic walls of the first turn of the guinea-pig cochlea. *J. Acoust. Soc. Am.* **40** 1398–1403.
5. Strelioff, D. (1973) A computer simulation of the generation and distribution of cochlear potentials. *J. Acoust. Soc. Am.* **54** 620–629.
6. Baden-Kristensen, K. and Weiss, T.F. (1983) Receptor potentials of lizard hair cells with free-standing stereocilia: Responses to acoustic clicks. *J. Physiol.* **335** 699–721.
7. Xue, S., Mountain, D.C. and Hubbard, A.E. (1995) Acoustic enhancement of electrically evoked otoacoustic emissions reflects basilar membrane tuning: A model. *Hear. Res.* **91** 93–100.

ELECTRICALLY EVOKED MICROMECHANICAL MOVEMENTS FROM THE APICAL TURN OF THE GERBIL COCHLEA

KIRIAKI D. KARAVITAKI, DAVID C. MOUNTAIN

Boston University Hearing Research Center, 44 Cummington Street,
Boston, MA 02215, USA
dkk@engc.bu.edu , dcm@enga.bu.edu

ALAN R. CODY

University of Queensland, Department of Physiology and Pharmacology
St. Lucia, 4072 QLD, Australia
a.cody@mailbox.uq.oz.au

A video microscopy system was used to measure electrically-evoked micromechanical movements in the apical turn of the excised gerbil cochlea. Motion synchronized to the stimulus frequency was frozen using stroboscopic illumination. Images were collected using a CCD camera and Fourier methods were then used to estimate the magnitude and phase of the radial displacements at the stimulus frequency. Motion was largest at the nucleus level of the outer hair cells and Hensen's cells where radial displacements reached 200-500 nm peak at low frequencies (<200 Hz). Outer and inner hair cell stereocilia, as well as the apical poles of outer and inner pillar cells, responded with small displacements of about 60 nm peak. At higher frequencies (2-3 kHz) motion for all cellular elements in the entire organ decreased. At low frequencies outer hair cell row 1 and row 2 nuclei were in phase with positive current into scala vestibuli and about 180 degrees out of phase with row 3 nuclei and Hensen's cell nuclei. Inner and outer hair cell stereocilia were in phase with each other for the stimulus frequency range used (20 Hz - 3 kHz).

1 Introduction

Experimental evidence suggests that the outer hair cells (OHC) of the mammalian cochlea are part of an electromechanical amplifier that greatly enhances hearing sensitivity and frequency selectivity. Most cochlear models, whether conceptual or computational, assume that the amplification process is the result of the voltage-dependent length changes observed in isolated OHCs. Beyond this assumption however, there is little agreement on the model parameters including such features as the micromechanical properties of cellular elements within the organ of Corti. In order to increase our understanding of cochlear micromechanics, we have used video microscopy to characterize the magnitude and phase of the motion of individual cells within the organ in response to electrical stimulation.

2   Methods

2.1 Surgical preparation of gerbil cochleas

Young female Mongolian gerbils were used in these experiments. The animals were deeply anaesthetized with an intraperitoneal injection of sodium pentobarbital (60mg/Kg). Following decapitation both temporal bones were excised and immersed in oxygenated culture medium. The tympanic membrane was removed and the cochlea was exposed. Most of the basal turn and the bone covering the apical turn were removed with a pair of forceps, and the organ of Corti was visualized in the apex. During this procedure care was taken not to break Reissner's membrane. The preparation was then mounted on the stage of an upright microscope and the organ of Corti visualized with a 40x water immersion lens. The condition of the preparation was assessed by the degree of swelling of the OHC nuclei and the level of current required to detect motion in the sensory epithelium.

2.2 Electrical stimulation

AC current was delivered near scala vestibuli of the apical turn with a low impedance ($<$30KΩ) glass pipette filled with a 3M NaCl. The pipette was sealed with agar at the tip to prevent any NaCl leakage. The return electrode was placed near the modiolus in the scala tympani of the second turn. The stimulus electrodes were connected to an optically isolated constant current source, which provided currents of up to 3 mA peak for frequencies ranging from 20 Hz to 3 kHz. The injected current was monitored by measuring the voltage across a 100 Ω resistor in the current return path.

Movements synchronized to the stimulus frequency were captured using stroboscopic illumination. The strobe consisted of a light emitting diode driven by a constant current source. The input pulses to the strobe system occurred at a fixed phase in each period of the stimulus with a duration equal to 10% of the stimulus period. Images were collected at five phases for each frequency using a CCD camera and stored on magnetic tape. These data were subsequently digitized and animations of the observed motion were created for each frequency.

2.3 Motion estimation

Fourier analysis was used to extract the magnitude and phase of the intensity changes for each pixel within the image for each stimulus frequency. In order to estimate radial displacement, the magnitude of the fundamental Fourier component of each pixel was divided by its intensity gradient. The pixel size was 0.32 μm and the reference

394

direction for motion was defined as radial displacement towards the modiolus. The measurement site was approximately 2 mm from the apex. The estimated characteristic frequency (CF) for this region is 600 Hz[2].

3 Results

Data from one of our best preparations are presented here. Fig. 1a shows the frequency response of the radial motion recorded at the level of the OHC nucleus for the three rows of OHCs. The plotted points in the figure represent the average of several cells from the same row. The noise level for this experiment was estimated to be below 10 nm.

For the OHC nuclei shown, radial displacement is maximal at low stimulus frequencies and shows a low-pass characteristic. For frequencies below 200 Hz the displacements of the first row OHC (OHC-1) nuclei are twice the displacements of the second (OHC-2) and third (OHC-3) row nuclei. At higher frequencies the displacements of the OHC-3 nuclei are greater than those of the OHC-1 and OHC-2.

The corresponding phase curves for these rows are shown in Fig. 1b. OHC-1 and OHC-3 are 180° out of phase while OHC-1 and OHC-2 are in phase up to about 600 Hz (estimated

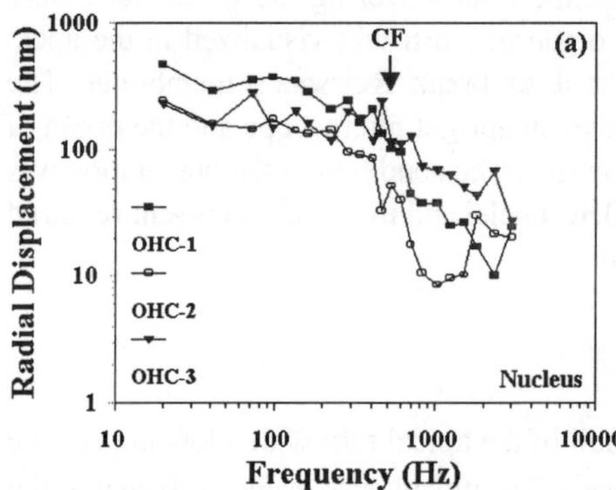

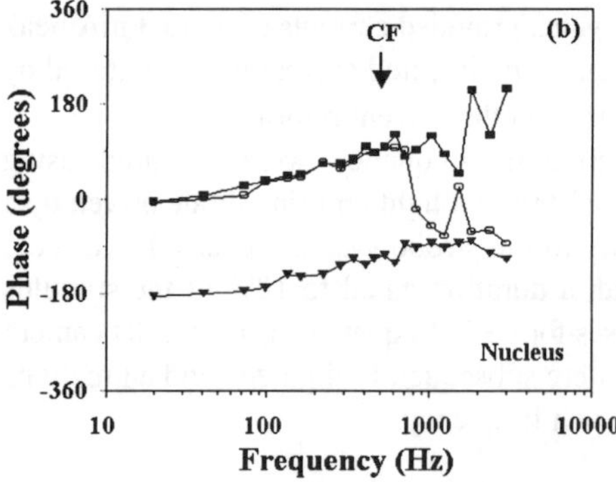

Fig. 1. Magnitude (a) and phase (b) response of the first, second and third row of OHC nuclei. The magnitude of the current stimulus was 2mA.

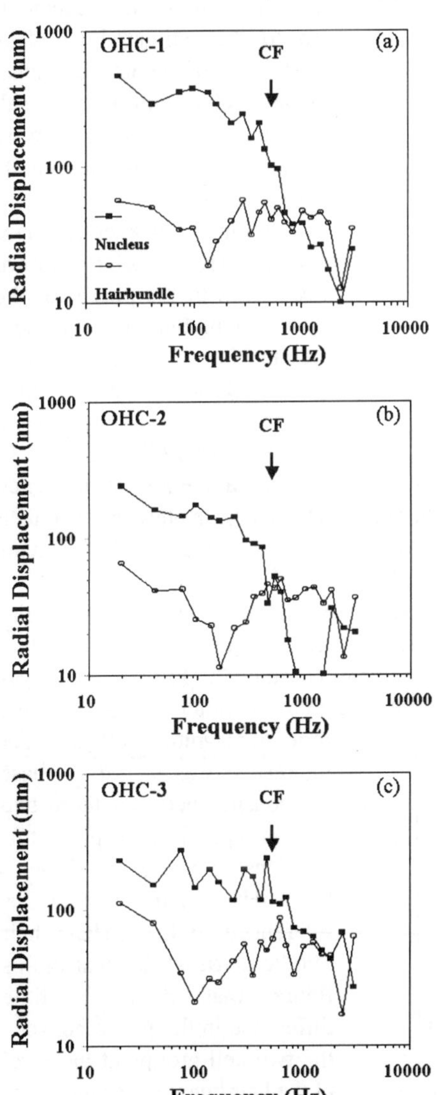

Fig. 2. Magnitude responses of the nucleus and the corresponding stereocilia of a (a) first row, (b) second row and (c) third row OHC.

CF) where they separate. Above CF OHC-2 is approximately in phase with OHC-3.

The Hensen's cell nuclei follow the OHC-3 nuclei both in magnitude and phase. The low-pass magnitude response and the increasing phase as a function of electrical stimulus frequency are consistent features across all of our excised cochlear data.

In comparison with motion at the level of the OHC nuclei, motion at the level of the hair bundles for both the OHCs and the inner hair cells (IHCs) is considerably less, particularly for low stimulus frequencies. This comparison is shown in Fig. 2 for the three OHC rows recorded in the same cochlea. For OHC-1 (Fig. 2a) the hair bundles show maximal radial displacements of approximately 60 nm at low stimulus frequencies which is an order of magnitude smaller than that recorded for the nuclei from the same cells. For the hair bundle, for all three rows, there is evidence for a notch in the magnitude of the motion around 100-300 Hz which recovers to a plateau for stimulus frequencies around CF. This relationship is repeated for OHC-2 (Fig. 2b) and OHC-3 (Fig. 2c) with the OHC nucleus radial displacements being larger than

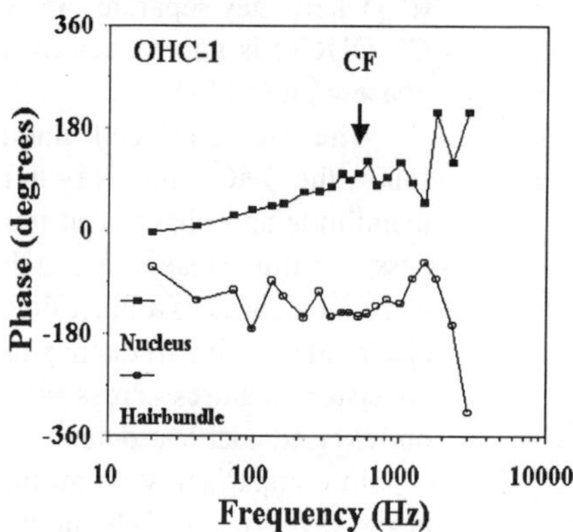

Fig. 3. Average phase response of the first row OHC nucleus and stereocilia.

the hair bundle displacements up to the estimated CF. The apical pole of the outer and inner pillar cells exhibited small displacements which were similar to the OHC hairbundle displacements.

In Fig. 3 the average phase for the OHC-1 nuclei is shown together with the phase for the OHC-1 hair bundles. At low frequencies the OHC-1 nuclei start in phase with the stimulus and accumulate phase reaching a lead of about 120° by 1 kHz. In contrast, at the lowest frequency (20 Hz) the OHC-1 hair bundle phase lags the stimulus by approximately -60° and then shifts to about -130° for frequencies up to 1 kHz. Above this frequency the behavior of the phase of both structures becomes complex.

For the IHC hair bundle, peak displacements approached 60 nm which is similar to that recorded for the hair bundles of the OHC. Although not shown, the notch that was observed for the OHC hair bundle displacement over the 100-300 Hz region was also seen in the IHC hair bundle motion and the depth of the notch was of the same

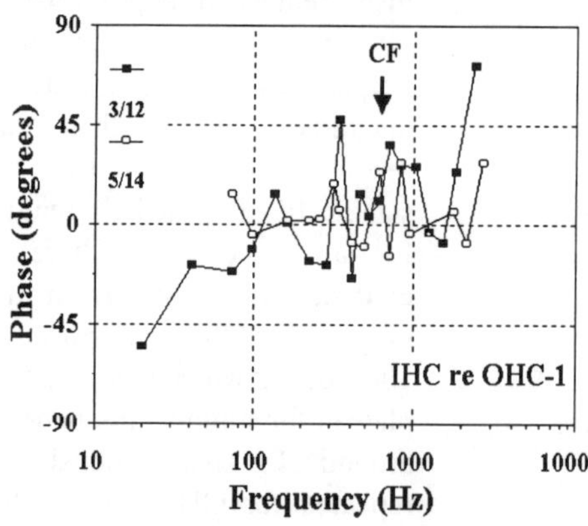

Fig. 4. Phase of IHC hair bundle referenced to the first row of OHC hair bundle for two different experiments.

order of magnitude. Of particular interest was the phase relationship between these two cell groups. Fig. 4 plots this relationship where the phase of the IHC hair bundle is referenced to the OHC-1 hair bundle phase. It is clear in this figure that there is little difference in the phase between the two cell groups at the level of the hair bundle over the range 70 Hz to 2 kHz. This relationship was seen in all four of the preparations for which both IHC and OHC hair bundle data were recorded.

In summary, the displacements of the OHC nuclei demonstrate a low-pass magnitude response and are larger than those of the hair bundles at low frequencies. For these frequencies the phase of the OHC nuclei leads the phase of the OHC hair bundles. Displacements of the IHC and the OHC hair bundles are very similar in magnitude and there is little difference in phase. In particular, OHC-1 nuclei exhibited the largest motion observed in the organ at low frequencies.

3 Discussion

Based on the data recorded in this study it is clear that electrical stimulation of the sensory epithelium of the isolated cochlear preparation results in motion within the organ of Corti. This motion is complex, stimulus frequency dependent and largest in the region of the OHC nuclei. It is also clear that electrical stimulation induces motion in the plane of the hair bundle and that this motion has the potential to excite the IHC hair bundles, a basic requirement for acoustic transduction.

Our finding that the radial displacements of the OHC-3 nuclei are out of phase with respect to the OHC-1 nuclei is predicted by the finite-element model of Zhang et al.[4] and is a characteristic of the first vibrational mode for both apical and basal turn geometries. If we assume that the frequency responses of the OHC nuclei are representative of the first vibrational mode, then we can estimate the natural frequency (NF_1) and the damping ratio of this mode in our preparation. The data suggest that the first mode is overdamped and that NF_1 is in the range of 300-400 Hz.

The finite-element model also predicts that the natural frequency of the second vibrational mode (NF_2) is 1.6 times NF_1 or about 600 Hz which corresponds well with our estimate of the characteristic frequency in our preparation. The notches observed in the magnitude of the hair bundle responses in the 100-200 Hz region (c.f. Fig. 2) may be the result of cancellation between the radial components of the first and second vibrational modes. In other experiments these notches are not as prominent in which case the IHCs and the OHCs hair bundles exhibit a low-pass response which has a slower roll-off than the OHC nuclei response. This difference between preparations may be due to the relative contribution of the first and second vibrational modes to the hair bundle motion. The slower roll-off observed for hair bundle motion may be the result of a stronger contribution of the second mode than in the case of the OHC nuclei.

One of the surprising findings in this study was that the displacements of the IHC and OHC hair bundles were in phase with each other over a wide frequency range. The published receptor potential data[1,3] suggest that the IHC hair bundle phase should lead the OHC hair bundle phase at low frequencies. In order to resolve this apparent discrepancy between our data and the receptor potential data it will be necessary to estimate hair bundle rotation.

Acknowledgments

The authors wish to thank Dr. Allyn Hubbard for his useful discussions on the phase data and help in editing the text. Special thanks go to Heidi and Ram for their help. This research was supported by NIDCD.

References

1. Dallos, P. J. Neurosci. **5**, 1591 (1985).
2. Müller, M. Hear. Res. **94**, 148 (1996).
3. Sellick, P.M. and Russell, I.J. Hear. Res. **2**, 439 (1980).
4. Zhang, L., Mountain, D.C. and Hubbard, A.E. (see this volume).

ELECTRICALLY-EVOKED EMISSION MAGNITUDE IS AN APPROXIMATELY LINEAR FUNCTION OF CURRENT LEVEL NEAR CHARACTERISTIC FREQUENCY AND VERY NONLINEAR AT LOW FREQUENCIES.

H.H. NAKAJIMA

Hearing Research Center and Department of Biomedical Engineering, Boston University, 44 Cummington St., Boston, MA 02215   hhn@buenga.bu.edu

D.C. MOUNTAIN

Hearing Research Center, Department of Biomedical Engineering, and Department of Otolaryngology, Boston University, 44 Cummington St., Boston, MA 02215 dcm@buenga.bu.edu

A.E. HUBBARD

Hearing Research Center, Department of Biomedical Engineering, Department of Electrical, Computer, and Systems Engineering, and Department of Otolaryngology, Boston University, 44 Cummington St., Boston, MA 02215   aeh@buenga.bu.edu

Many characteristics of the cochlear responses are nonlinear. To further our knowledge regarding outer haircell nonlinearities, we measured the dependence of the electrically-evoked otoacoustic emissions (EEOE) on current level for a wide range of frequencies. Alternating electrical current was delivered into the scala media of a gerbil's cochlea while the EEOE was measured with a calibrated probe-tube microphone. While the EEOE generally exhibited linear characteristics, notable exceptions occurred. For frequencies below 250 Hz and currents above 20-30 μA_{peak}, the gain (primary EEOE magnitude divided by the current level) increased abruptly, up to 30 dB for a $10\mu A_{peak}$ current increase. For higher frequencies, the gain often increased slightly with increasing current of up to 30-50 μA_{peak}, then decreased at even higher current. At frequencies and current levels where the gain was not constant, the waveforms of the EEOE exhibited distortion.

We also investigated acoustic enhancement of EEOE by introducing simultaneous acoustic stimuli. The effects of electrical current level on the enhancement of EEOE was investigated. Generally, the amount of enhancement remained constant for current levels up to $20\mu A_{peak}$. Above 45 μA_{peak}, the enhancement decreased slightly.

1   Introduction

The cochlea exhibits a variety of interesting nonlinear characteristics. Nonlinearities in the mechanoelectric and/or electromechanical transduction may underlie the nonlinear phenomena observed in acoustically-evoked and electrically-evoked basilar membrane motion and otoacoustic emissions.

We have studied electromechanical transduction *in vivo* by measuring the mechanical response to electrical current stimulation of the scala media.

Electrically-evoked otoacoustic emissions (EEOE) have been shown to originate from the area of the electrode location [1,2]. In the gerbil, they are largest for frequencies below the characteristic frequency (CF) of the electrode location and are smaller for frequencies near the CF. This may be due to phase cancellation at higher frequencies [2].

EEOE have been shown to exhibit an interesting non-linear phenomenon in which an acoustic stimulus at frequency F_A (introduced simultaneously with a sinusoidal electrical current at F_E) *enhances* the EEOE at F_E [3].

To further our knowledge regarding outer haircell (OHC) nonlinearities, we measured the EEOE gain as a function of current level for a wide range of frequencies. We also studied the effect of electrical stimulus levels on the ability of the acoustic stimuli to enhance the EEOE.

2 Methods

Mongolian gerbils, *Meriones unguiculatus,* anesthetized with sodium pentobarbital were used in the manner described previously [2]. A 2 to 4 µm tip glass microelectrode filled with 1.5 M KCl solution with 1 to 2 MΩ resistance was inserted into the scala media of the second turn of the cochlea. This electrode was used to measure electrical potentials and to deliver sinusoidal electrical current. The negative summating potential was used to estimate the CF of the micro electrode location. The compound action potential evoked by tone bursts was measured at the round window with a silver electrode to assess cochlear condition.

Otoacoustic emissions were evoked by electrical current injected into the scala media of turn 2, and were measured with a calibrated probe-tube microphone. The injected current stimulus was recorded and stored to confirm its stability and low distortion. Noise measurements without electrical stimulation and control measurements with electrical stimulation and the electrode tip on the bulla surface were made to verify electrical isolation and the lack of artifact.

EEOE measurements were made with simultaneous acoustic stimulation for electrical stimulation at 800 Hz and acoustic stimulation at 1.2 or 2.5 kHz. The order of presentation of different electrical and acoustic stimulus intensities was totally randomized. Control measurements without acoustic stimulus, and noise measurements without electrical stimulation were also made within the randomized presentation.

The data presented are characteristic of cochleas in good condition. These cochleas were characterized by high endocochlear potential (above 65 mV) throughout the experiment. The reference potential was reestablished at the surface

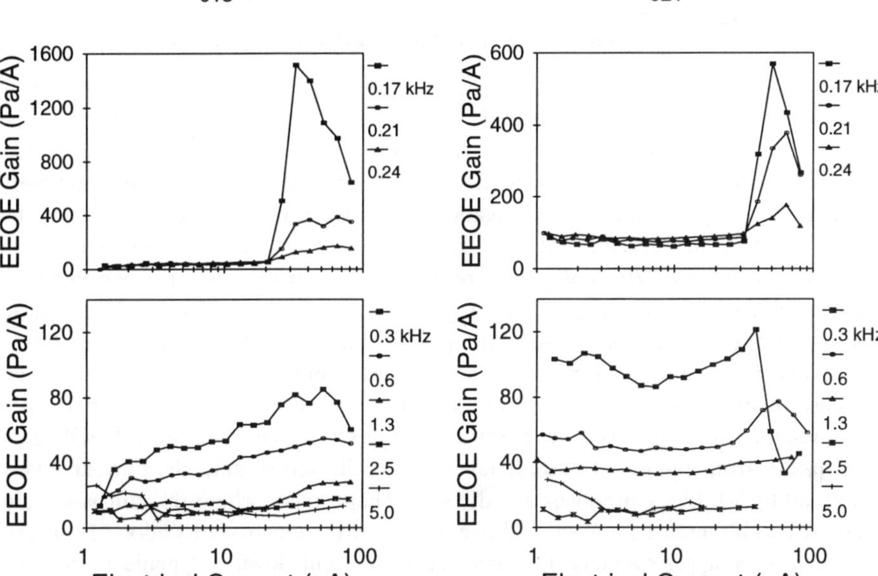

Figure 1 Each column represents a different cochlea. The top row plots the EEOE gains for low frequencies and the bottom row plots the high frequency gains.

of the cochlea at the end of the experiment. This was performed because the electrode can polarize over time.

Cochleas in good condition also exhibited sensitive N_1 responses to tone bursts, which remained stable throughout the experiment. The negative summating potential was also large for cochleas in good condition.

3 Results

3.1 Primary EEOE for various electrical stimulation intensities and frequencies

The EEOE linearity was assessed by calculating the emission gain. Emission gain is defined as the primary EEOE magnitude (at the frequency of the electrical stimulus) divided by the current level (Pa/A).

$$Gain = \frac{EEOE\ primary\ magnitude\ (\ \mu Pa\ rms\ )}{current\ stimulus\ magnitude\ (\ \mu A\ rms\ )}$$

Emission gains are plotted for several frequencies in Figure 1. Each column in the figure represents a different cochlea. The top row represents the low frequencies. For current levels below 10 to 30 μA_{peak}, the emission gain was approximately constant, thus representing a linear relationship between the stimulus current and the EEOE primary magnitude. At low frequencies, below 250 Hz, an increase in stimulus current over 20 to 50 μA_{peak} resulted in an abrupt large increase in gain. Further increase in current, over 50 μA_{peak}, resulted in decreased gain. The bottom row represents the higher frequencies plotted on a different scale. There was variability across animals for higher frequencies. Between 300 Hz and 1 kHz, an increase in stimulus current resulted in a slight increase then decrease in gain. We have assigned the term "self enhancement" to describe the increase in EEOE gain that results from increased current level. Overall, across animals, current levels above 20 to 50 μA_{peak} produces a 2 dB self enhancement where the emission gain increases with increased current. Above the CF of the electrode location (2.5 kHz), the gain was approximately independent of current level. Cochleas in poor condition were more linear, even for cochleas that originally exhibited such nonlinearity.

Linearity was also assessed by analyzing the waveforms of EEOE. Waveforms of the recorded emission magnitude were sinusoidal for currents below 20 to 30 μA_{peak}. In general, stimulus current levels and frequencies that resulted in non-linear behavior (as seen in the gain plots) corresponded to emission responses with distorted waveforms.

3.2 Acoustic enhancement of EEOE

The top panel of the left column of Fig. 2 shows the gain of EEOE at the electrical stimulus frequency ($F_E = 800$ Hz) as the function of acoustic stimuli ($F_A = 1.2$ kHz). The phase of the EEOE versus acoustic stimulus is plotted in the bottom panel. The different curves represent different electrical stimulus levels. EEOE enhancement is qualitatively similar for all current levels. However, the highest current level saturates at a lower gain. For $F_A = 1.2$ kHz, the threshold for acoustic enhancement of 2dB was approximately 45 dB SPL. The right column shows the same type of data as the left column for a higher acoustic stimulus frequency ($F_A = 2.5$ kHz, near the CF of the electrode). Again, the enhancement is fairly consistent for all current levels except for the highest current. Note that the threshold of enhancement occur at lower acoustic stimulus levels (approximately 20 dB SPL) than for $F_A = 1.2$ kHz.

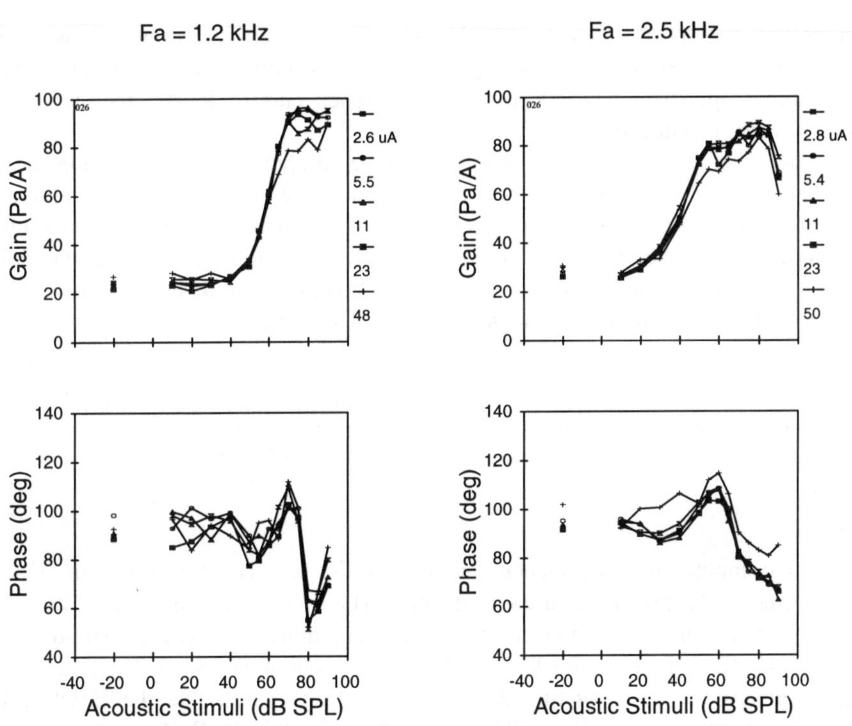

Figure 2   EEOE gain and phase evoked with current (F_E = 800 Hz) and simultaneous acoustic stimuli with frequency of F_A = 1.2 kHz (left column) and F_A = 2.5 kHz (right column) for various current intensities. Data points at -20 dB SPL correspond to EEOE gains with no acoustic stimuli.

4   Discussion

In this study we found that the second turn EEOE gain was relatively independent of current intensity for low currents. However, for low frequencies, below the CF of the electrode location, self enhancement occurred at approximately 20 to 50 µA. Self enhancement may be due to vibration produced by OHC motility, which may enhance the EEOE (similar to the enhancement effect by simultaneous acoustic stimulation). It is interesting to note that the threshold of acoustic enhancement starts at a lower acoustic stimulus for F_A = 2.5 kHz (which is near the CF of the electrode location) than for a lower frequency of acoustic stimulus (F_A = 1.2 kHz) with a threshold of approximately 45 dB SPL. The effect of stimulus current level on the acoustic enhancement of EEOE by simultaneous acoustic stimuli showed that the enhancement effect was generally independent of current level until the current was above approximately 40 μA_{peak}. At higher current levels, the maximum enhancement is reduced.

The enhancement data can be used to make an approximate calculation of the equivalence factor, relating the effect of electrical stimulation on partition motion to the effect of acoustic stimulation on partition motion. This calculation relies on the assumption that the electrical stimulus produces partition motion at the self-enhancement threshold which is equal to the motion produced by the acoustic stimulus at the acoustic-enhancement threshold. Defining

$$Equivalence\ Factor\ =\ \frac{acoustic - enhancement\ threshold}{self - enhancement\ threshold}$$

we can compute the equivalence factor as follows. The threshold for a self enhancement of 2 dB for electrical frequencies (F_E < CF) is approximately 20 to 50 μA_{peak}, while acoustic enhancement of 2 dB requires an acoustic stimulus of roughly 45 dB SPL (F_A = 1.2 kHz). This yields a computed equivalence factor of approximately 70 Pa/A for turn 2. It is interesting to note that the EEOE gain without acoustic stimulus (F_E = 800 Hz) is approximately 50 Pa/A, supporting the assumption of equal motion produced by high electrical stimulus or simultaneous acoustic stimulus.

This calculation can be compared to the results for turn 1 of Xue *et al.*[6], which are based on basilar membrane measurements. They reported that a 60 dB SPL acoustic stimulus would produce basilar membrane motion equivalent to that of a 25 μA_{peak} electrical stimulus. This yields an equivalence factor of approximately 1000 Pa/A, which is more than an order of magnitude larger than the one predicted using the turn 2 data, suggesting that the OHC force production is higher in the base than in the apex.

Because the EEOE gain and the equivalence factor are of similar magnitude, and current levels above the self-enhancement threshold interfere with acoustic enhancement, we hypothesize that EEOE self enhancement and acoustic enhancement involve a common mechanism. Previous studies have implicated saturation of mechanoelectric transduction in acoustic enhancement since the acoustic enhancement threshold corresponds to the level at which the cochlear microphonic saturates. We therefore hypothesize that EEOE self enhancement also involves saturation of the mechanoelectric transduction process.

We propose two alternative (but not mutually exclusive) hypotheses for the influence of mechanoelectric transduction on the EEOE. The first hypothesis is that the OHC's mechanoelectric transduction is coupled to the electromechanical transduction, forming a negative feedback loop which reduces EEOE gain for $F_E <$ CF[3,4]. Alteration of the feedback loop by saturating mechanoelectric transduction gain would then result in increased EEOE gain at low frequencies [5,4,2].

The alternative hypothesis is that the OHC mechanoelectric transducer exhibits asymmetric saturation. High level electrical or acoustic stimulation results in a mechanical input to the OHC which results in an increase in the average apical conductance. This increased conductance would result in an increase in the fraction of the electrical stimulus current flowing through the OHC. Thus, this increase in current would lead to an enhanced emission.

Acknowledgments

This work was supported by the National Science Foundation.

References

1. Xue,S. *et al.* (1993) Acoustic enhancement of electrically-evoked otoacoustic emissions reflects basilar membrane tuning: Experiment results. *Hearing Research* **70** 121.
2. Nakajima, H.H. *et al.* (1994) Electrically evoked otoacoustic emissions from the apical turns of the gerbil cochlea. *J. Acoust. Soc. Amer.* **96** 786.
3. Mountain, D.C. *et al.* *(1983)* Electromechanical processes in the cochlea. In: *Mechanics of Hearing*, 119, ed. E. De Boer and M.A. Viergever , Delft Univ. Press, Delft, Netherlands.
4. Mountain, D.C. and Hubbard A.E. (1989) Rapid force production in the cochlea. *Hearing Research* **42** 195.
5. Hubbard, A.E. and Mountain, D.C. (1990) Haircell forward and reverse transduction: differential suppression and enhancement. *Hearing Research.* **43** 269.
6. Xue, S.*et al.* (1993) Direct measurement of electrically-evoked basilar membrane motion. In: *Biophysics of Hair Cell Sensory Systems*, 361, ed. H. Duifhuis, J.W. Horst, P. van Dijk, and S.M. van Netten (World Scientific, New Jersey.

Part Four

Synthetic models of the organ of Corti

THE INVERSE PROBLEM FOR WAVES IN A TWO SUB-PARTITION COCHLEAR MODEL SUGGESTS AXIAL ELECTROMECHANICAL COUPLING OF OUTER HAIR CELLS

R. S. CHADWICK, E. K. DIMITRIADIS

Biomedical Engineering and Instrumentation Program, NCRR
National Institutes of Health, Bldg. 13/3N17
Bethesda, MD 20892
chadwick@helix.nih.gov

The electromechanical processes responsible for sharp tuning in the cochlea are still a matter of controversy. When independently acting outer hair cells (OHCs) are assumed to be the sole source of activity, the low-pass filter that characterizes isolated cells clearly proves to be insufficient. We address this problem using the WKB framework to solve an inverse problem for actively-controlled waves in a cochlear model having two degrees of freedom in a cross section representing the coupled transverse motions of the tectorial (TM) and basilar membrane (BM). That is, we seek the space-frequency map of the active filter that enables the model to reproduce experimentally determined tuning curves, requiring only that OHCs are activated by the motion of the TM and exert forces on both the reticular lamina (RL) and BM. We find that to a good approximation the active component of impedance is proportional to the local wavelength on the cochlear partition (CP). Furthermore, we can account for this behavior with an electromechanical circuit containing resistive coupling between OHCs, supporting cells, and extracellular spaces. When this activity mechanism is used together with a new poroelastic model for the passive impedance of the CP, very sharp waveforms can be computed.

1 Introduction

The model, as previously proposed and analyzed by Chadwick *et al.*[1] for the forward problem with independently acting OHCs, was developed with the criterion that controller elements be placed in a structurally realistic setting. The complete model allows different parts of the cross section of the organ of Corti (OC) to oscillate with different amplitudes and phases as the recent experiments of Hemmert *et al.*[2] suggest. The CP is divided into three subpartitions representing the TM, RL, and BM. OHC stereocilia are placed between the TM and RL to sense their motions, while somatic motility of the OHCs act between the RL and BM as in vivo. Axial elastic coupling is neglected within the OC but axial mass and frictional coupling exist due to fluid solid interaction. Three fluid channels, the scalae above and below the TM and BM, as well as the thin gap between the TM and RL contain incompressible viscous liquid to provide fluid loading of the subpartitions.

Mechanical properties such a mass, stiffness, and damping of the subpartitions were lumped into discrete components and allowed to slowly vary along the axial coordinate z. Locally, the masses were assumed to perform transverse piston-like oscillations displacing liquid in the adjacent channels. The WKB approximation was used to compute the response of the subpartitions to sinusoidal input at the stapes. The main findings of that study were: the RL and TM move in unison with essentially no squeezing of the thin gap, thus reducing the number of degrees of freedom from three to two; an active force level consistent with measurements on isolated OHCs can provide and 35 dB amplification by spatially delaying dissipation and allowing a greater structural resonance to occur before the wave is cut off; however, previously postulated activity mechanisms for single partition models cannot achieve sharp enough tuning in subpartitioned models. It was also suggested to further investigate the distribution of mass between the subpartitions and to consider other activation mechanisms.

2   Inverse Problem for a Model with Two Subpartitions

The mathematical problem is written in terms of time harmonic waves traveling along the CP, using the WKB approximation. This method is based on the fact that slowly varying geometry supports wave propagation with slowly varying wavenumbers. The problem is therefore cast in terms of the local wavenumber $k(\omega,z)$, and the displacement vector of the complete wave can be described in the form

$$\tilde{Y}(\omega,z) = Y(\omega,z)\,e^{i(\omega t - \varepsilon^{-1}\int_0^z k(\omega,z)\,dz)} \tag{1}$$

where the axial coordinate $z \in [0,1]$ is normalized by the cochlear length L; the inverse of the wavenumber is normalized by the BM width at the base, w_o, and ε is the slenderness ratio $w_o/L \ll 1$. The displacement vector $\tilde{Y}$ has components $\tilde{Y}_t$ and $\tilde{Y}_b$ denoting the transverse displacements of the TM and BM, respectively. The BM component of the amplitude vector Y has the explicit form

$$Y_b = \frac{c_o\,k(1 - k\sqrt{-i\upsilon/(\omega w_o^2)})\,y_{bt}}{\rho\,\omega^2\sqrt{w}}\,exp[-\int_0^z \frac{y'_{bt}\,\eta_{bt}\,dz}{1 + y_{bt}\,\eta_{bt}}] \tag{2}$$

where c_o is a constant of integration that can be found from the stapes input magnitude; υ and ρ are the kinematic viscosity and density of the fluid; w is the normalized variable width of the CP; y_{bt} is the mode ratio Y_b/Y_t and y'_{bt} is its z derivative; and η_{bt} is an adjoint mode ratio to be defined below. The wavenumber

k and the mode ratio Y_b/Y_t are determined by solving the coupled linear homogeneous system

$$\begin{bmatrix} Z_{11} & Z_{12} \\ Z_{21} & Z_{22} \end{bmatrix}\begin{bmatrix} Y_t \\ Y_b \end{bmatrix} = 0 \tag{3}$$

where the Z_{ij} are components of the impedance matrix for the system shown in Fig.1:

$$Z_{11} = -\omega^2(M_{tr} + M_f/k) + K_t + K_r + K_c + i\omega(C_t + C_r + C_f) - \alpha \tag{4a}$$

$$Z_{22} = -\omega^2(M_b + M_f/k) + K_b + K_r + K_c + i\omega(C_b + C_r + C_f) \tag{4b}$$

$$Z_{12} = -(K_r + K_c + i\omega C_r) \tag{4c}$$

$$Z_{21} = -(K_r + K_c + i\omega C_r) + \alpha \tag{4d}$$

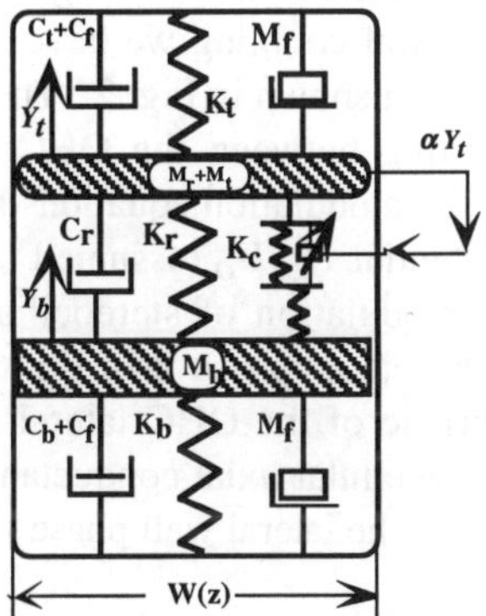

Figure 1: Cross sectional structural elements of cochlear model with two subpartitions. The Ms, Cs, and Ks denote the slowly varying mass, structural damping, and stiffness of the subpartions per unit axial length. M_f and C_f are wavelength-dependent fluid effective mass and damping. The OHC active control loop is denoted by α.

A nontrivial solution of Eq. 3 can exist only if $Det[Z_{ij}]=0$, which yields a quadratic equation for the wavenumber k. The two roots of the quadratic equation represent the wavenumber at a given frequency as a function of z for forward and reflected waves. Only the forward wave propagates in the present application. The mode ratio can then be expressed in terms of the wavenumber using Eq. 3. The adjoint mode ratio η_{bt} can also be obtained from Eq. 3 with Z_{ij} replaced by its transpose.

For the inverse problem we determine the k that solves Eq. 1 when the left-hand side is the measured response, e.g. using the treatment of Rhode's data by Zweig[3]. Differentiating Eq. 1 with respect to z yields the first approximation for k for $\varepsilon<<1$, which is sufficiently accurate for our purposes here.

$$k \cong i\varepsilon\frac{\tilde{Y}'}{\tilde{Y}} \tag{5}$$

When Eq. 5 is used in the relation $Det[Z_{ij}]=0$, we can determine the cochlear amplifier (CA) space-frequency map $\alpha(\omega,z)$, which happens to be numerically well approximated by

$$\alpha(\omega,z) \propto k(\omega,z)^{-1} . \tag{6}$$

This implies that OHCs apply an active force proportional to the local wavelength, which requires axial electromechanical coupling of OHCs. To investigate a possible mechanism for this axial coupling we have studied the transfer function characteristics of the cable circuit shown in Fig. 2. The essential new feature of the circuit is the resistive coupling between the OHCs, supporting cells, and the extracellular spaces. When the modulation equations for this circuit are solved for the OHC transmembrane potential U_c-U_o (assumed to be proportional to α) with the circuit driven by wave modulation of stereocilia resistance, we find that if $k^2R_m/r>>\omega R_mC_m$, for each $r=(r_m,r_g,r_o)$, then Eq. 6 can be well approximated. Thus the low pass characteristic of the OHC lateral membrane can be bypassed provided that the ratio of extracellular axial conductance to the conductance of the lateral wall is large compared to the lateral wall phase lag.

3 Forward Problem with a Poroelastic Organ of Corti

If we reconsider the passive impedance of the organ of Corti using a simplified poroelastic model then very sharp waveforms can be demonstrated with the approximation for the CA filter given by Eq. 6. Consider the cross sectional space bounded by the BM ($y=0$) and the RL ($y=H$) as a mixture of incompressible elastic solid and incompressible viscous fluid. For simplicity, assume that the fluid is confined to extracellular "pores" that can be characterized by vertical channels of width h. When the RL and BM move with different amplitudes and/or phases then the elastic component will deform and fluid will flow through the extracellular

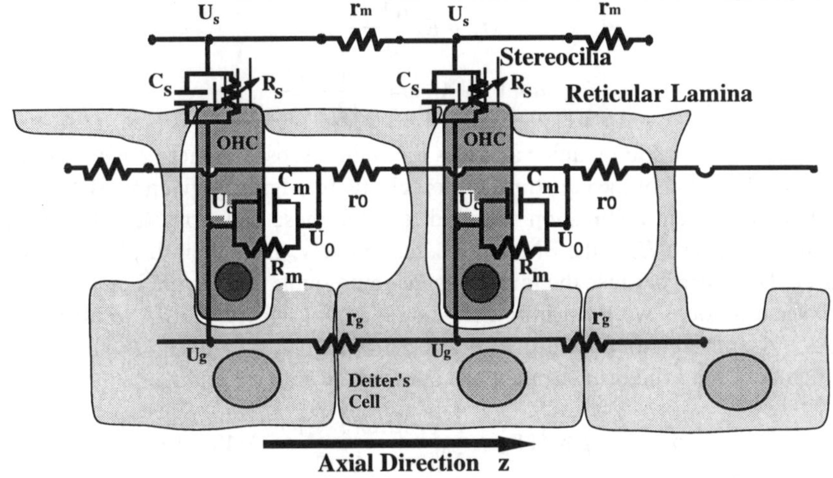

Figure 2: Proposed cable circuit of the CA with resistive axial coupling.

channels. If the cross sectional area fraction of the channels is denoted by Φ, then the effective stress σ of the mixture is

$$\sigma = (1-\Phi)\sigma_s - \Phi p \tag{7}$$

where σ_s is the local stress in the solid phase and p is the local pressure in both phases. When the local wavelength on the CP is large compared to H, motions of the CP in the axial direction can be neglected. Let $V_s(y)$ and $V_f(y)$ denote the averaged vertical transverse displacements of the solid and fluid phases. If the mixture is also incompressible then

$$\frac{d}{dy}[(1-\Phi)V_s + \Phi V_f] = 0 \ . \tag{8}$$

The equation of motion of the mixture for simple harmonic motion is

$$-\rho \omega^2 [(1-\Phi)V_s + \Phi V_f] = \frac{d\sigma}{dy} \ . \tag{9}$$

In addition we use Hooke's law for an incompressible elastic solid and Poiseuille's law for flow in the channels:

414

$$\sigma_s = E_s \frac{dV_s}{dy} - p \tag{10}$$

$$i\omega(V_f - V_s) = -\frac{h^2}{12\mu}\frac{dp}{dy} \tag{11}$$

where E_s is the elastic modulus and μ is the fluid viscosity. These equations are a specialized version of the equations of poroelasticity originally given by Biot[4].

For the present application we need to solve these equations for the mixture stresses $\sigma(0)$ and $\sigma(H)$ at the BM and RL, respectively, given their displacements Y_b and Y_t. However, because the mixture is incompressible and we are ignoring radial transverse motions we must introduce a sink at $y=l$, where $0{\leq}l{\leq}H$, to absorb the fluid. Assuming no pressure build-up in the sink, i.e. $p(l)=0$, along with continuity of the solid displacement and stress at the sink we find

$$\sigma(0) \cong -\rho\,\omega^2 l\,Y_b + \frac{1}{2}\sqrt{\frac{12\mu i\omega(1-\Phi)E_s}{h^2\Phi}}(Y_t - Y_b) \tag{12}$$

$$\sigma(H) \cong \rho\,\omega^2(H-l)\,Y_t - \frac{1}{2}\sqrt{\frac{12\mu i\omega(1-\Phi)E_s}{h^2\Phi}}(Y_t - Y_b). \tag{13}$$

These relations can be used to assign mass, stiffness, and damping components to the passive impedance matrix to replace the M_r, K_r, and C_r elements in Fig. 1.

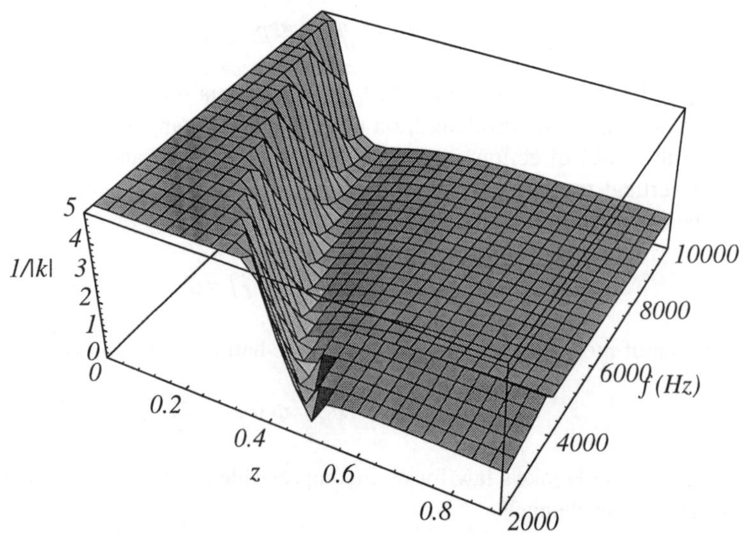

Figure 3: Calculated magnitude of CA space-frequency map using Eq. 6. Note figure is clipped in upper plateau region.

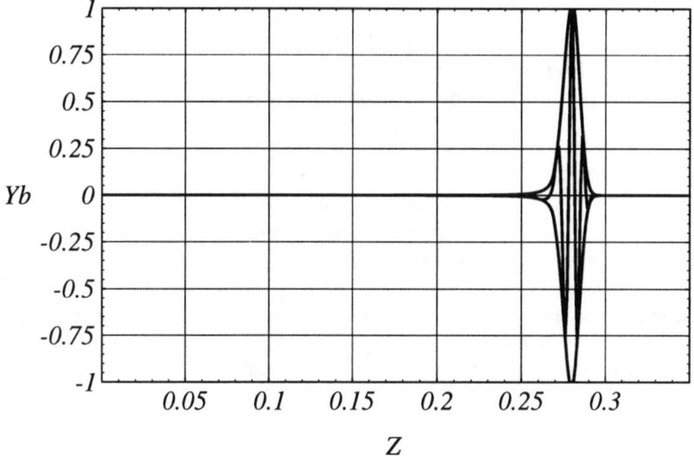

Figure 4: Calculated BM waveform and envelope at 5 kHz.

Computed results using this model are shown in Fig. 3 and Fig. 4. The CA space-frequency map in Fig. 3 indicates a small valley and a nonzero high-frequency plateau, which would not be present if OHCs were acting independently. Fig. 4 demonstrates a remarkable localization of the waveform on the BM.

References

1. Chadwick, R. S., Dimitriadis, E. K., and Iwasa, K.H. (1996) Active control of waves in a cochlear model with subpartitions, *Proc. Natl. Acad. Sci. USA* **93**(6) 2564-2569.
2. Hemmert, W., Zenner, H.-P., and Gummer, A.W. (1995) Three-dimensional vibration measurements on different locations of the cochlear partition, *18th Mid-winter Research Meeting of the ARO*, Abstract **448** 112.
3. Zweig, G. J. (1991) Finding the impedance of the organ of Corti, *J. Acoust. Soc. Am.* **89**(3) 1229-1254.
4. Biot, M., A. (1955) Theory of elasticity and consolidation for a porous anisotropic solid, *J. Applied Physics* **26**(2) 182-185.

A NEW ASSUMPTION FOR MECHANICAL OHC–IHC INTERACTION

A. DANCER

French-German Research Institute of Saint-Louis
68301 Saint-Louis, France
dancer@nucleus.fr

B. HAMONIC

Laboratoire d'Acoustique, ISEB
29200 Brest, France
iseb0586@eurobretagne.fr

A new kind of mechanical interaction between the outer and the inner hair cells is proposed. Combination of phasic (AC) and tonic (DC) displacements of different parts of the organ of Corti (basilar membrane, outer hair cells, tectorial membrane...) could induce an unidirectional and continuous deflexion of the stereocilia of the inner hair cells and provide a mechanical stimulation well-fitted to the specific electrical characteristics of the membrane of these cells.

1. Introduction

The organ of Corti is built to work in a transversal direction: from the outer hair cells (OHC) to the inner hair cells (IHC). It is now well known that the OHC and their active mechanisms are responsible for the sensitivity at threshold and for the frequency selectivity as recorded on the afferent fibers directly connected to a single IHC. How the mechanical excitation provided at the lowest levels by the OHC is transmitted to the IHC[1,2]? As the tips of the OHC stereocilia are embedded in the tectorial membrane (TM) which covers the IHC stereocilia, it is logical to think that the OHC movements are transmitted to the IHC by the TM. According to the stimulation frequency and to the degree of coupling between the IHC stereocilia and the TM, the IHC have been sought to be either amplitude or velocity sensitive[2].

However, because of the low pass characteristics of their membrane, the IHC are unable to respond linearly to phasic (AC) stimuli beyond a few tens Hertz[3,4], and are more sharply tuned as far as their tonic (DC) responses are concerned[5]. Therefore, the IHC are predisposed to receive and to transduce DC stimuli. It is then appealing to hypothesize that the DC responses of the OHC[6,7] correspond to the actual input signal to the IHC: tonic contraction of the OHC would bring the TM in close contact with the IHC stereocilia, force them to bend, and induce the mechano-electrical transduction.

We want to go further and put forward a new mechanism which takes advantage of both AC and DC components of the OHC displacements to stimulate the IHC.

2. An ultra-sonic-motor-like in the cochlea?

Zwislocki[8] and Allen[9] have shown that the organ of Corti can be modelled by two coupled oscillators (the first being composed of the basilar membrane and the hair cells, the second of the tectorial membrane). Close to the characteristic frequency of a given location, these oscillators move in perpendicular directions. Therefore, it is possible that the resulting displacement of the TM, (referring to the tips of the IHC stereocilia) is more or less elliptical. As a matter of fact, measurements performed by Khanna et al.[1] indicate that the relative displacements of the OHC, IHC and TM exhibit different directional components.

In an ultra-sonic-motor, a ring of piezo-electric ceramic is excited in quadrature and two standing waves combine to induce an elliptical displacement of the surface of the ring. If a second (passive) ring is pressed on top of the first, it will rotate (clockwise or anti-clockwise) because the surface elements of the first ring drive the second one during the upper part of their elliptical trajectory. Speed and torque of the rotating movement of the passive ring depend on the amplitude of the elliptical displacements of the piezo-electric ring and on the force pressing the two rings together.

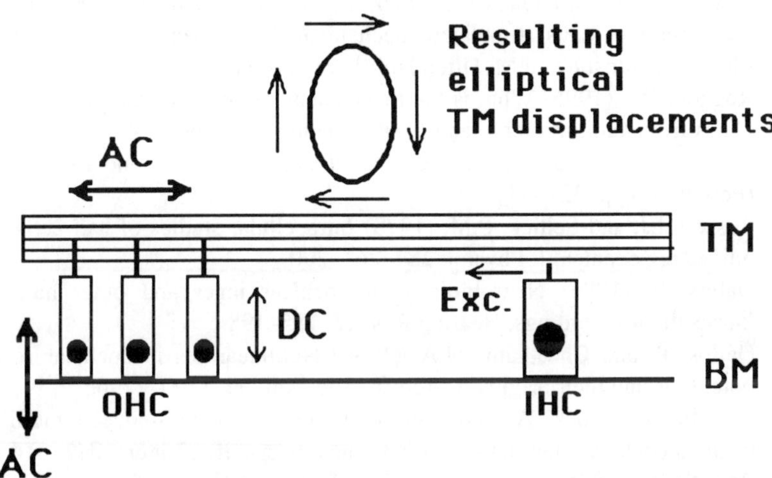

Figure 1: Schematic representation of the OHC-IHC interaction

Coming back to the cochlea and supposing elliptical displacements (AC induced) of the TM over the IHC stereocilia, we can imagine that the DC contractions of the OHC put the TM in contact with the tips of the IHC stereocilia and produce a continuous and unidirectional deflexion (in case of stimulation by a tone-burst for example) (fig. 1). Amplitude of the IHC stereocilia deflexion would be a function of the amplitude of the passive and active AC movements (resulting in elliptical displacements), and of the force (DC contraction of the OHC) pulling the TM on the tips of the IHC stereocilia.

If this hypothesis was verified, it could also explain the action of the medial efferent fibers which, by modulating the length of the OHC and thereby the force pulling the TM on the tips of the IHC stereocilia, might either increase or decrease the transmission of the excitation from the OHC to the IHC (at least at low and moderate stimulation levels).

3. Conclusion

The combination of phasic (AC) and tonic (DC) movements of the different parts of the organ of Corti (basilar membrane, outer hair cells, tectorial membrane...) could induce an unidirectional deflexion of the IHC stereocilia during the whole duration of the stimulation. This unidirectional deflexion would be well fitted to the electrical characteristics of the IHC membrane and would give rise to the "rectified" response of these cells.

References

1. Khanna, S.M., Ulfendahl, M., Flock, A. and Heneghan, C. (1995) How are the inner hair cells stimulated mechanically?, In: Active Hearing, eds. A. Flock, D. Ottoson and M. Ulfendahl (Pergamon) pp. 257–270.
2. Ruggero, M. (1995) What is the mechanical stimulus for the inner hair cell? Clues from auditory-nerve and basilar-membrane responses to low-frequency sounds, In: Active Hearing, eds. A. Flock, D. Ottoson and M. Ulfendahl (Pergamon) pp. 321–336.
3. Russell, I.J. and Sellick, P.M. (1978) Intracellular studies of hair cells in the guinea pig cochlea, J. Physiol. **284** 261–290.
4. Dallos, P. (1986) Neurobiology of cochlear inner and outer hair cells: intracellular recordings, Hearing Res. **22** 185–198.
5. Dallos, P. and Cheatham, M.A. (1989) Nonlinearities in cochlear receptor potentials and their origins, J. Acoust. Soc. Am. **86** 1790–1796.
6. Brundin, L., Flock, A. and Canlon, B. (1989) Sound-induced motility of isolated cochlear outer hair cells is frequency-specific, Nature. **342** 814–816.
7. Brundin, L. and Russell, I. (1994) Tuned phasic and tonic motile responses of isolated outer hair cells to direct mechanical stimulation of the cell body, Hearing Res. **73** 35–45.
8. Zwislocki, J.J. and Kletsky, E.J. (1979) Tectorial membrane: a possible effect on frequency analysis in the cochlea, Science **204** 639–641.
9. Allen, J.B. (1980) Cochlear micromechanics - a physical model of transduction, J. Acoust. Soc. Am. **68** 1660–1670.

ACTIVE NONLINEAR MODEL FOR A DAMAGED COCHLEA

M. FURST, A. COHEN and A. MATZA
Dept. of Electrical Engineering - Systems Faculty of Engineering,
Tel Aviv University, Tel Aviv 69978, Israel
mira@eng.tau.ac.il

In our previous studies, we have shown that an active nonlinear transmission line model with non-uniform amplification along the cochlear partition can account for many normal behavioral phenomena that are due to cochlear properties, such as combination tones and masking. Cochlear emission properties also were explained by the model, including the different emissions types, the relationship between them, and their effect on hearing.

In the present study, the same model is used to predict abnormal behavior as demonstrated by damaged cochleae. The most common cochlear damage is high frequency hearing loss due to age or noise trauma. In order to characterize hearing loss, we have defined a model audiogram. The cochlear displacement obtained as a response to 500 msec continuous sine wave at low level is integrated along the cochlear partition, and its value represents the threshold of normal cochlea at that frequency.

Hearing loss is defined as the increase in level required in order to obtain the normal threshold level. High frequency hearing loss usually interpreted as a loss of outer hair cells especially at the apical part of the basilar membrane. In the model, the amplification factor represents the outer hair cells population and their contribution to the basilar membrane displacement and velocity. The amplification factor at every point is proportional to the number of outer hair cells at that region along the cochlea. Outer hair cell loss is then modeled by reduction in the amplification factor. As a result, audiograms with high frequency loss are obtained, and the nonlinear properties are suppressed. For example, combination tones are not obtained, and less suppression is achieved. Another result of the model for damaged cochlea is a significant reduction in all cochlear emissions types. The model predictions for damaged cochlea will be presented and discussed.

A COCHLEAR TRAVELING-WAVE AMPLIFIER MODEL WITH REALISTIC SCALA MEDIA AND HAIRCELL ELECTRICAL PROPERTIES

A.E. HUBBARD, P. RAMACHANDRAN, D.C. MOUNTAIN

Boston University College of Engineering and Hearing Research Center, 44 Cummington St., Boston, MA 02215 ,USA

The traveling-wave amplifier (TWAmp) model of the cochlea has been augmented to contain a realistic representation of the electrical properties of the scala media. Now, rather than using direct coupling between two hydromechanical modes of propagation, simulated cochlear-partition displacement drives outer hair cell (OHC) transducers, which produce OHC transmembrane voltage changes, which produce force that couples to the second hydromechanical mode. The enhanced model produces basilar-membrane motion data that are similar to those previously demonstrated without the use of the scala media circuitry, plus it also produces cochlear microphonic. The model's electrically-evoked otoacoustic emissions (EEOE) share salient characteristics with experimental data. Moreover, the simulated electrically-evoked basilar-membrane velocity has characteristics similar to those found in the EEOE at lower frequencies and to those found in the acoustically-driven response at higher frequencies. Both of these model observations are in qualitative agreement with experimental findings.

1 Introduction

We previously [2,3] presented a unique model of cochlear hydrodynamics, the travelling wave amplifier (TWAmp). This model used two wave propagation structures that were coupled by sources that exchanged energy between the two modes. The first, linear version of the model was able to achieve magnitude and phase angle responses that were in close agreement with experimental data. A nonlinear version [1,3] of the model that used saturating force production produced good agreement with basilar membrane mechanical data for various frequencies and sound levels [9].

The bi-directional, distributed amplification model in its earliest formulation had several deficiencies. The second propagation mode was not assigned to a unique structure within the cochlea. The structure is either a small, fluid- filled tube or a highly-damped mechanical transmission line, depending on which analogy one uses to interpret the equations. Also, the progression of characteristic frequencies (CFs) with increasing sound level was such that growth curves of basilar membrane velocity versus sound level for frequencies at or above CF bent over or stayed constant with increasing sound level. Experimental evidence suggests that they, at most, flatten out for mid-range sound levels, but generally continue to grow for frequencies at or above CF. Finally, the model could only produce "pseudo-" EEOEs by driving the sources that coupled the modes, since the model had no scala media into which simulated current could be injected. Adding a scala media model to the existing TWAmp model made EEOE simulation possible, corrected the peak-shift problem, and also made the model more physiologically relevant.

2 Model

Figure 1 shows one section of the TWAmp model, which now includes the scala media electroanatomy. Although the symbols used (e.g. L, R, C) are similar, the top and bottom circuits represent the hydromechanics of the first and second mode, respectively; while the middle circuit represents the electroanatomy of scala media and the outer hair cells (OHC). The longitudinal resistance represents the conducting endolymph in the longitudinal cochlear dimension. The scala is shunted to ground by a RC network. The OHC model is comprised of apical and basal membrane portions that are both RC circuits. The apical conductance, however, is time-varying and controlled by the displacement variable of the upper hydrodynamic line. The displacement to conductance transfer characteristic results from a three-state Boltzman membrane model. The conductance at zero displacement is 32 nS and the maximum conductance is 97.5 nS. The sensitivity constants are 30 nm and 6nm. The intracellular and stria vascularis batteries cause dc offsets in the feedback loop that present severe computational difficulties, which we circumvented using a high-pass filter that cut off below 100 Hz. We used a middle ear model [1,4] that had infinite compliance in the portion representing the bulla cavity, to simulate the open-bulla condition used experimentally [6,7]. We modeled a blocked ear-bar condition [6] when simulating EEOE by open-circuiting the ear canal model at the 2 mm location.

3 Results

3.1 Mechanical responses to sound stimuli

The model's mechanical responses and comparable experimental data are shown in Figure 2. The appearance of the curves obtained for identical sound levels and frequencies in both the simulation and the experiment is quite similar. Indeed, input/output functions (Figure 3) in the experimental and simulated cases match very well.

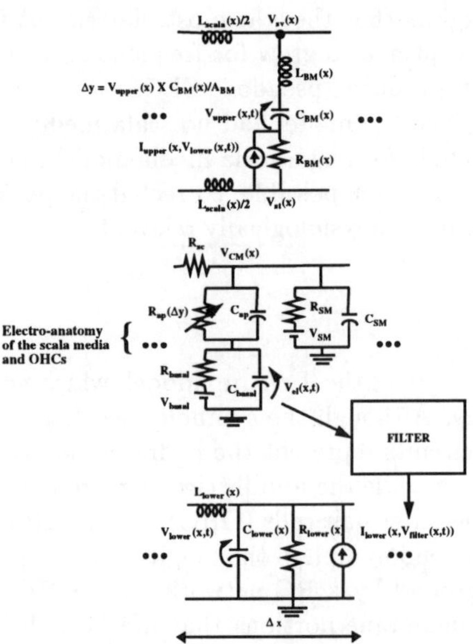

Figure 1: A circuit describing the TWAmp model that includes a representation of scala media. This section is repeated, with varying parameters, 400 times in the full model.

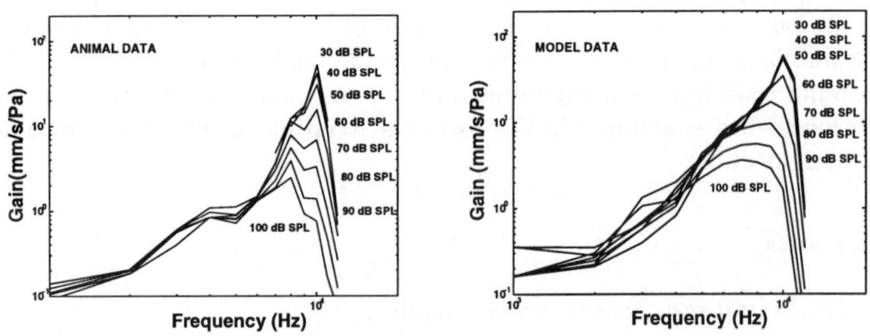

Figure 2: Comparison of model and experimental responses to tone stimuli. Both sets of responses have been scaled by the level of the corresponding input tones.

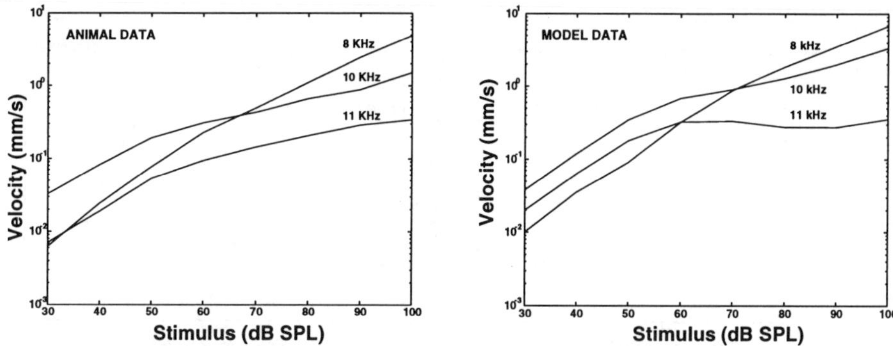

Figure 3: Basilar membrane input-output curves for several frequencies: This is a replot of experimental and model responses from Figure 2.

3.2 Cochlear microphonic responses to sound stimuli

The model's CM response is compared with experimental data[6,7] in Figure 4. Overall, the model and experimental CM data are fairly similar. The model and the experimental data show saturation of output in the 2.5 kHz region for sound inputs in the 50-60 dB SPL range. Both the model and the experimental data can show reduction in CM output following saturation (bendover). There are some general differences in shapes of the responses at low frequency, which are due to the middle-ear portion of the model.

3.3 Electrically-evoked emissions

The model's EEOE response is compared with experimental data[6,7] in Figure 5. In both the model result and the experimental data, the EEOE is a bandpass function, such that the emission drops off at low frequencies and also at a frequency below the CF of the current injection site. A large peak is not seen at CF. In general, the simulated EEOE magnitudes are too large to compare well with the experimental result.

3.4 Electrically-evoked emissions and basilar-membrane velocity

Figure 6 shows model EEOE and the electrically-evoked basilar membrane velocity (EEBMV) response alongside data from Xue et al.[11]. The experimental data are from the extreme base of the cochlea, for which the simulation failed to converge; and thus the model response was computed for the turn 2 location for which we have considerable emission data. When considered relative to CF

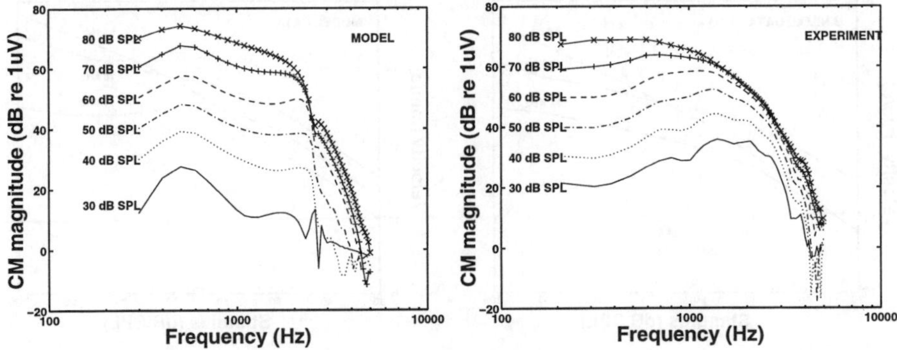

Figure 4: Model and experimental CM responses for various frequencies and sound levels. The model data is from the 2.5 kHz place. The experimental data is from turn 2 of the gerbil, whose tuned best frequency as determined using the summating potential is approximately 2.8 kHz.

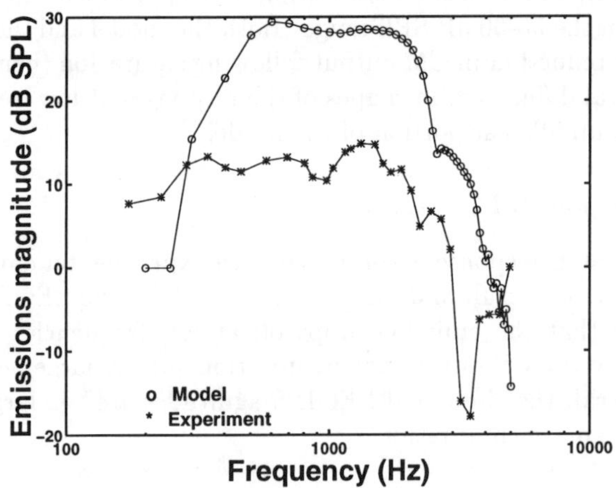

Figure 5: Model vs. experimental EEOE magnitudes from turn 2 of the gerbil. The CF of the model location is 2.5 kHz. The approximate experimental CF determined using the summating potential is 2.8 kHz

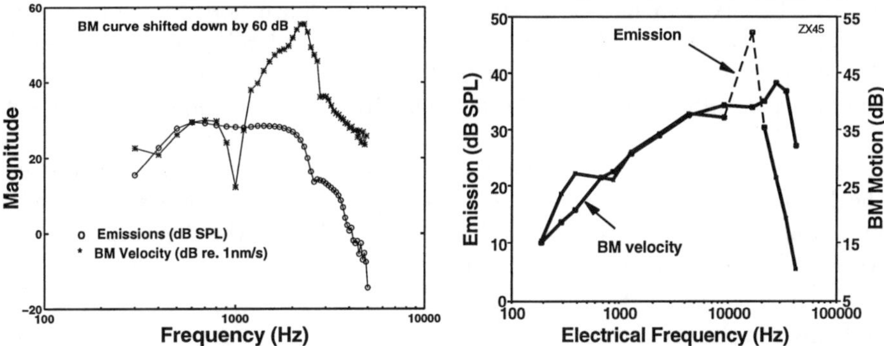

Figure 6: The left panel shows model results comparing EEOE and EEBMV. The right panel shows animal data from the gerbil. The dashed line indicates what is probably due to an ear-bar resonance, and thus the experimental EEOE do not peak as suggested by the dashed line. In the simulation, the EEBMV is referenced to nanometers, while the experimental data are referenced to micrometers. The simulation result was shifted so that a single ordinate can be used directly.

of the current injection location, there are general characteristics that both data share. At lower frequencies relative to the CF of the current injection site, EEBMV follows the profile of the EEOE. Also, in both data, the EEOE diminishes at a frequency less than CF. The detailed nature of the EEBMV response is not the same as would occur in the case of normal sound delivery in the ear canal, even though a peak is still present at CF. At a factor of 0.4 below CF in the model and from 0.3-0.7 below CF in the experimental data is a notch whose depth for the model is about 20 dB and in the case of the data ranges up to 20 dB. The notch both in the model and in the data is accompanied by a 180 degree phase shift.

4 Discussion

The traveling-wave amplifier model [1,2,3] augmented [8] with a model of scala media [10] is reasonably well validated against a broad range of experimental data. The basilar membrane mechanical data are almost ideal fits to the experimental data [9] across broad frequency and sound level ranges. The CM produced by the model lines up qualitatively well with data, although not perfectly for all frequencies and levels at the present time. In general, however, the model's frequency-dependence, level- dependence, phase angle, saturation, and bendover that characterize the CM are qualitatively close to physiological reality. The experimental and simulated EEOE shown here are quite similar in shape above 600 Hz, although they still differ considerably in absolute level. The drop-off in the model's emission at lower frequencies must occur due to the high-pass filter. The model also demonstrates salient points of agreement with EEBMV data [11], including the notch in magnitude that occurs roughly a factor of 0.5 below CF, the remnant of a CF-peak, and the similarities between the EEOE and EEBMV curves at lower frequencies. All this was achieved [8] by taking the scala media model [10] and joining it with the TWamp [1] model, without further parameter adjustment.

Acknowledgments

This work was funded by NIDCD and NSF.

References

1. Gonzales, D. (1994) *A nonlinear travelling wave amplifier model of the cochlea*, MS Thesis Boston University, Boston, MA .
2. Hubbard, A. (1993) *Science* **259** 68-71.
3. Hubbard, A. Gonzales, D. and Mountain D. (1993) *Proceedings of the International Symposium on the Biophysics of Hair Cell Sensory Systems*, 370-376.
4. Lutman, M. and Martin, A. (1979) *J. Sound and Vibration*, **64** 133-157.
5. Mountain, D. Hubbard, A. and McMullen,T (1983) *Mechanics of Hearing*, ed. E. deBoer and M. Viergever (Delft U.P. Delft).
6. Nakajima,H. (1996) *personal communication.*
7. Nakajima, H. Olsen, E. Mountain, D. and Hubbard ,A. (1994) *J. Acoust. Soc. Am,* **96** 786-794.
8. Ramachandran, P. (1996) *Investigations into a travelling wave amplifier model of the cochlea*, MS Thesis Boston University, Boston, MA.
9. Ruggero, M. Rich, N. and Recio, A. (1992) in *Auditory Physiology and Perception*, eds. Y. Cazals, L. Demany, and K. Horner (Pergamon Press, Oxford).
10. Shine, D. (1991) *The development and evaluation of an active model of the gerbil cochlea*, MS Theses Boston University, Boston, MA.
11. Xue, S. Mountain, D. and Hubbard, A. (1995) *Auditory Neuroscience*, in press.

POWER FLOW WITHIN THE ORGAN OF CORTI OF A THREE-DIMENSIONAL FINITE-ELEMENT COCHLEAR MODEL

P. J. KOLSTON

Department of Physiology, University of Bristol

Bristol BS8 1TD, United Kingdom.

paul.j.kolston@bristol.ac.uk

Three-dimensional finite-element modelling techniques make it possible to formulate a cochlear model without making assumptions regarding the number or types of degrees of freedom at each cross-section, and the number of modes of travelling-wave propagation. Here, analyses of longitudinal power flow within the organ of Corti of such a model are used to demonstrate that the cochlear amplifier produces a large and broad peak in the model's response using two mechanisms: (1) actively adding power to the travelling-wave and (2) reducing the stiffness of the basilar membrane.

1   Introduction

There can be little doubt that structures other than the basilar membrane (BM) and the outer hair cells (OHCs) are important to the integrity of the cochlear amplifier (CA). Many have shown that a mechanical system with two degrees of freedom (DOFs) at each cross-section of the cochlea[1-3] is able to account for cochlear amplification. Such lumped-element models exhibit a realistic response, but the verification of the assumptions made in the formulation of these models it is not possible *in vivo*, due to the extreme vulnerability of the CA to surgical insult. Although an isolated section of the organ of Corti (OC) appears to operate as a simple 2 DOF system[4] these *in situ* experiments do not provide the normal hydrodynamic loading that greatly affects the motion of the BM in the intact cochlea.[5] Extrapolations from such *in situ* experiments to the *in vivo* situation must therefore be exercised with great caution.

Three-dimensional finite-element (3-D FE) modelling techniques can be used to bridge the gaps in experimental data. These techniques remove the need for *a priori* assumptions in the formulation of a cochlear model regarding the number or types of DOFs at each cross-section, and the number of modes of travelling-wave propagation. Therefore, conclusions from studies utilizing 3-D FE methods are more general than those from studies using lumped-element models, and hence are more likely to be relevant to the real cochlea. Although finite-element models have enormous computational requirements, they can be implemented successfully in the frequency domain on inexpensive personal computers using specialized software; the implementation of a 3-D FE model has been described elsewhere.[6] Briefly, the cochlea is divided into a three-dimensional network of nodes, connected by branches representing the local mechanical properties.

The model system of simultaneous equations, obtained by applying continuity at each node, are solved iteratively using a variant of the conjugate gradient method.

The first simulations of a 3-D FE cochlear model have demonstrated that force generation by OHCs can indeed produce a large and broad peak in the BM response, presumably reflecting the role of the OHCs *in vivo*. It is the purpose of this paper to show how the model achieves this response, by looking at micromechanical power flow within the OC.

2   What does power flow tell us about the cochlear amplifier?

Sinusoidal motion of the stapes supplies the cochlea with mechanical power. This sets up a travelling-wave that propagates from base to apex, supported by the transmission-line formed by the mass of the cochlear fluid and the stiffness of the BM. The speed of propagation decreases as the wave travels through regions of lower BM stiffness. As the resistance of the BM becomes comparable to its stiffness, the energy in the travelling-wave is absorbed by the BM and a peak is produced in the envelope of the BM motion (the so-called tuning curve). An arbitrarily large peak in the tuning curve can be achieved by assuming a suitably small BM resistance, but the resulting peak is unrealistically sharp. Broadness can be added in the tuning curve either by also reducing the stiffness of the BM,[2] or by adding power to the travelling-wave as it nears its peak.[7]

Many of the current lumped-element models of the cochlea are formally equivalent.[8] Most rely on the same basic mechanism to achieve realistic tuning: the addition of power (i.e. activity) by OHCs. Some others achieve a realistic response by relying more on the OHCs reducing the stiffness of the BM[2,9]. Activity by OHCs is equivalent to the addition of *real* power to the cochlea, whereas BM stiffness reduction can be achieved via the addition of *reactive* power to the cochlea. The generalized flow of power in the cochlea is illustrated schematically in Fig. 1. The distinction between these two types of power flow is more than pedantic: the net flow of reactive power is always zero, so that electrochemical power sources to the cochlea (e.g. the stria vascularis) are only drained of real power. Indeed, the consideration of these two types of power may aid the identification of the components of the CA that are most vulnerable to surgical insult.

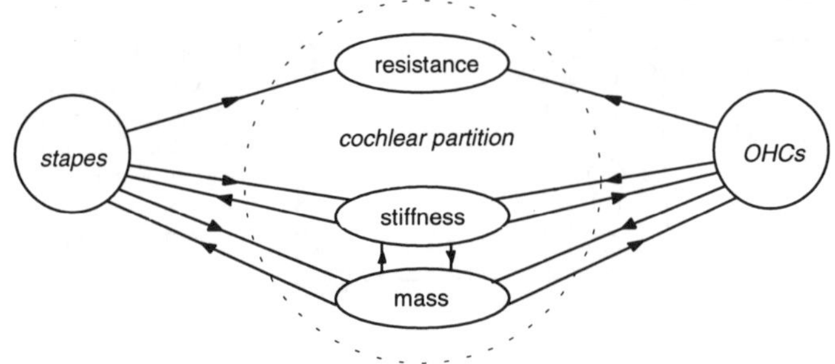

Figure 1. The generalized flow of power in the cochlea. Power flow is always *towards* a resistive component, where it is dissipated as heat. The power flow from a source to a reactive component (mass or stiffness) is *bi-directional*: during one half cycle of a sinusoidal stimulus the power flows to the component, to be returned on the opposite half cycle back to the source. Power flow between two reactive components is similarly bi-directional. By considering the flow of real and reactive power we can gain a more complete understanding of the operation of the cochlear amplifier.

3   Real and reactive power flow within the organ of Corti

The 3-D FE model allows us to visualize the flow of the two types of power anywhere within the cochlea. The model parameters used for the responses shown are given elsewhere.[6] The cochlea was discretized into 36000 nodes: 60 by 20 by 30 in length, height and width, respectively, representing the most basal 4.5mm portion of the cochlea. The stapes provided stimulation at 10kHz, and two sets of response data were obtained: with and without force generation by the OHCs.

Since analyses were performed in the frequency domain for sinusoidal excitation only, the time dependence of pressure and velocity at any position $\mathbf{x}=(x,y,z)$ within the 3-D FE model can be restated as $P(\mathbf{x},t)=P(\mathbf{x})e^{i\omega t}$ and $V(\mathbf{x},t)=V(\mathbf{x})e^{i\omega t}$, where $\omega=2\pi f$ and $i^2=-1$. The longitudinal flow of real power was calculated as $P(\mathbf{x})V_x(\mathbf{x})\cos(\phi)$, where $V_x(\mathbf{x})$ is velocity in the longitudinal direction and ϕ is the phase angle between pressure and velocity. Reactive power flow was calculated as $P(\mathbf{x})V_x(\mathbf{x})\sin(\phi)$.

Figure 2 shows the model OC with the four bead positions from where recordings have been made. The remaining figures shows the responses - vertical velocity and longitudinal power flow - at these points as a function of longitudinal position in the model. All ordinates are relative to the same arbitrary velocity (relative to stapes) or power reference.

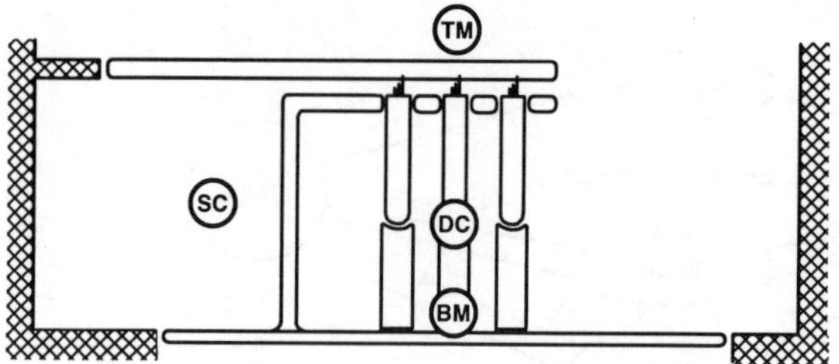

Figure 2. Positions in the organ of Corti (OC) from where recordings have been taken: vertical motion at BM and DC (Fig. 3), and real (Fig. 4) and reactive (Fig. 5) longitudinal power flow at all four positions.

When OHC force generation is present, the motion of the BM is less than the motion at the top of the DC (Fig. 3a). This is the result of the finite axial stiffness of Deiters' cells limiting the transmission of OHC forces to the BM. The removal of force generation by the OHCs causes a significant reduction in all motion. In agreement with experimental measurements,[10] the response phase (Fig. 3b) to the peak is little affected by OHC force generation. Close examination of Fig. 3b reveals that in the presence of OHC force generation there is a small phase difference between the motions at the top and the bottom of the Deiter's cell. This phase difference has been shown to play an important role in the operation of the CA.[6]

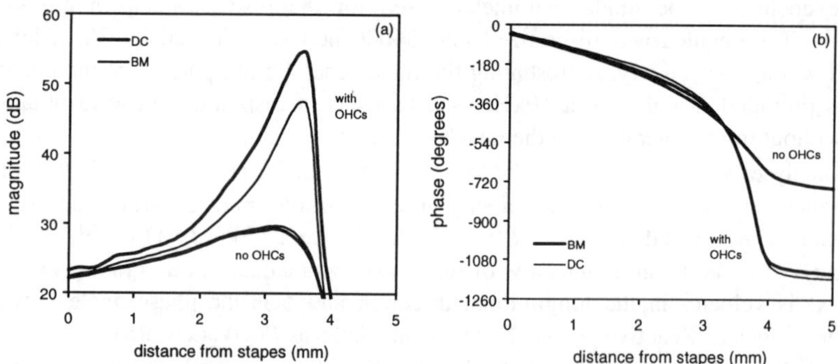

Figure 3. Magnitude (a) and phase (b) of the response on the basilar membrane (BM) and at the top of the Deiter's cell (DC). Force generation by the outer hair cells (OHCs) produces a large peak in the magnitude of the BM response but has little effect on the phase response to the peak, in agreement with experimental measurements *in vivo*. The finite axial stiffness of the DCs results in a smaller response on the BM than at the DC, and contributes to a small phase difference between the motions at each end of the DC.

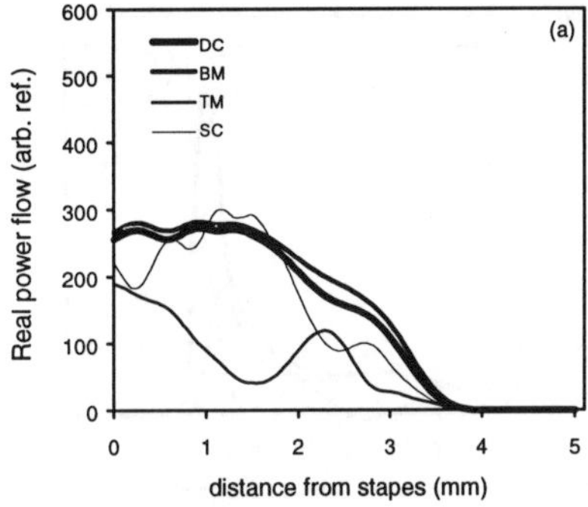
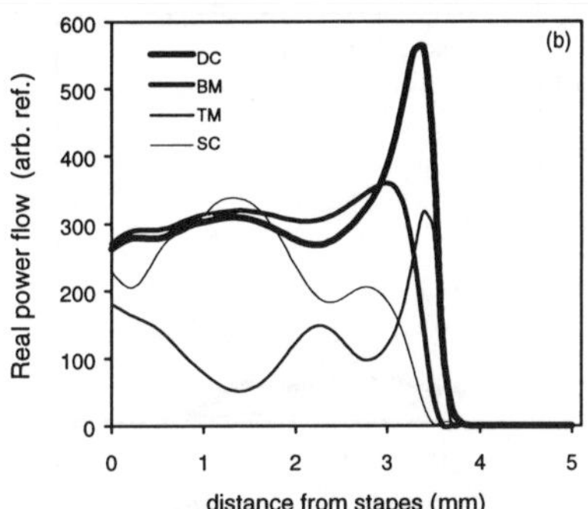

Figure 4. The longitudinal flow of real power at four positions within the OC, in the absence (a) and presence (b) of OHC force generation. In the absence of OHC force generation, the real power flows in the sulcus and near the tectorial membrane (TM) fluctuate, indicating a transfer of power from one region of the OC to the other. However, when integrated over each cross-section of the model, the net real power decreases monotonically. OHC force generation causes a large increase in real power at the DC near the peak of the tuning curve (Fig. 3a). This power is shared between the BM and the TM.

The longitudinal flow of real power near the BM decreases monotonically in the absence of OHC force generation (Fig. 4a), indicating that power injected by stapes motion is gradually absorbed along the length of the model. This absorption increases markedly near the peak of the tuning curve, where the speed of travelling-wave propagation is lowest. The real power flows in the sulcus and near the tectorial membrane (TM) fluctuate, indicating that power is transferred from one region of the OC to the other. This may be indicative of 2 modes of travelling-wave propagation in the model.[11] When integrated over each cross-section of the model, the net real power decreases monotonically (data not shown).

The presence of OHC force generation produces a sharp increase in the real power at the level of the Deiter's cells (Fig. 4b). This power is shared between the TM and the BM, due to the position of the OHCs within the OC. The small difference in the positions of the power flow maxima on the BM and TM further suggests that travelling-wave propagation in the real cochlea is not represented accurately in single-transmission-line cochlear models.

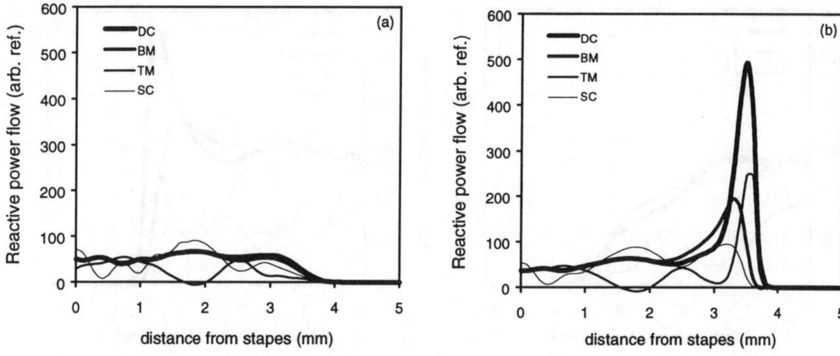

Figure 5. The longitudinal flow of reactive power at four positions within the OC, in the absence (a) and presence (b) of OHC force generation. Comparison with Fig. 4 reveals that the cochlear amplifier works by adding both real and reactive power to the travelling-wave.

Figure 4 shows clearly that in the presence of OHC force generation the model is active, with the CA adding real power to the travelling-wave. However, a similar enhancement occurs in the amount of reactive power flowing longitudinally (Fig. 5). This suggests that the two possible effects of force generation by OHCs - the addition of real power to the travelling-wave and the reduction of BM stiffness - are both important in the real cochlea.

4 Conclusion

Lumped-element models of cochlear mechanics produce realistic BM tuning curves in two ways: by adding power to the travelling-wave or by reducing the stiffness of the BM. The analyses presented here, of micromechanical power flow in a 3-D FE model, suggest that the operation of the CA relies on *both* mechanisms to achieve a large and broad enhancement of the BM tuning curve. In contrast to studies involving lumped-element models, in the 3-D FE model this conclusion is independent of either the number or types of DOFs at each cross-section, or the number of modes of travelling-wave propagation. The results presented here provide further support for the contention[12] that the term "active process" does not adequately describe the behaviour of the CA.

Acknowledgement

The author is a Royal Society University Research Fellow.

References

1. Neely, S.T. and Kim, D.O. (1986). A model for active elements in cochlear biomechanics. *J. Acoust. Soc. Am.* **79** 1472-1480.
2. Kolston, P.J., de Boer, E., Viergever, M.A. and Smoorenburg, G.F. (1990). What type of force does the cochlear amplifier produce? *J. Acoust. Soc. Am.* **88** 1794-1801.
3. Geisler, C.D. (1993). A realizable cochlear model using feedback from motile outer hair cells. *Hear. Res.* **68** 253-262.
4. Mammano, F. and Ashmore, J.F. (1993). Reverse transduction measured in the isolated cochlea by laser Michelson interferometry. *Nature* **365** 838-841.
5. Cooper, N.P. and Rhode, W.S. (1996). Fast travelling waves, slow travelling waves and their interactions in experimental studies of apical cochlear mechanics. *Auditory Neuroscience*, (In Press).
6. Kolston, P.J. and Ashmore, J.F. (1996). Finite element modeling of the cochlea in three dimensions. *J. Acoust. Soc. Am.* **99** 455-467.
7. Diependaal, R.J., de Boer, E. and Viergever, M.A. (1987). Cochlear power flux as an indicator of mechanical activity. *J. Acoust. Soc. Am.* **82** 917-926.
8. de Boer, E. (1995). On the equivalence of locally active models of the cochlea. *J. Acoust. Soc. Am.* **98** 1400-1409.
9. Geisler, C.D. (1995). A cochlear model using feed-forward outer-hair-cell forces. *Hear. Res.* **86** 132-146.
10. Ruggero, M.A. and Rich, N.C. (1991). Furosemide alters the organ of Corti mechanics: Evidence for feedback of outer hair cells upon basilar membrane. *J. Neurosci.* **11** 1057-1067.
11. Hubbard, A.E. (1993). A traveling-wave amplifier model of the cochlea. *Science* **259** 68-71.
12. Kolston, P.J. (1988). Sharp mechanical tuning in a cochlear model without negative damping. *J. Acoust. Soc. Am.* **83** 1481-1487.

A GENERATION OF DISTORTION PRODUCTS IN A MODEL OF COCHLEAR MECHANICS

S.T. NEELY, L.J. STOVER

Boys Town National Research Hospital, 555 North 30th Street
Omaha, NE 68131, USA
neely@boystown.org

Considerable evidence implicates outer hair cells (OHC) as being responsible for the generation of distortion products (DP) in cochlear mechanics. Forces exerted on the basilar membrane by OHCs must saturate at high levels and, thereby, become a major source of nonlinearity. Realistic growth of distortion products requires that the saturation of OHC forces (with increasing level) be gradual. The apparent band-pass filtering of the distortion product otoacoustic emission (DPOAE) observed in ear canal sound pressure can be explained as the combination of two effects. (1) The DPOAE becomes smaller as the primary frequencies are separated because the basilar membrane vibration becomes smaller at the place where the two tones interact. (2) The DPOAE becomes smaller as the primary frequencies are brought closer together because reflected energy from the DP place partially cancels the retrograde signal. This explanation does not require the presence of any "second filter" in the mechanics of the cochlear partition. With a nonlinear, active model of cochlear mechanics, we have explored whether a simulated hearing loss at the DP frequency can influence the apparent band-pass filtering of DPs, which are generated primarily at the f_2 place. Results of this simulation are compared with DP measurements from a subject with low-frequency hearing loss.

1 Introduction

Distortion product otoacoustic emissions (DPOAE) are generated within the cochlea when two tones interact at some place on the basilar membrane (BM). Distortion products (DP) are a consequence of nonlinear forces exerted on the BM by outer hair cells (OHC). These OHCs forces have the beneficial effect of extending the dynamic range of hearing because they provide greater gain at low levels than at high levels[1]. DPOAEs are a by-product of the OHC influence on cochlear mechanics. The most prominent DPOAE is observed at the frequency $f_d=2f_1-f_2$.

The DPOAE measured with f_1 swept and f_2 held constant is observed to have maximum amplitude when f_d is 0.25 to 0.75 octave below f_2. When DP amplitude is plotted as a function of DP frequency, it has a band-pass appearance because it decreases when f_d becomes either greater or smaller than the optimum f_d. It has been suggested that this so-called "DP filter" is due to resonant tuning of the tectorial membrane[2,3] or other, similar "second filter" mechanism in the micromechanics of the organ of Corti[4]. The model results presented in this paper require an alternative explanation.

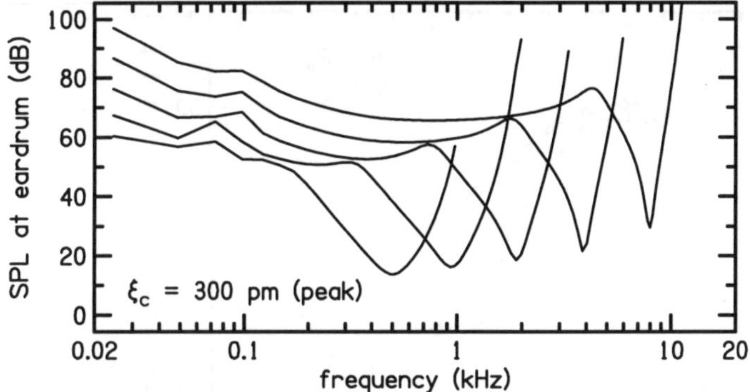

Figure 1: Isodisplacement tuning curves. The curves indicate the stimulus pressure at the eardrum required to produce a 300 pm displacement (1 pm = 10^{-12} m) in the shearing between tectorial membrane and reticular lamina at 5 places along cochlear partition, 6.8, 11.8, 16.7, 21.0, and 24.7 mm from the base. The frequency-place map resembles a human cochlea. These tuning curves were inferred from the response of the model to a very low level click, because the model is nearly linear at low levels.

2   Methods

DPOAEs were generated in a nonlinear, active model of cochlear mechanics. The major differences between the present model and the model described previously by Neely and Stover[4] are (1) the model parameters were adjusted to obtain the iso-displacement tuning curves shown in Fig 1 and (2) the saturating nonlinearity in the OHC mechano-electric transduction was modified to produce more gradual saturation.

The mechano-electric transduction stage of the OHCs in the model was made to be nonlinear by the introduction of a dimensionless multiplier γ which was a function of the displacement hair bundle (HB) at the top of the OHC. The HB displacement is equal to the shear displacement ξ_c between the tectorial membrane and reticular lamina.

$$\gamma = \left[1 + \left(\frac{\xi_c}{d_o} \right)^2 + \left(\frac{\xi_c}{d_o} \right)^4 \right]^{-\frac{1}{4}}$$

The form of this saturating nonlinearity, is similar, but more gradual, than the non-linear function described by Yates[5]. For the model results in this paper, the value of the parameter d_o was 10 nm.

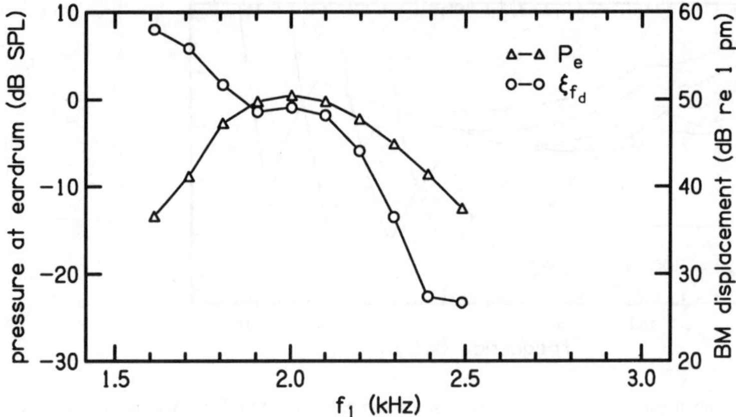

Figure 2: Simulated DPOAE and BM displacement with f_d constant. The f_2 frequency was chosen to keep the DP frequency, $f_d=2f_1-f_2$, constant at 1550 Hz. The primary tone levels were 60 and 55 dB SPL. The triangles indicate the amplitude of the DP in the pressure at the eardrum as a function of the f_1 frequency. This simulated DPOAE was separated from the total pressure at the eardrum by Fourier analysis. The circles show the amplitude of the DP component of BM displacement at the DP place, 18.1 mm from the base of the cochlea. Note that as f_1 approaches f_d below 1.9 kHz, the DPOAE decreases, whereas, the BM displacement continues to increase.

3   Results

3.1   DP generated with f_d held constant

In order to compare the frequency dependence of the DPOAE amplitude with BM displacement at the characteristic place for the DP frequency, it is convenient to vary the frequency of the primary tones in a manner that keeps the DP frequency (and thereby also the DP place) constant. Figure 2 shows results of DP generation as a function of the f_1 frequency. The f_2 frequency was adjusted to keep $f_d=2f_1-f_2$ constant at 1550 Hz. The level of the f_1 tone at the eardrum was 60 dB SPL and the level of the f_2 tone was 55 dB SPL. A band-pass characteristic is observed in the amplitude of the pressure at the eardrum, but not in BM displacement at the DP place. Unlike the pressure at the eardrum, the BM displacement continues to increase as f_1 approaches f_d.

The observation that the frequency dependence of the simulated DPOAE differs from that of the BM displacement suggests that the DPOAE represents the combination of signals from multiple sources. Apparently, the DP generation is distributed over multiple points on the BM. Evidence to support this interpretation is

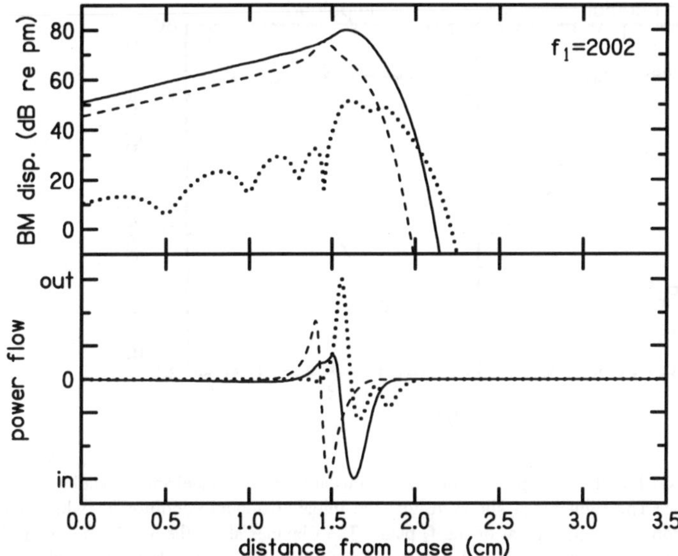

Figure 3: BM displacement and power flow as a function of place. The primary frequency components for these model results were $f_1=2002$ and $f_2=2490$. The solid, dashed, and dotted lines represent the f_1, f_2, and f_d frequency components, respectively, obtained by Fourier analysis. The upper panel shows BM displacement in dB re 1 pm. Each power flow curve in the lower panel was normalized so that its maximum value (positive or negative) is at full scale. Positive values of power flow for the primary frequencies indicate places along the cochlear partition where signal energy is generated due to OHC forces. The positive peak in the power flow for f_d indicates the place where the DP is generated. Negative power flow values indicate places where that frequency component is absorbed by the cochlear partition.

provided in upper panel of Fig. 3 where the f_1, f_2, and f_d components of BM displacement are plotted as a function of place along the BM for one particular choice of primary frequencies. The notches observed in the f_d component suggest "standing waves" due to interference between the DP generated at the f_2 place and the reflected signal from the DP place. The power flow plot (in the lower panel of Fig. 3) shows the site of DP generation between the f_1 and f_2 places.

3.2 DP generated with f_2 held constant

Although, the DP is generated near the f_2 place, the DPOAE is apparently also influenced by the region of the cochlea apical to the f_2 place. This question was further investigated by altering OHC forces in the cochlear model at all points apical to the f_2 place. DP were generated with a paradigm that kept the f_2 frequency constant

438

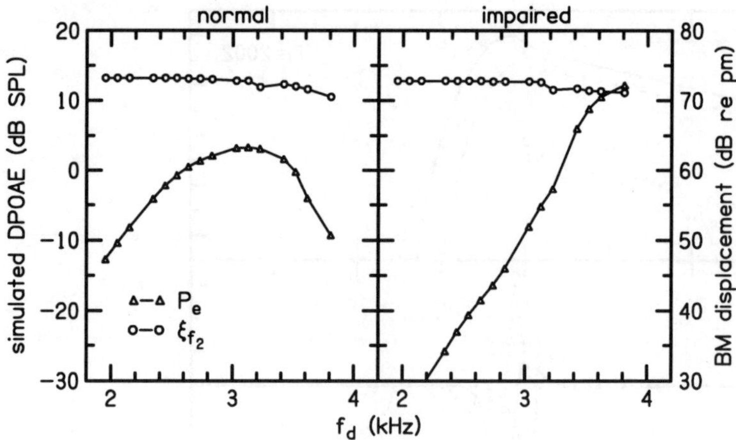

Figure 4: Simulated DPOAE and BM displacement with f_2 constant. The left panel shows results from the normal model condition. The right panel shows results the impaired model condition in which OHC forces are eliminated from all points apical of the f_2 place. The triangles show the amplitude of the DP component of the pressure at the eardrum, i.e. the simulated DPOAE. The circles show the amplitude of BM displacement at the f_2 place. The primary tone levels were 55 and 60 dB SPL. Note that the impaired DPOAE does not have the band-pass characteristic observed in the normal DPOAE.

in order to monitor the effect of the simulated cochlear impairment on BM vibration at the f_2 place.

Figure 4 shows results of DP generation as a function of the $f_d = 2f_1 - f_2$ frequency. The f_1 frequency was adjusted to keep f_2 constant at 4004 Hz. The level of the f_1 tone at the eardrum was 60 dB SPL and the level of the f_2 tone was 55 dB SPL. The left panel shows the normal state of the model; the same nonlinear, active model used to generate the results shown in Figs. 1-3. A band-pass characteristic is observed in the amplitude of the pressure at the eardrum, the simulated DPOAE. BM displacement at the f_2 place (11.3 mm from the base) is almost constant, but shows some evidence of suppression as f_1 approaches f_2.

The right panel of Fig. 4 shows an impaired cochlear model. Low-frequency hearing loss was simulated in the model by eliminating OHC forces at all points apical of the f_2 place (12 to 35 mm from the base). BM displacement at the f_2 is essentially unaffected by this alteration to the model. In contrast, however, the simulated DPOAE loses its band-pass characteristic. The amplitude of the DPOAE in the impaired model condition continues to increase as f_1 approaches f_2.

Measurements of the DPOAE in ears with normal hearing threshold at f_2 and elevated threshold at lower frequencies do not have the same band-pass appearance

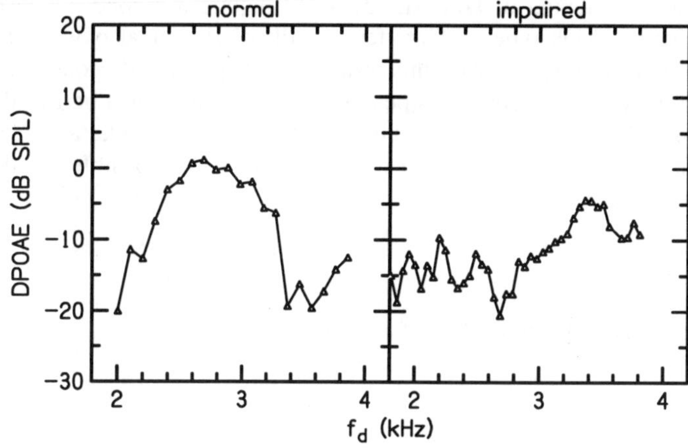

Figure 5: DPOAE measurements from normal and impaired ears. The right panel shows DPOAE amplitudes as function of f_d (with f_2 held constant) in an ear with normal hearing thresholds. The primary tone levels were 50 and 60 dB SPL. The left panel shows the results of similar measurements in an ear with low-frequency hearing loss showing the loss of the band-pass filter shape that is observed in the normal ear. The primary tone levels were 70 and 60 dB SPL.

observed in normal ears. Examples of DPOAE frequency response from a normal hearing subject and a subject with low-frequency hearing loss are show in Fig. 5. The DP filter shape in the impaired ear appears to be more high-pass than band-pass. The change from band-pass to high-pass is similar to the trend observed in the model.

Inevitable differences in tuning-curve shape and growth of BM displacement between the model and the subjects' ears may account observed between Figs. 4 and 5. The impaired subject had normal hearing at 4 kHz (f_2) and moderate hearing loss at 3 and 2 kHz (within the range of f_d), but the extent and severity of the cochlear damage is not know and probably less extensive than the simulated impairment.

4   Conclusions

The model results support the interpretation that the apparent band-pass characteristic of the DP frequency response is due to two separate mechanisms. (1) As the primary tones come closer together, the DPOAE is reduced by out-of-phase contributions coming from either near the f_2 place or reflected from the DP place. (2) As primary tones are separated further apart, the DPOAE is reduced because the amplitude of basilar membrane (BM) vibration at the place where the primary tones interact becomes smaller. This observation was first reported by Matthews and Molnar[6] who showed that the band-pass tuning of DPOAEs does not require a second-tuning in cochlear micromechanics. This type of "interference filter" should also work for higher-order distortion products; however, this result has not yet been demonstrated. Although, the model used in this paper does possess a second tuning as a part of the OHC feedback system, the "spectral zero" is about an octave below the characteristic frequency (as can be seen in Fig. 1) and, therefore, cannot be responsible for the band-pass tuning of the DPOAE.

Acknowledgments

We thank Michael Gorga and Douglas Keefe for helpful comments.

References

1. Allen, J.B. and Neely, S.T. (1992) Micromechanical models of the cochlea, Physics Today **45** 40-47.
2. Allen, J.B. (1990) Modeling the noise damaged cochlea. In: The Mechanics and Biophysics of Hearing, ed. P. Dallos, C.D. Geisler, J.W. Matthews, M.A. Ruggero, and C.R. Steele (Springer-Verlag, New York) pp. 324-332.
3. Brown, A.M. and Gaskill, S.A. (1992) Can basilar membrane tuning be inferred from distortion measurement? In: The Mechanics and Biophysics of Hearing, ed. P. Dallos, C.D. Geisler, J.W. Matthews, M.A. Ruggero, and C.R. Steele (Springer-Verlag, New York) pp. 164-169.
4. Neely, S.T. and Stover, L.J. (1993) Otoacoustic emissions from a nonlinear, active model of cochlear mechanics. In: Biophysics of Hair Cell Sensory Systems, ed. H. Duifhuis, J.W. Horst, P. van Dijk, and S.M. van Netten (World Scientific, Singapore) pp. 64-71.
5. Yates, G.K. (1990) Basilar membrane nonlinearity and its influence on auditory nerve rate-intensity functions, *Hearing Research* **50** 145-162.
6. Matthews, J.W. and Molnar, C.E. (1986). Modeling intracochlear and ear canal distortion product ($2f_1-f_2$). In: Peripheral Auditory Mechanisms, ed. J.B. Allen, J.L. Hall, A. Hubbard, S.T. Neely, and A. Tubis (Springer-Verlag, New York) pp. 258-265.

ENERGY TRANSFER AMONGST COUPLED OSCILLATING MODES IN THE NONLINEAR COCHLEA: THE PHYSICAL BASIS OF THE BASILAR MEMBRANE RESPONSE TO TRANSIENTS

R. NOBILI

Dipartimento di Fisica "G.Galilei", via Marzolo 8,
35100 Padova, Italy

F. MAMMANO

International School for Advanced Studies
Laboratory of Biophysics, via Beirut 9
34014 Trieste, Italy

In two previous papers (Mammano and Nobili [1], Nobili and Mammano [2]) we presented a frequency–domain analysis of cochlear mechanics, aiming at clarifying stationary phenomenology both in the linear approximation and in nonlinear regimes. In this paper we further the analysis by solving the motion equation of the cochlear partition in the time domain and report some results on transient responses which we deem relevant for understanding the role of nonlinearity in cochlear sound processing. In particular, we found that traveling wave propagation, combined with compressive nonlinearity of forward transduction, results in immediate energy transfer between cochlear partition oscillating modes during rapid changes of input frequency. The consequences of this may be relevant for signal processing applications.

1 The time–domain motion–equation of the cochlear partition

Referring, both for contents and notation, to the papers quoted in the Abstract, we transcribe in shorthand the cochlear partition motion equation

$$\partial_t^2 \vec{\xi} = -\left(\mathbf{G} + \mathbf{M}\right)^{-1}\{\vec{g}_s\, \partial_t^2 \sigma(t) + \mathbf{K}\vec{\xi} + \mathbf{H}\, \partial_t \vec{\xi} + \vec{u}[\vec{\eta}]\}. \tag{1}$$

solved for the second partial time derivative (acceleration) $\partial_t^2 \vec{\xi}$ of the array of basilar membrane (BM) displacements $\vec{\xi}$. These are compactly represented here as a vector each element of which is the local BM displacement $\xi(x,t)$ at site x and time t. As in Ref.2 Appendix, $\sigma(t)$ is the stapes displacement, $\vec{g}_s$ is the vector representation of the stapes acceleration propagator $G_s(x)$, $\mathbf{G}$ is the matrix representations of the Green's function $G(x,x')$ and $\mathbf{M}$, $\mathbf{K}$, $\mathbf{H}$ are diagonal matrix representations of the BM mass $m(x)$, stiffness $k(x)$ and viscosity coefficient $h(x)$, respectively. $\vec{u}[\vec{\eta}]$ is the vector representation of the nonlinear undamping functional $U[x,t;\xi]$, which depends on ξ through the outer hair cell (OHC) stereocilia displacement $\eta(x,t)$ (Ref.2, Eq.22), represented here

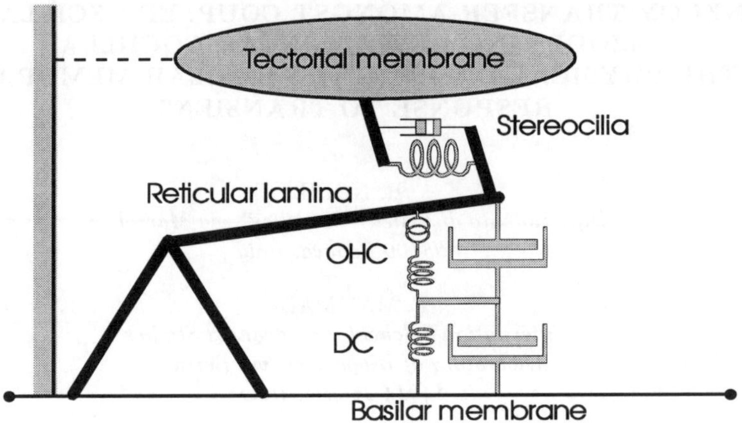

Figure 1: Viscoelastic characteristics of cochlear partition sections.
The outer hair cell (OHC) motor (crossing circles) is represented as a displacement
generator in series with finite source stiffness (spring). OHCs and Deiters' cells (DCs)
are assumed to have similar viscosity–dominated viscoelastic parameters, here represented in spring dash–pot notation. Thus the reticular lamina (RL) to basilar membrane (BM) coupling acts as a mechanical high–pass filter whose transfer–function
pole cancels the electrical low–pass zero filtering the OHC receptor potential. The
stereocilia–TM coupling, which is mechanically effective because of the RL tilt, is
supposed to be stiffness–dominated. Thus the TM resonates locally at frequencies
approaching BM characteristic frequencies (CFs) from below. Dashed line represents
ineffective TM attachment to limbus.

as a component of the array $\vec{\eta}$. As the stereocilia displacement is caused by
the shearing motion of the tectorial membrane (TM) relative to the reticular
lamina (RL), $\vec{\eta}$ satisfies the time domain representation of Ref. 2 Eq.12

$$\partial_t^2 \vec{\eta} = -\partial_t^2 \vec{\xi} - \bar{\mathbf{M}}^{-1}\{\bar{\mathbf{K}}\,\vec{\eta} + \bar{\mathbf{H}}\,\partial_t\vec{\eta}\}\,, \tag{2}$$

where $\bar{\mathbf{M}}$, $\bar{\mathbf{K}}$, $\bar{\mathbf{H}}$ are diagonal matrix representations of the TM mass $m_{TM}(x)$
stiffness $k_{TM}(x)$ and viscosity coefficient $h_{TM}(x)$, respectively. For the sake
of simplicity we ignored the longitudinal shearing viscosity coupling amongst
adjacent BM sections in Eq. 1, as well as the viscoelastic coupling of the TM
attachment to the limbus in Eq. 2 (see Fig.1).

The elements $u(x,t)$ of $\vec{u}$ depend locally on $\eta(x,t)$ according to the expression

$$u(x,t) = A(x)\,S[B(x)\,\eta(x,t)]\,, \tag{3}$$

where $S(y)$ is the normalised Boltzmann's partition function of OHC mechano–electrical transducer channels (Ref.2, Fig.1 and Eq.9), $A(x) \approx h(x)/B(x)$, $B(x)$ being a geometrical form factor which accounts for TM–stereocilia coupling.

The simultaneous system of Eqs. 1 and 2 was solved numerically using Euler's method (Press *et al.*[3]) and assuming

$$B(x) \approx \beta(x)\frac{m(x)}{h(x)} \, .$$

Explicit expressions for all the above functions are found in Ref.2 Appendix.

Two points are worth emphasising in Eq. 1. Firstly, were $\mathbf{G}$ zero, the equation would describe a system of uncoupled harmonic oscillators with non-linear damping. Actually, the rows of the inverse mass–added Green's function matrix $(\mathbf{G} + \mathbf{M})^{-1}$ have zero–mean Mexican–hat profiles like the one sampled in Fig.2a. Therefore Eq. 1 describes a system of nonlinear oscillators linearly interacting through a sort of medium–range negative inverse–mass coupling.

Secondly, product $(\mathbf{G} + \mathbf{M})^{-1}\vec{g}_s$ is the effective contribution to the local BM acceleration $\partial_t^2 \xi(x,t)$ coming from the direct action of the stapes. As evidenced in Fig.2b, this term decays rapidly moving away from the base of the cochlea and becomes negligible within 1/5 of the BM length. This clearly implies that traveling waves are excited in close proximity to the base and propagate towards the apex by virtue of the BM–BM hydrodynamic coupling alone.

Another point concerns the relationship between Eq.1 and Eq.2. Considering that IHCs respond to $\vec{\eta}$ rather than $\vec{\xi}$, from Eq.2 it is appearent that waves traveling on the BM work merely as carriers for the TM resonances, which localise in the proximity of the wave peaks and enhance the frequency selectivity of the input to the VIII nerve.

As discussed in Ref.2, the shape of the nonlinear undamping term $U[x, t; \xi]$ follows from the assumptions that: *i*) the OHC receptor potential rolls off with frequency as expected for a simple RC circuit with local cut-offs much lower then the corresponding BM characteristic frequencies (CFs); *ii*) the TM resonates locally at frequencies approaching CFs from below; *iii*) Deiters' cells transmit OHC forces to the BM primarily through viscous coupling, thus acting as mechanical high–pass filters which compensate for the electrical low–pass filtering of the OHC membrane (pole–zero cancellation). These properties combine to produce a force term which, at low sound pressure levels (SPLs), acts as a negative viscous resistance only over a BM tract

whose length is comparable to the width of the TM resonant peak. These concepts are summarised schematically in Fig.1.

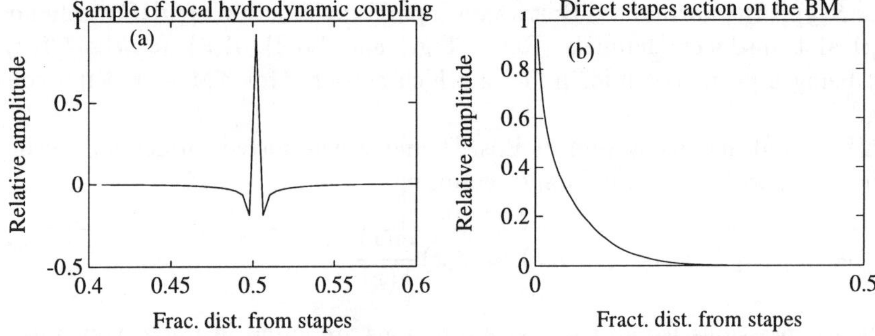

Figure 2: Hydrodynamic BM–BM and stapes–BM coupling.

(a) Typical row profile of $(\mathbf{G}+\mathbf{M})^{-1}$, the inverse mass-added Green's function in matrix notation, appearing in Eq.1. All matrix rows exhibit the same Mexican–hat–like behaviour, varying only slightly in size. All row profiles peak on the principal diagonal, the only subset of positive matrix elements. The triangular shape of the peak is an artefact due to the limited number of BM sections used (245). Increasing matrix dimension increases both positive and negative peak heights and causes the peak width to shrink. The height of each pea
k represents the inverse of the local effective self–mass of the corresponding cochlear section. The positive peak is sided by negative regions representing the strength of the coupling to adjacent cochlear partition sections. Singularly, the hydrodynam
ic effect does not correspond to a sort of distributed mass loading the cochlear partition, as the integral over the whole Mexican–hat curve vanishes. (b) The curve represents normalised product $(\mathbf{G}+\mathbf{M})^{-1}\vec{g}_s$ which enters Eq.1 as
a distributed proportionality constant of the input signal. Hence, curve ordinates are point–by–point proportional to the contribution to the BM acceleration from the stapes motion. Notice rapid decay moving away from the base of the cochlea. Approxim
ation of the profile in (a) by a differential operator and that in (b) by a function vanishing everywhere except in zero, yields a differential equation version for Eq.1 with input injected as a boundary condition at the cochlear base. This forms the mathematical substrate for transmission–line models of the cochlea.

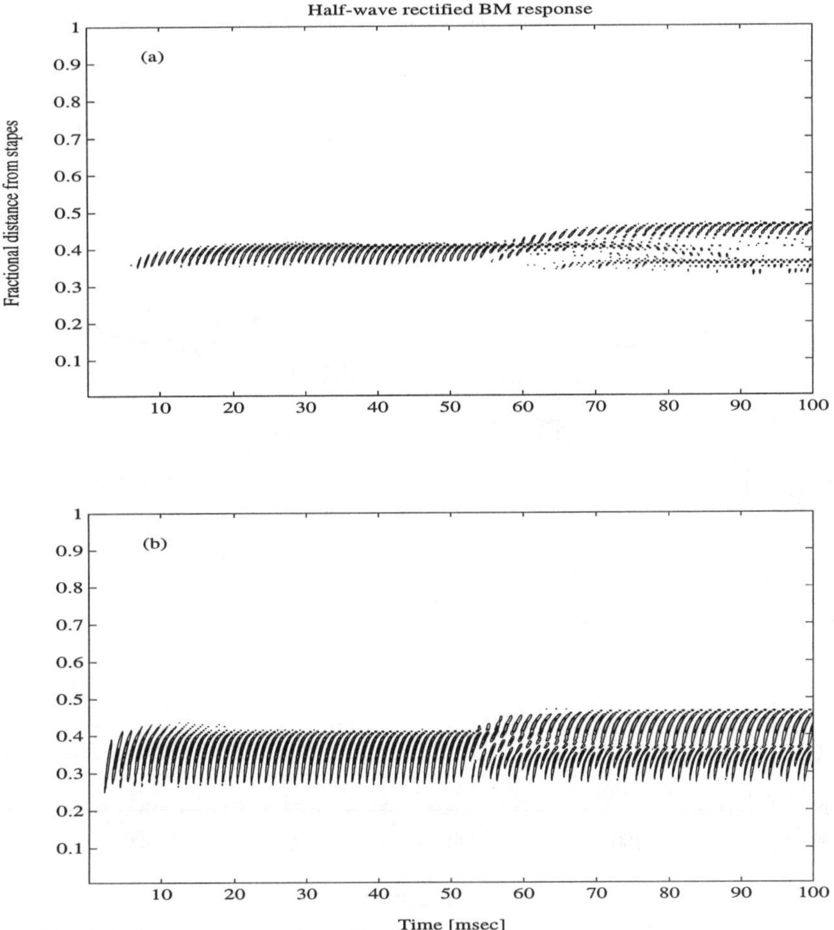

Figure 3: Energy transfer during tone bifurcation

A 1 kHz input tone bifurcates abruptly into the superposition of 1.2 kHz and 0.8 kHz
tones whose amplitudes are half that of the initial signal. Contours show half–wave
rectified BM responses. Amplitude in (a), which is 20 dB less than (b), falls
within the lower linearity range of the BM input/output function. Notice that in (a)
the response to the initial tone continues to ring while the side tone responses are
slowly growing in amplitude. By contrast, in (b) the initial response does not ring b
ut transfers continuously its energy to the lower-frequency tone while the higher–
frequency response rises somewhat independently and beats slightly with the other.

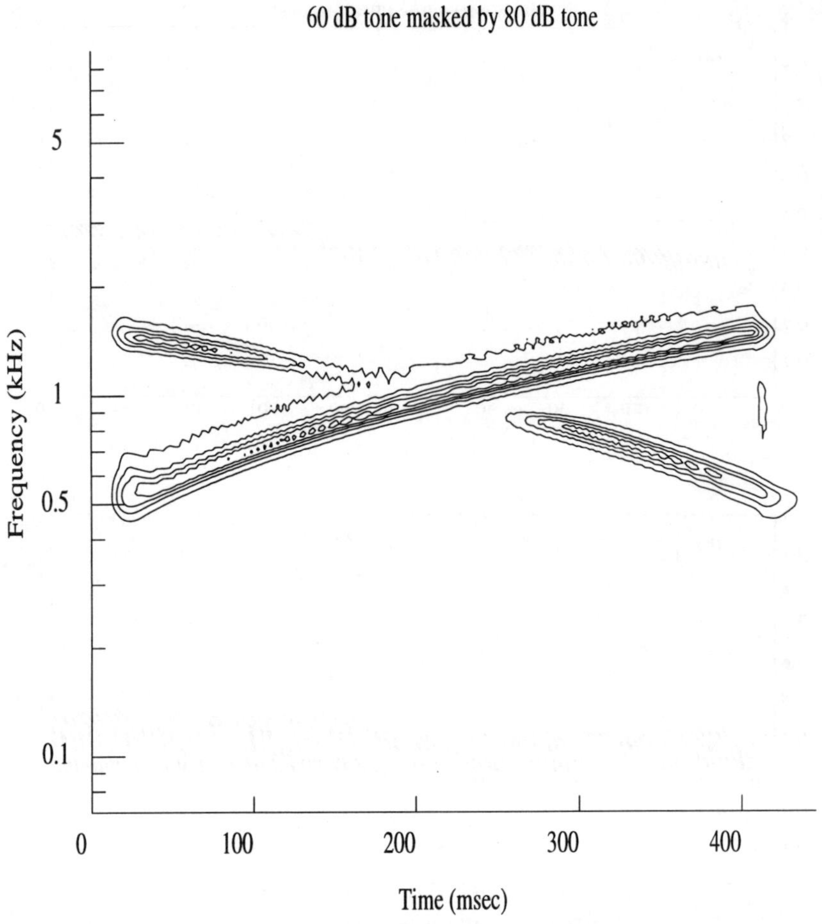

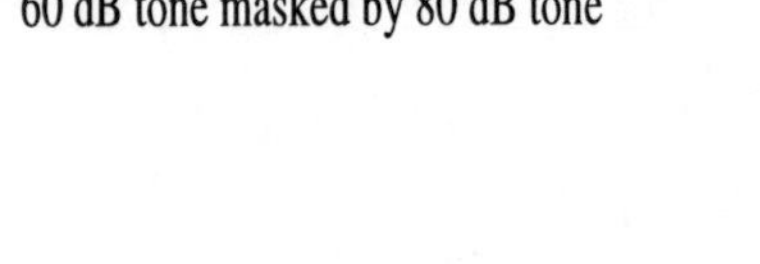

Figure 4: Dynamic masking.

Contour plot of BM squared amplitude responses, averaged over one period of local oscillation, to a pair of saturating tones with 20 dB amplitude ratio. Tone frequencies vary with time and cross at 1kHz. Notice that, far from the crossing region, the am plitude of the 60 dB tone response is comparable to the 80 dB tone response because of the BM compressive nonlinearity. This simulation is representative of amplitude response information putatively detectable at the acoustic ganglion level.

2 How nonlinearity affects BM transient responses

In the active cochlea, harmonic distortions are negligible relative to the fundamental (Ref.2 Fig.4) below ≈ 30 dB SPL, where BM responses are finely tuned, and above ≈ 90 dB SPL, where the responses are broadly tuned (Ref.2 Fig 3). As in both these conditions the linear approximation holds, the BM oscillation modes can be decomposed into an orthogonal system of independent vibrations. This implies that, in these conditions, the cochlea is equivalent to a Fourier filter bank. However, in normal speech communication, SPLs fall just between these two regimes, precisely where distortion is maximal, implying that non linearity is strategic for sound processing.

Fig.3 shows computer simulations of the half–wave rectified BM responses at low (a) and saturating (b) SPLs for an input tone bifurcating abruptly from a given frequency f into two tones with half amplitude, one tone of lower frequency and the other higher. These results indicate that nonlinearity combines with the underlying hydrodynamics so as to favour intermodal energy transfer during rapid frequency changes, such as those occurring at consonant–vowel formant transitions.

Fig.4 shows the masking effect produced by an 80 dB SPL tone of linearly increasing frequency, crossing a 60 dB tone of decreasing frequency. This result is particularly interesting as it shows that the same properties we found for steady–state masking (Ref.2 Fig.6) apply also to dynamic conditions.

References

1. Mammano F. and Nobili R. (1993) "Biophysics of the cochlea: Linear approximation", *J. Acoust. Soc. Am.*, **93** 3320–3332.
2. Nobili R. and Mammano F. (1996) "Biophysics of the cochlea II: Stationary nonlinear phenomenology", *J. Acoust. Soc. Am.*, **99** 2244–2255.
3. Press W.H., Flannery B.P., Teukolsky S.A., Vetterlin W.T. (1988) *Numerical Recipes in C*, Cambridge University Press, Cambridge, U.K.

AN ANALYSIS OF MECHANICAL INTERACTION BETWEEN THE OUTER HAIR CELL AND TWO ADJACENT COCHLEAR MEMBRANES

S. M. NOVOSELOVA

Russian Academy of Sciences,
Steklov Mathematical Institute, St. Petersburg Department,
Fontanka 27, St. Petersburg 191011, Russia

E-mail: smn@pdmi.ras.ru

Introduction

Discovery of outer hair cells motility gave a rise to a certain reconsideration of basic principles of cochlear mechanics. The active models became recognized as received fact. Contrary to widely accepted beliefs, vibrations of complex cross section of cochlear partition is examined here in terms of mechanics of multi-degree-of-freedom systems.

1   Statement of the eigenvalue problem

Consider a cross section of a coupled system made up of two thin elastic plates linked with a raw of springs (Fig. 1).

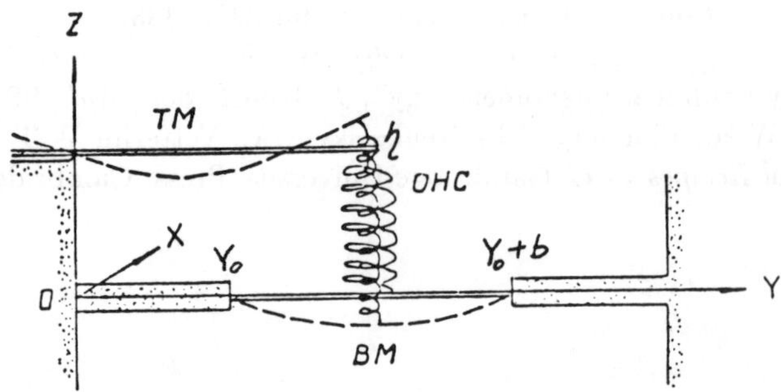

Fig. 1. A model of cochlear complex cross section. TM – tectorial membrane; BM – basilar membrane; OHC – outer hair cell.

For simplicity and brevity of derivations, the energy dissipation is neglected here without loss of generality; the fluid media is provisionally removed for the same sake. A possibility to describe the tectorial membrane with a flat thin anisotropic plate is examined by Novoselova[1].

The free vibrations of both membranes obey the plate equations:

$$D_t \frac{\partial^4 U_t}{\partial y^4} + \mu_t \frac{\partial^2 U_t}{\partial t^2} = 0, \quad D_b \frac{\partial^4 U_b}{\partial y^4} + \mu_b \frac{\partial^2 U_b}{\partial t^2} = 0, \tag{1}$$

where D_t and D_b are the bending stiffnesses of tectorial and basilar membranes respectively, μ_t and μ_b are the surface mass densities, $U_t(y,t)$ and $U_b(y,t)$ are the normal displacements of the membranes.

The boundary conditions for the basilar membrane are the traditional hinged edges:

$$U_b(y_0) = U_b(y_0 + b) = 0, \quad \frac{\partial^2 U_b(y_0)}{\partial y^2} = \frac{\partial^2 U_b(y_0 + b)}{\partial y^2} = 0. \tag{2}$$

Consider the boundaries of the tectorial membrane. Its left edge is supported onto the immovable limbus, so:

$$U_t(0) = \frac{\partial^2 U_t(0)}{\partial y^2} = 0. \tag{3}$$

The marginal edge of the tectorial membrane experiences a load from the spring restoring force $F(t)$, so the shear force Q_t is equal to this load, related to unit of length:

$$Q_t(\eta) = D_t \frac{\partial^3 U_t(\eta, t)}{\partial y^3} = \frac{F(t)}{\Delta x}, \tag{4}$$

here Δx is the distance between two neighboring OHCs in longitudinal direction.

The forth boundary condition for the tectorial membrane concerns the bending moment M_t, that is a product of the force by its arm:

$$M_t(\eta) = Q_t(\eta) \cdot \eta. \tag{5}$$

The force $F(t)$ that compresses and elongates OHC is proportional to variation of distance between the membranes:

$$F(t) = S(U_t - U_b)\big|_{y=\eta} + m \frac{\partial^2 (U_t - U_b)}{\partial t^2}\bigg|_{y=\eta} \tag{6}$$

Here m denotes the mass of OHC and S is the restoring spring constant.

The force F also affects the basilar membrane, causing a break of shear force under the line of OHCs:

$$Q_b(\eta + 0) - Q_b(\eta - 0) = -\frac{F}{\Delta x}. \tag{7}$$

2 Solution

The Fourier method is a good approach for solving of system (1)–(7). Suppose displacements U_t and U_b be the products of functions dependent only on any one of variables:

$$U_i(y,t) = W_i(y) \cdot T(t), \qquad i = t,b \tag{8}$$

Substituting of (8) into Eqs. (1) provides the equations with left part dependent only on y, while the right-hand part depends only on t. So, both are constant relatively these variables:

$$\frac{D_i}{\mu_i} \cdot \frac{W_i''''(y)}{W_i(y)} = -\frac{T''(t)}{T(t)} = \text{const} \equiv \omega_0^2. \tag{9}$$

Then $T = \exp(i\omega_0 t)$, and this expression indicates the physical meaning of ω_0: it is an eigenfrequency of the complex cross section.

Let k_i be a wave number of each membrane:

$$k_i^4 \equiv \frac{W_i''''(y)}{W_i(y)}, \quad \text{then} \quad \omega_0^2 = k_i^4 \frac{D_i}{\mu_i}, \quad i = t,b \tag{10}$$

The classical solution to the first of Eq. (2.4) has a form:

$$W_i = a_{1i} \sin k_i y + a_{2i} \cos k_i y + a_{3i} \sinh k_i y + a_{4i} \cosh k_i y \tag{11}$$

From the conditions (3) and (4), it follows:

$$W_t(y) = a_{1t} \left(\sin k_t y + \frac{\sin \lambda_t - \lambda_t \cos \lambda_t}{\sinh \lambda_t - \lambda_t \cosh \lambda_t} \sinh k_t y \right), \tag{12}$$

$$\lambda_t = k_t \eta. \tag{13}$$

W_t is the general form of eigenfunction of the tectorial membrane vibrations; the wavenumber k_t has to be determined from Eqs. (4) and (6).

Now return to the basilar membrane. The concentrated force F applied along the line of OHCs causes a break in the third derivative of $W_b(y)$. Let us define the part of cross section to the left from the line as W_l, and the part to the right as W_r. Application of conditions (2) to Eq. (11) yields:

$$\begin{aligned}
W_l &= a_{1l}\sin k_b(y - y_0) + a_{3l}\sinh k_b(y - y_0)\\
W_r &= a_{1r}\sin k_b(y_0 + b - y) + a_{3r}\sinh k_b(y_0 + b - y).
\end{aligned} \qquad (14)$$

Displacement $W_b(y)$ and two its derivatives are continuous through over the cross section. Continuity in $y = \eta$ provides three equations allowing to eliminate a_{3l}, a_{1r} and a_{3r}. For the sake of simplicity and without loss of generality we assume the approximate relationships:

$$\eta = b, \qquad y_0 = \eta/2. \qquad (15)$$

Then:

$$a_{1r} = a_{1l}, \qquad a_{3r} = a_{3l}, \qquad a_{3l} = -a_{1l}\frac{\cos\lambda_b}{\cosh\lambda_b}, \qquad \lambda_b = \frac{k_b b}{2}. \qquad (16)$$

The solution for basilar membrane vibrations is then described with expression:

$$W_b = a_{1b}\begin{cases}
\sin k_b(y - y_0) - \dfrac{\cos\lambda_b}{\cosh\lambda_b}\sinh k_b(y - y_0) & \text{if } y_0 \leq y \leq \eta\\[2ex]
\sin k_b(y_0 + b - y) - \dfrac{\cos\lambda_b}{\cosh\lambda_b}\sinh k_b(y_0 + b - y) & \text{if } \eta \leq y \leq y_0 + b
\end{cases}$$

$$(17)$$

Now consider the shear forces Q_t and Q_b; let the explicit factor $T(t)$ be omitted:

$$Q_t = D_t W_t''' = \frac{S - m\omega_0^2}{\Delta x}(W_t - W_b)\big|_{y=\eta}$$

$$Q_b(\eta + 0) - Q_b(\eta - 0) = \pm D_b(W_r''' - W_l''') = \frac{S - m\omega_0^2}{\Delta x}(W_b - W_t)\big|_{y=\eta} \qquad (18)$$

The double sign $\pm$ indicates a possibility of synphase and counterphase vibrations of two membranes; formally, it arises from equal probabilities to write $W_r''' - W_l'''$ or $W_l''' - W_r'''$.

Substituting of (12) and (17) into (18) yields the system:

$$\begin{aligned}
a_{1t}\{Q_t(\eta) - qW_t(\eta)\} + a_{1b}qW_b(\eta) &= 0\\
a_{1t}qW_t(\eta) + a_{1b}\{\pm\Delta Q_b(\eta) - qW_b(\eta)\} &= 0,
\end{aligned} \qquad (19)$$

where

$$\Delta Q_b(\eta) = 4D_b k_b^3 \cos\lambda_b, \qquad q = \frac{S - m\omega_0^2}{\Delta x} = \frac{m}{\Delta x}(\omega_c^2 - \omega_0^2). \qquad (20)$$

Here $\omega_c^2 = S/m$ is the eigenfrequency of isolated outer hair cell.

System (19) has an untrivial solution if its determinant is zero. Following relationships then hold:

$$\omega_0^2 = \omega_c^2 \pm \frac{\Delta x}{m} \frac{Q_t \Delta Q_b}{W_b Q_t \pm W_t \Delta Q_b}, \quad a_{1t} = a_{1b} \frac{qW_b \mp \Delta Q_b}{qW_t} \tag{21}$$

The first is a nonlinear equation for the eigenfrequency of the complex cross section. The double sign indicates effect of splitting eigenfrequency which is specific to multi-degree-of-freedom systems. Substitution of (20) into (21) yields:

$$\omega_+^2 = \omega_c^2 + \frac{\Delta x}{m} \frac{1}{r_b^+ + r_t^+}, \quad \omega_-^2 = \omega_c^2 - \frac{\Delta x}{m} \frac{1}{r_b^- - r_t^-} \tag{22}$$

where

$$r_b = \frac{\tan \lambda_b - \tanh \lambda_b}{4 D_b k_b^3}, \quad r_t = \frac{2 - \lambda_t (\cotan \lambda_t + \cotanh \lambda_t)}{D_t k_t^3 (\cotan \lambda_t - \cotanh \lambda_t)}. \tag{23}$$

We may conclude that the higher of eigenfrequencies (22) is associated with a counterphase movement between the marginal edge of tectorial membrane and the basilar membrane, because resistance of linkage is higher in this case. Due to that λ_t and λ_b are the arguments of periodic functions and related to $\omega_\pm$ through Eqs. (10), (13) and (16), we have two infinite sets of eigenfrequencies and two infinite sets of each membrane eigenfunctions. Usually, the eigenfrequencies of the linked system are named 'normal frequencies'.

Consider some special cases. Suppose $\omega_\pm = \omega_c$. The second term of Eq.(2.16) equals to zero, if either r_b, or r_t are infinite. This occurs, if either $\tan \lambda_b = \infty$, or $\cotan \lambda_b = \cotan \lambda_t$, otherwise, if either $\lambda_b = \pm(\pi/2 + n\pi), n = 0, 1, 2 \ldots$, or $\lambda_t = \pm(5\pi/4 + n\pi)$. But these eigenvalues are also the eigenvalues of free vibrations of the uncoupled membranes. Hence, if the partial eigenfrequency of the isolated outer hair cell equals to any of partial eigenfrequencies of any of uncoupled membranes, it is also the normal frequency of the cross section. It is the only case, when the synphase and counterphase vibrations have one and the same frequency.

3 Forced vibrations

To study the forced vibrations in cochlea, the cochlear hydrodynamics and longitudinal coordinate should be taken into account. Such expansion exceeds the scope of the present paper. However, some essential information on the specific features of resonance in the coupled system under examination can be obtained from the considered matters.

Let the complex cross section be subject to a periodic force $P_0 e^{i\omega t}$ applied, for example, from below. The vibrations of two coupled membranes then obey the equations:

$$D_b \frac{\partial^4 U_b}{\partial y^4} - \mu_b \omega^2 U_b = P_0 e^{i\omega t}, \quad D_t \frac{\partial^4 U_t}{\partial y^4} - \mu_t \omega^2 U_t = 0. \tag{24}$$

It can be verified, that the eigenfunctions W_{bm} and W_{tm} are not orthogonal to each other at least in the conventional sense. So, the traditional method of expansion into the eigenfunctional series is not applicable here in general form. However, in close vicinities of $\lambda_{bn} = \pm(\pi/2 + n\pi)$, $n = 0, 1, 2\ldots$, the eigenfunctions (17) are very close to sines. In these narrow regions, the approximate equality is justified:

$$U_b(y,t) \approx \sum_{n=0}^{\infty} c_{bn} \sin k_{bn}(y - y_0) \exp(i\omega t), \qquad k_{bn} = \pm(2n+1)\pi/b. \tag{25}$$

Substituting of (25) into (24) and decomposing constant P_0 into the sine series yields:

$$c_{bn} \approx \frac{2P_0(1 - (-1)^n)}{n\pi\mu_b(\omega_{0n}^2 - \omega^2)}$$

Application of Eq.(22) results:

$$c_{bn} \approx \frac{2P_0(1 - (-1)^n)}{n\pi\mu_b(\omega_c^2 \pm \frac{\Delta x/m}{r_{bn} - r_{tn}} - \omega^2)} \tag{26}$$

To determine the tectorial membrane displacement, we represent it as a sum of tectorial membrane eigenfunctions with indeterminate coefficients, and equate the shear forces of two membranes. This yields:

$$U_t(y,t) = \frac{D_b}{D_t} \sum_{n=0}^{\infty} c_{bn} \left(\frac{k_{bn}}{k_{tn}}\right)^3 \frac{W_{tn}(y)}{W_{tn}(\eta)} \exp(i\omega t) \tag{27}$$

Conclusions

Consider the last factor of denominator of (26). It is seen that a resonance of complex cross section is the most pronounced, if any of partial eigenfrequencies of uncoupled basilar membrane and the eigenfrequency of isolated outer hair cell both coincide with the applied frequency.

Similarly, if the force is applied from above to the tectorial membrane , its displacement may be decomposed into the series of orthogonal eigenfunctions of uncoupled tectorial membrane in the points $\lambda_{tn} = \pm(5\pi/4 + n\pi)$, $n = 0, 1, 2 \ldots$ Hence, the second probable resonance appear, if the partial eigenfrequency of the outer hair cell coincides with any of partial eigenfrequencies of the tectorial membrane .

Through the slow motility, the outer hair cell is capable to vary its partial eigenfrequency, either moving it closer to that of a membrane, or drifting apart. By this way the shape, sharpness and shift of the tuning curve can be modified. Such experimental data are in focus of attention.

Of particular interest is the leading eigenfunction of the tectorial membrane in the vicinity of its resonance. The eigenfunction has a node near the marginal edge, hence the marginal part of the tectorial membrane moves in the opposite direction to the middle portion. At resonance of a cross section, when the middle part of tectorial membrane moves downwards, it pushes out of sulcus some fluid, which streams through the opened subtectorial gap. In counterphase, the exit from the gap is closed by dropped marginal edge. Away of the resonance, the distance between the marginal edge and basilar membrane remains almost constant. Such mechanics of subtectorial streaming is strikingly similar to that supposed by Steele in 1973[2]. If so, the resonance of tectorial membrane seems to be more important for excitation of inner hair cells then that of the basilar membrane, if the leading partial eigenfrequencies of two membranes do not coincide.

Mechanics of multi-degree-of-freedom systems can serve as a key that puts a great deal of experimental findings into a mutually associated series, as demonstrated by Novoselova[1].

Acknowledgments

The author is very grateful to Professors V.M.Babich and Egbert de Boer for fruitful discussions. This work is supported by Russian Basic Research Foundation, Grant 93-011-16148.

References

1. S. M. Novoselova (1994) "The transversal modes of tectorial membrane free vibrations and origin of the outer hair cells oscillations." Zap. Nauchn. Semin. POMI **218**, 138–148 (1994). English translation has to appear in J. of Mathematical Sciences.
2. C. R. Steele (1973) "A possibility for subtectorial fluid motion," in: *Basic mechanisms in Hearing*, ed. A. R. Møller (Academic press, New York) pp 69–94.

THREE-DIMENSIONAL MECHANICAL MODELING OF THE COCHLEA

CHARLES R. STEELE
Stanford University
Stanford, CA 94305, USA
chas@am-sparc7.stanford.edu

The response of diverse auditory organs is carried out with the program Fast4. The actual geometry and elastic properties of the tissue can be taken into consideration. The resonance modes in the organs of the Tokay gecko and the bobtail lizard show the effects of hair cell support, tectorial membrane and sallets. Interesting response is also found in the tectorial membrane of the bird and the mustached bat..

1 Introduction

We begin with the premise that the elaborate mechanical apparatus found in the mammalian cochlea has a relation to the function. Because of the complexity, however, modeling has been restricted to rather crude approximation and distortion of the actual anatomy. For a proper resolution of the fluid-elastic behavior of the cochlea, the computational problem is severe. We report on some preliminary results with an approach to the problem which combines asymptotic and numerical methods, implemented in the computer program Fast4[1]. With this approach, the cochlea is modeled as a shell of revolution, Fig. 1. The details can be taken just as they are on a micrograph, for the fiber reinforced basilar membrane, the wall and supporting structure, Reissner's membrane, and the components of the organ of Corti, including the attachments of the cilia to the tectorial. Particularly important are the inclinations of the receptor cells, fibers and phalangeal processes in both the radial and longitudinal directions. The goal is to understand the functional significance of the mechanical features of the "normal" mammalian cochlea and those of specialized cochleas, such as in certain bats, whales, and moles. It is also important to study the nonmammalian auditory organs.

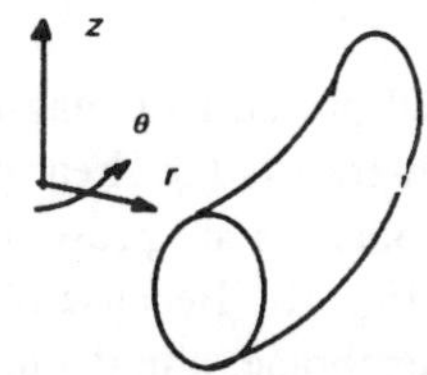

Figure 1: Shell of revolution.

2   Bobtail Lizard

What appears to be a simple organ of hearing is found in the bobtail lizard *Tiliqua rugosa*[2]. There is no tuning of the basilar membrane, since it is thick and not very long, while auditory neurons have reasonable sharpness of tuning. There is also no tectorial membrane in the basal region. Instead the cilia are covered by sallets. It appears likely that the tuning is largely in the resonance of the cilia and sallets, as indicated by a mechanical analysis[3]. Fig. 2 shows results from the Fast4 analysis of this organ. The radius of curvature in Fig. 1 is taken very large, so the behavior is essentially plane. Only the behavior of one section is computed. The anatomy for the model is taken from the cross section[2], at 45% of the basal segment, at which the neural tuning is about 1500 Hz. The elastic properties are taken to be: basilar membrane 50% collagen $E = 0.5$ GPa, tectorial membrane $E = 30$ kPa, layer of cilia matrix $E = 73.2$ Pa, longitudinal $E = 73.2$ kPa, hair cell layer $E = 30$ kPa, very soft layer between hair cells and fundus $E = 1$ kPa. The density is taken as 2, to account for the surrounding fluid.

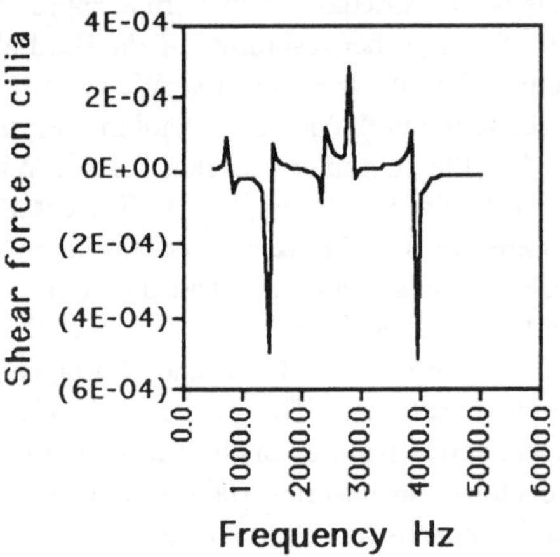

Fig. 2a: Response of model for Bobtail lizard.

The loading consists of a fixed pressure of magnitude 1 Pa acting on the basilar membrane. The response of interest is the shear stress acting on the cilia which is shown in Fig. 2a. Several resonances are present. The deformation mode for the first resonance at 800 Hz is in Fig. 1b. Because of a small asymmetry in the size of the two edges of the basilar membrane, a uniform pressure causes a rocking of the fundus. The first mode consists of all the soft structure moving in phase. The second mode is at 1420 Hz and is shown in Fig. 2c. For this the tectorial membrane and hair cells are out of phase. This mode is closest to that in[3], who assume that the cells remain fixed while the cilia and TM move. Since the nerves in this region are tuned to about this frequency, it is tempting to relate this mode to the primary excitation of the nerves, while the lower first mode may be significant for the combination tones[4]. More modes are present. Figs. 2d,e show the modes for 2.1, which involves a compression of the soft layer, and 2.79 kHz, which is a combination of flexing and shear. Since the gradient of properties and damping due to viscosity of fluid and materials are not taken into consideration, it is not clear which of these modes will be significant in the actual organ.

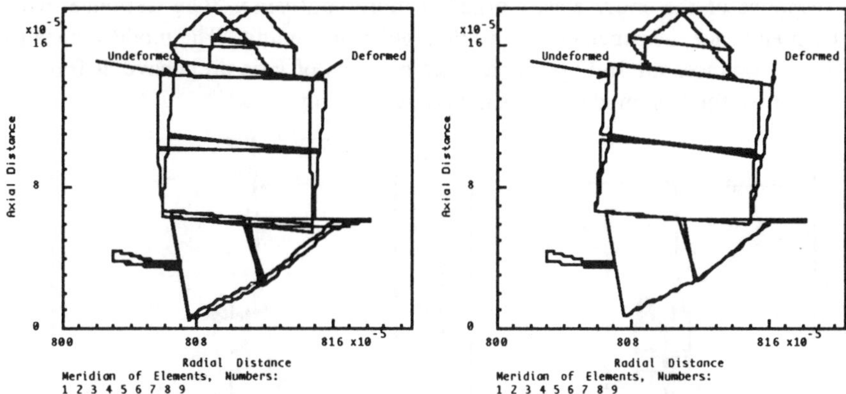

Fig. 2b,c : Resonance mode shapes for model of bobtail lizard at (b) 800 Hz and (c) 1420 Hz.

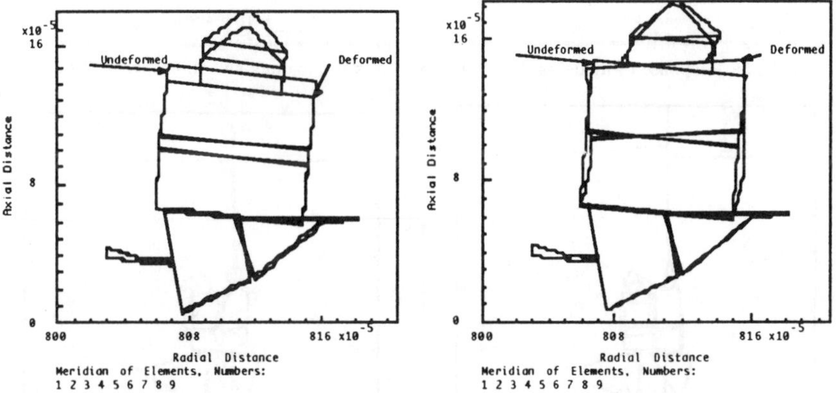

Fig. 2d,e : Resonance mode shape for model of bobtail lizard at (d) 2100 Hz and (e) 2788 Hz.

3   Tokay gecko

The lizard Tokay gecko is of interest because the apical region consists of two sets of cilia. In Fig. 3a is the model representing the transverse section 75% from the

458

basal end[5]. As in all lizards, the basilar membrane consists of a very thick portion (fundus) and thin connections on the sides. This is modeled by five elements in Fig. 3. Attached to the fundus above are elements representing: in order from bottom to top, a layer of soft material, the hair cells, and the cilia. On the left (preaxial or neural side), the cilia are covered with a small tectorial membrane, while on the right side (postaxial or abneural), the cilia are covered with sallets. Nerves from this region have CF from 1.1 to 5.2 kHz. It is shown[6] that the gradient in size of covering and lengths of cilia correspond well to a tonotopic arrangement. The response of the entire elastic organ is more confusing. The response of the basilar membrane, as expected, shows no significant tuning. The mode shapes for the first resonances are in Figs. 3a–d. The two sets of cilia do behave differently, but except for the first mode there is not an uncoupling.

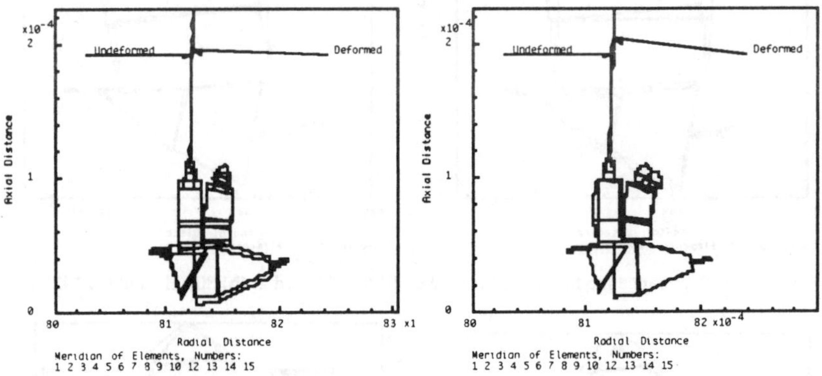

Fig. 3a,b: Response of model of Tokay gecko at (a) static loading and at resonance (b) 2 kHz.

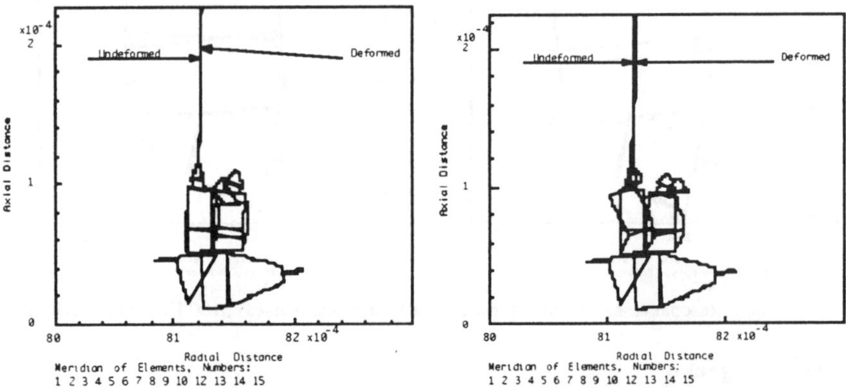

Fig. 3c,d: Response of model at (c) 2.426 kHz and (d) 3.155 kHz.

4   Bird

The bird hearing organ is of considerable interest, since it seems to represent an intermediate stage between lizard and mammal. There is an extensive tectorial membrane which most likely is a very soft material, with little protein. The abneural (short) hair cells must have a motor function, but cannot have the electromotility of the mammalian outer hair cells[7]. Furthermore the neural (tall) hair cells are located above the limbus and there is no inner sulcus. It is suggested[8] that the short hair cells may beat and generate waves which travel to the tall cells. A premininary calculation for the organ is shown in Fig. 4. The hair cells and the attachment to the basilar membrane are represented by the single lower layer. The cilia and tectorial membrane are represented by the single tapered layer above. The left portion of the lower surface is attached to the basilar membrane. The neural side is to the right, where the majority of tall hair cells with afferent enervation are located. The short hair cells to the left are without afferent enervation. In the calculation the possible beating of the short hair cells is simulated with forces at the interface. The response shown is for a higher resonance at 1800 Hz, for which the waves propagate well into the region of the tall hair cells. The elastic modulus for tectorial membrane and cell layer for this calculation is the low value of $E = 100$ Pa. for such a low value, short wave length resonance modes occur, such as shown in Fig. 4, that would correspond to the suggestion[8].

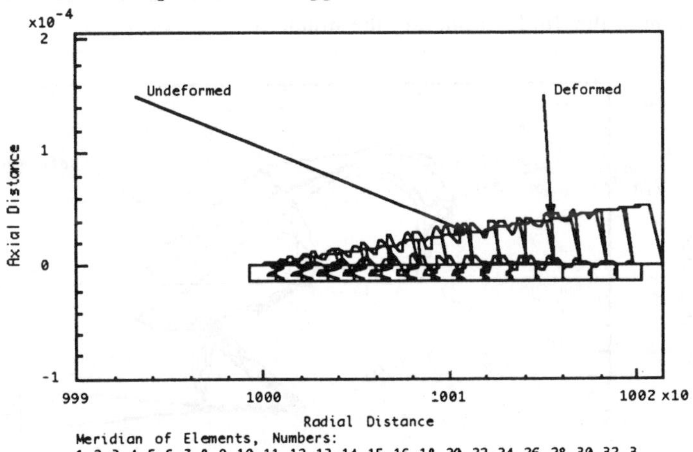

Fig. 4 : Model for hair cells and tectorial membrane in bird, resonance at 1800 Hz,.

460

5   Mustached bat

In some bats, there is a contrast to the very soft tectorial membrane in bird. Particularly the mustached bat (*Pteronotus parnellii*) has a tectorial membrane that is very stiff and of unusual form. There is sharp neural tuning at the frequencies around 60 and 90 kHz [9]. The basilar membrane shows sharp resonances at these frequencies[10]. However, the thickness and attachment of the basilar membrane preclude this from being the source of such a resonance. In the region from 20 to 40% of the distance from the base, the tectorial membrane has a substantially different form[11]. The limbal attachment is much smaller, the membrane protrudes upward from the limbus, and has a surface layer of 50% collagen. There is in addition an intermediate support layer of high collagen content. This structure is modeled as indicated in Fig. 5. Not included are the hair cells and Deiter cells. The lower surface consists of, from left to right, the arcuate and pectinate zones of the basilar membrane and the attachment to the secondary spiral osseus lamina. The high protein layers of the tectorial membrane are shown. The softer interior is not included. The elastic modulus used is 50% collagen, $E = 0.5$ GPa, and the density taken as 4, to account for the enclosed material as well as the external fluid. The first resonance from the model occurs at 73 kHz and the corresponding mode of displacement is shown in Fig. 5. So this special tectorial membrane does have a resonance in the correct range. Of course, inclusion of the hair cells and proper consideration of the fluid will modify the situation.

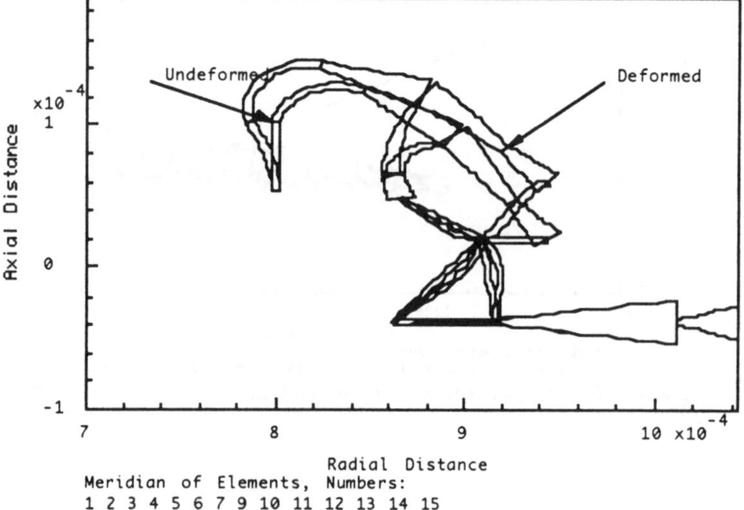

Fig. 5 : Model for tectorial membrane in fovea of mustached bat, resonance at 73 kHz,.

6 Conclusion

The Fast4 program can be applied to the diverse hearing organs, often with unexpected results. Next is the computation of the traveling waves.

Acknowledgments

The development of the Fast4 program was under support of NIH DC 00108. This application is enabled by a Humboldt Senior Fellowship Award, which made possible a visit to the laboratory of G.A. Manley. The helpfulness of Dr. Manley and all his associates is greatly appreciated.

References

1. Steele, C.R., and Shad, K.R. (1995). Asymptotic-numeric solution for shells of revolution, *Applied Mechanics Reviews*, **48** (11, part 2).

2 Köppl, C. (1988) Morphology of the basilar papilla of the bobtail lizard *Tiliqu rugosa. Hearing Research* **35**: 209–228.

3. Manley, G.A., Köppl, C., and Yates, G.K. (1989). Micromechanical basis of high-frequency tuning in the bobtail lizard. in *Cochlear Mechanisms*, J.P. Wilson and D.T. Kemp, eds, (Plenum): 143–151.

4. Taschenberger, G., Gallo, L., and Manley, G.A. (1995) Filtering of distortion-product otoacoustic emissions in the inner ear of birds and lizards. *Hearing Research* 91: 87-92.

5. Köppl, C., and Authier, S. (1995) Quantitative anatomical basis for a model of micromechanical frequency tuning in the Tokay gecko, *Gekko gecko. Hearing Research* **82**: 14-25.

6. Authier, S. and Manley, G.A. (1995) A model of frequency tuning in the basilar papilla of the Tokay gecko, *Gekko gecko. Hearing Research* **82**: 1-13.

7. Fischer, F.P. (1994) General pattern and morphological specializations of the avian cochlea. *Scanning Microscopy* **8** (2): 351-364.

8. Manley, G.A. (1995) The avian hearing organ: A status report. in *Advances in Hearing Research*, G.A. Manley, G.M. Klump, C. Köppl, H. Fastl, and H. Oeckinghaus, eds. (World Scientific) 219-232.

9 Kössl, M. and Vater, M. (1995) Cochlear structure and function in bats. in *Hearing by Bats*, A.N. Popper, R.F. Fay, eds. Springer Handbook of Auditory Research, Vol 5; 191-234.

10. Kössl, M. and Russel, I.J. (1995) Basilar membrane resonance in the cochlea of the mustached bat. *Proc. Natl. Acad. Sci. USA*, 92:276-279.

11. Kössl, M., and Vater, M. (1995) A tectorial membrane fovea in the cochlea of the mustached bat. Manuscript.

MODELING OTOACOUSTIC EMISSION FINE STRUCTURE

C. L. TALMADGE, A. TUBIS AND P. PISKORSKI

Department of Physics, Purdue University
West Lafayette, IN 47907

G. LONG

Department of Audiology and Speech Sciences,
Purdue University, West Lafayette, IN 47907

A comprehensive model of otoacoustic emissions based upon cochlear reflection is summarized. It can account for a large collection of observations, including the fine structures of distortion product and synchronous evoked emissions, the frequency spacing between adjacent spontaneous emissions and the microstructure of hearing thresholds.

1 Introduction

The similarities in the: 1) frequency spacing of spontaneous otoacoustic emissions[1] (SOAEs); 2) fine structure of synchronous evoked[2] and distortion production otoacoustic emissions[3,4] (SEOAEs and DPOAEs); and 3) threshold microstructure[5] suggest a common cochlear origin for these features. We summarize here the relationships between these experimental measures which follow from a general class of cochlear models[6,7,8] with: 1) tall/broad activity patterns; and 2) a random component of the parameters of the organ of Corti.

2 Cochlear Model

A. Time Domain Model

Our cochlear model is based on 1-dimensional flow and an inviscid incompressible perilymph, and gives the standard set of equations governing the time evolution of the pressure difference $P_d(x,t)$ between the scala vestibuli and scala tympani and the displacement of the basilar membrane (BM), $\xi(x,t)$:

$$\frac{\partial^2 P_d(x,t)}{\partial x^2} = k_0^2 \ddot{\xi}(x,t), \tag{1}$$

$$\ddot{\xi}(x,t) + \gamma(x,t,\xi,\dot{\xi})\dot{\xi}(x,t) + \omega_{bm}^2(x,t,\xi,\dot{\xi})\xi(x,t) = \frac{1}{\sigma_{bm}(x)}P_d(x,t). \tag{2}$$

In this system of equations, $k_0 = \sqrt{2\rho W_{bm}/\sigma_{bm}S} \cong 10 - 30\,\mathrm{cm}^{-1}$ is a geometric constant, and $\gamma(\cdots)$ and $\omega_{bm}(\cdots)$ are the local damping and natural frequency constants for the organ of Corti. We also assume that the mass density $\sigma_{bm}(x) \cong \sigma_{bm}$ (a constant). The other physical quantities used in these equations are defined in the Appendix. The form of the boundary equations assumed in this model are given by Eqs. (2.1) – (2.4) of Talmadge and Tubis.[7]

Zweig[6] has suggested the phenomenological use of delayed stiffness to obtain physiologically reasonable "tall and broad" BM activity patterns (AP). This modification is included in the present analysis as,

$$\omega_{bm}^2(x, ...)\xi(x,t) = \omega_0^2(x)\xi(x,t) + \rho_f(x)\omega_0(x)\xi(x, t - \psi_f(x)/\omega_0(x))$$
$$+ \rho_s(x)\omega_0(x)\xi(x, t - \psi_s(x)/\omega_0(x)). \tag{3}$$

Here f, s refer to fast, slow feedback contributions. The fast feedback will behave like a negative damping (energy source), and the slow feedback gives rise to a broad BM AP. The fast stiffness feedback of Eq. (3) can be associated with a rapid outer hair cell stiffness change, whereas the slow feedback should be viewed as a parametrization necessary to obtain realistic "tall and broad" APs, and whose origin may arise from effects such as multidimensional fluid flow, viscous flow, and the micromechanics of the organ of Corti.

We use a simple "Van der Pol-like" damping for the BM nonlinearity,

$$\gamma(x, \xi) = \gamma_0(x) + \gamma_x(x)\xi^2(x, t). \tag{4}$$

This nonlinearity is the simplest form which gives rise to cubic distortion products. However, the nonlinearity in the real organ of Corti is likely to be much more complicated.

B. Linear Frequency Domain Approximation

In the analysis that follows, we further simplify the model of Eqs. (1), (2), (3) and (4) by considering only the frequency response of the linearized model, where, when necessary, the nonlinear component is treated perturbatively. The linearized system of equations is,

$$P_d''(x) + k^2(x)P_d(x) = 0, \qquad k^2(x) \equiv \frac{k_0^2\omega^2}{\Delta(x)}, \tag{5}$$

$$\xi(x) = \frac{P_d(x)}{\sigma_{bm}\Delta(x)}, \tag{6}$$

$$\Delta(x) = \omega_0^2(x) - \omega^2 + i\omega\gamma_0(x) + \rho_f\omega_0(x)e^{\frac{-i\psi_f\omega}{\omega_0(x)}} + \rho_s\omega_0(x)e^{\frac{-i\psi_s\omega}{\omega_0(x)}}, \tag{7}$$

where we follow the convention of writing, e.g., $P_d(x)$ in place of $P_d(x, \omega)$. Any linearized model consistent with the general assumptions of our model *must* gives rise to Eqs. (5) – (6), with only $\Delta(x)$ open to modification. Since the place impedance $Z_{bm}(x) \equiv P_d(x)/\dot{\xi}(x) = \sigma_{bm}\Delta(x)/i\omega$, this assertion is consistent with de Boer's observation[9] that the differences between all local micromechanical cochlear models reduce to a choice of $Z_{bm}(x)$.

From the model of Ref. [7], the boundary conditions are (see Appendix)

$$P'_d(0) + k_{ow}P_d(0) = G_{me}k_{ow}P_{dr}, \tag{8}$$

$$k_{ow} = \frac{\sigma_{bm}}{\sigma_{ow}}\frac{k_{ow,0}\,\omega^2}{\omega^2_{ow} - \omega^2 + i\omega\gamma_{ow}}, \tag{9}$$

$$P_d(L_{bm}) = 0. \tag{10}$$

The pressure in the ear canal P_e is given by

$$P_e = P_{dr} - \frac{a_d}{\omega^2}P'_d(0), \qquad a_d = \frac{SP_a}{2\rho V_e}G_{me} \tag{11}$$

where the "calibrated driving pressure" P_{dr} would be the pressure in the ear canal in the case of a rigid ear drum.

C. Cochlear Basis Functions

Eq. (5) is the so-called pressure wave equation and characterizes the "free-field" propagation of traveling waves in the cochlea. Since this equation is second-order, it gives rise to two independent solutions, which can be characterized as "right" or apically traveling waves, $\psi_r(x)$, and "left" or basally traveling waves, $\psi_\ell(x)$. Any solution $P_d(x)$ of Eq. (5) can be then written as

$$P_d(x) = a_\ell(x)\psi_\ell(x) + a_r(x)\psi_r(x), \tag{12}$$

where we take $\psi_\ell(0) = \psi_r(0) \equiv 1$, and $a_{r,\ell}(x)$ carry the dimension of pressure (leaving $\psi_{r,\ell}(x)$ dimensionless). Since $a_{\ell,r}$ are over-specified, we write

$$P'_d(x) = a_\ell(x)\psi'_\ell(x) + a_r(x)\psi'_r(x), \tag{13}$$

We also define $\psi_r(x)$ as the cochlear response to an input tone in the ear canal at frequency ω, with $\psi_\ell(x)$ given by

$$\psi'_\ell(x)\psi_r(x) - \psi_\ell(x)\psi'_r(x) = W_0, \tag{14}$$

The Wronskian W_0 is independent of x and can be obtained by taking $\psi'_\ell(0) \cong [\psi'_r(0)]^*$.

Note that $\psi_{r,\ell}(x)$ depend only on the cochlear model *in the absence of any BM sources*, and are therefore independent of these sources. The $a_{r,\ell}(x)$ are constant *except in BM regions containing source terms*. Thus the parameters $a_{r,\ell}(x)$ contain only local information about the presence of sources and are constant otherwise, whereas $\psi_{r,\ell}(x)$ are independent of sources and describe only how the effects of local sources are propagated along the BM.

In the absence of an ear canal driver, we have in the vicinity of the stapes,

$$P_d(x) = a_\ell[\psi_\ell(x) + r_b\psi_r(x)] \qquad r_b \equiv a_r/a_\ell, \tag{15}$$

where r_b depends only on the properties at the base of the cochlea and on the properties of the middle and outer ear. Also, the phase of r_b varies slowly with frequency, and the magnitude of r_b is close to unity except near the middle ear resonance.

D.   Effect of BM Roughness

The model presented so far is based on the (unphysical) assumption that the BM parameters vary smoothly. Consequently the effects of a small random variation in the BM parameters ("roughness") must be included. The discussion that follows is based on Ref. [8]. The effect of a small BM roughness is to modify Eq. (5) by having $k \to \tilde{k}$, where the tilde indicates that $\tilde{k}$ now contains a random component. We assume for simplicity that the dominant source of roughness comes from $\tilde{\omega}_0(x) = [1 + \tilde{r}(x)]\omega_0(x),$ [a] so that

$$\tilde{k}^2(x) = k^2(x) + \delta\tilde{k}^2(x), \qquad \delta\tilde{k}^2(x) \cong -\frac{2k_0^2 w^2\omega_0^2(x)\tilde{r}(x)}{\Delta^2(x)}. \tag{16}$$

We consider the effect of roughness on an unperturbed apically moving wave $P_r(x) = a_r\psi_r(x)$ by applying perturbation theory to find,[8,10]

$$\tilde{P}_d(x) = a_r(x)[\psi_r(x) + r_a(x)\psi_\ell(x)], \qquad r_a \equiv a_\ell(x)/a_r(x), \tag{17}$$

$$r_a(x) \cong \frac{2k_0^2\omega^2}{W_0} \int_x^\infty dx' \left[\frac{\omega_0(x')\psi_r(x')}{\Delta(x')}\right]^2 \tilde{r}(x'). \tag{18}$$

If the BM AP is sufficient tall and broad,[8] then $\omega_0(x)\psi_r(x)/\Delta(x)$ can be approximated in the integral by $\sigma_{ap}A_{ap}^2\delta(x - \hat{x})$, where $\delta(x)$ is the usual Dirac δ-function, A_{ap} and σ_{ap} are the amplitude and full-width half maximum of the AP peak, and $\hat{x}$ is the BM location of AP peak. It follows that,[8,10]

$$\tilde{r}_a(x) \propto r_0(x)\sigma_{ap}A_{ap}^2e^{+2ik\hat{x}}\Theta(\hat{x} - x), \tag{19}$$

---

[a] However, randomly varying almost any cochlear parameter gives rise to similar effects.

where $\hat{k} = k(\hat{x})$, $r_0(x) \equiv \sqrt{\langle \tilde{r}^2(x) \rangle}$ and $\Theta(x)$ is the Heaviside Θ-function. The presence of the $\sigma_{ap} A_{ap}^2$ term signifies that the AP must be *both* tall and broad in order to get significant reflection.[8] In the analysis that follows, we include the effect of roughness on the BM, and further assume that the effects of this roughness are localized in the manner described by Eq. (19).

We note that r_a depends *only* on sources that are *apical* to x. Also, $|r_a|$ may be regarded as a phenomenological parameter depending on the local pattern of roughness on the basilar membrane as well as on the amplitude and width of the activity pattern. However, the phase of r_a is taken from Eq. (19),

$$\arg(r_a) \cong +2\hat{k}\hat{x} \cong (-2\hat{k}/k_\omega) \log(\omega/\omega_0) \equiv -\phi_0 \log(\omega/\omega_0). \tag{20}$$

3 Traveling Wave Model of Fine Structure

A. Synchronous Evoked Otoacoustic Emissions

SEOAEs can be modeled by considering a pressure wave transmitted through the middle ear into the cochlea, where it undergoes multiple reflections, so that

$$P_d(x) = a_r [\psi_r(x) + r_a(x)\psi_\ell(x)], \tag{21}$$

where a_r is determined by applying Eq. (8) to (21),

$$a_r = \frac{G_{me} k_{ow}}{k_{ow} + \psi_r'(0)} \cdot \frac{P_{dr}}{1 - r_a r_b}, \tag{22}$$

and P_e is obtained by combining Eqs. (11), (21) and (22),

$$P_e = P_{dr} \left[1 - \frac{a_d}{\omega^2} \frac{G_{me} k_{ow} \psi_r'(0)}{k_{ow} + \psi_r'(0)} \frac{1 + r_a \mathcal{R}_s}{1 - r_a r_b} \right], \qquad \mathcal{R}_s \equiv \frac{\psi_\ell'(0)}{\psi_r'(0)}. \tag{23}$$

B. Threshold Microstructure

The hearing threshold is modeled by assuming a fixed detection threshold ξ_{th}, which characterizes the minimum detectable BM amplitude for a given frequency ω. The hearing threshold is then the calibrated ear canal pressure level $P_{dr} = P_{th}$ necessary to generate a BM amplitude of ξ_{th}. We start by combining Eqs. (6) and (21) evaluated at $\hat{x}$:

$$P_d(\hat{x}) = a_r [\psi_r(\hat{x}) + r_a(\hat{x})\psi_\ell(\hat{x})]. \tag{24}$$

Since $\psi_r(\hat{x}) \gg \psi_\ell(\hat{x})$,[10] the combining of Eq. (24) with (6) and (22) gives

$$P_{th} = \frac{k_{ow} + \psi_r'(0)}{G_{me} k_{ow} \psi_r'(0)} \cdot (1 - r_a r_b) \cdot \sigma_{bm} \Delta(\hat{x}) \xi_{th}. \tag{25}$$

C. DPOAE Fine Structure

The two external tones of frequencies f_1 and f_2 will give distortion products with frequencies $f_{dp} = f_1 - n(f_2 - f_1)$, $n = 0, \pm 1, \pm 2, \cdots$. We consider the case $f_{dp} < f_1 < f_2$, and for purposes of simple exposition also assume that the interaction region of the two primaries can be approximated as a single δ-function source located at the DP energy generation site x_s (assumed near f_2). The traveling wave equation for frequency ω_{dp} then becomes

$$P_d''(x) + k^2(x)P_d(x) = \Gamma_s \delta(x - x_s), \tag{26}$$

where Γ_s parametrizes the level and phase of the DP source. This equation gives rise to the additional boundary conditions,[10]

$$P_d(x_s - \delta x) = P_d(x_s + \delta x), \qquad P_d'(x_s - \delta x) = P_d'(x_s + \delta x) + \Gamma_s, \tag{27}$$

where $\delta x \to 0^+$. Eq. (27) implies $P_d(x)$ varies continuously through the interaction region but $P_d'(x)$ is discontinuous at $x = x_s$. We find

$$P_e = -\frac{a_d}{\omega^2} \frac{k_{ow}}{k_{ow} + \psi_r'(0)} \frac{1 + r_a \mathcal{R}_d(x_s)}{1 - r_a r_b} \Gamma_s \psi_r(x_s), \qquad \mathcal{R}_d(x) \equiv \frac{\psi_\ell(x)}{\psi_r(x)}. \tag{28}$$

D. SOAE Spacing

SOAEs correspond to cochlear model instability modes of the linear active cochlear model,[7] and are studied by considering the conditions necessary to obtain energy in the ear canal in the absence of an external tone. Eq. (23) suggests that $P_e = 0$ whenever $P_{dr} = 0$. However, whenever $1 - r_a(\omega)r_b(\omega) = 0$, the expression becomes indeterminate.[b] The values of $\omega = \omega_R + i\omega_I$ (with ω_R and ω_I real) that are necessary for $r_a(\omega)r_b(\omega) = 1$ correspond to the so-called eigenfrequencies of the cochlear model. Modes with $\omega_I < 0$ are unstable, and modes with $\omega_I \geq 0$ are stable.

The modal eigenstructure can be estimated by studying the phase behavior of $r_a(\omega)$ and $r_b(\omega)$ in the neighborhood of some real frequency ω_1. We write $r_a(\omega) \cong |r_a(\omega_1)|e^{-i\phi_0 \log(w/w_0)}$, and expand $r_b(\omega)$ to get $r_b(\omega) \cong |r_b|e^{-iw\tau_b}$ where $|r_a(\omega_1)$ and $|r_b(\omega_1)|$ are assumed to be approximately constant. We find[7]

$$\omega_I \cong -\frac{\omega_1}{\phi_0 + \omega_1 \tau_b} \log\left(|r_a(\omega_1)|\,|r_b(\omega_1)|\right), \qquad \frac{\Delta \omega_R}{\omega_1} = \frac{2\pi}{\phi_0 + \omega_1 \tau_b}, \tag{29}$$

where $\Delta \omega_R$ is the frequency spacing between neighboring eigenmodes.

---

[b]The frequency dependence of r_a and r_b is made explicit to clarify this discussion.

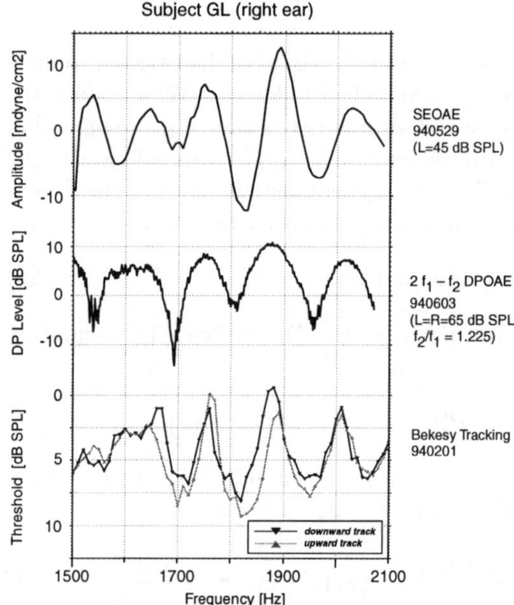

Figure 1: Comparison of SEOAE, DPOAE, and threshold microstructure for subject GL.

4 Analysis and Discussion

The strong experimental evidence that the frequency spacing characteristics of SOAEs and SEOAEs, DPOAEs, and threshold microstructure are very similar suggests a strong connection between the underlying mechanisms that gives rise to these phenomena. This connection has a natural explanation in terms of cochlear reflections of traveling waves, as we show below.

The dominant contribution to the frequency spacings in all of these measures comes from the rapid phase variation of r_a. This rapid phase variation is a consequence of the long round trip travel time of a traveling wave from the stapes to the AP peak. The delay varies from approximately 10 ms for a 1500 Hz tone to 3 ms for a 5000 Hz tone. The delays coming from the other experimental parameters are generally much smaller, and are typically no larger than 0.5 ms. For the experimental measures considered above, it is only necessary to consider the contributions arising from terms involving r_a. Assuming

$|r_a| \ll 1$, we find

$$\left(\frac{\Delta\omega}{\omega}\right)_{SEOAE} = \frac{2\pi}{\phi_0 + \omega\tau_s}, \qquad \tau_s = -\frac{d}{d\omega}\arg(r_b + \mathcal{R}_s), \quad \text{(SEOAE)}, \quad (30)$$

$$\left(\frac{\Delta\omega}{\omega}\right)_{DPOAE} = \frac{2\pi}{\phi_0 + \omega\tau_d}, \qquad \tau_d = -\frac{d}{d\omega}\arg(r_b + \mathcal{R}_d), \quad \text{(DPOAE)}, \quad (31)$$

$$\left(\frac{\Delta\omega}{\omega}\right)_{SOAE} = \frac{2\pi}{\phi_0 + \omega\tau_b}, \qquad \tau_b = -\frac{d}{d\omega}\arg(r_b), \quad \text{(SOAE, threshold)}. \quad (32)$$

There are a number of qualitative predictions that can be made from these equations. First of all, $\phi_0 \cong 30\pi \gg \omega\tau_s, \omega\tau_d, \omega\tau_b$, so $\Delta\omega/\omega$ will be approximately equal for the four types of phenomena, a result supported by Fig. 1.

A prediction of the formalism that the frequency spacings for SOAE and threshold microstructure will be equal, but a deviation is expected for the spacings of both SEOAEs and DPOAEs. However, the *sign* of the shift in $\Delta\omega/\omega$ for SEOAEs and DPOAEs depends sensitively on the underlying model, since it arises from the addition of two slowly varying terms.

A second prediction is that the only source of DP reflection is around the DP tonotopic place, in disagreement with a suggestion by Engdahl and Kemp.[4] A consequence of this is that the fine structure of DPOAEs is rooted in the tonotopic location of the DP and not in the interaction region of the primaries. This implies that DPOAE fine structure will have nearly equal spacing (but *not* necessarily the same phase of oscillation), *independent of the experimental paradigm* (e.g., fixed ratio, fixed f_1 or fixed f_2) and *independent of DP order*, when the DP level is plotted versus DP frequency. However, if the level is plotted versus either f_1 or f_2, a strong dependence of the frequency spacing on the paradigm used and DP order can be observed. A special exception is the fixed ratio paradigm, in which the fine structure spacing remains independent of DPOAE order regardless of whether the level is plotted versus f_{dp}, f_1 or f_2. This result is a consequence of the approximately exponential scaling of the place-frequency map.

Other predictions of the formalism include 1) a modulation of DPOAE group delay with frequency that is correlated to amplitude fine structure (now observed); and 2) the observed phase shift of π in the $2f_1 - f_2$ DPOAE when the frequency ratio of fixed ratio measurements is shifted from 1.225 to 1.12.

In summary, we have developed and applied a general formalism for studying a large collection of experimental phenomena. Although this formalism is currently restricted to low level BM excitations, it offers the hope of a unifying framework for describing and predicting most of the essential features of otoacoustic emissions.

470

Appendix: Summary of Notation

Parameter	Description
$\omega_0(x)$	$\omega_0 e^{-k_\omega x} + \omega_1$, place-frequency map
$\gamma_0(x)$	$\gamma_0 e^{-k_\gamma x} + \gamma_1$, passive linear damping
$\rho_{f,s}; \psi_{f,s}$	fast, slow stiffness feedback magnitude and delay constants
σ_{bm}, W_{bm}	BM mass density, average width
S	cross-sectional area of cochlea
$\omega_{ow}; \gamma_{ow}$	middle ear resonance frequency, damping constant
$\sigma_{ow}; S_{ow}$	effective mass density, area of oval window
$k_{ow,0}$	$2\rho S_{ow}/\sigma_{bm} S$, middle ear coupling strength
G_{me}	mechanical gain of ossicles
P_a	adiabatic bulk modulus of air
ρ	density of perilymph

References

1. Long, G. R., Talmadge, C, and Tubis, A. (1993) New off-line method for detecting spontaneous otoacoutic emissions in human subjects. *Hear. Res.*, **71**:170–182.
2. Zwicker E. (1990) On the frequency separation of simultaneously evoked otoacoustic emissions' consecutive extrema and its relation to cochlear traveling waves. *J. Acoust. Soc. Am.*, **88**:1639–1941.
3. He, N. J. and Schmiedt, R. A.(1993). Fine structure of the $2f_1 - f_2$ acoustic distortion product: Changes with primary level. *J. Acoust. Soc. Am.*, **94**:2659–2669.
4. Engdahl, B. and Kemp, D. T.(1996). The effect of noise exposure on the details of the distortion product emissions in humans. *J. Acoust. Soc. Am.*, **99**:1573–1588.
5. Kemp, D. T. (1979). The evoked cochlear mechanical response and the auditory microstructure - evidence for a new element in cochlear mechanics. *Scand. Audiol.*, Supp 9:35–47.
6. Zweig, G. (1991). Finding the impedance of the organ of Corti. *J. Acoust. Soc. Am.*, **89**:1229–1254.
7. Talmadge, C. and Tubis, A.(1993). On modeling the connection between spontaneous and evoked otoacoustic emissions. In: Duifhuis, H., Horst, J. W., van Dijk, P, and van Netten, S. M., eds., *Biophysics of Hair Cell Sensory Systems*, pages 25–32, Singapore, World Scientific.

8. Zweig, G. and Shera, C. A. (1995) The origins of periodicity in the spectrum of evoked otoacoustic emissions. *J. Acoust. Soc. Am.*, **98**:2018–2047.

9. de Boer, E. (1995). On equivalence of locally active models of the cochlea. *J. Acoust. Soc. Am.*, **98**:1400–1409.

10. Talmadge, C., Tubis, A., Long, G., and Piskorski, P. Reflection model of distortion product otoacousitc emission fine structure. *in preparation*.

SHAPE AND STIFFNESS CHANGES OF THE ORGAN OF CORTI FROM BASE TO APEX CANNOT PREDICT CHARACTERISTIC FREQUENCY CHANGES: ARE MULTIPLE MODES THE ANSWER ?

L. ZHANG, D.C. MOUNTAIN, A.E. HUBBARD

Hearing Research Center, Boston University, 44 Cummington Street, Boston MA 02215, USA

The size and shape of the architecture of the mammalian organ of Corti varies from base to apex. Based on two different basal and apical cross sections, two finite element models were created. Both clamped and hinged inner pillar cell boundary conditions were used in each model. Material parameters for each region were estimated by matching the basal turn basilar membrane stiffness vs. radial position profile to experimental data by Naidu and Mountain[5]. Using these material properties, the fundamental natural frequencies (NF1) of the basal model are 23.88 kHz and 23.83 kHz for clamped and hinged inner pillar cell boundary conditions, respectively. For the apical model, using the same material parameters, NF1s are at 16.12 kHz and 10.27 kHz. The effects of changing the stiffness of each cellular component were also investigated. No single component has the ability to reduce the NFs of the apex significantly without changing the mode shape substantially.

1 Introduction

The mammalian organ of Corti changes considerably from its base to its apex. The mammalian cochlea spans a wide range of characteristic frequencies (CF), which vary by a factor of perhaps 300, from apex to base[4]. Cochlear models have typically used stiffness ranges on the order of 9×10^4, due to the square law relation between stiffness and resonant frequency in a spring-mass system. This is in spite of the fact that von Békésy[6] found only differences on the order of a factor of 100 from base to apex. Because there are also large differences in the appearance of the organ of Corti from base to apex, we explored the extent to which organ of Corti shape differences might account for the range of CFs.

2 Method

We constructed an anatomically-based representation of the organ of Corti of the gerbil and used the finite element method (FEM) to solve for the natural modes of vibration. We used a commercially-available CAD system, IDEAS. The three-dimensional organ of Corti representation uses solid brick, solid tetrahedron, solid wedge, and thin shell elements. The solid representation was meshed into parabolic triangular shell elements. We collapsed the three-dimensional representation to a two-dimensional equivalent of a slice that was 25 μm in longitudinal thickness.

The cellular representation of the organ of Corti was comprised of elastic components. We used two different boundary conditions at the foot of the inner pillars. In one case it was attached firmly (clamped) to the bony shelf. In the other case, it was allowed to rotate (hinged). We used two different organ of Corti cross-sections. One shown in Figure 1 (a) is similar to that found in the approximately 4-7 mm (from the base) region of the gerbil cochlea, while the other one depicts a more apical region. Each cochlear cross-section has ten different components, each having different physical characteristics. The model regions are: outer hair cells (OHC), Dieters' cells, Henson's cells, basilar membrane (BM) arcuate region, BM pectinate region, pillar cells, reticular lamina (RL), tectorial membrane (TM), inner hair cell (IHC) region and spiral ligament (SL). For the modal analysis, the TM was omitted and the natural modes of vibration calculated are those of the organ itself, without hydrodynamic load. We chose model parameters that allowed a match to static deflection data from Naidu and Mountain[5] measured at 17 kHz place. Table 1 shows the material parameters that were used for the basal model.

We explored the effect of stiffness changes on the natural frequency (NF) of the first and second natural mode of vibration, NF1 and NF2 respectively. This was done by varying the elastic parameter relative to the value fixed for the basal model, as listed in Table 1. In the apex, for each inner pillar boundary condition, clamped and hinged, parameter values were changed. All stiffnesses were reduced to 7.43% of the basal value. The reduction in stiffness is consistent with Naidu and Mountain's[5] estimate at a location 12 mm from the base, where the CF is around 300-800 Hz [4]. Then, each stiffness was reduced by 1% instead of 7.43% while keeping all other values constant at the estimated stiffness at the 12 mm location. This reduction was used in order to study the sensitivity to parameter variation in the vicinity of the estimated physiological stiffness.

3   Results

For both the clamped and hinged IPC boundary conditions, the fundamental mode shapes (Figure 1 a, c) are similar in both the base and apex. The undeformed geometry is given in solid lines, while the exaggerated (to aid visualization) deflection characteristic of the fundamental mode is shown using dashed lines. The data shown here, in which the clamped and hinged basal NF1s are 23.88 kHz and 23.83 kHz, respectively, were computed using the

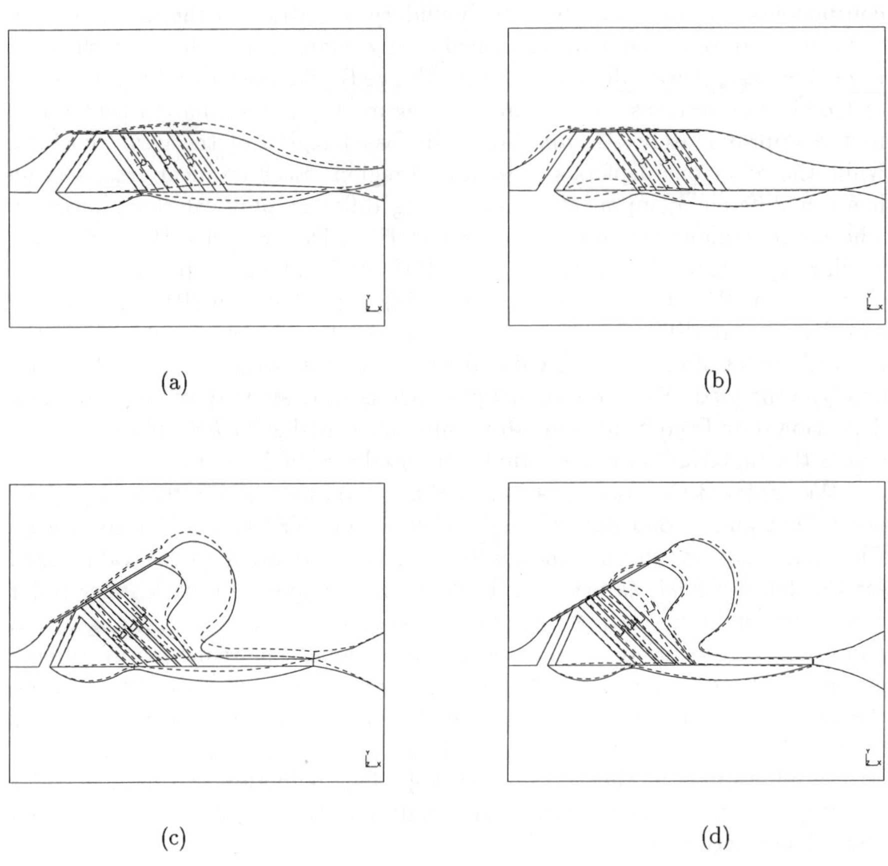

(a)

(b)

(c)

(d)

Figure 1: Base and Apex first two vibrational modes : Clamped IPC Boundary Conditions.

Table 1: Basal model material parameters.

Components	Elastic Modulus (Pa)		Poisson Ratio	Mass Density (kg/m^3)
	Clamped IPC	Hinged IPC		
Pillar Cells	4.67×10^8	4.00×10^8	0.45	1000
Basilar Membrane (Arcuate Zone)	5.00×10^5	7.50×10^5	0.29	1000
Basilar Membrane (Pectinate Zone)	1.58×10^7	5.00×10^6	0.29	1000
Outer Hair Cells	2.50×10^5	2.50×10^6	0.45	1000
Deiters' Cells	6.67×10^6	2.50×10^6	0.45	1000
Henson's Cells	1.83×10^7	1.75×10^7	0.45	1000
Reticular Lamina	1.58×10^6	2.00×10^7	0.29	1000
Inner Hair Cell Region	2.50×10^5	5.35×10^5	0.45	1000
Spiral Ligament	1.75×10^6	2.00×10^6	0.29	1000
Tectorial Membrane	6.00×10^4	6.00×10^4	0.29	1000

parameter values listed in Table 1. The same parameter values were used for the apical geometry, and the NF1s were 16.12 kHz and 10.27 kHz, respectively. The second mode shapes (Figure 1 b, d) are quite different. In the base, there are larger motions in the arcuate region of BM and at the first row OHCs. In the apex, there are larger motions at the third row OHC and Henson's cell region. Additionally, various portions of the arcuate and pectinate regions move out of phase. The NF2s are 46.77 kHz and 51.17 kHz in the base and 26.57 kHz and 38.59 kHz in the apex for the clamped and hinged cases, respectively.

Since shape changes caused little change in NFs relative to the known tuning characteristics in the base and apex, we reduced every apical component's stiffness to 7.43% of their basal turn values. Naidu and Mountain[5] estimated the stiffness vs. the distance from the base follows $\ln(k_2/k_1) = \alpha \times (x_1 - x_2)$, where α is about 0.325. This stiffness reduction produced NF1s of 4.4 kHz and 2.8 kHz and NF2s of 7.25 kHz and 10.52 kHz in the clamped and hinged IPC cases respectively. We further reduced each element's stiffness to 1% of their basal values to study the sensitivity of NFs to individual parameter variations. Table 2 shows that most such reductions had little effect on the NF1. The pa-

Table 2: Effect on apical model NF1 and NF2 of reducing stiffness parameters from 7.43% to 1% of the basal value. %Δ is the percentage of the original NFs achieved for a particular stiffness reduction.

Stiffness Reduced	Clamped IPC case				Hinged IPC case			
	NF1		NF2		NF1		NF2	
	kHz	%Δ	kHz	%Δ	kHz	%Δ	kHz	%Δ
Basilar Membrane (Arcuate)	4.38	99.7	4.93	68.06	2.79	99.68	5.96	56.62
Basilar Membrane (Pectinate)	2.86	65.14	6.40	88.28	2.00	71.42	8.58	81.57
Deiters' Cells	4.31	97.95	4.82	66.46	2.78	99.39	6.14	58.35
Henson's Cells	3.87	88.03	6.75	93.07	2.04	73.03	9.43	89.58
Inner Hair Cell Region	4.39	99.84	6.60	91.05	2.65	94.68	9.92	94.27
Outer Hair Cells	4.35	99.02	5.90	81.33	2.79	99.57	7.10	67.44
Pillar Cells	3.53	80.34	7.11	98.07	2.77	97.03	10.42	99.01
Reticular Lamina	4.25	96.59	4.53	62.43	2.72	97.03	8.63	82.02
Spiral Ligament	2.67	60.66	6.41	88.47	1.95	69.56	7.89	75.00
Every Component	1.61	36.63	2.66	36.66	1.03	36.80	3.86	36.67

rameter that had the largest effect on NF1 was the SL, which caused NF1 to be reduced to 60.66% and 69.56% of its initial value for the clamped and hinged cases, respectively. The next most important parameter was the stiffness of the BM pectinate region. The stiffness of the arcuate region plays almost no role in the determination of NF1, given the baseline parameters used. When the elastic modulus of every element was concurrently reduced from 7.43% to 1%, the NF1 in the clamped and hinged boundary cases was changed by 36.63% and 36.80% respectively. Note that the square root of 1/7.4 is 0.367 or 36.7%. We also investigated the effects of parameter variation (both one at a time and concurrently) on NF2 as shown in Table 2, and found changes in NF2 quite different from those found for NF1. The parameters that had the

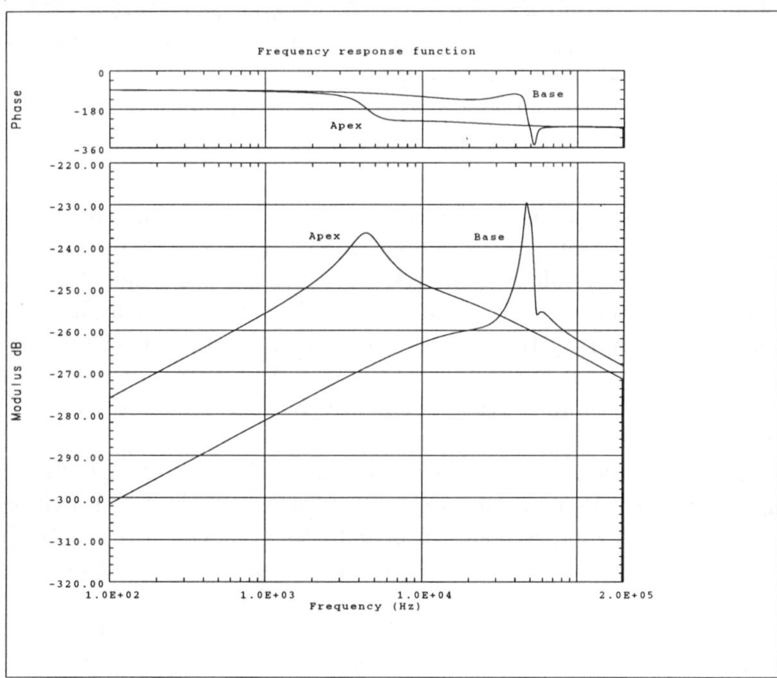

Figure 2: Frequency responses of IHC radial motion under uniform excitation in on the underside of arcuate and pectinate BM for the base and apex in clamped IPC case.

maximum effect on NF2 are the arcuate region of the BM, the RL, Deiters' cells and the OHC. Again the maximum change in NF2 was when all stiffnesses were changed, and the result was proportional to the square root of structure stiffness. We observed the mode shapes of both first and second modes when stiffnesses were changed. In most cases, they were quite similar in their appearance. However, in some cases, local motions become significantly different. For example, when the stiffness of OHCs or Deiters' cells were reduced, the junction between them showed a large radial motion. And when the stiffness of the RL was reduced, its vibrating motion increased considerably.

Because the radial motion of the RL at IHC location is an important factor for auditory nerve excitation, we obtained the response at that location to uniform excitation across the arcuate and pectinate regions of the BM, using a damping factor of 1 for NF1 and 0.03 for NF2 in the basal model and 0.2

478

for NF1 and 1 for NF2 for the apical model. The apical stiffness were 7.43% of the stiffness values used in the basal turn. The results (Figure 2) somewhat resemble auditory nerve tuning curves.

4 Discussion

Subject to the assumptions used in the model, geometry differences can only account for about a factor of two change in NF1 from base to apex. Moreover, physiological stiffness change estimates[5] do not change NF1 enough to account for changes in auditory nerve tuning. The IPC boundary condition has an influence in determining the relative importance of different cellular regions on NF1. Irrespective of the IPC, the SL and BM pectinate zone are of major importance in determining NF1. The ratio NF2/NF1 is less than 2 in the clamped case and nearly 4 in the hinged case.

These observations coupled with the shapes of Figure 2 suggests the following hypothesis. Perhaps the cochlear region where the basal architecture applies, namely 0-7 mm, responds principally to NF2, while the apex responds principally to NF1. If this were true, the range of frequencies spanned could be roughly 51.17 kHz down to 2.8 kHz. Suppose further that fluid mass loading reduced each number by 33% to 17 kHz and 900 Hz. Such CFs would be physiologically reasonable and can be achieved with a stiffness gradient of 13.5. This hypothesis may also fit well with one in which multiple wave propagation modes also exist[1-3].

References

1. Hubbard, A.E. (1993) A traveling wave amplifier model of the cochlea. *Science* **259** 68-71.
2. Hubbard, A.E., Gonzales, D. and Mountain, D.C. (1993) A nonlinear traveling-wave amplifier model of the cochlea. *Proceeding of the international symposium on biophysics of hair cell sensory system* 370-376
3. Hubbard, A.E., Ramachandran, P. and Mountain, D.C. (1996) A cochlear traveling-wave amplifier model with realistic scala media and hair cell electrical properties: Comparison between electrically-evoked emissions and basilar membrane velocity. This volume.
4. Miller, M. (1996) The cochlear place-frequency map of the adult and developing mongolian gerbil. *Hearing Research* **94** 148-156.
5. Naidu, R.C. and Mountain, D.C. (1996) Multiple stiffness gradients in the cochlea? This volume.
6. Von Békésy, G. (1960) Experiments in hearing. McGraw-Hill, New York.

Part Five

Descriptive models of cellular elements

THE INTRINSIC LIMIT FOR ACTIVE COCHLEAR MECHANICS

J.F. ASHMORE[*], J.E. GALE[‡]

Department of Physiology, School of Medical Sciences, University of Bristol
Bristol BS8 1TD, England
j.ashmore@ucl.ac.uk

The limiting frequency response of the outer hair cell motor is investigated in single isolated patches of membrane. In cell attached and in inside-out patches we find that the mean charge movement is approximately 5 fC with a limiting voltage dependent relaxation of 10 µs, a figure which agrees with measurements from single patch capacitance. This suggests that this OHC motor mechanism is restricted to cochlear designs operating up to about 25 kHz at 37°C.

1 Introduction

There are many direct and indirect lines of evidence which indicate that the outer hair cell (OHC) generates sufficient force to affect the mechanics of the cochlear partition. Economy of design suggests that it might be desirable to have a single cellular mechanism along the full length of the mammalian cochlea, but there remain questions about the details of tuning in the high frequency cochlear region and it has been argued that it may be necessary to include other mechanisms of cell force excitation[1].

A further question which has been apparent from an early stage in the investigation of OHC motility is whether the motor protein can operate fast enough[2,3]. As an integral membrane protein undergoing a conformational change, the OHC motor molecule has a rate of conformational change that is determined by its lipid environment it as well as by its own intrinsic dynamics. The OHC motor presents similar kinetic issues to those which have been raised in understanding fast transporter systems in many cells[4].

We describe here experiments which attempt to detect the limiting conformation rate change of the outer hair cell motor as measured by the charge displaced during the change. Although this issue has been addressed before in OHCs[2,5], those data were based on whole-cell recording where the large membrane capacitance of the cell becomes an obstacle to the rate at which patch clamp recording can resolve fast events. By using small patches, we show that there is a limiting time constant of about 10 µs measured at room temperature.

---

*Present address: *Dept of Physiology, University College London, Gower Street, London WC1E 6BT, UK and ‡Dept of Otolaryngology & Neuroscience, University of Virginia, Charlottesville, VA 22908, USA*

2 Methods

Conventional preparation and recording methods were employed[6]. Cells were isolated from the guinea pig cochlea and kept in artificial perilymph in a continuously perfused chamber. Large recording pipettes (inside diameter 2-3 μm) were employed to make wide bandwidth recordings in the cell attached and detached modes from the lateral cell membrane. The recording amplifier (Axon 200A) was used with a bandwidth extending to 60kHz. Data was collected at 330kHz sampling rates (CED 1401plus) and up to 4000 records were usually averaged.

The capacitance of single patches was measured by solving the equivalent cell circuit of the cell membrane for a given sinusoidal input[7]. A lock-in amplifier (Stanford Research, SR530) was used to detect the amplitude and phase of current in response to a sinusoidal voltage command signal at frequencies between 500Hz and 90kHz. The sinusoidal command was summed with a pipette potential which stepped the cell membrane from -130mV to +50mV over 30s (to ensure a good signal to noise ratio of the signal). In some cases, the patch was detached into the inside-out configuration. In these cases the patch could be recorded with stability for up to 60 minutes and the membrane potential calibrated.

3 Results

3.1 Charge movement in single patches

The potential across the membrane in cell attached patches was stepped rapidly for 1 ms and the current at onset and offset measured. As with whole cell recording protocols, it was necessary to subtract residual currents using either a P/4 or a P/2 protocol. The results of averaging such a response is shown in Figure 1. The residual current transients at ON and OFF were voltage dependent and were reversibly reduced by introducing 10mM salicylate into the bath[8]. The transients are characteristic of the charge movement associated with the OHC motor. The difference here, however, is that the relaxation time constants were significantly smaller (typically between 10 μs and 16 μs) than found for whole cell recording.

Patch movement was recorded by projecting a small laser photodiode beam perpendicularly through the membrane at the tip of the pipette. It was found that the patch movement followed the movement of charge closely with only a short delay which could have arisen from fluid drag within the pipette.

We have attempted to measure fluctuations of charge moving across the membrane as a way of restricting the possible candidates for the motor. For ion channels, macropatch recordings show that the fluctuation of a single e⁻ crossing.

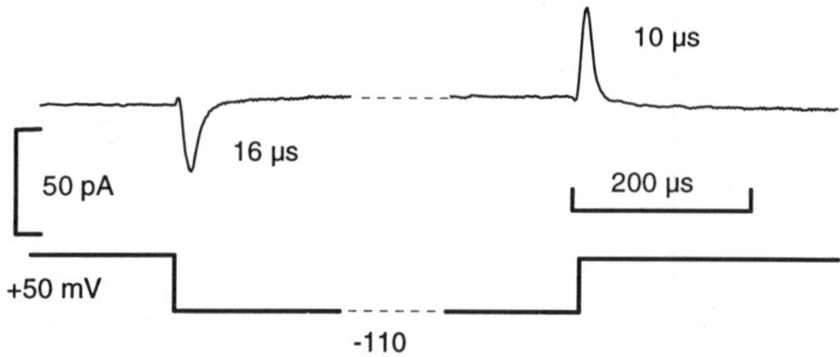

Figure 1. Charge displacement in single cell attached membrane patches from lateral OHC membrane when the pipette potential was stepped for 1ms to the potentials shown. A P/4 averaging protocol to remove residual leak [2]. Time constants adjacent to OFF and ON indicate best exponential fits to the charge relaxation.

the membrane can be detected[9]. No such fluctuations were observed in outer hair cell membranes, either in the patches or in whole cell recordings

3.2   Capacitance of single patches

The frequency response of the charge movement was measured from the patch membrane capacitance. The voltage dependent capacitance was measured as the membrane potential was ramped from -130mV to +50mV. The resulting capacitance was well fitted by the derivative of a Boltzmann function, $d\Phi/dV$[2,3], where the Boltzmann function $\Phi(V)$ is given in Eqn (A3). To fit the data at low frequencies, we found that $\beta = 1/30$ mV^{-1} (corresponding to 0.8-0.9 elementary charges) and $Q = 5$ fC in typical patches (corresponding to about 30000 elementary charges moving in the entire patch).

The precise value of the maximum nonlinear capacitance depended upon the frequency that was used as stimulus. Above 8kHz, there was a pronounced decrease in the value of β, so that as frequency increased the non-linear capacitance became progressively less voltage dependent (Figure 2) and we have interpreted this to mean that above a limiting frequency the charge no longer followed the command potential across the membrane.

The data of Figure 2 can most economically be described by a maximum voltage dependent capacitance which has a form

$$C_{max} = C_o \frac{1}{(1+(f/f_m)^2)^{1/2}} \cdot \frac{1}{(1+(f/f_2)^2)^{1/2}} \cdot \frac{1}{(1+(f/f_3)^8)^{1/2}}$$

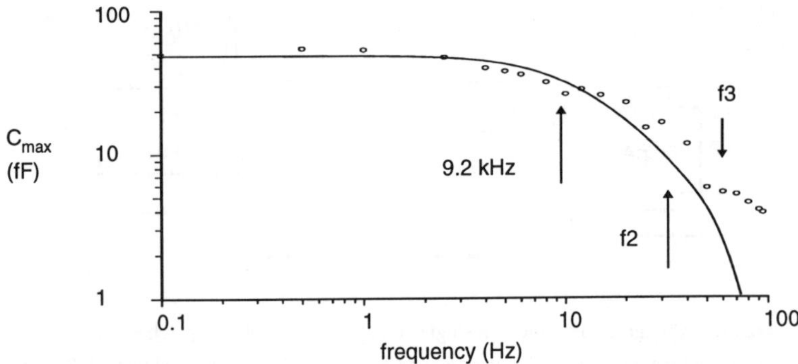

Figure 2. Maximum patch capacitance as a function of sinusoidal frequency for a typical patch. The continuous line is the fit is described in the text with the parameters f_1=9.2 kHz, f_2=30 kHz and f_3=62 kHz. The patch holding potential was -20mV and the asymptotic patch capacitance 49 fF at 0Hz.

which contains three low pass filters. The last term, with cut-off at f_3, represents the properties of the patch amplifier electronics and is given as a 4-pole filter. The middle term, with cutoff at f_2, represents the filtering effect of the stray capacitance of the pipette. The first term, characterised by a cut-off f_m, is interpreted as arising from the charge movement kinetics and can be most easily understood from the following considerations. Consider the movement of charge across the membrane as a two state model[11]

$$q_{in} \longleftrightarrow q_{out} \tag{1}$$

governed by forward (k_f) and backward (k_b) rate constants and where the process of the transfer obeys first order kinetics:

$$\frac{dq_{out}}{dt} = k_f q_{in} - k_b q_{out} \tag{2}$$

and where $Q = q_{in} + q_{out}$ is the total moved charge. As will be apparent, higher order kinetic schemes, as well as being unnecessarily complex, are not consistent with the experimental roll-off. Choosing the simplest exponential form for the rate constants, $k_f(V) = K\exp(\beta(V-Vo)/2)$ and $k_b(V) = K\exp(-\beta(V-Vo)/2)$, where K is a numerical constant, then the probabilty distribution is a Boltzmann function:

$$\Phi(V) = q_{out} / Q = 1/ (1 + \exp(-\beta(V-V_o))) \tag{3}$$

and the approach to equilibrium (from all the charge on the inside) is given by

$$q_{out} = Q \, \Phi(V) \, (1 - \exp(-t/\tau)) \tag{4}$$

where $\tau(V) = (k_f + k_b)^{-1}$ is the voltage-dependent relaxation time constant. This model predicts that the time constant of the charge relaxation should be maximum at $V=V_o$.

With these assumptions, the effective capacitance $C_{eff}(V) = dq_{out}/dV$ will have an apparent frequency dependence given by

$$C_{eff}(V,f) = C_{eff}(V,0) / (1 + j\, f/f_1) \tag{5}$$

where $f_1 = 1/2\pi\tau$ and $j = \sqrt{-1}$. Eqn 5 predicts that the capacitance will progressively develop an asymptotic phase lag of 90 degrees above f_1, i.e. appear as a reactance. The effect of a finite charge relocation time is equivalent to a conductance of about 0.16pS in series with the voltage dependent capacitance.

4 Discussion

The data suggest that there is a limiting rate at which the OHC motor operates. In the time domain, this is set by the relaxation time constant of the charge movement following a voltage step. It has a value of close to $\tau = 10$ µs at a membrane potential of -50mV corresponding in the frequency domain to $1/2\pi\tau = 16$ kHz. With a correction for temperature[10] the limiting frequency would be approximately 24 kHz at 37°C. Thus we conclude that the motor appears to operate rapidly enough to cope with the frequency amplification requirements of all but the cochleas of extreme design.

Simple kinetic schemes involving the two charge states of the motor can give rise to the observed frequency dependence if the reaction rates are of the order 10^5 s^{-1}. These transition rates are within the range inferred for translocation processes inferred for a variety of transporters[4], and provide circumstantial evidence at least that the OHC motor may have molecular similarities more with a transporter than with a modified ion channel. In other ion channels which have been investigated by means of fluctuation analysis[9], the transition rates are smaller by an order of magnitude. In contrast, the highest resolution measurements of the Na/Ca and Na/K transporters suggest that there charge movements are limited by diffusion of the cations down a deep access pore.

Acknowledgements

This work was supported by the Wellcome Trust and the Royal Society. JEG was a Hearing Research Trust / Colt Foundation postdoctoral research fellow.

486

References

1. Dallos, P. and Evans, B. (1995). High frequency motility of outer hair cells and the cochlear amplifier. *Science.* **267** 2006-2009.
2. Santos-Sacchi, J. (1991). Asymmetry in voltage dependent movements of isolated outer hair cells from the organ of Corti. *J. Neurosc*i. **9** 2954 (1991).
3. Ashmore, J.F. (1992). Mammalian hearing and the cellular mechanisms of the cochlear amplifier. In: *Sensory Transduction,* eds. D. Corey and S.Roper, Rockefeller Press, New York.
4. Hilgemann, D.W. (1994). Channel-like function of the Na,K pump probed at microsecond resolution in giant membrane patches. *Science* **263** 1429-1432.
5. Ashmore, J.F. (1987) A fast motile response in guinea-pig outer hair cells: the cellular basis of the cochlear amplifier. *J. Physiol.* **388** 323-347.
6. Housley, G. and Ashmore, J.F. (1992). Ionic currents of outer hair cells isolated from the guinea pig. *J. Physiol.* **448** 73-98.
7. Neher, E. and Marty, A. Discrete changes of cell membrane capacitance observed under conditions of enhanced secretion in bovine adrenal chromaffin cells. *Proc. natl. Acad. Sci. USA* **79** 6712-6716.
8. Tunstall, M.J. Gale, J.E. and Ashmore, J.F. (1995). Action of salicylate on membrane capacitance of outer hair cells from the guinea pig cochlea. *J. Physiol.* **485** 739-752.
9. Conti F. and Stühmer, W. (1989). Quantal charge redistributions accompanying the structural transitions in sodium channels. *Eur. Biophys. J.* **17** 53-59.
10. Ashmore J.F. and Holley, M.C. (1988). Temperature-dependence of a fast motile response in isolated outer hair cells of the guinea pig cochlea. *Q. J. Exp. Physiol.* **73** 143-145.
11. Iwasa, K..H. (1994). A membrane motor model for the fast motility of the outer hair cell. *J. Acoust. Soc. Am.* **96** 2216-2224.

MECHANICALLY INDUCED SHORTENING IN ISOLATED GUINEA PIG OUTER HAIR CELLS

E. CHAN and M. ULFENDAHL

Department of Physiology & Pharmacology
Div. Physiology II, Karolinska Institute
S - 171 77 Stockholm
Sweden

An anti-phasic shortening at the base was frequently observed when the apex of isolated outer hair cells was compressed with the tip of a quartz fibre. Shortenings could also be seen at both the apex and base by poking the lateral wall of the cell. The behaviour was instantaneous and reversible upon withdrawal of the compression from the cell.

1. Introduction

Outer hair cells are capable of maintaining their elongated shape even after isolation from the hearing organ. The physiological features that have been observed in isolated conditions have provided important clues about the function of sensory hair cells. External factors such as mechanical[1,2], chemical[3,4] and electrical[5] stimuli have been reported to elicit length changes in isolated outer hair cells. These features indicate a motile response of outer hair cells in the intact inner ear. We were concerned about the structural changes that appeared during stiffness measurements from isolated outer hair cells. Therefore the cells were continuously monitored throughout the manipulation. Here we observed an anti-phasic and reversible shortening at the base of isolated outer hair cells when they were compressed at the apex. Poking the lateral wall of the cells could also induce a shortening behaviour at the apical and basal ends. The shortenings were clearly detectable when visualized with the microscope.

The extent of the anti-phasic shortening at the base was found to be related to the force of the compression at the apex. The position where the lateral wall was poked produced different amount of shortening at the two ends.

2. Methods

Pigmented guinea-pigs were decapitated and detached cochleae were placed in a culture medium, Eagle's Minimal Essential Medium with Hanks' salts (without L-glutamine). The organ of Corti was dissected with a fine stainless steel blade. The coils were treated with collagenase (0.5mg/ml) for 3min and were rinsed several times. Cells were dissociated by trituration and were transferred to a Cell-Tak coated glass chamber containing the culture medium. Experiments were carried out at room temperature.

The cells were viewed at 40x magnification with water-immersion objective lens using an upright microscope (Zeiss ACM) equipped with a CCD camera (Hamamatsu).

Isolated outer hair cells were manipulated with quartz fibres (2-3μm in diameter and 1mm in length) of known stiffness. The stiffness of the quartz fibre was calibrated using glass microbeads. Movement of the quartz fibre was controlled using a micromanipulator (Narishige). In order to compress a cell, the quartz fibre was positioned so that it was just touching the site. The experiments were divided into two groups - 1. compression at the apex was increased in small steps resulting in increased bending of the quartz fibre or force of compression, and possible shortenings were observed; 2. the tip of the quartz fibre was pointed towards and poked gently on the lateral wall for observation of shortenings at the two ends of the cell. The experiments were recorded using the CCD camera and a video tape recorder (Panasonic).

In addition to observation of shortenings, the compression stiffness of the isolated outer hair cells under examination was measured. The cells were compressed at the apex by the tip of a quartz fibre of known stiffness. The compression stiffness of the cell could then be calculated by the amount of bending of the quartz fibre. Mechanically induced shortenings and other shape changes were analysed from the video images using a frame grabber (Matrox Magic) and an image analysis software (Image-Pro Plus).

3. Results

3.1 Apical compression and induced shortening

The extent of the induced shortening at the basal end of the isolated outer hair cells was increased as the force of the compression at the apical end increased. Fig. 1 shows the pattern of the response of an isolated outer hair cell (cell length = 72.6μm). The force of the apical compression by the quartz fibre was increased in small steps of about 0.2nN. The resulting induced shortening at the base was increased in a step-like manner. A plateau of 0.2μm was finally reached and there was no further shortening with increase in force. This response pattern was typical of the cells (n=26) studied.

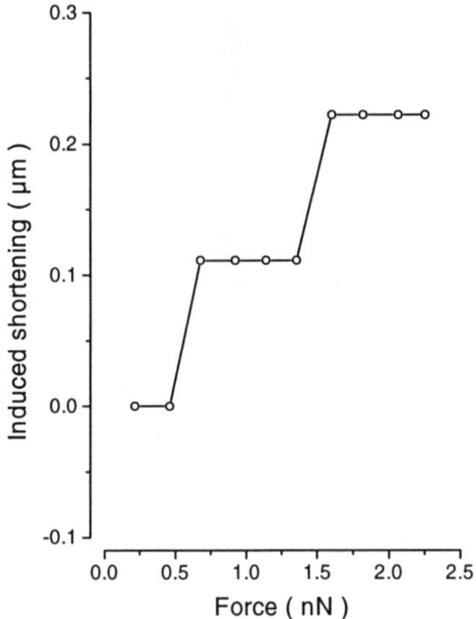

Figure 1: An isolated outer hair cell (cell length = 72.6μm) was compressed at the apex with increasing force and the induced shortening at the base was measured. The force of the compression was increased in steps of about 0.2nN. The symbols represent the measurements made at each step.

3.2 Lateral wall compression and shortening

Poking the lateral wall of the isolated outer hair cells (n=11) could also induce shortenings at the apical and basal ends. The diagrammatic illustration in fig. 2a shows the amount of shortenings at the apex and base of a cell (cell length = 70.1μm) when the lateral wall was poked by the tip of a quartz fibre. The depth of the indentation was 1.4μm and the position was 51.4μm from the apex along the longitudinal axis of the lateral wall. The resulting shortenings were 0.11μm at the apex and 0.09μm at the base. However, as the indentation moved to other positions along the lateral wall, the shortenings at the two ends changed. Fig. 2b shows an example of this typical response. The amount of shortening at the two ends became equal when the cell was poked midway between the apex and base (fig. 2b).

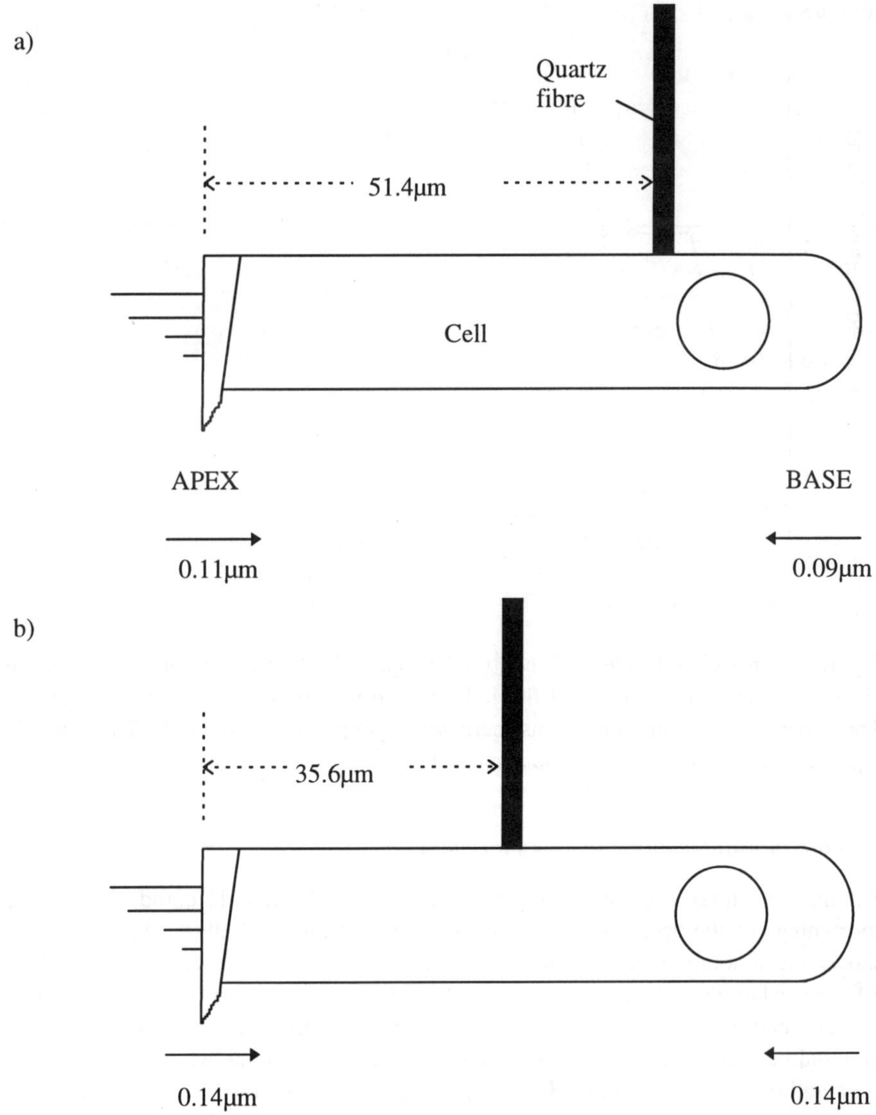

Figure 2: Diagrams illustrating induced shortenings at the apex and base of an isolated outer hair cell (cell length = 70.1µm) when the lateral wall was probed by the tip of a quartz fibre. The indentations were at positions a) 51.4µm and b) 35.6µm from the apex. The amount of shortenings in µm are indicated below the solid arrows.

4. Discussion

Out of the population of cells being tested, approximately 70% of which showed visually detectable compression induced anti-phasic shortenings. Even a higher percentage (about 80%) of cells was observed to respond to lateral wall compression with shortenings at the apex and base. The responding cells had healthy appearance and there were no signs of cellular damage. The cells in this study ranged from 60 to 80μm in length. Care was taken not to choose those cells that had a large proportion of the cell body adhered to the glass of the chamber, preferably with less than half of the cell attached. The induced shortenings were not likely to be due to the chemical effect of Cell-Tak because cells settled on uncoated glass also responded to the compression. In addition, cells held by suction pipettes showed this shortening behaviour. Therefore, it was apparent that the anti-phasic shortenings of the cells were induced mechanically by compression. The results have also shown that poking at different regions of the lateral wall produced different amount of shortenings at the apex and base. Structural features along the lateral wall might be related to the difference in the shortenings.

Preliminary experiments have been carried out to study the effects of salicylate on the compression induced shortenings in the cells. Previous studies have shown administration of salicylate caused tinnitus and auditory threshold shifts[6,7,8]. Outer hair cells as the site of salicylate action has been implicated[9,10]. Salicylate has been shown to cause decrease in cell stiffness and electromotile response[11]. Our preliminary results have shown that perfusion with salicylate (5mM) caused a decrease in cell stiffness but an enhancement of the induced anti-phasic shortenings. Experiments were also carried out to study whether the enhanced response was due to the change in cell stiffness or other toxic effects of salicylate. Therefore, the cells were exposed to hypertonic media to test the effect on the compression induced shortenings. During exposure to hypertonic media, the cells became less stiff, and this was comparable to the previous results by others[12]. However, the decrease in cell stiffness by exposure to hypertonic media did not lead to an increase in the compression induced anti-phasic shortening response. Therefore, other cellular effects of salicylate on the shortening response could be involved.

The described shortening behaviour in isolated outer hair cells is interesting in the way that it could be induced by slow compression. It has previously been shown[1,2] that anti-phasic length changes of isolated outer hair cells can be elicited in response to acoustical (mechanical) stimuli applied to the cell body by means of a 200Hz oscillating water-jet. This is probably qualitatively similar to the shortening response induced by slowly poking the lateral wall. However, the maximal magnitude of the acoustically induced shortening was up to more than 3μm and this is considerably more than what we report here. The difference in the magnitude of the responses may be related to the difference in the area of the cell membrane being stimulated or the frequency of the stimulation. The response to axial compression is possibly of greater functional importance in that it may link the observed phenomenon to stimuli readily occurring in the hearing organ. The mechanical stimulation acting on the cell bodies in the intact hearing organ during sound stimulation is not known in detail. It is however likely that the up-and-down motions of the basilar membrane and the reticular laminar will cause compression and stretching of the sensory cells. It is thus suggested that this may be the physiological stimulus for the shortening response. The mechanism of the anti-phasic shortening behaviour of isolated outer hair cells remains, however, to be investigated.

Acknowledgements

Supported by the Swedish Medical Council, the Swedish Work Environment Fund, a Guest Scholarship of the Swedish Institute and Stiftelsen Einar Lundströms Minne.

References

1. Canlon, B., Brundin, L. and Flock, Å. (1988) Acoustic stimulation causes tonotopic alterations in the length of isolated outer hair cells from the guinea pig hearing organ, *Proc. Natl. Acad. Sci.* **85** 7033-7035.
2. Brundin, L., Flock, Å and Canlon, B. (1989) Sound-induced motility of isolated cochlear outer hair cells is frequency-specific, *Nature* **342** (No. 6251) 814-816.
3. Zenner, H.P. (1986) Motile responses in outer hair cells, *Hearing Res.* **22** 83-90.
4. Flock, Å., Flock, B. and Ulfendahl, M.(1986) Mechanisms of movement in outer hair cells and a possible structural basis, *Arch. Otorhinolaryngol.* **243** 83-90.
5. Brownell, W.E., Bader, C.R., Bertrand, D. and de Ribaupierre, Y. (1985) Evoked mechanical responses of isolated hair cells, *Science* **227** 194-196.
6. Myers, E.N. and Berstein, J.M. (1965) Salicylate ototoxicity. A clinical and experimental study, *Arch. Otolaryngol.* **82** 483-493.
7. McCabe, P.A. and Dey, F.L. (1965) The effects of aspirin upon auditory sensitivity, *Ann. Otol. Rhinol. Larygol.* **74** 312-325.
8. Ramsden, R.T., Latif, A. and O'Malley, S. (1985) Electrocochleographic changes in acute salicylate overdosages, *J. Laryngol. Otol.* **99** 1269-1273.

9.   Shehata, W.E., Brownell, W.E. and Dieler, R. (1991) Effects of salicylate on shape, electromotility and membrane characteristics of isolated outer hair cells from guinea pig cochlea, *Acta Otolaryngol. (Stockholm)* **111** 707-718.

10.   Kössl, M. and Russell, I.J. (1992) The phase and magnitude of hair cell receptor potentials and frequency tuning in the guinea pig cochlea, *J. Neuroscience* **12** 1575-1586.

11.   Russell, I. and Schauz, C. (1995) Salicylate ototoxicity: effects on the stiffness and electromotility of outer hair cells isolated from the guinea pig cochlea, *Auditory Neurosci.* **1** (No. 3) 309-319.

12.   Chertoff, M.E. and Brownell, W.E. (1994) Characterization of cochlear outer hair cell turgor, *Am. J. Physiol.* **266** C467-C479.

RECONSIDERATION OF THE INFLUENCE OF EXTRACELLULAR VOLTAGES ON IHC TRANSMITTER RELEASE

M.A. CHEATHAM AND P. DALLOS

Auditory Physiology Laboratory (The Hugh Knowles Center)
Department of Communication Sciences and Disorders
Northwestern University, Evanston IL 60208-3550 USA
m-cheatham@nwu.edu

We encourage reconsideration of a proposal[10,15,18] which suggests that extracellular voltages, reflecting outer hair cell receptor currents, can influence inner hair cell (IHC) transmitter release at low frequencies. This, along with the velocity sensitivity of IHCs, may explain paradoxical results in the single unit literature with respect to the timing of suppression at best frequency and the timing of excitation for low frequency suppressors.

1 Introduction

Comparisons at the mechanical, hair cell and single unit levels provide insights into underlying nonlinearities with respect to sites of origin and mechanisms of operation. Of interest here is the phase of suppression at best frequency (BF) versus the phase of excitation for low-side suppressors since single unit results have presented opposing observations. In some cases, the time of excitation for the suppressor coincides with the time of maximum suppression[16,18]. Alternatively, the phase of suppression can be displaced by either 1/4 or 1/2 cycle relative to the time of excitation for the low frequency suppressor alone[3,22]. Although these results are yet to be reconciled, it has been suggested that extracellular, organ of Corti (OC) voltages can contribute to the potential gradient across the IHC's basolateral membrane thereby influencing transmitter release[10,15,18]. Thus, it is possible that electrical interactions underlie differences in the phases of suppression versus excitation. Evaluation of two-tone responses in IHC receptor potentials (RP) and in extracellular responses measured nearby in the OC may shed light on these temporal relationships.

2 Methods

Recordings are made from second turn of the guinea pig cochlea where BF is approximately 3500 Hz. Responses from IHCs and from the OC fluid space are collected for two-tone inputs consisting of a BF probe and a second tone at 40 Hz. Since the cochlear microphonic (CM) recorded in the OC reflects outer hair cell (OHC) receptor currents and since OHCs respond in phase with basilar membrane (BM) motion at low frequencies, the positive phase of this extracellular ac response is associated with BM displacement to scala vestibuli (SV). Thus, position shifts of the BM produced by the low frequency input can be determined locally in the same general area as the IHC and no corrections are required to compensate for traveling wave or synaptic delays. This makes correlating the phases of excitation and/or suppression with displacements of the BM more accurate than if one relies on measures of the CM measured at the round window. Further details are available in a previous publication[4].

3 Results and Discussion

Waveforms at the top of Fig. 1 show IHC RPs for a near BF probe measured in the presence of a second tone at 40 Hz. To better illustrate modulations in the probe response, the two-tone waveform has been high-pass filtered, thereby removing the response at 40 Hz and any dc potentials associated with either input. The low frequency tone alone is plotted using the ordinate on the right. The middle panel provides a similar portrait for measures in the OC fluid space. Comparisons between the two-tone response and that at 40 Hz alone reveal that the BF probe is reduced during the negative phase of the CM response which is associated with BM displacement to scala tympani (ST). This relationship is thought to reflect asymmetries in the OHC transducer[7,13] such that BM displacements to ST bias the transducer in the off position. As the operating point moves along the hair cell's transfer function, the associated changes in gain influence probe responses.

In the bottom panel, the OC response is subtracted from that measured in the IHC. This subtraction process[5] illustrates two important features. First, the IHC response to 40 Hz alone leads that measured in the OC[6,11] reflecting the velocity sensitivity of IHCs at low frequencies. Second, the waveforms also reveal that amplitude modulations appear during the negative phase of the CM response and not during the negative phase of the IHC response to 40 Hz, as indicated by vertical lines at 80 msec. Since the phase of excitation for the low frequency tone is shifted roughly 90° relative to the phase of maximum suppression for the BF probe, this feature may underlie the observation that the time of maximum suppression in neural responses can be displaced 1/4 cycle relative to the excitatory response to the suppressor alone[3,22].

Additional single unit results, obtained using suppressors with slightly higher frequencies where IHCs no longer respond to BM velocity, indicate that the excitatory response phase of the low frequency suppressor alone can be displaced by approximately 1/2 cycle relative to the phase of maximum rate decrease for BF inputs[3,22]. This temporal disparity is represented on the left in Fig. 2 where hypothetical relationships between BM displacement, hair cell depolarization and single unit rate responses are displayed. When intracellular RPs control transmitter release, BM displacements to SV (row 1) depolarize IHCs (row 2) and increase rate for single tone inputs (row 4). Since the IHC RP exceeds that in the OC (row 2), the voltage gradient across the IHC's basolateral membrane (row 3) is virtually identical to the IHC RP and subtraction of the OC response has little effect. In the two-tone case, rate decreases are recorded during displacement to ST (bottom row) probably because of asymmetries in the OHC transducer[7,13]. Thus, the phase of excitation for the low frequency tone alone is shifted roughly 1/2 cycle relative to the phase of maximum two-tone rate reduction observed at BF.

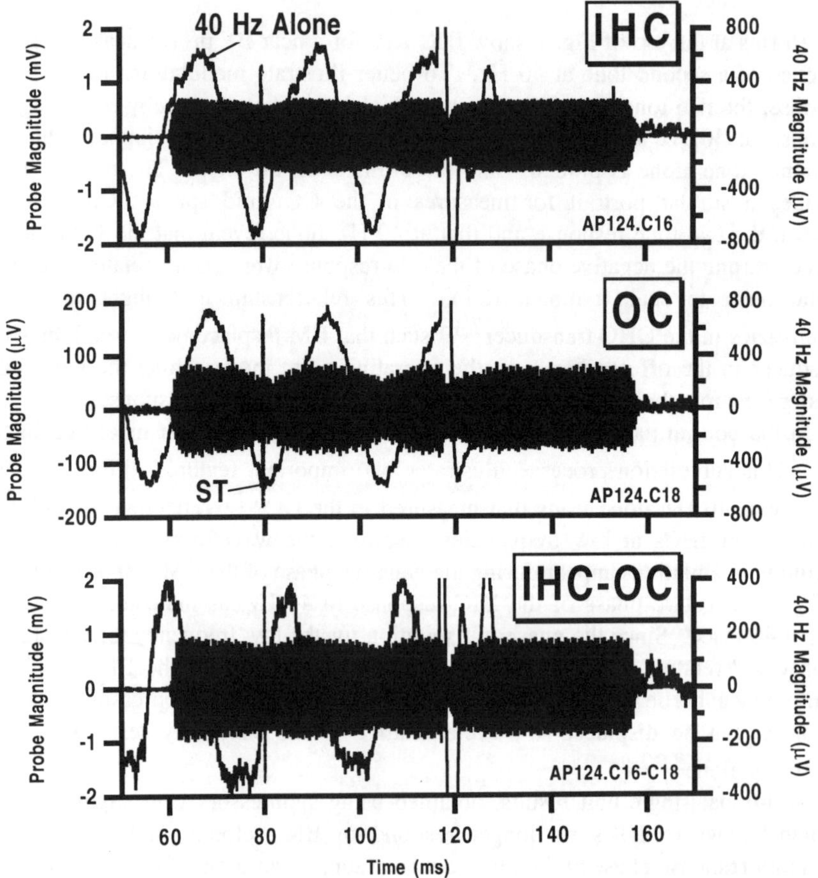

Fig. 1. Response waveforms are shown for the IHC ac RP (top) and for the OC response (center). High-pass filtered, two-tone waveforms are presented in combination with those for 40 Hz alone (75 dB). The 3500 Hz probe (40 dB) is plotted on the left ordinate. At the bottom, the OC response is subtracted from that measured inside the IHC for both the 40 Hz alone and the two-tone conditions.

There are, however, other studies where this 1/2 cycle relationship was not seen[16,18]. For example, Sachs and Hubbard[16] reported that the phase of the low frequency suppressor that produced a rate increase when presented alone produced a rate decrease when presented with a BF probe. This behavior was recorded in single units with high BFs and for suppressor tones introduced at their lowest effective levels. Although this relationship may not be a general feature of two-tone interactions[3], it could relate to the observation that extracellular voltages, measured in the OC and reflecting OHC receptor currents, can exceed intracellular responses measured inside IHCs[12,15]. While a model incorporating extra-synaptic influences has been proposed[8], we are here considering a presynaptic influence rather than a direct effect on the spike generator itself[2,9,21]. In other words, it is argued below that extracellular rather than intracellular voltages can, under certain conditions, influence and/or control transmitter release from individual IHCs[10,14,15,18,20], thereby affecting the magnitude and phase of postsynaptic responses.

When evaluating this proposal, it is important to note that transmitter release from IHCs is dependent on transmembrane voltage. At BF it is generally accepted that the dc RP, produced by asymmetries in the IHC transducer, drives postsynaptic communication. However, for low frequency inputs on the tails of tuning curves, extracellular potentials reflecting OHC receptor currents could be larger than those provided by intracellular sources. In other words, OHCs in the base of the cochlea could generate voltages for low frequency inputs at levels below those that induce IHCs to produce RPs large enough to excite auditory nerve fibers directly[12,15].

In order to contrast the effects of intracellular versus extracellular voltages on transmitter release, additional schematics are provided on the right in Fig. 2. Since OHC receptor currents are reflected in the OC fluid space, these variations can potentially influence voltage gradients across the IHC's basolateral membrane. For example, when the BM moves to ST (row 1), and OHC and OC responses become more negative (row 2), the voltage gradient "seen" by the IHC becomes relatively more positive (row 3). Thus, low frequency inputs can increase rate in high BF fibers during the ST-phase of BM motion (row 4) when extracellular voltages exceed those produced intracellularly. In the two-tone case, rate decreases due to suppression also occur for displacements to ST (row 5) but because the OHC transducer is driven into saturation[7]. Although extracellular dc voltages can influence this synaptic transmission directly, ac variations can also effect communication via rectification at the synapse[1,17,19] thereby providing a form of electrical interaction between the two populations of hair cells.

498

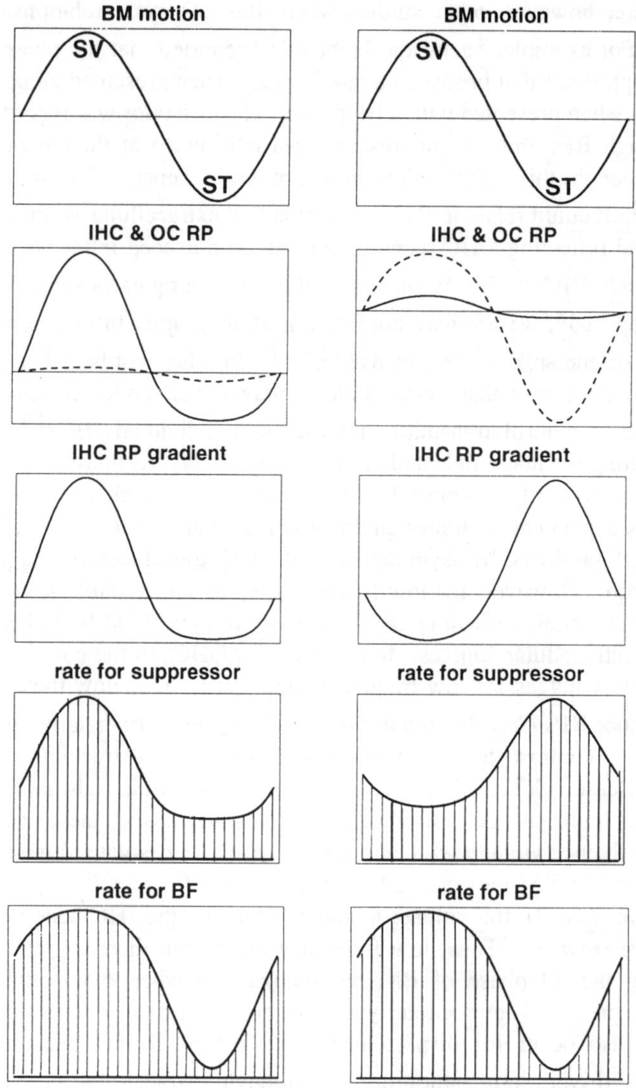

Fig. 2. This figure demonstrates the effects of basilar membrane displacement on hair cell and single unit responses. In all panels the abscissa represents one period of a low frequency sinusoid that is well below the BF of this basal location. The representation on the left (right) illustrates the case where the potential gradient across the IHC's basolateral membrane is dominated by intracellular (extracellular) voltages. Organ of Corti responses are plotted with dashed lines.

Figure 2 demonstrates that when low level, low frequency suppressors are paired with near-BF probes, maximum rate suppression occurs for BM displacement to ST. If IHC RPs control transmitter release as shown on the left, then the phase of excitation for the suppressor alone will be displaced by approximately 1/2 cycle relative to the phase of suppression when the velocity dependence of the IHC is not a contributing factor. In contrast, the right column depicts the case where the phase of excitation for the suppressor alone coincides with the phase of maximum suppression possibly because transmitter release is controlled by extracellular voltages that are roughly 180° out of phase with intracellular IHC responses. Since voltage gradients across the IHC's basolateral membrane can be influenced by extracellular potentials reflecting OHC receptor currents[15,18], electrical interactions between the two hair cell populations may be possible but only in the basal half of the cochlea.

Acknowledgment

Work supported by research grant 5 R01 DC00089 from the NIDCD, NIH.

References

1. Allen, J.B. (1983) A cochlear micromechanical model of transduction, in *Mechanics of Hearing,* eds. E. de Boer and M.A. Viergever (Delft University Press, The Netherlands) pp. 85-92.
2. Brownell, W.E. (1982) Cochlear transduction: an integrative model and review, *Hear. Res.* **6**, 335-360.
3. Cai, Y. and Geisler, C.D. (1996) Suppression in auditory-nerve fibers of cats using low-side suppressors: I. Temporal aspects, *Hear. Res.*, in press.
4. Cheatham, M.A. and Dallos, P. (1992) Physiological correlates of off-frequency listening, *Hear. Res.* **59**, 39-45.
5. Cody, A.R. and Mountain, D.C. (1989) Low-frequency responses of inner hair cells: evidence for a mechanical origin of peak splitting, *Hear Res.* **75**, 103-113.
6. Dallos, P. and Santos-Sacchi, J. (1983) AC receptor potentials from hair cells in the low-frequency region of the guinea pig cochlea, in *Mechanisms of Hearing,* eds. W.R. Webster and L.M. Aitkin (Monash University Press, Clayton, Australia) pp. 11-16.
7. Geisler, C.D., Yates, G.K., Patuzzi, R.B. and Johnstone, B.M. (1990) Saturation of outer hair cell receptor currents causes two-tone suppression, *Hear. Res.* **4**, 241-256.
8. Hill, K.G., Stange, G., Gummer, A.W. and Mo, J. (1989) A model proposing

synaptic and extra-synaptic influences on the responses of cochlear nerve fibres, *Hear. Res.* **39**, 75-90.

9. Honrubia, V., Strelioff, D. and Sitko, S.T. (1976) Physiological basis of cochlear transduction and sensitivity, *Ann. ORL* **85**, 697-711.

10. Ingvarsson, K. (1981) Dynamics of Cochlear Hair Cells as Inferred from Cochlear Potentials and Responses from Auditory Nerve Fibers. Ph.D. Dissertation, Northwestern University, Evanston IL 60208.

11. Nuttall, A.L., Brown, M.C., Masta, R.I. and Lawrence, M. (1981) Inner hair cell responses to velocity of basilar membrane motion in the guinea pig, *Brain Res.* **211**, 171-174.

12. Patuzzi, R.B. and Sellick, P.M. (1984) The modulation of the sensitivity of the mammalian cochlea by low frequency tones. II. Inner hair cell receptor potentials, *Hear Res.* **13**, 9-18.

13. Patuzzi, R.B. Sellick, P.M. and Johnstone, B.M. (1989) Outer hair cell receptor currents and sensorineural hearing loss, *Hear. Res.* **42**, 47-72.

14. Ruggero, M.A. and Rich, N.C. (1983) Chinchilla auditory-nerve responses to low frequency tones, *J. Acoust. Soc. Am.* **73**, 2096-2108.

15. Russell, I.J. and Sellick, P.M. (1983) Low-frequency characteristics of intracellularly recorded receptor-potentials in guinea-pig cochlear hair cells, *J. Physiol.* **338**, 179-206.

16. Sachs, M.B. and Hubbard, A.E. (1981) Responses of auditory-nerve fibers to characteristic-frequency tones and low-frequency suppressors, *Hear Res.* **4**, 309-324.

17. Schroeder, M.R. and Hall, J.L. (1974) Model for mechanical to neural transduction in the auditory receptor, *J. Acoust. Soc. Am.* **55**, 1055-1060.

18. Sellick, P.M., Patuzzi, R.B. and Johnstone, B.M. (1982) Modulation of responses of spiral ganglion cells in the guinea pig cochlea by low frequency sound, *Hear Res.* **7**, 199-221.

19. Smith, R.L. and Brachman, M.L. (1982) Adaptation in auditory nerve fibers: A revised model, *Biol. Cybern.* **4**, 107-129.

20. Strelioff, D. (1986) Physiological basis of low-frequency biasing, *Abs. Assoc. Res. Otolaryngol.*, p. 41.

21. Strelioff, D., Sitko, S.T. and Honrubia, V. (1976) Role of inner and outer hair cells in neural excitation, *Trans. Acad. Ophth. & Otol.* **82**, 322-327.

22. Temchin, A.N., Rich, N.C. and Ruggero, M.A. (1994) The effect of low-frequency tones on the responses of auditory-nerve fibers to characteristic-frequency tones, *Abs. Assoc. Res. Otolaryngol.*, p. 97.

EFFERENT CONTROL OF COCHLEAR MECHANICS: OUTER HAIR CELLS

P. DALLOS, D.Z.Z. HE, X. LIN, B.N. EVANS

Auditory Physiology Laboratory (The Hugh Knowles Center), Departments of Neurobiology and Physiology and Communication Sciences and Disorders,
Northwestern University, Evanston, IL 60208 USA
p-dallos@nwu.edu

I. SZIKLAI

Department of Otorhinolaryngology, Semmelweis University Medical School, H–1083
Budapest, Hungary

Here we examine the effect of ACh upon the OHC's electromotile response, i.e., upon somatic shape changes under control of the cell's membrane potential. Cells are electrically stimulated in a microchamber or under whole-cell voltage-clamp and length and radius changes are measured. We show that ACh increases the axial, while reduces the radial motile response. This suggests that the dominant mechanism is consistent with ACh acting on the mechanical load to the motors, but not exclusively via membrane potential and conductance changes. As both fast and slow efferent actions are known to be inhibitory *in vivo*, while slow action of ACh increases electromotility *in vitro,* the present results suggest that slow efferent effects are not mediated by somatic length changes. Stiffness changes are possibly of greater consequence.

1 Introduction

Acetylcholine (ACh) is the principal efferent neurotransmitter in the cochlea (for review see Ref. 1). Efferent modulation of outer hair cell (OHC) motility *in vivo* may be a means for the central nervous system to control the state of the cochlea[2]. ACh binds to receptors at the cell's synaptic pole, increases the cell's input conductance and hyperpolarizes the cell membrane[1,3]. Second messenger activation[4] may also occur. The ACh receptor of the OHC is an unusual type, having both muscarinic and nicotinic features (see e.g., Refs. 1,5).

The OHC's electromotile response is probably mediated by membrane-bound voltage-sensing motor proteins, distributed over the basolateral cell membrane. As the OHC's electromotile response is membrane potential dependent[6], ACh-mediated channel openings could modulate electromotility. Indeed, as the cell's input conductance increases, the receptor-current-induced voltage drop on the basolateral (motor-bearing) membrane should decrease, along with the amplitude of the electromotile response. Thus the *a priori* expectation is that ACh should reduce electromotility, in harmony with the inhibitory influence attributed to cochlear efferents[7]. However, in previous experiments we observed that this is not the case[8], suggesting that factors other than conductance change may be important in the control of electromotility by the efferents.

There have been two principal approaches to the study of isolated OHC electromotility. One is to use whole-cell patch techniques which afford good control over the cell's membrane potential and the ionic content of the cytoplasm, but the cell's mechanical integrity is compromised. The microchamber technique maintains the cell's mechanical state, it, however, does not allow the accurate determination of either membrane potential or effective command voltage. We use both techniques in this work to assure that the unexpected result of increased motile response[8] in the presence of ACh is indeed real.

The electromotile response of OHCs consists of axial (δL) and radial components (δr). In a whole-cell stimulation mode the axial and radial components are antiphasic, as the cell maintains constant volume. In a whole-cell stimulation mode, measuring both δL and δr gives no more information than measuring either variable alone. However, in the microchamber configuration[9] length and radius changes are antiphasic for both respective partitioned cell segments (inside and outside of the microchamber), with the cell *in toto* maintaining constant volume. Thus any one variable does not constrain its covariant since compensatory movements can occur in the other partitioned cell segment. Consequently, as discussed below, joint measurement of two variables (δL and δr) can produce revealing information.

It is reasonable to assume that any influence (by ACh) that occurs *prior* to the activation of the motility motors is expressed similarly in δL and δr. Thus the constancy of the length change to radius change ratio before and after application of the ligand signifies that all effects occur prior to motor action, whereas non-constancy of the ratio indicates effects that happen in or after motor action. This heuristic notion is developed analytically below. We measure the $\delta L/\delta r$ ratio before and after application of ACh to the cell's synaptic pole and examine its constancy or change. In the whole-cell patch experiment we investigate whether the ACh effects persist when the cell is voltage-clamped. In order to identify the mechanism of ACh action, we also measure its effect on the cell's axial stiffness.

2 Methods

OHCs were obtained from the cochleas of euthanized albino guinea pigs (care and maintenance of animals was according to institutional guidelines). After removing segments of the organ of Corti, cells were transferred following enzymatic incubation to the experimental bath containing Leibovitz's L-15 medium, supplemented with 15 mM Hepes, 5 mM bovine serum albumin, and adjusted to 300 mOsm, and pH 7.35. OHCs were bathed in a Hanks' balanced salt solution. We have provided detailed descriptions of microchamber techniques[10] and they need no repeating. In the whole cell recording mode membrane potentials were clamped using the standard whole cell voltage-clamp technique. Zero current potentials of OHCs, measured after equilibration with the pipette internal solution, had to be at least -50 mV in order for the cell to be used. Pipette internal solution contained (in mM): KF 120; KCl 20; $MgCl_2$ 2; EGTA 10 and HEPES 10. The solution was buffered to pH 7.4 with Trizma Base (Sigma) and osmolarity adjusted to 300 mOsm with glucose. Whole cell currents and the photodiode signals were acquired by software clampex (Pclamp version 6, Axon Instruments Inc.) with the aid of a 12 bit A/D converter. Calibration of the photodiode system was accomplished by moving the slit in front of the photodiode over a fixed distance.

3 Results

3.1 Microchamber experiments

24 cells were examined with the microchamber paradigm. The example shown in Fig. 1 is representative of the entire data set. Contraction half-cyles of longitudinal motility increase fairly linearly, while elongation half-cycles rapidly saturate. Diameter changes are much smaller. At the largest signal level the $\delta L/\delta r$ ratio is approximately 10 for the example shown. We see a dramatic, approximately three-fold increase in δL with ACh. At the same time, δr is reduced. The range of length increases was between 12% and 440%. Length change increases due to ACh are in accordance with previous observations[8,11]. In most cases it is possible to completely reverse the effect of ACh by exchanging the medium in the experimental chamber to one not containing ACh (wash-out).

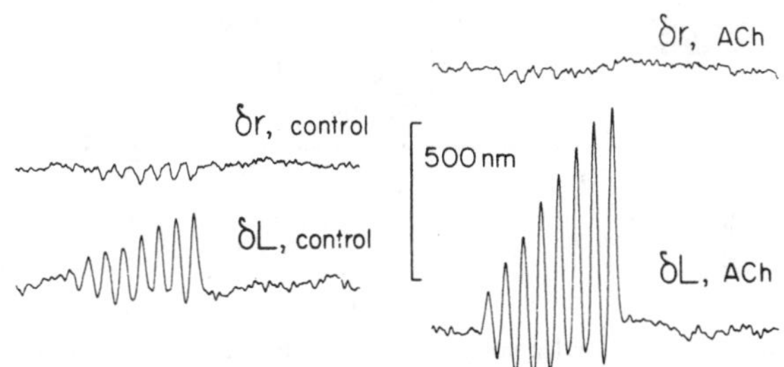

Figure 1: Motile responses to 10 Hz linear voltage ramp stimulus. Shown are diameter changes (δr) and length changes (δL) without and with 30 µM ACh in the bath. Contraction is plotted upwards.

Results presented here and before[8,11] are unequivocal. ACh in concentrations of 10-30 µM has a profound and reversible effect on the cell's fast electromotile response. Atropine, when applied together with ACh, completely suppresses the effect[11]. The ACh–effect is also eliminated when the external medium is Ca^{2+}–free. There is no effect on motility if ACh is applied to the cell anywhere but at the synaptic pole. The effects are not accompanied by measurable slow motile responses, in other words, the cell does not change shape appreciably in response to the ACh itself, as reported before[12]. The effect of ACh is greater on short (basal) cells than on long (apical) ones[11].

504

3.2 Voltage clamp experiments

We examined 15 cells in a whole-cell voltage-clamp configuration. Pressure ejection of ACh onto the cells' synaptic pole produced a large effect on electromotile response in 8 cases. Figure 2 depicts a sequence of responses to bi-polar square-pulse stimuli.

The time patterns of the whole-cell current and I-V curves (not shown) are as expected. The δL-V curves are Boltzmann functions, indicating larger response with saturation in the depolarizing (cell contraction) direction. When ACh is applied, the δL-V curves are significantly affected in that the small-signal gain (slope at holding potential) and the maximum responses are both increased approximately three-fold. After removal of ACh from the medium, both the response gain and magnitude revert to their original size.

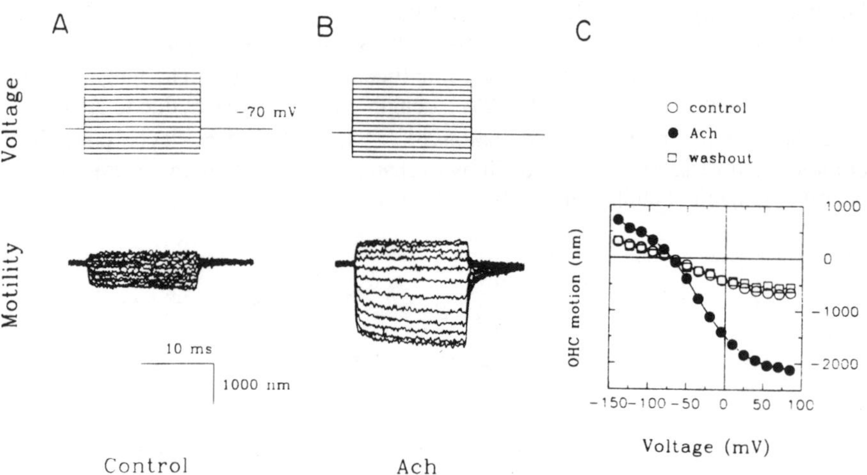

Figure 2: Motile responses under voltage clamp. In Fig. 2A and B we show the time patterns of representative motile responses. The membrane potential was stepped from a holding value of -70 mV over the range between -140 and +85 mV in 15 mV increments. Control conditions are depicted in column A, while column B shows responses obtained with ACh in the bath. In Fig. 2C displacement-voltage curves (δL-V), derived from the steady-state portions of the traces in panels A and B are shown. Contraction is plotted downward.

3.3 Stiffness measurements

In Fig. 3 axial stiffness measurements of the cell are shown. Similar experiments were performed on 14 cells. The cells were inserted into the microchamber with their ciliated pole first, so that approximately 80-90% was outside the chamber. A piezo-driven glass fiber was brought up against the synaptic pole. Unloaded and loaded fiber motion was measured with and without ACh in the bath. First we note that, in this example, upon pushing the fiber against the cell, its amplitude decreased to about 25%. Consequently, here the fiber's stiffness is approximately 33% of that of the cell. Upon application of ACh the amplitude increased by 75% (the range was from 50 to 114%). This implies that the cell's axial stiffness decreased due to ACh to about 40% of its original value.

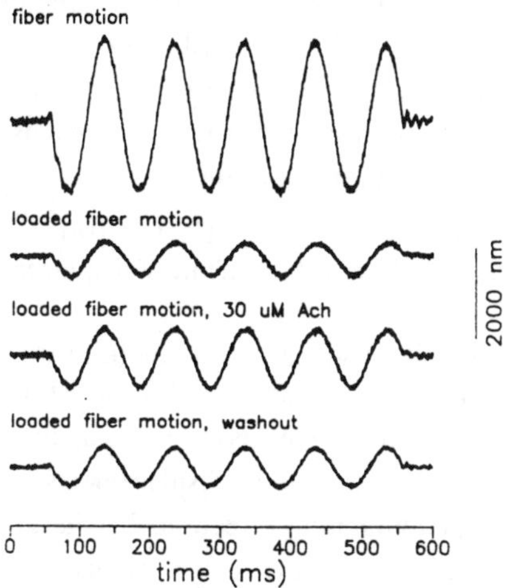

Figure 3: Displacement of a fiber driven by a piezoelectric actuator at 10 Hz, when the fiber is not in contact with the hair cell (top), after pushing against synaptic pole (second from top), after application of ACh (third from top) and after washout (bottom trace).

3.4 Time course of effects

In order to identify relations between ACh-induced modulation of somatic motility and previously described efferent effects, we examined the time course of a range of variables. Outward current and hyperpolarization were elicited approximately 100 msec after arrival of ACh at the synaptic pole (time values are to 63% of maximum response). Increase of OHC electromotility occurred after approximately 20 seconds. Thus the phenomena discussed here are akin to "slow" efferent effects[13].

4   Discussion

4.1 Mode of action of ACh

These experiments show that there is a significant influence on electromotile response by the binding of the ligand ACh, such that the axial electromotile response increases at all stimulus levels. In voltage-clamp experiments, at the same membrane potential, the motile response could be up to four times larger in the presence of ACh. It is thus apparent that ACh-action is not via voltage changes, but that it is an indirect effect on the motors proper or on their mechanical load. Conductance changes are unlikely to be of significance above the cutoff frequency of the cell membrane filter, at most 1 kHz.

506

We previously proposed a simple stochastic model for the electromotility of OHCs in the microchamber[9]. The model assumes that motility is powered by a large number of voltage-sensing protein molecules in the cell membrane. The motor is anisotropic in that its displacement in the axial direction $[d_a=\Phi(\delta V)\cos\gamma]$ is different from that in the circumferential direction $[d_c=\Phi(\delta V)\sin\gamma]$. $\Phi(\delta V)$ is the displacement of the motor along its hypothetical principal direction γ, where $\cot\gamma=d_a/d_c$. The motor displacement stochastically depends on the change in membrane potential δV, a Boltzmann relationship:

$$\Phi(\delta V) = d_0\{[1+ Exp(-a\,\delta V +b)]^{-1} - [1+ Exp(b)]^{-1}\}: \tag{1}$$

where a and b are constants and d_0 is the elementary displacement of the motor in the γ direction.

Denote the length of the cell's segment whose motility was monitored in these experiments as L, the global axial stiffness as K_a, while the elementary axial stiffness (connecting individual motor elements) as k_a. The linear density of motors is N, the number of motors summing their axial displacements is LN. Take k_c as the elementary stiffness in the circumferential direction, K_c the global stiffness in the circumferential direction, while r is the cell's radius. For the linear case, displacements of the cell segment (δL and δr) can be approximated:

$$\delta L \approx \frac{2\pi LNk_a \cos\gamma}{2\pi k_a + LK_a}\Phi(\delta V) ; \qquad \delta r \approx \frac{rLNk_c \sin\gamma}{Lk_c + 2\pi rK_c}\Phi(\delta V) \tag{2}$$

The ratio of length and radius changes:

$$\frac{\delta L}{\delta r} \approx 2\pi \frac{L + 2\pi r\dfrac{K_c}{k_c}}{2\pi r + L\dfrac{K_a}{k_a}}\cot\gamma \tag{3}$$

In line with our heuristic argument, the ratio $\delta L/\delta r$ is independent of the actual motor displacement function, $\Phi(\delta V)$ and of δV, at least in this linear treatment. Moreover, the $\delta L/\delta r$ ratio is independent of parameters N, a, b and d_0. Voltage drop on the cell segment is determined by the reactive voltage divider formed by the included and excluded cell membranes. ACh–gated channel openings modulate the resistance of the synaptic pole and motor action is thought to modulate the capacitance of both cell segments[3]. *None of these electrical changes matter: the δL/δr ratio is independent of them.* We conclude that changes in the length-to-radius change ratio cannot be due to direct electrical influences (impedance or membrane potential changes). This agrees with the results of the voltage-clamp experiments.

Expressed in terms of the elementary and global axial stiffnesses, the total longitudinal stiffness of the cell:

$$K_L = K_a + \frac{2\pi r}{L} k_a \tag{4}$$

Our experimental results indicate that $\delta L/\delta r$ and δL increase, δr decreases and K_L decreases when ACh is applied. These conditions can be jointly fulfilled if K_a/k_a decreases and γ decreases. The constraint on K_L shows that it is necessary for K_a to decrease. Thus the large changes in motile response due to application of ACh may be obtained by a decrease in the cell's global axial stiffness, coupled with redirection of the principal motor action in a more axial direction (possibly a reorientation of cortical lattice domains). It is as if ACh increased the cell's anisotropy. All slow ACh effects are eliminated if the external medium is calcium–free. Consequently, it is our assumption that the mechanical changes are brought about by a Ca^{2+}–dependent second messenger process, possibly culminating in protein phosphorylation which might influence the cortical lattice structure or its coupling to the motor molecules. Decreased axial stiffness is not a consequence of altered turgor, at least not such that can be measured by static length changes.

4.2 Efferents and the cochlear amplifier

Finally, let us consider that an *increased* motile response due to the action of the neurotransmitter ACh appears to be contrary to available data on the influence of the medial efferent system on cochlear response, which is inhibitory. Moreover, it is the consensus that efferent inhibition occurs by the reduction in the gain of the cochlear amplifier[1,2]. A majority assume that somatic length change of OHCs (producing "negative damping") is the effective feedback variable. The minority view is that basilar membrane reactance (stiffness) changes can account for cochlear amplification[14,15]. Both the classical fast effects and newly described "slow" efferent effects[13] are inhibitory and both are assumed to result from conductance changes in OHCs. While our data do not address fast effects, it is clear that the slow effects need to be differently interpreted: they are due to OHC stiffness change.

If the cell is seen by the organ of Corti as a driven spring, then the dynamic force, from Hooke's law is:

$$df = K_L \frac{dL}{dt} + L \frac{dK_L}{dt} \tag{5}$$

where L is the cell length and K_L is the cell's axial stiffness (from Eq. 4). In the organ of Corti the cell is somewhat constrained and the organ sees both length and stiffness changes. It is thus possible that *in situ*, when the cell's motion is restrained by the organ of Corti matrix, cochlear amplification, or "electromotility" is a combined somatic length and stiffness change, affecting both resistive and reactive components of basilar membrane impedance[14]. We are now investigating such voltage-dependent stiffness of OHCs.

Acknowledgments

Supported by the National Institute of Deafness and Other Communication Disorders, NIH

References

1. Guinan, J.J., Jr. (1996) The physiology of olivocochlear efferents, in *Handbook of Auditory Research Vol. 8, The Cochlea* eds. P. Dallos, A.N. Popper and R.R. Fay. (Springer-Verlag, New York) in press
2. Kim, D.O. (1986) Active and nonlinear cochlear biomechanics and the role of outer-hair-cell subsystem in the mammalian auditory system, *Hearing Res.* **22**, 105–113.
3. Ashmore, J.F. (1992) Mammalian hearing and the cellular mechanisms of the cochlear amplifier, in *Sensory Transduction* Eds. D.P. Corey, S.D. Roper (Rockefeller University Press, New York) pp. 395412.
4. Schacht, J., Fessenden, J.D. and Zajic, G. (1995) Slow motility of outer hair cells, in *Active Hearing* eds. Å. Flock, D. Ottoson, M. Ulfendahl (Pergamon, London) pp. 209–220.
5. Elgoyhen, A.B., Johnson, D.S., Boulter, J., Vetter, D.E. and Heinemann, S. (1994) a9: An acetylcholine receptor with novel pharmacological properties expressed in rat cochlear hair cells, *Cell* **79** 705–715.
6. Santos-Sacchi, J. and Dilger, J.P. (1988) Whole cell currents and mechanical responses of isolated outer hair cells, *Hear. Res.* **35** 143–150.
7. Galambos, R. (1956) Suppression of auditory activity by stimulation of efferent fibers to the cochlea, *J. Neurophysiol.* **19** 424-437.
8. Sziklai, I. and Dallos, P. (1993) Acetylcholine controls the gain of the voltage-to-movement converter in isolated outer hair cells, *Acta Otolaryngol. Stockholm* **113** 326–329.
9. Dallos, P., Hallworth, R. and Evans, B.N. (1993) Theory of electrically-driven shape changes of cochlear outer hair cells, *J. Neurophysiol.* **70** 299–323.
10. Evans, B.N., Hallworth, R. and Dallos, P. (1991) Outer hair cell electromotility: The sensitivity and vulnerability of the DC component, *Hear. Res.* **52** 288–304.
11. Sziklai, I., He, D.Z.Z. and Dallos, P. (1996) Effect of acetylcholine and GABA on the transfer function of electromotility in isolated outer hair cells, *Hear. Res.* in press.
12. Bobbin, R.P., Fallon, M., Puel, J-L., Bryant, G., Bledsoe, S.C., Zajic, G. and Schacht, J. (1990) Acetylcholine, charbacol and GABA induce no detectable change in the length of isolated outer hair cells, *Hear. Res.* **47** 39–52.
13. Sridhar, T.S., Liberman, M.C., Brown, M.C. and Sewell, W.F. (1995) A novel cholinergic "slow effect" of efferent stimulation on cochlear potentials in the guinea pig, *J. Neurosci.* **15** 3667-3678.
14. Kolston, P.J., de Boer, E., Viergever, M.A. and Smoorenburg, G.F. (1990) What type of force does the cochlear amplifier produce? *J. Acoust. Soc. Amer.* **88** 1794–1801.
15. Allen, J.B. (1990) Modeling of the noise damaged cochlea, in *The Mechanics and Biophysics of Hearing* eds. P. Dallos, C.D. Geisler, J.W. Matthews, M.A. Ruggero and C.R. Steele (Springer-Verlag, New York) pp. 324-331 .

RESPONSE OF THE OUTER HAIR CELL TO PROLONGED HYPO-OSMOTIC PERFUSION

D.H. EHRENSTEIN, K.H. IWASA

Biophysics Section, NIDCD, NIH
Bethesda, MD 20892-0922
david-e@nih.gov

Outer Hair Cell (OHC) motility is strongly influenced by passive mechanical properties of the membrane. In previous theoretical work, the membrane was assumed to be purely elastic,[1] but we show here that it has some viscoelastic properties as well. We exposed isolated cells to a hypo-osmotic solution for varying durations and then punctured them, to immediately release the osmotic stress. Using video records of the cells, we determined both the imposed length strain and the strain after puncturing, when stress was reset to zero. The strain data were described by a simple rheological model consisting of two springs and a dashpot, and the fit to this model gave a time constant of 40 ± 19 s for the relaxation (reduction) of tension during prolonged strain. For time-scales much shorter or longer than this we would expect essentially elastic behavior. A further test with Ca-free perfusate showed that the viscoelasticity is not significantly affected by Ca. This relaxation process affects the membrane tension of the cell, and since it has been shown that membrane tension has a modulatory role in the OHC's motility, this relaxation process may be part of an adaptation mechanism, with which the motility system of the OHC can adjust to changing conditions and maintain optimum membrane tension.

1 Introduction

Outer hair cell (OHC) motility[2–5] is thought to be largely responsible for the exquisite sensitivity and tuning in mammalian hearing.[6,7] The motility mechanism is located at the plasma membrane[8–10] and is strongly influenced by membrane tension, as shown by measurements of the non-linear membrane capacitance.[11–13] Membrane tension is determined by both the motors themselves and by passive mechanical properties of the membrane, so the mechanical properties are important for the OHC's function.

The purpose of this study is to clarify the limits of the purely elastic treatment of the OHC that has been used in modeling. We found that the cell membrane (including the plasma membrane together with the underlying cytoskeleton) is viscoelastic,[14–17] although the elastic approximation is valid for time-scales much longer or shorter than the time-constant for viscoelastic relaxation. We determined the time dependence of membrane tension in response to an applied strain by measuring strain immediately after stress was released. This *release strain* was a probe of the stress that existed before the release. We used hypo-osmotic perfusion as the means of applying measurable strains to the cell, and puncturing it was our method of releasing osmotic stress. We found the characteristic time for viscoelastic changes in the cell membrane to be about 40 s.

2   Results

When perfused with the hypo-osmotic medium, cells swelled, decreasing in length and increasing in diameter simultaneously. Figure 1 shows strain kinetics with an exponential fit for a typical cell.

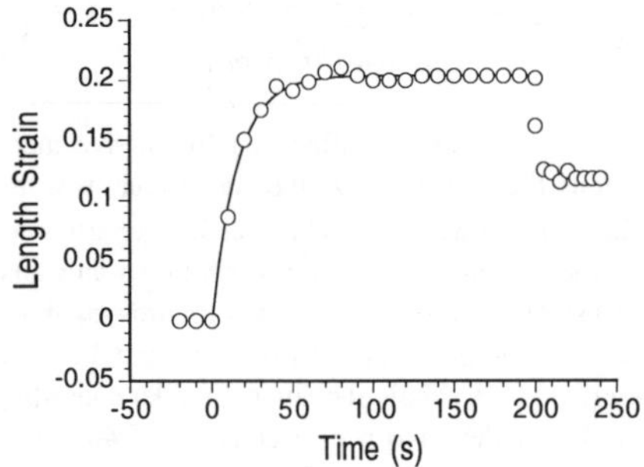

Figure 1: Strain kinetics. Curve is an exponential fit (eq. 3). Length strain was defined as fractional length change, $(L_0 - L)/L_0$, where L is the length at any time, and the reference length L_0 is taken before perfusion. Perfusion starts at $t = 0$, and the pressure is released by puncturing the cell membrane after 198 s (the *perfusion time* in this case). For this cell the release strain is 0.11, and the time constant for swelling is 16 s. A non-zero release strain indicates that the system has non-elastic components, so it must be described with a viscoelastic theory. **Conditions** Perfusion medium osmolarity 165 mOs/kg; standard bathing medium osmolarity 305 mOs/kg. Osmotic pressure was released using a patch pipette to puncture the cell with a short pulse of suction.

Making a small hole in the cell membrane releases the pressure and causes an immediate elongation, which is completed within about 10 s, followed by a much slower elongation. Since this slower recovery may take place with the cell interior exposed to the bathing medium, we did not study it closely, except to note that it is slow and clearly distinguished from the fast recovery. (Only the fast recovery phase is shown in Figure 1.)

If the perfusion time was sufficiently short (compared with 40 s), the fast recovery after pressure release brought cells close to their pre-perfusion lengths. In other words, the release strain was small. This behavior is consistent with pure elasticity. If the perfusion time was longer than 3 min, cells recovered only slightly from their pre-release strains. This larger release strain after a long perfusion time is a manifestation of membrane viscoelasticity; it implies that membrane tension relaxed during perfusion.

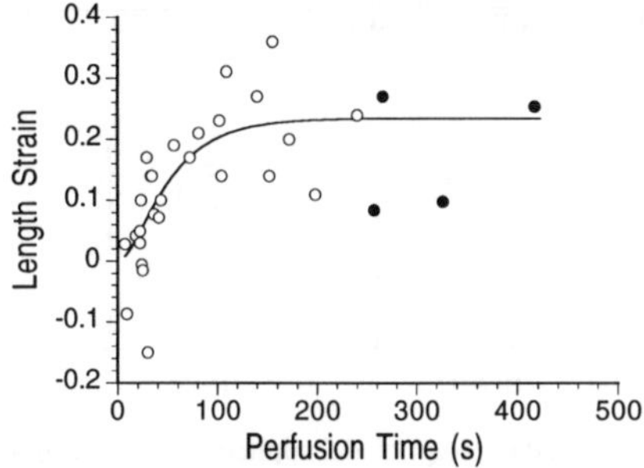

Figure 2: Release strain. The release strain is the strain after pressure release and is plotted against perfusion time for each cell. Filled circles represent cells perfused with a Ca-free medium, while the rest of the cells were perfused with a hypo-osmotic medium containing a normal Ca concentration (1.5 mM). These data are fit to eq. 7 holding ε_z^0 and τ_0 fixed at 0.35 and 16 s, respectively (determined from kinetics data). The curve shows the two-parameter fit, which yields $\tau = 40 \pm 19$ s and $p = 0.5 \pm 0.2$.

To examine the possible involvement of Ca with the viscoelasticity, we perfused some cells with a Ca-free medium. Ca may have important effects on cytoskeletal elements and may be involved in the osmotic response of OHC's.[18] We found no significant effect of the Ca-free perfusion medium (Figure 2).

The release strains for the cells examined are plotted against perfusion time in Figure 2. Although there is some scatter in the data, showing the variability among cells, the plot shows that the release strain is significant for cells with perfusion times longer than 40 s.

3 Theory

We assume the cell to be cylindrical and that the shape of the cell is supported by the lateral membrane (including cytoskeleton). As in the previous analyses, this system can be described with the axial strain, ε_z, circumferential strain, ε_c, axial tension σ_z, and circumferential tension σ_c.[19,20] We use the terms "membrane tension" and "membrane stress" interchangeably. The area strain ε_a, shear strain ε_s, area stress σ_a, and shear stress σ_s are defined by these equations:

$$\begin{cases} \varepsilon_a = \varepsilon_z + \varepsilon_c \\ \varepsilon_s = \varepsilon_z - \varepsilon_c \end{cases} \qquad \begin{cases} \sigma_a = \tfrac{1}{2}\left(\sigma_z + \sigma_c\right) \\ \sigma_s = \tfrac{1}{2}\left(\sigma_z - \sigma_c\right) \end{cases} \tag{1}$$

A general two-dimensional strain has components of both area strain and shear strain.[14] With these variables, the membrane elasticity equations are

$$\begin{cases} \sigma_a = K\varepsilon_a \\ \sigma_s = \mu\varepsilon_s \end{cases},$$

512

where K is the area modulus, and μ is the shear modulus.

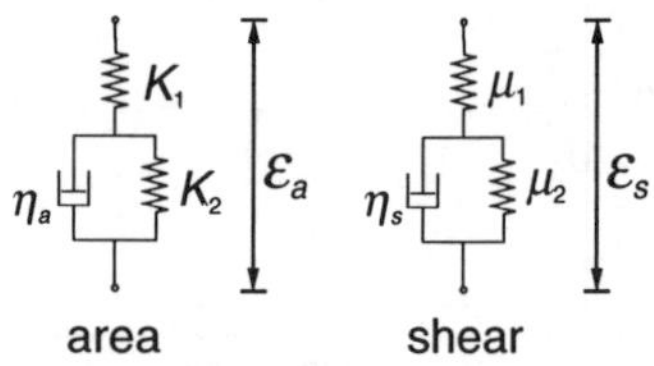

Figure 3: Three-parameter Voigt model applied to a viscoelastic membrane.

A simple consideration of the force balance between the pressure and tensions for a cylinder leads to this equation for the lateral membrane:[19]

$$\sigma_s = -(1/3)\sigma_a \tag{2}$$

In our experiments, the length strain was well described by an exponential time dependence (Figure 1), and we assume the same time dependence applies to the volume strain (the direct result of osmotic stress), and therefore area and shear strains as well (we only show the area component, but the shear strain is analogous):

$$\varepsilon_a(t) = \varepsilon_a^0 (1 - e^{-t/\tau_0}), \quad \text{for } t \geq 0. \tag{3}$$

The simplest viscoelastic model which is consistent with our observations is a series connection of a spring and Voigt element (Figure 3), called a *three-parameter Voigt model* by Tschoegl.[15,21] Using the fundamental equations for springs and dashpots, and the schematic of Figure 3, we derive this differential equation for area stress and strain (an analogous one applies to shear stress and strain):

$$\frac{d\sigma_a}{dt} + \frac{K_1 + K_2}{\eta_a}\sigma_a = K_1 \frac{d\varepsilon_a}{dt} + \frac{K_1 K_2}{\eta_a}\varepsilon_a . \tag{4}$$

Using eqs. 3 and 4 (along with the analogous shear equations) and the initial conditions $\sigma_a(0) = \sigma_s(0) = 0$, we solve for the stresses, $\sigma_a(t)$ and $\sigma_s(t)$. Putting these results together with eq. 2 we find relationships between several parameters for the two directions, with this resulting area stress (shear stress is analogous):

$$\sigma_a(t) = K_1 \varepsilon_a^0 \left[1 - e^{-t/\tau_0} - \frac{1}{1+p}\left(1 - \frac{\tau}{\tau - \tau_0}e^{-t/\tau} + \frac{\tau_0}{\tau - \tau_0}e^{-t/\tau_0}\right)\right],$$

$$\text{where } \tau = \frac{\eta_a}{K_1 + K_2} = \frac{\eta_s}{\mu_1 + \mu_2}, \quad p = \frac{K_2}{K_1} = \frac{\mu_2}{\mu_1}, \quad \text{and } \varepsilon_s^0 = -\frac{K_1}{3\mu_1}\varepsilon_a^0. \tag{5}$$

Eq. 5, which is plotted in Figure 4, shows the relaxation of tension resulting from prolonged strain and represents the main affect our experiments were designed to measure.

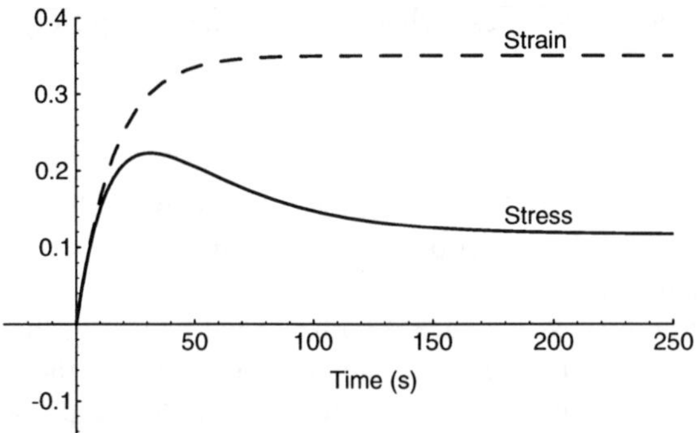

Figure 4: Calculated stress (see eq. 5). The stress relaxation $\sigma_a(t)/K_1$ determined from the fit in Figure 2 (scaled so that $\varepsilon_a^0 = \varepsilon_z^0$,). The dashed line is the typical (axial) strain applied. At short times, where the curves overlap, a purely elastic description is reasonable.

If the stresses maintaining the strains are released and reset to zero at time t_r, the strains due to the pure spring elements instantly return to zero, leaving the Voigt elements unchanged. The axial release strain ε_{zr} then consists only of the Voigt elements' strain (transformed to the axial direction) immediately before the release:

$$\varepsilon_{zr}(t_r) = \frac{1}{2}\left(\varepsilon_a(t_r) + \varepsilon_s(t_r) - \frac{\sigma_a(t_r)}{K_1} - \frac{\sigma_s(t_r)}{\mu_1} \right) . \tag{6}$$

Using eqs. 1, 3, and 5 (and their shear counterparts) in eq. 6 we obtain the axial release strain:

$$\varepsilon_{zr}(t_r) = \frac{\varepsilon_z^0}{1+p}\left(1 - \frac{\tau}{\tau - \tau_0} e^{-t_r/\tau} + \frac{\tau_0}{\tau - \tau_0} e^{-t_r/\tau_0} \right) . \tag{7}$$

We present the release strain in eq. 7 as a function of t_r, rather than t, because it only applies at a single time to a given cell. For the fit in Figure 2, perfusion time was used for t_r.

Two assumptions upon which the analysis relies are that the cell is cylindrical and that the strains are small enough that linearized elasticity theory applies. A test of the former assumption is a rough calculation of the typical volume strain of our cells, which agrees closely with the swelling expected based on the osmolarity of our perfusion medium. The latter assumption is justified because an earlier study,[19] in which brief pressure stresses were applied under voltage clamp, did not show a systematic deviation from linearity up to the range used in this study.

The linearity of the stress-strain relationship also suggests that the osmotic stresses were not large enough to cause irreversible damage. Further evidence comes from our observation that cells re-exposed to the regular saline after hypo-osmotic

514

perfusion for up to ten minutes (without puncturing) completely returned to their original lengths.

4   Conclusions

We have shown that the OHC membrane has a viscoelastic relaxation time of about 40 s. Therefore, theoretical descriptions of fast OHC motility may safely assume a purely elastic membrane.

The relaxation process we have described could be one of the mechanisms by which the cell adjusts to slowly changing conditions in the cochlea, such as fluctuations in osmolarity. The relaxation tends to keep membrane tension relatively constant and could prevent external factors from interfering with the cell's ability to generate force.

References

1. Iwasa, K.H. (1994) A membrane model for the fast motility of the outer hair cell, *J. Acoust. Soc. Am.* **96** 2216–2224.
2. Brownell, W., Bader, C., Bertrand, D. and Ribaupierre, Y. (1985) Evoked mechanical responses of isolated outer hair cells, *Science* **227** 194–196.
3. Ashmore, J.F. (1987) A fast motile response in guinea-pig outer hair cells: the molecular basis of the cochlear amplifier, *J. Physiol. (Lond.)* **388** 323–347.
4. Santos-Sacchi, J. and Dilger, J.P. (1988) Whole cell currents and mechanical responses of isolated outer hair cells, *Hearing Res.* **35** 143–150.
5. Iwasa, K. and Kachar, B. (1989) Fast *in vitro* movement of outer hair cells in an external electric field: effect of digitonin, a membrane permeabilzing agent, *Hearing Res.* **40** 247–254.
6. Lieberman, M.C. and Dodds, L.W. (1984) Single neuron labeling and chronic cochlear pathology. III. Stereocilia damage and alterations of threshold tuning curves., *Hear. Res.* **16** 55–74.
7. De Boer, E. (1991) Auditory physics. Physical principles in hearing theory III, *Phys. Rep.* **203** 125–231.
8. Dallos, P., Evans, B.N. and Hallworth, R. (1991) Nature of the motor element in electrokinetic shape changes of cochlear outer hair cells, *Nature* **350** 155–157.
9. Kalinec, F., Holley, M.C., Iwasa, K., Lim, D. and Kachar, B. (1992) A membrane-based force generation mechanism in auditory sensory cells, *Proc. Natl. Acad. Sci. USA* **89** 8671–8675.

10. Huang, G. and Santos-Sacchi, J. (1993) Mapping the distribution of the outer hair cell motility voltage sensor by electrical amputation, *Biophys. J.* **65** 2228–2236.

11. Iwasa, K. (1993) Effect of stress on the membrane capacitance of the auditory outer hair cell, *Biophys. J.* **65** 492-498.

12. Gale, J.E. and Ashmore, J.F. (1995) Non-linear capacitance in isolated patches of the lateral membrane of cochlear outer hair cells, *Biophys. J.* **68** A392.

13. Kakehata, S. and Santos-Sacchi, J. (1995) Membrane tension directly shifts voltage dependence of outer hair cell motility and associated gating charge, *Biophys. J.* **68** 2190–2197.

14. Evans, E.A. and Skalak, R. (1980) *Mechanics and thermodynamics of biomembranes* (CRC Press, Baca Raton, FL).

15. Poznanski, J., Pawlowski, P. and Fikus, M. (1992) Bioelectrorheological model of the cell. 3. Viscoelastic shear deformation of the membrane, *Biophys. J.* **61** 612–620.

16. Sung, K.-L.P. and Chien, S. (1992) Influence of temperature on rheology of human erythrocytes, *Chinese J. Physiol.* **35** 81–94.

17. Hochmuth, R.M. (1993) Measuring the mechanical properties of individual human blood cells, *J. Biochem. Eng.* **115** 515–519.

18. Harada, N., Ernst, A. and Zenner, H.P. (1994) Intracellular calcium changes by hyposmotic activation of cochlear outer hair cells in the guinea pig, *Acta Otolaryngol.* (Stockh) **114** 510–515.

19. Iwasa, K. and Chadwick, R. (1992) Elasticity and active force generation of cochlear outer hair cells, *J. Acoust. Soc. Am* **92** 3169–3173.

20. Iwasa, K.H. and Chadwick, R.S. (1993) Factors influencing the length change of an auditory hair cell in a tight-fitting capillary, *J. Acoust. Soc. Am.* **94** 1156–1159.

21. Tschoegl, N.W. (1989) *The Phenomenological Theory of Linear Viscoelastic Behavior* (Springer-Verlag, Berlin).

MECHANICALLY AND ATP-INDUCED CURRENTS OF MOUSE OUTER HAIR CELLS ARE ADDITIVE AND BLOCKED BY D-TUBOCURARINE

E. GLOWATZKI*, A. RÜSCH[#], J.P. RUPPERSBERG* & R.A. EATOCK[#]

* Univ. of Tübingen, Dept. of Sensory Biophysics, Röntgenweg 11
72076 Tübingen, Germany
Elisabeth.Glowatzki@uni-tuebingen.de
[#] Dept. of Otolaryngology and Communicative Sciences
Baylor College of Medicine, Houston, TX 77030, USA

Two recent observations have let to speculations that ATP-receptors might be related to mechano-electrical transducer (MET) channels of hair cells:

(1) Brändle et al.[1] found a cloned P_{2X}-ATP receptor[2] in cochlear hair cells, and (2) Housley et al.[3] localized ATP-induced inward currents to the apical cell pole. To test for a possible identity, we looked for any interference of mechanically and ATP-induced currents in outer hair cells of the cultured mouse cochlea.

Using standard solutions[4], we voltage clamped outer hair cells at -84 mV in whole cell mode. Hair bundles were stimulated by a fluid jet every 500 ms in bursts of 10 cycles of a 60 Hz sine wave. Transducer currents of up to 500 pA were elicited (n = 9). Saturating transducer currents could reversibly be blocked (about 95 %) by application of 100 µM d-tubocurarine (n = 2).

In 9 cells, 100 µM ATP elicited inward currents between 20 and 400 pA. 100 µM d-tubocurarine reversibly suppressed the ATP-induced currents by 50 % (n = 3).

When 100-300 µM ATP was applied during saturating mechanical stimulation in three hair cells, transducer currents and ATP-activated currents were additive. In two cases no interference of both currents with each other was observed, in one case the transducer current was irreversibly reduced by about 10 %. This finding is inconsistent with the view that MET channels and ATP-activated channels are identical, but it suggests that they form two distinct channel populations in hair cells.

References

1. Brändle, T.U., Glowatzki, E., Wild, K., Zenner, H.P. and Ruppersberg, J.P. (1995) Expression of P_{2X}-receptor sequences in different cell populations of the organ of Corti: detected by single-cell RT-PCR, *Mol. Biol. of Hearing and Deafness, abstract* **168**.
2. Brake, A.J., Wagenbach, M.J. and Julius, D. (1994) New structural motif for ligand-gated ion channels defined by an ionotropic ATP receptor, *Nature* **371** 519-523. 3.
3. Housley, G.D., Greenwood, D. and Ashmore, J.F. (1992) Localization of cholinergic and purinergic receptors on outer hair cells isolated from guinea pig cochlea, *Proc. R. Soc. Lond. B* **249** 265-273.
4. Kros, C.J., Rüsch, A. and Richardson, G.P. (1992) Mechano-electrical transducer currents in hair cells of the cultured mouse cochlea, *Proc. R. Soc. Lond. B* **249** 185-193.

STEREOCILIARY ULTRASTRUCTURE IN RELATION TO MECHANOTRANSDUCTION: TIP LINKS AND THE CONTACT REGION

C.M. HACKNEY, D.N. FURNESS, Y. KATORI

Department of Communication and Neuroscience, Keele University
Keele, Staffs. ST5 5BG
c.m.hackney@keele.ac.uk

Recent immunocytochemical experiments have suggested that the mechanotransduction channels in hair cells may be located in a contact region between the stereocilia rather than being directly associated with the tip link. Ultrastructural studies have shown that this region contains pillar-like structures which detergent extraction reveals as connecting the actin cores of the adjacent stereocilia via transmembrane domains. The tip links and their attachment sites also survive detergent extraction, indicating that they too are connected to the cytoskeleton. The upper insertional plaque of the tip link contains a regular array of ring-like subunits suggestive of anchoring or motor proteins. These results indicate that there are structures in the contact region which could operate transduction channels. If this is the case, the tip link could be acting along with the lateral linkages to maintain the precise position of the stereocilia in relation to each other, or to adjust it via tension changes induced by movements of the upper insertional plaque as suggested previously.

1 Introduction

Hair cells respond to displacements of their apical bundle of stereocilia by becoming depolarised during deflections towards the tallest row and hyperpolarized during deflections in the opposite direction. This is thought to be the result of the direct operation of mechanoelectrical transduction channels by a 'gating spring'.[1] One candidate for the gating spring is the tip link which connects the tip of each shorter stereocilium to the sides of the taller stereocilium in the row behind.[2] According to the tip link hypothesis, deflections towards the taller stereocilia would stretch the tip link, resulting in an increased probability of opening of channels located at one or both ends of the link, whilst deflections in the opposite direction would reduce tension and decrease channel opening (see e.g.[3]). During sustained displacements of the bundle, the initial transduction current produced slowly declines.[4] This adaptation has been attributed to a reduction in tension in the tip link based on slippage[4,5] of the electron-dense plaque found at its upper end[6] along the actin filaments of the stereociliary core. It has been suggested that this plaque contains myosin which, by climbing the actin core, increases the tension on the link and resets the operating point (see e.g.[7]).

Recent immunocytochemical experiments aimed at localising the transduction channels are not, however, in full accord with the tip-link hypothesis. The fact that transduction channels are amiloride-sensitive led to polyclonal antibodies to the epithelial Na+ channel from kidney, another amiloride-sensitive channel, being used in an attempt to localise them. Labelling with these antibodies is not directly associated with the tip link but occurs predominantly in a region below the tips of shorter stereocilia where the membranes of adjacent stereocilia appear to be very closely apposed.8 This labelling has been shown to be associated with an amiloride-binding site by experiments which used amiloride to prevent destruction of such sites by trypsin, and is also reduced by the aminoglycoside antibiotic dihydrostreptomycin which is a potent blocker of the transduction channels.9

Preliminary ultrastructural examination has revealed a junction-like structure in the region of apposition between the stereocilia.8 The ultrastructure of the interstereociliary connections in this contact region and their relationship to the stereociliary cytoskeleton has therefore been investigated further using electron microscopy of both conventionally prepared and detergent-extracted tissue. The connection of the tip link to the electron-dense plaque has also been examined. Understanding these structures better may help distinguish the different functions of the components of the transduction apparatus.

2   Materials and Methods

2.1 Preparation for scanning and transmission electron microscopy

For fixation for both scanning (SEM) and transmission electron microscopy (TEM), guinea-pig cochleas and utricles were perfused with, and immersed for 2 h in, 2.5% glutaraldehyde in 0.1 M sodium cacodylate buffer containing 2 mM calcium chloride then postfixed for 1 h in 1% osmium tetroxide in the same buffer. To enhance membrane features, some cochleas were fixed in glutaraldehyde containing 1% tannic acid.

The OTOTO technique was used for SEM.10 Cochleas were dissected into segments and incubated alternately in saturated aqueous thiocarbohydrazide solution followed by thorough washing in distilled water and immersion in 1% osmium tetroxide. This procedure was repeated and the segments were then washed, dehydrated, critical-point dried and mounted on specimen stubs for examination in a Hitachi S-4500 field emission scanning electron microscope at 5 kV.

For TEM, cochleas were either left whole or dissected into segments, dehydrated and embedded in Durcupan resin. Some utricles were also embedded for comparative ultrastructural studies. Ultrathin radial sections were cut, stained with uranyl acetate and lead citrate and examined in a JEOL 100 CX transmission electron microscope.

2.2 Detergent extraction of stereocilia

Detergent extraction was performed either before or during a preliminary fixation, using Triton-X 100 at concentrations of 0.1% to 2.5%. Cochleas were either pre-incubated for 10 min in HEPES-buffered salt solution containing detergent or fixed in 4% paraformaldehyde in 0.1 M phosphate buffer containing detergent, and subsequently fixed in glutaraldehyde and osmium tetroxide as described above.

3   Results

3.1   Ultrastructure of the contact region

With conventional preparation for TEM, pillar-like connections can be observed between the membranes in the contact region (Fig. 1a).

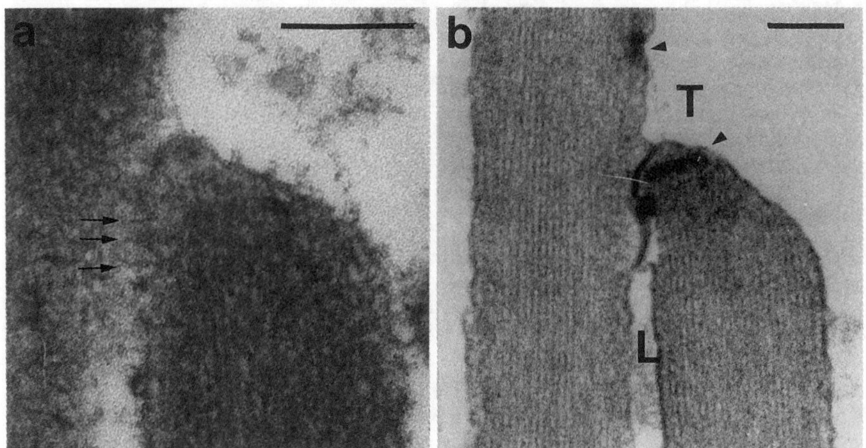

Figure 1: (a) Transmission electron micrograph of utricular stereocilia showing pillar-like connections in the contact region (arrows). (b) Transmission electron micrograph of the contact region in a cochlear hair cell following tannic acid preparation. Note the closely apposed, densely stained membranes. Lateral links (L) are also visible below the contact region, along with the tip link (T) and the dense material associated with its upper and lower insertions (arrowheads). Scale bars = 100 nm.

When tannic acid is included in the fixatives, the membranes appear denser and are specifically enhanced in the contact region. The membranes of the adjacent stereocilia appear to be almost fused, and shrinkage during the preparation procedure causes them to pull away from the actin core above and below these regions in a manner which suggests a strong coupling between the membranes. Dense material is also found associated with the region of contact (Fig. 1b).

3.2   Effects of detergent extraction on the contact region

In the contact region, pillar-like structures are retained following extraction with detergent indicating that they are attached to the actin cores (Fig. 2a, b). Electron-dense material associated with the contact region is also still present (Fig. 2b).

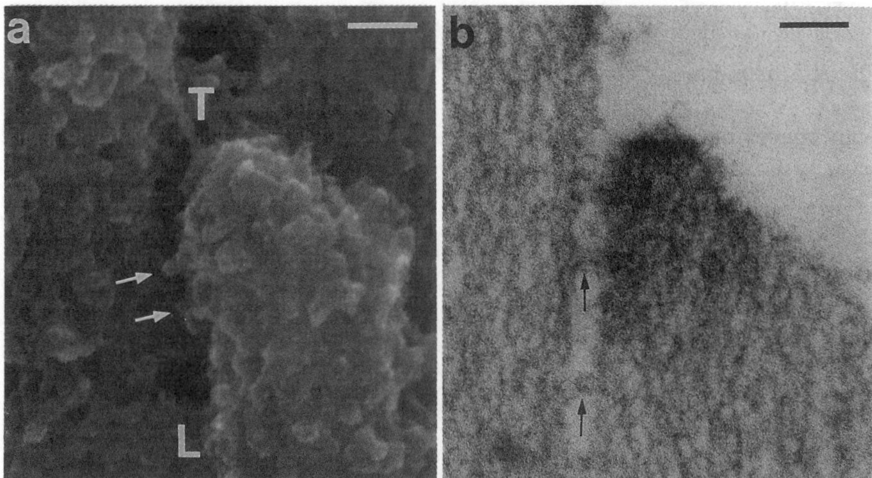

Figure 2: (a) Scanning and (b) transmission electron micrographs of detergent-extracted cochlear hair-cell stereocilia. Pillar-like structures (arrows), lateral links (L) and tip links (T) all survive treatment with 2.5% Triton-X 100 during fixation. Scale bars = 50 nm.

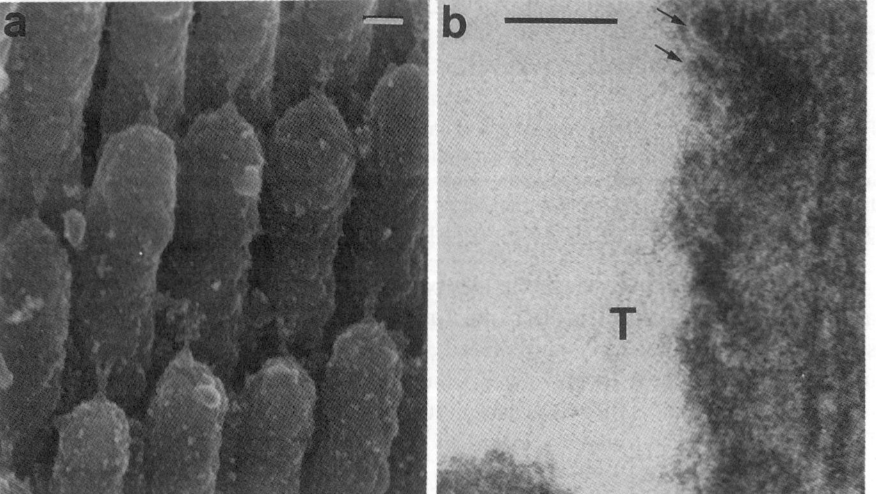

Figure 3: (a) Scanning electron micrograph of stereocilia after mild detergent treatment which does not produce substantial removal of the membrane. The majority of the tip links can be seen to branch to form two strands attaching to the taller stereocilium. (b) Transmission electron micrograph of a tip link (T) and its attachment points. Note the rows of ring-like subunits in the upper insertional plaque (arrows). Scale bars = 50 nm.

3.3 Ultrastructure of the tip link and its upper insertional plaque

The tip links usually consist of apparently one strand near their lower attachment point and two or more near their upper attachments (Fig. 3a). The branch point varies in its position usually occurring at least half way along the length or closer to the upper attachment. In TEM the upper insertional plaque can be seen to contain a regular array of 10 nm diameter, ring-like subunits (Fig. 3b).

3.4 Effects of detergent extraction on the tip link and insertional plaque

Following sufficient treatment with detergent to expose the actin cores, tip links and both their upper insertional plaques and lower attachments are still present (Fig. 4b).

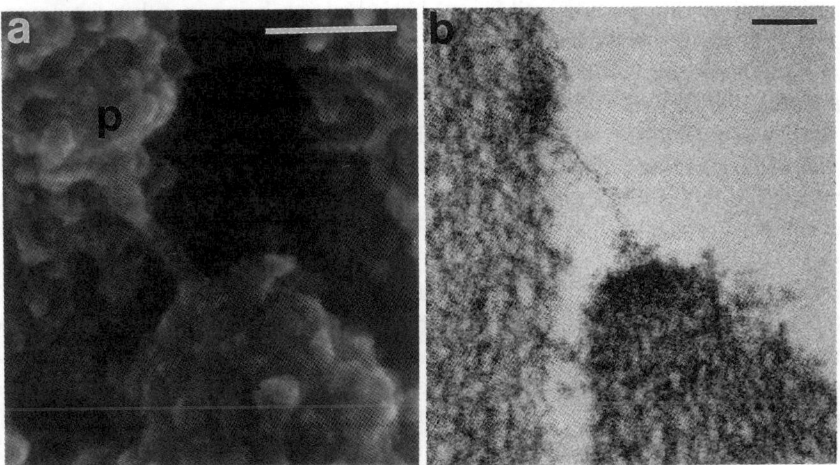

Figure 4: (a) Scanning electron micrograph of stereocilia following treatment with Triton-X 100 during fixation showing the presence of a tip link and its upper insertional plaque (P). (b) Transmission electron micrograph of detergent-treated stereocilia. The link appears to separate into strands at both ends where it inserts into dense material on the actin core. Scale bars = 50 nm.

4 Discussion

The pillars and electron-dense material in the contact region indicate that it is a specific structure rather than just a close approach of adjacent membranes. Coupled with the immunolabelling for amiloride-sensitive channels in the contact region, these findings may suggest that this region is involved in mechanotransduction.

Because the pillars survive detergent extraction, it appears that they are connected to the cytoskeleton and that they have transmembrane domains. The linkage to the cytoskeleton may represent mechanical ties which fix the transduction channels in place, whilst the extracellular domains could represent the 'gating springs'.1 Shear displacements parallel with the lateral wall of the stereocilia could then operate the channels via these structures, although the mode of operation would have to be assymetric to achieve the polarity of the hair-cell response.

A recent kinematic analysis of relative movement of stereocilia during deflections in the physiological range has shown that the amount of shear displacement in the contact region would be as great or greater than the predicted elongation of the tip link.11 This suggests that the contact region is as plausible a location for the channels as the tip link insertions. Moreover, the results of all the physiological experiments to date which have suggested that the channels are near the stereociliary tips are compatible with their location being in either the contact region or at the tip-link insertions (see12). Unfortunately, even the latest calcium imaging experiments have not had the resolution to distinguish between the two sites.13,14

Like the pillars in the contact region, the tip link and electron-dense plaque also survive detergent extraction. Hence the link appears to have transmembraneous domains connecting it to the actin core at the upper end via the insertional plaque. The subunits of the plaque may represent adhesion or anchoring proteins; this suggests the possibility that the tip link acts to maintain the apposition of the stereocilia in the contact region. The lateral links may perform a similar function.12 In this model, it is still possible that the subunits of the plaque could represent some form of motor protein, such as myosin, through which tension on the link could be modulated to adjust the position of the stereocilia during transduction as has been suggested previously.4,5,7

Alternatively, if the immunolabelling is revealing some other form of channel, and not transduction channels, then the latter could in fact be associated with the tip-link insertions. Indeed, the ring-like subunits of the electron-dense plaque could themselves represent channels. If this is so, the converse arrangement to that suggested above may be the case, i.e., the contact region may help to couple the stereocilia together to prevent excessive movements from breaking the tip links.

Acknowledgements

This work has been supported by grants from the Wellcome Trust and Hearing Research Trust. YK is supported by a bursary from Tohoku University, Sendai, by kind arrangment of Prof. T. Takasaka.

References

1. Corey, D.P. and Hudspeth, A.J. (1983) Kinetics of the receptor current in bullfrog saccular hair cells, *J. Neurosci.* **3** 962-976.
2. Pickles, J.O., Comis, S.D. and Osborne, M.P. (1984) Cross-links between stereocilia in the guinea-pig organ of Corti, and their possible relation to sensory transduction, *Hear. Res.* **15** 103-112.
3. Pickles, J.O. and Corey, D.P. (1992) Mechanoelectrical transduction by hair cells, *TINS* **15** 254-259.
4. Howard, J. and Hudspeth, A.J. (1987) Mechanical relaxation of the hair bundle mediates adaptation in mechanoelectrical transduction by the bullfrog's saccular hair cell, *Proc. Natl. Acad. Sci. USA* **84** 3064-3068.
5. Assad, J.A. and Corey, D.P. (1992) An active motor model for adaptation by vertebrate hair cells, *J. Neurosci.* **12** 3291-3309.
6. Furness, D.N. and Hackney, C.M. (1985) Cross-links between stereocilia in the guinea-pig cochlea, *Hear. Res.* **18** 177-188.
7. Jaramillo, F. (1995) Signal transduction in hair cells and its regulation by calcium, *Neuron* **15** 1227-1230.
8. Hackney, C.M., Furness, D.N., Benos, D.J., Woodley, J.F. and Barratt, J. (1992) Putative immunolocalization of the mechanoelectrical transduction channels in mammalian cochlear hair cells, *Proc. R. Soc. Lond. B.* **248** 215-221.
9. Furness, D.N. Hackney, C.M. and Benos, D.J. (1995) The binding site on cochlear stereocilia for antisera raised against renal Na+ channels is blocked by amiloride and dihydrostreptomycin, *Hear. Res.* **93** 155-165.
10. Furness, D.N. and Hackney, C.M. (1986) High resolution scanning electron microscopy of stereocilia using the osmium-thiocarbohydrazide coating technique, *Hear. Res.* **21** 243-249.
11. Zetes, D.E. (1995) Mechanical and morphological study of the stereocilia bundle in the mammalian auditory system. Ph.D thesis, Department of Mechanical Engineering, University of Stanford.
12. Hackney, C.M. and Furness, D.N. (1995) Mechanotransduction in vertebrate hair cells: structure and function of the stereociliary bundle, *Am. J. Physiol.* **268** C1-C13.
13. Denk, W., Holt, J.R., Shepherd, G.M.G and Corey, D.P. (1995) Calcium imaging of single stereocilia in hair cells: localization of transduction channels at both ends of tip links, *Neuron* **15** 1311-1321.
14. Lumpkin, E.A. and Hudspeth, A.J. (1995). Detection of Ca2+ entry through mechanosensitive channels localizes the site of mechanoelectrical transduction in hair cells, *Proc. Natl. Acad. Sci. USA* **92** 10297-10301.

OUTER HAIR CELL STIFFNESS AND FORCE AND THEIR MODULATION BY AGENTS KNOWN TO AFFECT HEARING

R. HALLWORTH

Department of Otolaryngology, U.T.H.S.C.S.A., 7703
Floyd Curl Drive, San Antonio, Texas 78284
hallworth@uthscsa.edu

Outer hair cells are imperfect generators of length change, that is, their length change due to electrical stimulation is reduced when cell deformation is opposed by a load. The length change generated by outer hair cell motility *in vivo* depends on both the stiffness of the organ of Corti at that location and the cell's internal stiffness. In consequence, outer hair cell motility may be affected directly, by action on the motility motor, or indirectly, by changing the cell's mechanical properties. Examples of experimental manipulations that illustrate both types of action are given.

1   Introduction

If the role of outer hair cell (OHC) motility in cochlear function is unknown, it is at least in part because the capabilities of the outer hair cell under load, as must be the case *in vivo*, are also unknown. The first direct measurements of forces generated by OHCs have been published recently[1-3]. In these studies, the mechanical properties of, and force generation by, isolated outer hair cells have been studied using a glass fiber as a test load. Here I introduce some new results and extend the concepts introduced in one of those initial publications. In addition, I discuss the effects of modulating agents on OHC mechanical properties.

2   Methods

The methods used in these experiments were as described elsewhere[1-2]. In brief, isolated OHCs from albino guinea pigs, immersed in L-15 medium, were held by a suction pipette at their basal (synaptic) poles. Calibrated glass fibers (stiffness 0.3-3.0 mN/m) were apposed orthogonally to the cell's apex. The fibers were mounted on a piezoelectic driver such that the fiber could be deflected in the direction of the cell's long axis. Fiber motion was detected by a photodiode system. Motion signals were averaged by computer and calibrated using an optical lever method[4]. Motility was evoked by voltage commands applied to the suction pipette.

Cell compliance was measured by observing the difference in the motion of the fiber tip relative to the fiber base when the base was moved in the compression direction. Force was computed from the fiber tip motion evoked by voltage commands delivered to the cell, knowing the fiber stiffness. Perfusion experiments were performed by washing in modified solutions.

3 Results

3.1 Force Generation Increases with Increasing Load

That the *in vitro* OHC is not a perfect extension generator, but is significantly affected by applied load, is demonstrated by the following experiment (Figure 1). An OHC, stimulated by a sinusoidal voltage command, was first positioned at the fiber tip, and then at several locations closer to the fiber base, thus increasing the load stiffness. Figure 1B shows that the effect of increased fiber stiffness is a reduction of fiber motion amplitude. The length change of the unloaded cell is included in Figure 1B for comparison.

The effect of load stiffness on OHC motility suggests that the cell has an internal stiffness that must be taken into account when computing the cell extension under load. A model of the OHC as an inelastic voltage-dependent extension generator (unloaded length change β) in series with an internal stiffness is shown in the figure. The equations governing cell extension and force generation are also given in Figure 2A. Simulations of the effects of increasing load stiffness k on length change and force for constant internal stiffness k', and for constant load stiffness when internal stiffness is varied, are depicted in Figure 2B. Note that, for constant internal stiffness, the extension declines to zero with increasing load, but the force increases to an asymptotic limit, the isometric force F_∞. The extension falls precipitously as the external load is increased from zero, so much so that, when the external load k equals the internal stiffness k', the extension is only one half the unloaded extension (and the force is one half the isometric force). When the internal

Figure 1: A) Method of applying increasing load stiffness to outer hair cells. B) Effect of increasing stiffness on fiber tip motion. The voltage command was a 120 mV peak sinusoid. The estimated load stiffness is shown on each waveform.

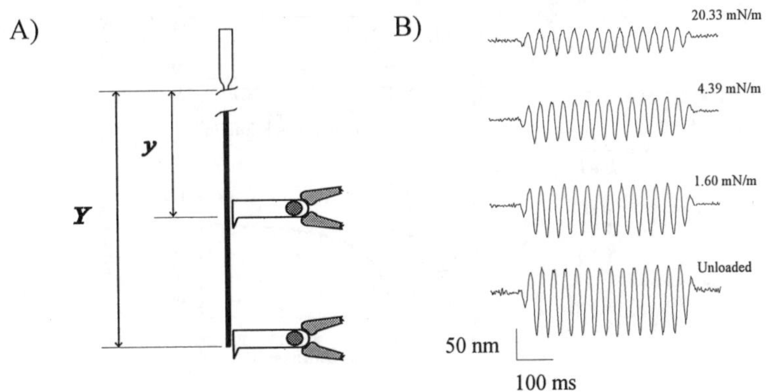

526

stiffness is varied with the load stiffness constant, the cell extension and the force both increase to asymptotic limits of β and $k\beta$, respectively.

3.2 Compliance and Force Generation are Increasing Functions of Cell Length

Given that the internal stiffness of OHCs may have a substantial influence on the ability of the OHC to generate length change *in vivo*, it is reasonable to ask how much the internal stiffness may change with cochlear position (and therefore cell length). Figure 3A shows the compliances of a series of 81 cells. As previously observed[1-3], the compliance increases with cell length. The longest cells are 4-6 times more compliant than the shortest cells. This suggests that OHCs may be made of a material of uniform specific compliance, consistent with the uniform diameters and appearance of OHCs[5]. The force for sinusoidal voltage commands was measured and the force per mV of voltage at the cell membrane was estimated for the same cells, and is plotted (for a narrow range of fibers stiffnesses) in Figure 3B. The force per mV was also an increasing function of cell length.

Assuming axial stiffness to be a measure of internal stiffness[3] then, using the relationships specified above, the unloaded extension β and the isometric force F_∞ can be estimated for the cells in Figure 3A. The results are shown in Figure 3C and D. β is an increasing function of length, that is, unloaded long cells generate more

Figure 2: A) Model of the OHC as an ideal inelastic extension generator with an internal spring. Formulae are given for extension, force and isometric force B) Simulation of the effects on extension and force generation of increasing load stiffness k for constant internal stiffness k' (β=50, k'=2) C) Simulation of the effects on extension and force generation of increasing internal stiffness k' for constant load (β=50, k=2).

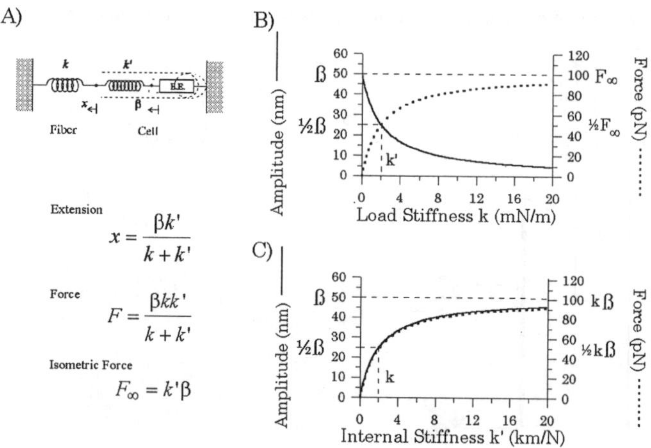

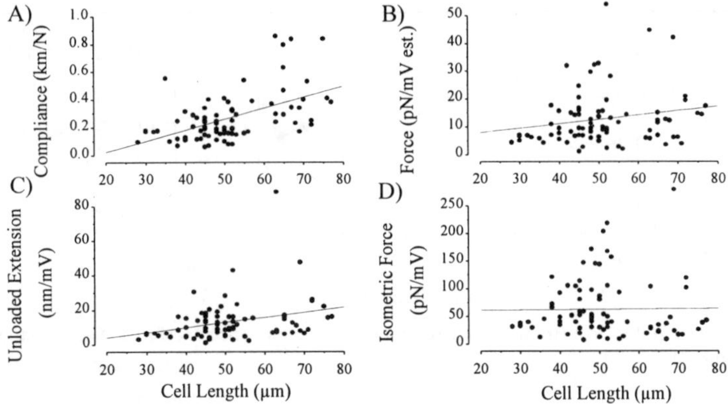

Figure 3: A) Compliance as a function of cell length for 81 cells. B) Calculated force per mV at approximately constant load stiffness. C) Calculated unloaded extension β per mV based on the data in A) and B). D) Calculated isometric force F_∞ for the same cells.

length change than unloaded short cells, an unsurprising result but not one that is been demonstrated previously. However, F_∞ was found to be independent of cell length, consistent with a view of the cell as a stacked series of force-generating elements. The isometric force generated by such an arrangement is independent of the number of elements.

3.3   *Effect of Mechanical Stimulation on Cell Length and Compliance*

Several interventions that affect hearing are thought to act via outer hair cells. If OHC motility is important to normal hearing, it may be that these interventions act

Figure 4: Effects of overstimulation on compliance, force, length and diameter. Test stimulus was a 120 mV voltage command. Damaging stimulus was a 240 mV command.

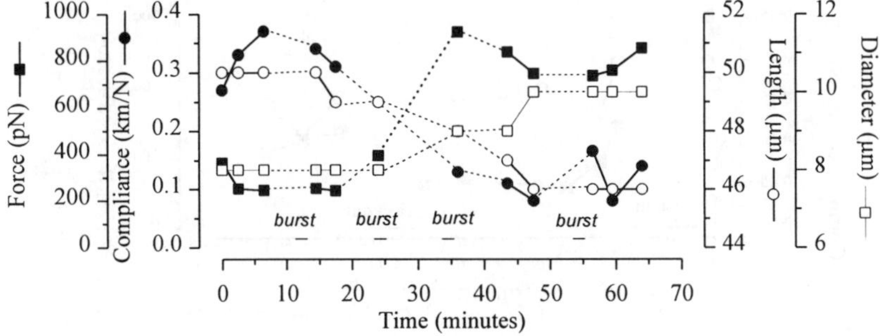

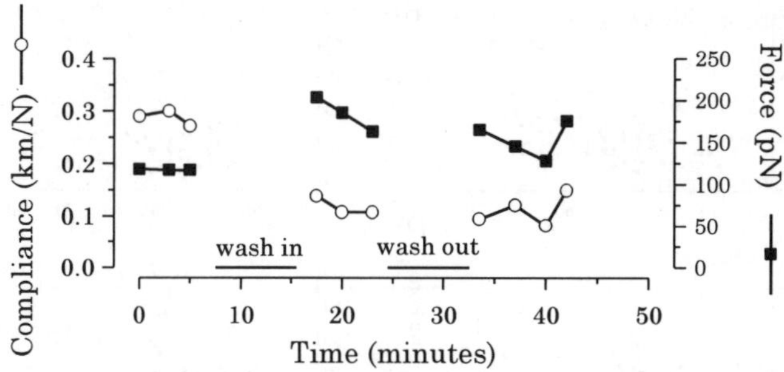

Figure 5: Effect of 260 mOsm (from normal 300 mOsm) on compliance and force. The test stimulus was a 120 mV sinusoid.

through an effect on OHC motility. Agents that affect OHC motility *in vivo* may in turn affect either the cell stiffness or the motor itself. One example of an intervention that acts through OHCs is the reduction in hearing sensitivity after overstimulation known as temporary threshold shift (TTS). To simulate overstimulation, the length and diameter of cells were monitored, along with the compliance and the force generated, with bursts of high voltage electrical stimulation to provoke overstimulation. As shown in Figure 4, the cell shortened and widened, and the compliance went down and the force went up. Compliance decreases were always observed to accompany cell shortening and were not usually observed without it. Sustained compliance increase was not observed. The force usually increased with shortening, but sometimes decreased or remained approximately the same.

3.4 Effect of Osmotic Challenge

OHCs may be subjected to osmotic shifts *in vivo*, especially during the hydrops consequent to Menieres disease. In several experiments, cell were exposed to

Figure 6: Effect of salicylate (5 mM) on compliance and force. The test stimulus was a 120 mV sinusoid.

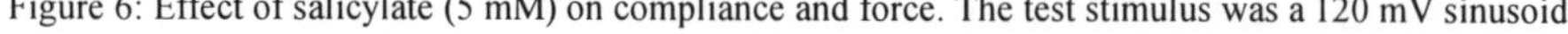
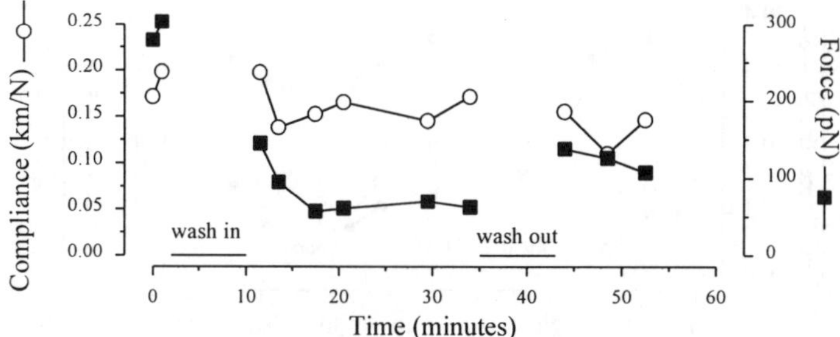

hypoosmotic media (260 mOsm from 300 mOsm in the standard medium). In all cases, of which Figure 5 is a representative example, the cell length decreased and the diameter increased. As with the overstimulation experiments, the compliance decreased along with the length decrease, and the force usually increased. Partial recovery was often but not always seen. The same changes were seen for 200 mOsm solutions. The opposite effects were usually observed for hyperosmotic stimulation (340 mOsm), although cell collapse sometimes made it impossible to complete the experiment.

3.5 Effect of Salicylate on Compliance and Force Generation

Salicylate is known to cause hearing loss, tinnitus, and a reversible hearing loss at high doses. At 5 mM and 1 mM, a substantial loss of force was observed with little change in compliance (Figure 6). Changes in compliance, when observed, were always decreases, and were accompanied by length decreases, but were not a consistent feature of these experiments. The reduction in force was typically 80% at 5 mM and 50% at 1 mM, but was very small or absent at 0.5 mM.

4   Discussion

It is apparent from the foregoing observations that the isolated cell data of previous years must be treated with caution. Not only must the external load on the OHC be understood before computing cell extension in response to voltage stimuli, but also the internal stiffness of the cell needs to be taken into account. This is of particular importance in comparing the roles of OHCs in basal versus apical turns, for which the OHCs may be four times as stiff, but the applied loads are probably 100 times as stiff. The data above and elsewhere are beginning to give a clear picture of the OHCs force generating capabilities under defined loads. However, the loads experienced by OHCs *in vivo* remain as yet undefined.

The effects of mechanical stimulation and hypoosmotic challenge were notably similar, in that the cell always decreased in length and increased in diameter. There was also similarity in the effects on OHC compliance and force of these two treatments. This suggests a common mechanism of an increase in internal pressure. The effects on force exhibited less consistency. An internal stiffness increase, on its own, should lead to a force increase at constant load (as demonstrated in Figure 2C), and this was usually the case. The variability may be the result of the pressure change directly affecting the motor state via a change in membrane tension[6-8].

The effect of salicylate demonstrated here is inconsistent with some results reported earlier[2,9]. However, there are considerable methodological differences between the studies, and the results may therefore be capable of resolution after further experimentation.

Acknowledgments

I thank Peter Dallos for the generous gift of data acquisition software and Kris Scott and Cindy Wright for technical assistance. This work was supported by NIH grant DC 02053.

References

1. Hallworth, R. (1995) The biomechanics of outer hair cell motility, in *Active Hearing*, eds. A. Flock, D. Ottoson and M. Ulfendahl (Pergamon, Oxford) pp. 155-166.
2. Russell, I.J. and Schauz, C. (1995) Salicylate ototoxicity: effects on the stiffness and electromotility of outer hair cells isolated from the guinea pig cochlea, *Aud. Neurosci.* **1** 309-320.
3. Hallworth, R (1995) Passive compliance and active force generation in the guinea pig outer hair cell, *J. Neurophysiol.* **74** 2319-2328.
4. Clark, B.A., Hallworth, R. and Evans, B.N. (1990) Calibration of photo-diode measurements of cell motility by a transmission optical lever method, *Pflugers Archives* **415** 490-493.
5. Pujol, R., Lenoir, M., Ladrech, S., Tribillac, F. and Rebillard, G. (1992) Correlation between the length of outer hair cells and the frequency coding of the cochlea, in *Auditory Physiology and Perception. Advances in the Biosciences*, eds. Y. Cazals, L. Demany and K. Horner (Pergamon, Oxford, UK) pp. 45-51.
6. Gale, J.E. and Ashmore, J.F. (1994) Charge displacement induced by rapid stretch in the basolateral membrane of the guinea-pig outer hair cell, *Proc. Roy. Soc.* **255** 243-249.
7. Iwasa, K.H. (1993) Effect of stress on the membrane capacitance of the auditory outer hair cell, *Biophys. J.* **65** 492-498.
8. Kakehata, S. and Santos-Sacchi, J. (1995) Membrane tension directly shifts voltage dependence of outer hair cell motility and associated gating charge, *Biophys. J.* **68** 2190-2197.
9. Brownell, W.E., Ratnanather, J.T., Popel, A.S., Zhi, M. and Sit, P.S. (1995) Labyrinthine lateral walls: cochlear outer hair cell permeability and mechanics, in *Active Hearing*, eds. A. Flock, D. Ottoson and M. Ulfendahl (Pergamon, Oxford) pp. 167-179.

FORCE GENERATION AND MECHANICAL IMPEDANCE OF OUTER HAIR CELLS

W. HEMMERT, C. SCHAUZ, H.-P. ZENNER, A.W. GUMMER
Section of Physiological Acoustics and Communication
Department of Otolaryngology
University of Tübingen, Silcherstr. 5, D-72076 Tübingen, Germany
werner.hemmert@uni-tuebingen.de

A novel technique was developed to measure the mechanical impedance and the electromotile force of isolated outer hair cells (OHC) up to frequencies in the kHz-range. The OHC behaved like an ideal spring only for frequencies below 200 Hz; for higher frequencies, the mechanical impedance decreased with 3 dB/oct. and the phase was about -45°. The mechanical impedance of Hensen cells and red blood cells also showed this behavior, indicating that membrane mechanics is probably viscoelastic. The electromotile force of OHC increased at 3 dB/oct for frequencies above 200 Hz. The displacement response was constant up to about 5 kHz. The results suggest that the motor proteins act as area-motors in series with viscoelastic elements in the cell membrane.

1 Measurement of Outer Hair Cell Mechanics

Isolated outer hair cells possess the unique ability to perform fast length changes.[1] With previous techniques it has been only possible to measure the OHC stiffness[2] and force[3-5] under quasi-static conditions. The present experiments were designed to measure both quantities up to 5 kHz.

2 Methods

OHC were mechanically isolated from the cochleae of young guinea pigs and maintained in Hanks´ balanced salt solution (Sigma, supplemented with sodium bicarbonate and 10 mM HEPES buffer, adjusted to 300 mOsm and pH 7.4). OHC were viewed with a fixed stage microscope (Leitz Labovert FS, Olympus 50x long distance objective, NA: 0.55) mounted on a translation stage. Only healthy looking cells with a bifringent membrane, the nucleus located near their basal pole and no apparent Brownian movement of their organelles were used. OHC were sucked partially into a heat polished borosilicate capillary (figure 1) by means of either a precision manometer or a syringe under micrometer-control.[1,3] The capillary was mounted on a piezoelectric stack (Pickelmann, PSt 150/7/15) to mechanically stimulate the OHC. The apical end of the OHC was positioned on the back of an atomic force cantilever (AFL), which served as a fast force to velocity transducer. The velocity of the AFL was measured with a laser-Doppler velocimeter (Polytec, OFV 302 and OFV 3000); the laser beam was focused with a Zeiss immersion objective (40x, 0.75 NA) on the cantilever. The force acting on the AFL is the product of the velocity of the AFL and its mechanical impedance. The mechanical impedance of the AFL (Z_{AFL}) was calculated from its stiffness, which was calibrated by the manufacturer, and from its mass and resistance in HBSS, which were calibrated by gluing the AFL with its substrate on a piezoelectric stack (Pickelmann, PSt 150/4/5, resonant frequency: 50 kHz). For frequencies up to 5 kHz the AFL behaved like a simple mass-spring-damper system; above this frequency range higher vibration modes occurred. Not all cantilevers were calibrated with this procedure because they were often destroyed by the gluing procedure. However, because all cantilevers of the same batch were equal in their mechanical properties, it was convenient to determine resistance and mass values for one cantilever from a batch.

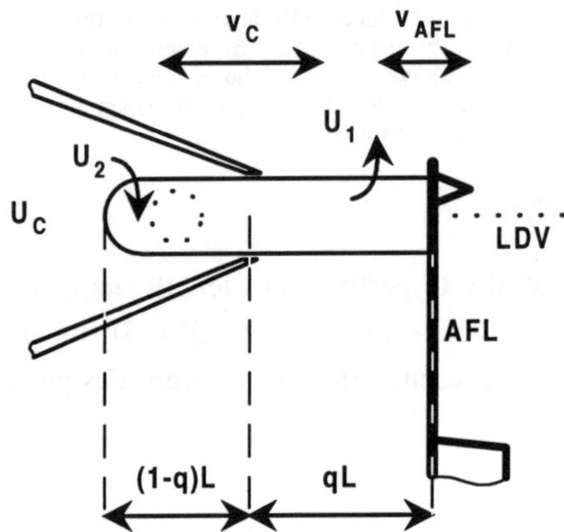

Figure 1: Measurement set-up. OHC were held in a capillary which allowed both electrical (U_C) and mechanical (v_C) stimulation. Force was measured by focusing a laser Doppler interferometer (LDV) on an atomic force cantilever (AFL) placed on the apical end of the OHC. q denotes the extrusion factor. Only part of the command voltage ($U_1 = U_C (1-q)$) appears across the extruded section of the cell.

To determine the axial force, the OHC was electrically stimulated in the microchamber[1] and the velocity of the AFL was measured. Since the AFL was an order of magnitude stiffer than the OHC, force was measured under nearly isometric conditions. The axial mechanical impedance of the OHC (Z_{OHC}) was measured by vibrating the microchamber with the piezoelectric stack and measuring the velocity of both AFL (v_{AFL}) and microchamber (v_C). The mechanical impedance was calculated as:

$$Z_{OHC} = Z_{AFL} \frac{v_{AFL}}{v_C - v_{AFL}} \tag{1}$$

The axial mechanical impedance and force describe the mechanical properties of the OHC, as if held between basilar membrane and reticular lamina.

A spectrum analyzer (AND 3525, AND Co., Japan) was used for producing stimuli, averaging (200x) and storing data. Command voltages for electrical and mechanical stimulation were multi-tone complexes with 38 frequencies (50-18000 Hz, 1024 points, repeated every 20 ms). All frequencies were harmonics of 50 Hz but logarithmically spaced at approximately 5.3 spectral points per octave. For electrical stimulation, the command voltage to the microchamber was 5.5 mV per spectral point. For the mechanical stimulation, the voltage delivered to the piezoelectric stack was low-pass filtered at -6 dB/oct to yield a capillary velocity which was approximately constant (10-40 µm/s). Compared with white noise, the total energy of the multi-tone signal is a factor of 10 less to provide the same signal-to-noise ratio. It is important to reduce the energy of the input signal because the non-linear electromotile properties of the OHC would otherwise cause distortions in the frequency response data. Another advantage of the multi-tone signal is that the distortion products fall in between its logarithmically spaced frequency components and thus distort the frequency response data less compared with white noise.

3 Results

Measurement of the dynamic properties of the OHCs showed that they behave as ideal springs only for frequencies below 200 Hz. The magnitude of the mechanical impedance fell with about 6 dB/oct and the phase tended to -90° (figure 2). The compliance, calculated from the measured impedance of the extruded cell part and extrapolated for the whole cell, ranged from 95-876 m/N (mean: 369 m/N, N=34). Irrespective of the origin of the OHC in the cochlea, above 200 Hz the amplitude of the mechanical impedance decreased over a wide frequency range with 3 dB/oct and the phase was at -45°. Above several kHz, fluid dynamics dominated OHC mechanics. This was demonstrated by measuring the impedance of the fluid after having ejected the OHC from the capillary, but with the same position of AFL and capillary. The mechanical impedance of Hensen cells and red blood cells showed the same mechanical properties, whereas the phalangeal processes of Deiters cells behaved as ideal springs up to high frequencies (data not shown).

OHC force ranged from 1.6-53 pN/mV (mean: 12.5 pN/mV, N=26, determined at 500 Hz and corrected for the voltage drop V_l over the extruded cell part). At frequencies above 200 Hz the electromotile force F of the OHCs increased with a slope of about 3 dB/oct (figure 3). Phase was positive for a positive command voltage and for force directed toward the AFL. The phase of the electromotile force was between -135° and -180°, indicating contraction when the extruded cell part was depolarized. The noise floor was below 1 pN from 500 to 5000 Hz, indicating the exquisite sensitivity of the measurements. Together with the mechanical impedance data, the displacement x of the OHC may be calculated by the formula $F/j\omega Z_{OHC}$, where j is $\sqrt{-1}$ and ω is the radial frequency. Then, the increasing force compensates the mechanical impedance of the OHC, so that the displacement amplitude was constant up to about 5 kHz (data not shown).

Mechanical impedance

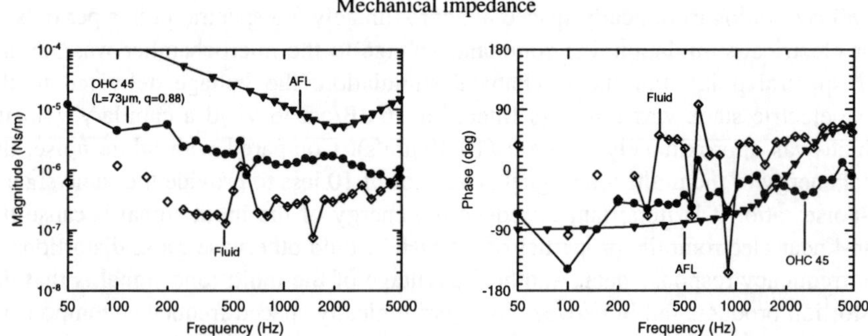

Figure 2: Dynamic properties of an isolated outer hair cell, left: amplitude and right: phase of mechanical impedance of the extruded partition of the cell (circles), atomic force cantilever (triangles) and fluid (diamonds). The diameter of the microchamber in this experiment was slightly smaller than the OHC providing a support of the basal pole of the OHC similar to a Deiters cell. Resonances in the fluid curve at 600 and 1300 Hz are due to transverse vibration modes in the microchamber. Notice that the mechanical impedance of the AFL is an order of magnitude higher than that of the OHC, implying that the AFL was acting as a true force transducer.

Force

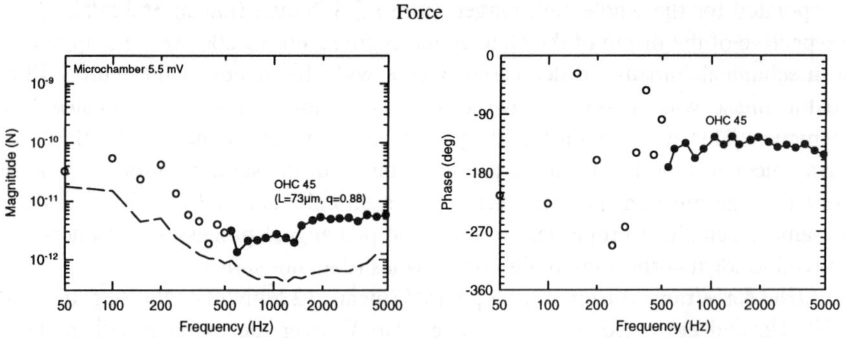

Figure 3: Force of the same outer hair cell as in figure 2. Left: amplitude and right: phase of the extruded partition of the cell. Dashed line: noise floor. The command voltage in the microchamber was 5.5 mV, the voltage over the extruded part of the cell was approximately 0.75 mV per frequency point (13 mV peak amplitude).

4   Model

As a first step in understanding the mechanics of the OHC, the mechanics of the subsurface cisternae (SSC) were modeled. The system of subsurface cisternae consists of straight, continuous and tightly packed lipid membranes, which lie underneath the plasma membrane. The intracisternal lumen is approximately 25 nm, the intercisternal space is 15-20 nm[6,7] and the distance to the cell membrane is about 50 nm. [8,9] At least one cistern seems to extend from the cell's apex to its basal end.[8,9] The thin fluid layers (viscosity η, thickness t) between the lipid membranes provide friction (R) which can not be neglected (l_{OHC} denotes OHC length, d_{OHC} diameter).[10]

$$R = \frac{\pi d_{OHC} l_{OHC} \eta}{t} \tag{2}$$

A very simple mechanical model of a circumferential section of an OHC showed that the subsurface cisternae are successively coupled by friction to the cell membrane with increasing frequency. As a consequence, at high frequencies the stiffness of the OHC is proportional to the number of lipid membranes parallel to the cell membrane. However, if the total stiffness of the cell is placed in the outer cell membrane[2], the corner frequency (determined from cell compliance and SSC friction) is in the range of a few Hertz. Additionally, if a displacement motor is introduced in the cell membrane, the model predicts constant force under isometric conditions and that the displacement amplitude under isotonic conditions decreases at very low frequencies. In summary, SSC mechanics do not explain the observed behavior of OHC for frequencies above 200 Hz.

The mechanical impedance data obtained from Hensen cells and red blood cells suggest that the viscoelastic properties might be a common feature of lipid membranes. Then the model of Dallos et al.[11] can be modified by replacing the elastic coupling of the motor elements in the outer cell membrane with viscoelastic elements (compare figure 4). This model predicts both constant motility and an increasing force as a function of frequency measured under isometric conditions.

5   Discussion

Combining an atomic force cantilever (AFL) as a fast force transducer with a laser-Doppler velocimeter (LDV) allowed precise and sensitive measurements of the mechanical properties of OHCs up to frequencies in the kHz-range. OHC force increased with a slope of about 3 dB/oct. Irrespective of their origin in the cochlea, OHCs behaved as springs only for frequencies below 200 Hz. Fluid forces dominated OHC mechanics above about 5 kHz. Our compliance data lie between previously measured values[2-5] and theoretical values.[12] From recordings from different cell types we conclude that cell membranes are generally viscoelastic. However, the viscoelastic membrane properties can not be described by a single time constant, instead, the magnitude of the mechanical impedance fell with 3 dB/oct. and its phase was -45° from 200 Hz to several kHz. As a consequence, the motor proteins in the outer membrane of the OHC are coupled in series by viscoelastic elements. The result that OHC motility is constant up to high frequencies requires that the motor proteins act as area-motors. Together, this model (figure 4) also explains the 3 dB/oct. increase in OHC force.

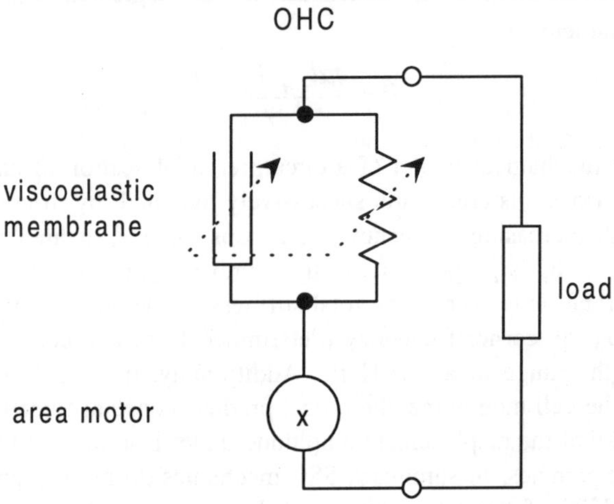

Figure 4: Mechanical model of an OHC. To model the -3 dB/oct. and -45° of the impedance of the OHC, the impedance of the resistive and compliant components of the cell membrane must be of equal magnitude above 200 Hz. The only way to yield constant displacement amplitude over a wide frequency range and a force increasing with 3 dB/oct., is to place a displacement source in series with the viscoelastic membrane impedance.

Our values of OHC force at low frequencies were higher than previous data[3-5] and are in the range of theoretical values.[12-14] Since the OHC force increases with frequency, the force estimated at high frequencies was underestimated by previous investigations by at least one order of magnitude.

Acknowledgments

Supported by the DFG, Klinische Forschergruppe "Hörforschung", Projekt A.

References

1. Dallos, P. and Evans, B.N. (1995) High-frequency motility of outer hair cells and the cochlear amplifier. *Science* **267** 2006-2009.
2. Holley, M.C. and Ashmore, J.F. (1988) A cytoskeletal spring in cochlear outer hair cells. *Nature* **335** 635-637.
3. Gitter, A.H., Rudert, M., and Zenner, H.-P. (1993) Forces involved in length changes of cochlear outer hair cells. *Pflügers Arch.* **424** 9-14.
4. Hallworth, R. (1995) Passive compliance and active force generation in the guinea pig outer hair cell, *J. Neurophysiol.* **74** 2319-2328.
5. Russell, I. and Schauz, C. (1995) Salicylate ototoxicity: Effects on the stiffness and electromotility of outer hair cells isolated from the guinea pig cochlea, *Aud. Neurosci.* **1** 309-319.
6. Slepecky, N.B. and Ligotti, P.J. (1992) Characterization of inner ear sensory hair cells after rapid-freezing and freeze-substitution, *J. Neurocytol.* **21** 374-381.
7. Brownell, W.E., Ratnanather, J.T., Popel, A.S., Zhi, M. and Sit, P.S. (1996) Labyrinthine lateral walls: Cochlear outer hair cell permeability and mechanics, in *Active Hearing*, eds. Å. Flock, D. Ottoson and M. Ulfendahl (Elsevier Science Ltd., Oxford) pp. 167-179.
8. Dieler, R., Shehata-Dieler, W.E., and Brownell, W.E. (1991) Concomitant salicylate-induced alterations of outer hair cell subsurface cisternae and electromotility, *J. Neurocytol.* **20** 637-653.
9. Forge, A. (1991) Structural features of the lateral walls in mammalian cochlear outer hair cells, *Cell Tiss. Res.* **265** 473-483.
10. Kuchling, H. (1985), *Taschenbuch der Physik* (Harry Deutsch, Thun, Frankfurt/Main).
11. Dallos, P., Hallworth, R. and Evans, B.N. (1993). Theory of electrically driven shape changes of cochlear outer hair cells. *J. Neurophysiol.* **70**, 299-323.
12. Iwasa, K.H. (1994) A membrane motor model for the fast motility of the outer hair cell, *J. Acoust. Soc. Am.* **96** 2216-2224.
13. Tolomeo, J.A. and Steele, C.R. (1995) Orthotropic piezoelectric properties of the cochlear outer hair cell wall, *J. Acoust. Soc. Am.* **97**, 3006-3011.
14. Mountain, D. C. and Hubbard, A. E. (1994). A piezoelectric model of outer hair cell function. *J. Acoust. Soc. Am.* **95**, 350-354.

THE EFFECT OF STATIC HAIR-BUNDLE DISPLACEMENT ON THE MECHANOELECTRIC TRANSDUCTION IN ISOLATED COCHLEAR HAIR CELLS

J. MEYER, S. PREYER, H.-P. ZENNER, A.W. GUMMER

Section of Physiological Acoustics and Communication, Dept. of Otolaryngology
University of Tübingen, Silcherstr. 5, 72076 Tübingen, Germany
e-mail: jens.meyer@uni-tuebingen.de

A movement of the hair bundle from its resting position led to a decreased receptor current without spontaneous recovery, indicating the absence of adaptation. Application of ATP results in a strong depolarizing inward current, but had no effect on the recovery of mechanoelectrical transduction.

1   Introduction

Auditory mechanoreceptors have evolved for the highly sensitive detection of vibrations and for the transformation of mechanical stimuli into receptor currents. According to current hypothesis mechanoelectrical transduction (MET) is achieved by a direct coupling of an elastic element, called a tip link, connecting two adjacent stereocilia with a mechanoelectrical transducer channel(s)[1]. The hair cells of the mammalian cochlea are reported to detect vibration amplitudes of atomic dimensions. As a consequence of the extremely high sensitivity and the very limited dynamic range, the system is also susceptible to mechanical disturbances. In order to increase the dynamic range and to protect against disturbances, an adaptation mechanism has evolved in hair cell stereocilia of lower vertebrates. Based on the tip-link hypothesis, hair cells adapt by an active re-tensioning of the tip links by an actin-myosin interaction[2,3]. Consequently the receptor current declines when stimulated with a constant bundle deflection[4]. However it is still unclear whether mammalian hair cells show an adaptation as described above.

According to the adaptation hypothesis, the stereocilia of outer hair cells (OHCs) should be able to reset their operating point. Therefore, the OHCs should be able to compensate the effect of static hair bundle deflections that normally would saturate the receptor current and make the cell insensitive to additional mechanical stimulation. Our experiments were performed to discover how the MET reacts following this kind of "mechanical disturbance". Nevertheless the time course of adaptation investigated in our experiments has to be seperated from that in other studies. For example, Hudspeth[3] described experiments on frog vestibular hair cells which show a spontaneous adaptation of the receptor current in response to rectangular deflections of the hair bundle with a time constant of about 25 ms. The aim of our study was to describe the response of the MET following a relatively slow shift of the resting point of the stereocilia.

It has been shown that purinergic receptors (P_{2X}) are located in the stereocilia of mammalian OHCs[5]. Until now, almost nothing is known about the role of these purinoceptors in OHCs. Extracellular binding of ATP to these receptors causes a nonselective ion-channel to open, resulting in a depolarizing inward curent, carried by an influx of Ca^{2+}-ions[6]. Because calcium is necessary for actin-myosin interaction this might be a factor for the regulation of hair-cell adaptation.

2   Methods

Experiments were performed with mechanically isolated OHCs prepared from the adult guinea-pig cochlea. The isolation procedure was described in detail by Preyer et al.[7] The whole cell potential and current were measured with the patch-clamp technique under video control. The hair bundles of the cells were stimulated by a fluid-jet driven by a piezoelectric crystal. The stimulus pipette was filled with extracellular fluid (Hanks` balanced salt solution, Seromed). The stimulus frequency was 8 Hz.

Drugs (ATP, Sigma; suramin, Bayer AG) were applied to the hair bundle region by pressure injection (Eppendorf Transjector 5246) through a double-barrel micropipette (tip diameter 10 μm). Care was taken not to cause movement of the hair bundle by drug application.

A static deflection of the hair bundle was achieved by varying the resting pressure of the fluid-jet. An increase of internal pressure led to a constant outflow of Hanks` solution resulting in a static deflection of the hair bundle. The movement of the stereocilia bundle was detected with a photodiode attached to the microscope. The photodiode showed a linear characteristic in the complete range we investigated.

3   Results

3.1   Influence of static hair-bundle deflection on mechanoelectrical transduction

The dynamic range of an OHC is limited to about 400 nm. This means that the cell will not respond with maximum sensitivity to mechanical stimulation when the position of the hair bundle is shifted away from the resting point. If stereocilia are capable of adaptation they should be able to reset their operating range when the hair bundle is displaced from its position by a static deflection. To test this, the stereocilia were deflected statically during sinusoidal mechanical stimulation (8 Hz). The recording of stereocilia movement showed that the peak-to-peak displacement of the hair bundle elicited by fluid-jet stimulation was identical in the resting position and during static deflection.

Strong static deflections (up to 3°) led to a total abolition of the response. This was observed for deflections in positive and in negative directions. No spontaneous recovery of the transduction current was seen, indicating that adaptation did not occur. Removal of the static deflection led to a total recovery of the response.

3.2   *Influence of extracellular ATP*

When ATP (300 μM) was applied during voltage clamp experiments (holding potential -60 mV) to the hair bundle region, a strong depolarizing inward current of several hundred pA could be seen for the time of application. ATP applied together with the purinoceptor blocker suramin (250 μM) led to a decreased (50-70%) inward current, indicating that extracellular ATP binds to purinoceptors (P_{2X}) causing a nonselective ion-channel to open.

In following experiments we wanted to test a possible effect of the activation of purinoceptors on the adaptation behaviour of OHCs. For that reason we carried out experiments which showed the expected ATP-induced current during mechanical stimulation and static deflection of the hair bundle. However, these data gave no indication that extracellular ATP has any effect on the dynamic response of the OHC. The deflection of the stereocilia in the negative direction led to a reduced transduction current that did not increase again. Application of ATP (300 μM) in this situation led to a strong inward current, much larger than the transduction current. Application of ATP did not effect the receptor current. Only a movement of the hair bundle back to its resting position led to a recovery of MET.

4   Conclusion

A movement of the stereocilia of guinea-pig OHCs from their resting position led to a reduced transduction current. No evidence of adaptation to a static deflection of the hair bundle was found. Dynamic responses could not be influenced by ATP.

Acknowledgments

This work was supported by DFG, Klinische Forschergruppe, Hörforschung, Projekt A.

References

1. Hudspeth, A.J. (1988) How the ear's works work, *Nature* **341** 397-404.
2. Gillespie, P.G. (1995) Molecular machinery of auditory and vestibular transduction, *Curr. Opin. Neurobiol.* **5** 449-455.
3. Hudspeth, A.J. and Gillespie P.G. (1994) Pulling springs to tune transduction: adaptation by hair cells, *Neuron* **12** 1-9.
4. Shepherd, G.M.G. and Corey, D.P. (1994) The extent of adaptation in bullfrog saccular hair cells, *J. Neurosci.* **14** 6217-6229.

5. Mockett, B.G, Housley, G.D. and Thorne, P.R. (1994) Fluorescense imaging of extracellular purinergic receptor sites and putative ecto-ATPase sites on isolated cochlear hair cells, *J. Neurosci.* **14** 6992-7007.

6. Nakagawa, T., Akaike, N., Kimitsuki, T., Komune, S. and Arima, T. (1990) ATP-induced current in isolated outer hair cells of guinea pig cochlea, *J. Neurophysiol..* **63** 1068-1074.

7. Preyer, S., Renz, S, Hemmert, W., Zenner, H.-P. and Gummer, A.W. (1996) Receptor potential of outer hair cells isolated from base to apex of the adult guinea-pig cochlea: implications for cochlear tuning mechanisms, *Aud. Neurosci.* **2** 145-157.

MULTIPLE STIFFNESS GRADIENTS IN THE COCHLEA ?

RAM C.NAIDU and DAVID C.MOUNTAIN

Boston University Hearing Research Center
44 Cummington Street,Boston, MA 02215

The point stiffness of the cochlear partition was measured at various locations along its length in the excised basal and second turns of the gerbil cochlea. The experiments were performed with a piezoelectric force probe from the side of basilar membrane while the organ of Corti was viewed from the side of the tectorial membrane using a CCD camera on a inverted microscope. The data indicate that the stiffness increases towards the hook region of the basilar membrane. Also, multiple stiffness gradients are present and these are significantly larger in the hook region than over the rest of the cochlea.

1   Introduction

The cochlear frequency map is believed to depend on the progressive increase in stiffness from apex to base. Previous measurements on cochleae from human cadavers[1] have suggested that the elasticity of the partition increases by a factor of 100 from the stapes to the helicotrema. However, a factor of nearly 10000 may be required to support the frequency range of normal hearing if entirely determined by partition stiffness. In this study, we investigated the nature of the stiffness gradients along the cochlea in an attempt to understand how cellular elements contribute to the passive tonotopicity of the cochlear partition. These results can give us an idea of the loads against which outer hair cell motility must work as well as provide data for model parameter estimation.

2   Methods

Young female mongolian gerbils were deeply anesthetized and then decapitated. The temporal bones were quickly excised and transferred into oxygenated culture medium (Leibovitz L-15). Following dissection to expose the cochlea, most of the bone around the round window was removed to expose the basilar membrane upto the hook region. The round window membrane was carefully removed and the bone above the basal turn was cut removing the higher turns. This enabled access to the organ of Corti from the side of the tectorial membrane. For measurements in the second turn, the basal and apical turn were both removed.

Point stiffness was obtained from the basilar membrane side by measuring the restoring force in response to a sinusoidal displacement of the partition over a range of static deflections. The measurements were performed using a piezoelectric probe[2] with a glass tip of diameter 10μm. Data was obtained at various longitudinal positions relative to the hook of the cochlear partition. At each location, stiffnesses were measured at radial positions spanning the width of the organ. The organ of Corti was simultaneously viewed from the tectorial membrane side using a CCD camera mounted on an inverted microscope. Images from the camera were recorded and subsequently digitized to determine probe location and organ of Corti deformation.

Typical stiffness curves showed an initial plateau of low magnitude, an abrupt rise to a second plateau followed subsequently by a region of increasing stiffness. (Fig. 1). The function $k = k_o + k_2(x-x_0)^2$ was used fit to the data obtained when the probe was retracting. The plateau stiffness, k_0, is predicted for bending for an edge-attached structure while the quadratically increasing stiffness is predicted when the structure is deflected to the stage that stretching becomes dominant. The value of k_o is a measure of the second plateau which is considered the physiological relevant stiffness for cochlear mechanics[3,4]. The restoring force due to a pure stiffness is theoretically 180° out of phase with the displacement stimulus. Hence the fit included only those data points for which the phase of the force fell within 3-4° of 180°.

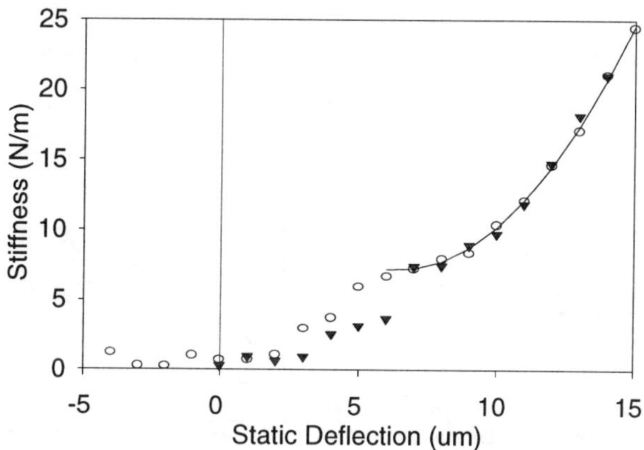

Figure 1: Typical stiffness-versus-deflection curve. The inverted triangles (▾) represent the data collected as the probe was advancing. The function $k = 7.13 + .24(x-6.4)^2$ was fit to the data taken as the probe was retracting (○).

3   Results

Video images from adjacent static positions of the probe were subtracted to estimate the extent of organ deformation during measurements. The data indicate that the partition is displaced mainly in the region local to the probe. The partition thus deflects in a manner different from a simple beam. The measurements must therefore characterize local , rather than global, stiffness.

The radial profile of k_o varies according to the cellular anatomy of the partition. The pillar cells form a region of high stiffness in contrast with the more compliant tunnel of Corti. The region of the outer hair cells and Hensen's cells is characterized by an intermediate stiffness that rises with positions approaching the spiral ligament. The spiral lamina and spiral ligament are much stiffer than positions in between and serve as landmarks on either side.

Values from the corresponding regions at the more basal location (Fig 2A, 1.28mm) show a higher stiffness than those obtained more apical (Fig 2B, 3.67mm). This is evident especially in the region of the outer pillar cell and in the pectinate zone. Also, the width of the basilar membrane is different at the two locations (basal = 90μm, apical = 190μm). The differing stiffness magnitudes clearly indicate the presence of gradients along the length of the cochlea.

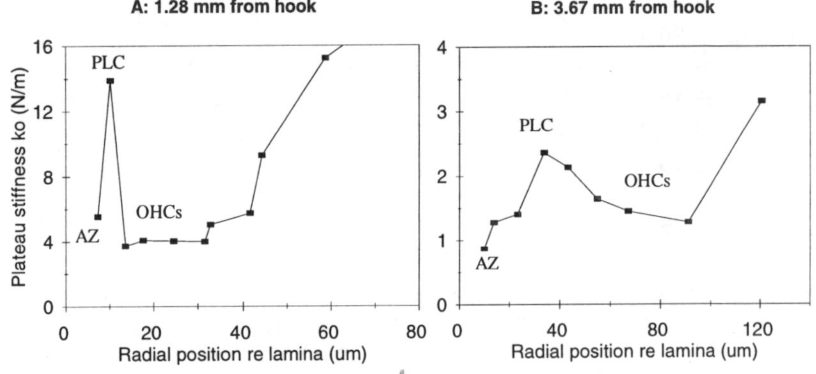

Figure 2: Plateau stiffness, k_0, is plotted against radial position at two longitudinal locations (A and B) measured from the hook of the basilar membrane. Note that the scales are different. The width of the partition is different at the two locations (A = 90μm and B = 190μm).

Data was pooled across animals to study the variation of k_0 with longitudinal position. This data is plotted in Fig. 3 for different locations within the organ of Corti. Since the outer hair cells span multiple radial measurement locations, three-point spatial averaging was used to obtain a representative value for the stiffness of this region. The data in each region was fit using the function $\ln[k_0] = c_1 + c_2\, x$ where x is the distance from the hook.

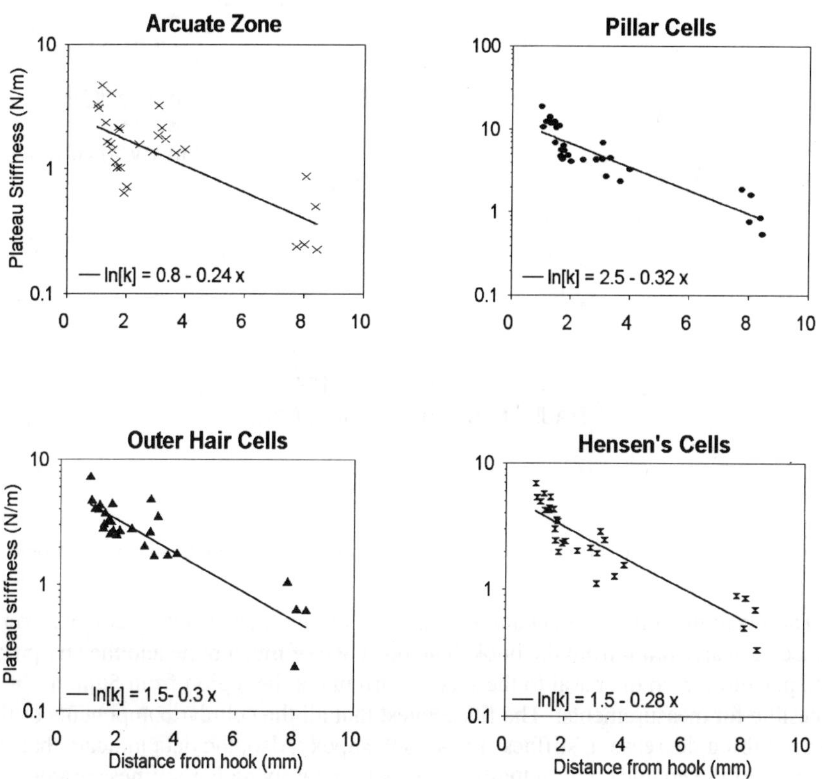

Figure 3: Pooled longitudinal data demonstrate stiffness gradients. Note that the pillar cell stiffness is represented on a larger scale.

4   Discussion

The excised cochlea preparation allows great flexibility and manipulation. However, it is important to understand if the data thus obtained is really representative of the micromechanical properties of the cochlea within the intact animal. Fig. 4 compares the values of k_o obtained *in vitro* with those obtained *in situ*[4,5]. Given the variability across animals and measurement locations, our data show a remarkable agreement which suggests that our excised preparations are representative of the intact cochlea.

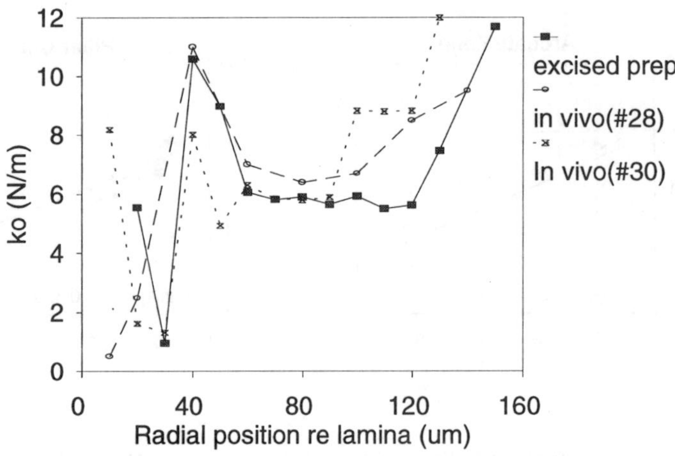

Figure 4: Stiffness as a function of radial position from an excised cochlea and from two *in situ* experiments.

The fits to the longitudinal data were used to obtain the stiffness gradients over a distance of nearly 8mm from the hook. The presence of much bone and the sharp rise of the partition from the basal to the second turn made the region from 5mm to 7mm inaccesible for measurements. The fits suggest that all the cellular components of the organ exhibit a decrease in stiffness towards the apex. Also, the data indicate that the first 2mm of the cochlea may actually have a significantly higher stiffness gradient.

The narrowness of the arcuate zone in the basal turn makes accurate positioning of the probe under the centre of the tunnel of Corti difficult. The increased variability in the data from the arcuate zone may therefore be due to a partial contact with the pillar cell during some measurements, resulting in a seemingly higher stiffness. The stiffness gradient in this region being close to the value in the pillar cells suggest that they may influence the arcuate zone mechanics to some extent.

To compare these longitudinal results to the gerbil frequency map[3], we assumed that the mass of organ remained constant so that the characteristic frequency would vary as the square root of the stiffness. The data was averaged over 500μm bins, normalized by the most basal stiffness and compared to the square of the normalized characteristic frequency that was estimated from the corresponding frequency-place map (Fig. 5). As is evident, the measured stiffness gradients alone cannot account for the range of frequencies observed in the gerbil.

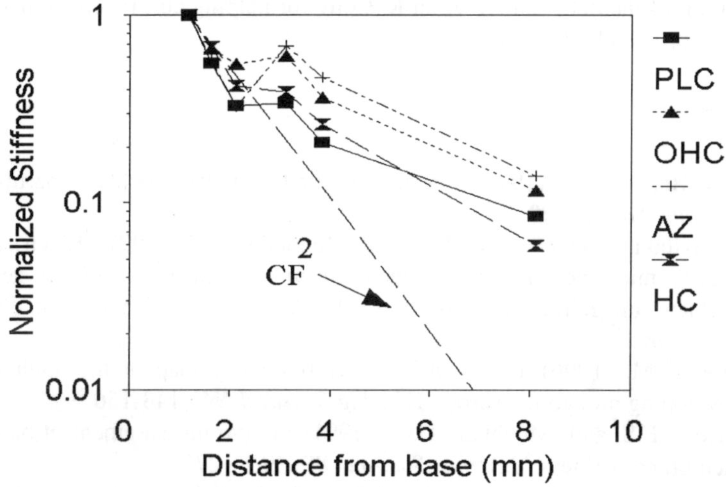

Figure 5: Comparing the stiffness with the square of the characteristic frequency. All values were normalized by the values at the hook. Assuming a constant mass for the partition, the stiffness should have followed the square of the characteristic frequency at each location.

The natural frequencies of predicted for beams and plates with distributed mass and elasticity for bending modes are proportional to the square root of their elasticity and inversely proportional to the squares of their lengths [7]. This suggests that the width of the partition, which increases from base to apex , could play a significant role in determining the characteristic frequency at a given longitudinal location along the cochlea.

In the first 2mm or 'hook' region of the basilar membrane, the width of the organ increases dramatically. The stiffness gradients local to this region are also much larger than in the rest of the cochlea. This specialization may be present to boost the frequency range to allow the representation of the highest frequency octave in the gerbil cochlea.

Based on the stiffness measured in the current study, it is possible to estimate the force produced by outer hair cells at locations in the in the apical turn where electromotility data is available[2]. It is assumed that the 10µm probe measures the stiffness of a single outer hair cell. For an average electrically evoked displacement of 300 nm and a predicted stiffness of 0.16 N/m at a location 11mm from the base, the force generated would be of the order of 50 nN.

Acknowledgements

We wish to thank Dr. Dimitrije Stamenovi_ for his valuable discussion regarding the interpretation of the data and Dr. Alan R. Cody for helping edit this document.This work was supported by NIDCD

References

1. von Békésy, G. (1948) On the elasticity of the cochlear partition. *J.Acoust.Soc.Am.* **20** 227-241.
2. Karavitaki, K.D., Cody, A.R. and Mountain, D.C. (1997) Electrically evoked micromechanical movements from the apical turn of the gerbil cochlea. In: *Diversity in Auditory Mechanics. World Scientific Publ. Singapore.*
3. Müller, M. (1996) The cochlear place-frequency map of the adult and developing mongolian gerbil. H*earing Research* **94** 148-156.
4. Olson , E.S. and Mountain, D.C. (1991) In vivo measurement of basilar membrane stiffness. *J.Acoust.Soc.Am.* **89** 1262-1275.
5. Olson, E.S. and Mountain, D.C. (1993) Probing the cochlear partition's micromechanical properties with measurements of radial and longitudinal stiffness variations. In: *Biophysics of hair cell sensory systems*, ed. H. Duifhuis, J.W. Horst, P. van Dijk and S. von Netten (World Scientific, Singapore)
6. Olson , E.S. and Mountain, D.C. (1994) Mapping the cochlear partition's stiffness to its cellular architecture. *J.Acoust.Soc.Am.* **95** 395-400.
7. Stokey, W.F. (1976) Vibration of systems having distirbuted mass and elasticity. In: *Shock and Vibration Handbook*, ed. C.M. Harris and C.E. Crede (McGraw-Hill, U.S.A.

SODIUM CURRENTS IN HAIR CELLS OF THE MOUSE UTRICLE

A. RÜSCH AND R.A. EATOCK

Department of Otorhinolaryngology and Communicative Sciences
Baylor College of Medicine, Houston, TX 77030, USA
eatock@bcm.tmc.edu

Whole-cell, tight-seal recordings were made from hair cells in excised mouse utricular epithelia. 42% of type II hair cells, but just one of 94 type I cells, expressed sodium current. There were no clear changes in size or incidence of sodium currents with age after birth. The currents had fast activation and inactivation kinetics and activated positive to - −60 mV. They were less sensitive to tetrodotoxin and had a more negative voltage range of inactivation than the sodium channels of nerve. They were inactivated at the mean resting potential of type II cells, −65 mV. If this is the case *in vivo*, the sodium currents would be activatable only after hyperpolarizing inputs.

1 Introduction

Voltage-gated sodium channels are crucial to the firing of action potentials, or spiking, of nerve fibers. Until a decade ago, hair cells were generally viewed as non-spiking and were therefore not expected to express voltage-gated sodium channels. Since then, however, reports of spiking by select populations of hair cells isolated from various organs have accumulated. Where the cells' region of origin is known, spiking is correlated with low characteristic frequencies (< 500 Hz)[1]. Some of the spikes appear to be calcium-based[2-4], while others are thought to be mixed calcium/sodium[1,5,6]. Tetrodotoxin (TTX)-sensitive sodium current (I_{Na}) is found in certain auditory hair cells from alligator[1], guinea pig[7] and immature mouse[6] cochleas and the goldfish saccule[5], and in vestibular hair cells from the semicircular canal organs of chicks[8] and rats[9].

Mammalian vestibular organs transduce head movements, which are generally low-frequency (<10 Hz)[10], providing the input to reflexes that maintain balance and gaze. These organs have two kinds of hair cell, type I and type II, which differ morphologically[11] and in their potassium conductances. Type I cells, but not type II cells, have a large delayed rectifier conductance ($g_{K,L}$) that is appreciably activated at the cells' resting potentials[12-14], conferring upon them a low input resistance. As a consequence, the voltage response to a given injected current is much smaller and more linear in type I cells than in type II cells[15].
Here we report that type I and II hair cells of the mouse utricle also differentially express voltage-gated sodium channels.

2 Methods

2.1 Preparations

Utricles were excised from albino mice and either studied acutely or put into organotypic culture. Utricles that were studied acutely were excised from mice ranging in age from one day to adult. Utricles that were cultured were excised on postnatal day (PD) 1 and maintained for between one and eight days before being used for experiments. Culturing techniques are described elsewhere[14]. Data from cultured and acutely studied utricles did not appear to differ and were pooled.

2.2 Recordings

Whole-cell tight-seal recordings were done as previously described[14]. The basolateral membranes of the hair cells in the epithelium were exposed for patch clamping by making a tear in the epithelium. Data were recorded in whole-cell voltage-clamp mode using the ruptured-patch method. Patch pipettes contained (in mM): 140 KCl, 0.1 $CaCl_2$, 5 EGTA-KOH, 3.5 $MgCl_2$, 2.5 Na_2ATP, 5 HEPES-KOH, pH 7.4. Series resistances were between 2.5 and 11 $M\Omega$, 70 - 90% of which was compensated. Data were low-pass filtered at 10 - 25 kHz and sampled at 10μs. Voltages were corrected off-line for uncompensated series resistances and liquid junction potentials (−4 mV). Values are expressed as means ± standard deviations.

The utricular epithelia were superfused at 23-25°C with a solution containing (in mM): 144 NaCl, 0.7 NaH_2PO_4, 5.8 KCl, 1.3 $CaCl_2$, 0.9 $MgCl_2$, 5.6 D-glucose, 10 HEPES-NaOH; pH 7.4. TTX was dissolved in the extracellular solution and applied to the cells via a gravity-fed micropipette.

2.3 Cell type classification

As previously described[14], we used the strong correlation between type I morphology and the presence of $g_{K,L}$[16] to classify the hair cells. Cells with $g_{K,L}$ have large input conductances at a holding potential of −64 mV, typically in excess of 20 nS, because $g_{K,L}$ is substantially activated at − 64 mV. We classified cells with input conductances >20 nS as type I and cells with conductances <4 nS as type II. Cells with intermediate input conductances were discarded.

3   Results

The standard voltage-step protocol that we have used was from a holding potential of 64 mV, near the mean resting potential of type II hair cells in our sample[14]. When the holding potential was −84 mV instead, steps positive to −64 mV activated small transient inward currents. We examined these currents in 94 type I cells and 123 type II cells, using 200-ms prepulses to −104 or −124 mV from holding potentials of either 64 or 84 mV.

3.1 Voltage dependence of sodium currents

Figure 1A shows a representative family of inward current traces that were activated by depolarizing voltage steps following a prepulse to −104 mV. Peak values of these current traces and additional traces are plotted against the membrane potential in Figure 1B. The inward currents in this cell activated positive to −60 mV and were maximal (−427 pA) at −29 mV. The time to peak decreased from 1.1 ms at −49 mV to 630 µs at −29 mV. Inactivation followed an exponential time course, with time constants varying from 1.1 ms at −49 mV to 0.7 ms at −29 mV. The inactivation at −29 mV was essentially complete before the delayed rectifier conductance had appreciably activated[14]. The voltage dependence and kinetics of these inward currents are consistent with those of sodium currents from other hair cells[1,5,7].

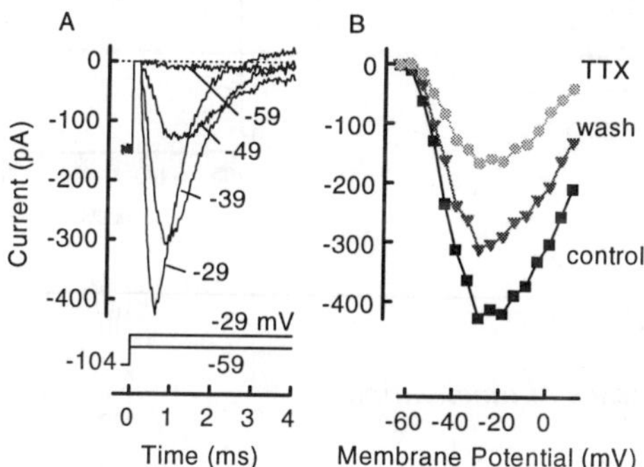

Figure 1.

3.2 Tetrodotoxin sensitivity and sodium dependence of transient inward current

For the cell in Figure 1, 500 nM TTX in the external medium reduced the peak current at −29 mV to −170 pA, 40% of the control current (Fig. 1B). Similar experiments were done on five other cells using six other TTX concentrations. The ratio of the peak currents in the presence and absence of TTX was plotted against TTX concentration and fitted with Equation 1:

$$\frac{I}{I_{control}} = \frac{1}{1 + \dfrac{[TTX]}{K_D}} \tag{1}$$

The best least-squares fit was produced by a K_D of 348 nM, in between the value for sodium channels from rat brain (~10 nM) and values for cardiac sodium channels from various mammalian tissues (650 nM - 1.3 μM) [17].

Two cells were superfused with an extracellular solution in which the impermeable cation N-methyl-D-glucosamine (NMDG) was substituted for sodium and potassium. The transient inward currents disappeared as soon as the NMDG solution displaced the control solution (data not shown). The effect was readily reversed. Thus, the transient inward currents were carried by sodium through TTX-sensitive channels.

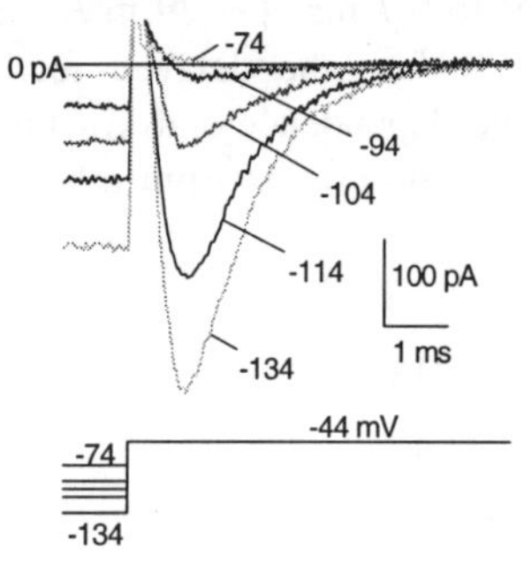

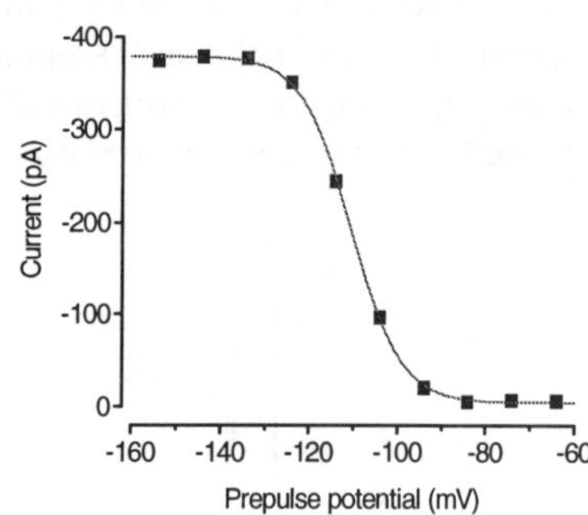

Figure 2.   Figure 3.

3.3 *Voltage dependence of inactivation*

Figures 2 and 3 show the voltage dependence of inactivation of the sodium conductance, g_{Na}. g_{Na} was activated by stepping to −44 mV after 16-ms prepulses at potentials between −154 and −64 mV from a holding potential of −84 mV (Fig. 2). Peak I_{Na} was plotted against the prepulse potential (Fig. 3). The resulting inactivation curve was well-fitted by a first-order Boltzmann function:

$$I(V_m) = \frac{I_{max}}{1 + e^{\frac{(V_m - V_{1/2})}{S}}} \tag{2}$$

I_{max} is the membrane current with g_{Na} fully activated; V_m is the prepulse potential; $V_{1/2}$ is the potential at which half the current is activated; S is the voltage that evokes an e-fold change in g_{Na}. For five type II cells, the mean $V_{1/2}$ and S values were -104 ± 8.2 mV and 6.2 ± 1.6 mV. This voltage range of inactivation is similar to that of sodium channels in other hair cells, but more negative than that of axonal sodium channels[18].

3.4 Current size and distribution

We examined the size and distribution of I_{Na} as functions of age from PD 1 to adult. Using the voltage protocol of Figure 1A, we found that 52 type II cells (42%) had I_{Na}. The mean value between -30 and 20 $-$mV was -212 ± 180 pA. There was no significant change with age either in current amplitude or in the percentage of type II cells with I_{Na}. Of the 94 type I cells in the sample, only one showed a transient inward current (-116 pA at -24 mV) when the voltage protocol of Figure 1A was applied.

4   Discussion

A voltage-gated, TTX-sensitive g_{Na} is present in a large fraction of type II hair cells of the mouse utricle, but not in type I cells. Its properties are consistent with those described for other hair cells. Relative to axonal g_{Na}, the hair cell conductance has a more negative voltage range of inactivation and reduced sensitivity to TTX.

The relatively negative voltage range of inactivation raises doubts about the physiological role of these channels. From the average inactivation curve described in Results, only 0.2% of the cell's sodium channels would be activated at steady state at the mean resting potential of mouse utricular type II cells (-65 mV[14]). If these conditions hold *in vivo*, sodium channels would contribute only in the event of depolarizing inputs that follow hyperpolarizing inputs such as efferent-evoked ipsp's. Consistent with this, in current clamp experiments on the mouse utricular cells, we have not observed spiking at the resting potential or in response to depolarizing current steps. However, either the resting potential or the inactivation curve may differ *in vivo*. If some type II cells have a resting potential *in vivo* that is close to the potassium equilibrium potential, say -84 mV, then ~4% of the channels would be available at steady state. Given the high input resistances of some type II cells (>1 GΩ), even this small number of channels could significantly boost the onset of the depolarizing response to positive current. For a cell with an input resistance of 1 GΩ , 4% of the mean maximal I_{Na} (212 pA) would contribute close to 10 mV depolarization. The sodium channels might therefore boost the responses of cells with relatively negative resting potentials into the voltage range of activation of the calcium channels that mediate transmitter release (positive to −60 or −50 mV in hair cells [19]). Hair cells that produce spikes with a sodium component do have resting potentials more negative than −70 mV[1,5,9].

Another possibility is that the voltage range of the inactivation curve is less negative *in vivo*. In the whole-cell recording method used here, soluble intracellular second messengers will wash out with time. I_{Na} inactivation may reside in the intracellular loop connecting membrane-spanning domains III and IV, which has a phosphorylation site[20]. Second messengers affect I_{Na} inactivation in other cell types[20,21].

Acknowledgments

This research was supported by NIDCD grant RO1-DC02290.

References

1. Evans, M.G. and Fuchs, P.A. (1987) Tetrodotoxin-sensitive, voltage-dependent sodium currents in hair cells for the alligator cochlea, *Biophys. J.* **52** 649-652.
2. Hudspeth, A.J. and Corey, D.P. (1977) Sensitivity, polarity, and conductance change in the response of vertebrate hair cells to controlled mechanical stimuli, *Proc. Natl. Acad. Sci. USA.* **74** 2407-2411.
3. Fuchs, P.A., Nagai, T., and Evans, M.G. (1988) Electrical tuning in hair cells isolated from the chick cochlea, *J. Neurosci.* **8** 2460-2467.
4. Fuchs, P.A. (1992) Ionic currents in cochlear hair cells, *Progress in Neurobiology.* **39** 493-505.
5. Sugihara, I. and Furukawa, T. (1989) Morphological and functional aspects of two different types of hair cells in the goldfish sacculus, *J. Neurophysiol.* **62** 1330-1343.
6. Kros, C.J., Rüsch, A., Richardson, G.P., and Russell, I.J. (1993) Sodium and calcium currents in cultured cochlear hair cells of neonatal mice, *J. Physiol.* **473** 231P- (Abstract).
7. Witt, C.M., Hu, H.-Y., Brownell, W.E., and Bertrand, D. (1994) Physiologically silent sodium channels in mammalian outer hair cells, *J. Neurophysiol.* **72** 1037-1040.
8. Sokolowski, B.H.A., Stahl, L.M., and Fuchs, P.A. (1993) Morphological and physiological development of vestibular hair cells in the organ-cultured otocyst of the chick, *Dev. Biol.* **155** 134-146.
9. Chen, W.-Y. and Eatock, R.A. (1993) Voltage-dependent conductances in hair cells isolated from the semicircular canal organs of rats, *ARO Abstr* **16** 20. (Abstract).
10. Wilson, V.J. and Melvill Jones, G. (1979) In: Mammalian Vestibular

Physiology, (Plenum Press, NY)

11. Wersäll, J. (1956) Studies on the structure and innervation of the sensory epithelium of the crista ampullares in the guinea pig, *Acta Otolaryngol.* **126** (Suppl.) 1-85.

12. Correia, M.J. and Lang, D.G. (1990) An electrophysiological comparison of solitary type I and type II vestibular hair cells, *Neurosci. Lett.* **116** 106-111.

13. Rennie, K.J. and Correia, M.J. (1994) Potassium currents in mammalian and avian isolated type I semicircular canal hair cells, *J. Neurophysiol.* **71** 1 1-13.

14. Rüsch, A. and Eatock, R.A. (1996) A delayed rectifier conductance in type I hair cells of the mouse utricle, *J. Neurophysiol.* **76** (In Press).

15. Rüsch, A. and Eatock, R.A. (1996) Voltage responses of mouse utricular hair cells to injected currents, *Ann. N Y Acad. Sci.* **781** 71-84.

16. Eatock, R.A., Chen, W.Y., and Saeki, M. (1994) Potassium currents in mammalian vestibular hair cells, *Sensory Systems* **8** 21-28.

17. Krafte, D.S. (1994) Cardiac sodium channel expression in *Xenopus* oocytes, In: Handbook of Membrane Channels: Molecular and Cellular Physiology, ed. C. Peracchia (Academic Press, San Diego) pp. 115-120.

18. Hodgkin, A.L. and Huxley, A.F. (1952) A quantitative description of membrane current and its application to conduction and excitation in nerve, *J. Physiol.* **117** 500-544.

19. Zidanic, M. and Fuchs, P.A. (1995) Kinetic analysis of barium currents in chick cochlear hair cells, *Biophys. J.* **68** 1323-1336.

20. Catterall, W.A. (1992) Cellular and molecular biology of voltage-gated sodium channels, *Physiol. Rev.* **72** S15-S48.

21. Fraser, D.D., Hoehn, K., Weiss, S., and MacVicar, B.A. (1993) Arachidonic acid inhibits sodium currents and synaptic transmission in cultured striatal neurons, *Neuron* **11** 633-644.

THE FUNCTION OF THE CYTOSKELETON IN DETERMINING THE MECHANICAL PROPERTIES OF EPITHELIAL CELLS WITHIN THE ORGAN OF CORTI

J.A. TOLOMEO, M.C. HOLLEY

Dept. of Physiology, University of Bristol

Bristol, BS8 1TD, England

J.Tolomeo@bris.ac.uk

M.C.Holley@bris.ac.uk

The mechanical properties of the cytoskeletal components of outer hair cells and pillar cells were measured. The cortical lattice in outer hair cells has a circumferential resultant stiffness modulus of 3×10^{-3} N/m, similar to that of the intact cell cortex. The axial stiffness modulus of the lattice is only 5×10^{-4} N/m. Thus, the lattice circumferentially reinforces the cell cortex and directs motility along the longitudinal direction. The stiffness of pillar cells was found to be dominated by the microtubule bundles. The measured Young's modulus for the microtubules was 6.5×10^9 N/m^2 which is similar to reported values of isolated single microtubules. This result implies that the total axial cell stiffness of a pillar cell is approximately four orders of magnitude greater than that of an outer hair cell. Predictive results for Dieiters' cells indicate that they are also significantly stiffer than outer hair cells. These relatively stiff supporting cells may transfer motion and forces between the basilar membrane and reticular lamina in a nearly rigid manner.

1 Introduction

Epithelial cells within the mammalian cochlea have developed very specialized cytoskeletal structures. It is reasonable to assume that this specialization is directly related to their contribution to the mechanical properties of the cochlea. It should be possible to predict mechanical properties based on a knowledge of cell morphology and constituent material properties. In this present work, the correlation between morphology and mechanical properties is tested for outer hair cells and pillar cells from the guinea pig organ of Corti. These cells have geometrically distinct cytoskeletal networks which facilitate this kind of 'bottom-up' approach to structural analysis. The function of these cells and cytoskeletal structures are subsequently discussed in terms of their measured mechanical properties

Outer hair cells are believed to enhance frequency discrimination within the cochlea. They accomplish this through a biophysical mechanism which allows them to change length in response to transmembrane electrical potential.[1] The three distinct layers that make up the cell cortex are the plasma membrane, the cytoskeletal lattice, and the lateral cisternae. The cytoskeletal lattice consists of an array of thick circumferential filaments, possibly actin, and small longitudinal cross-linking filaments thought to be spectrin.[2] It has been proposed that the cytoskeletal lattice mechanically reinforces the lateral wall and directs motility along the longitudinal axis of the cell.[3] This hypothesis is based on the clear visual anisotropy of the lattice.

Pillar cells form the arch of Corti which separates the inner hair cells from the outer hair cells. The central portion of each pillar cell is a long slender rod packed with a continuous bundle of parallel microtubules and actin filaments.[4] The apex and base of each pillar cell contains a large actin dense cap where the microtubules terminate.[5] The triangular form of the arch of Corti gives the impression of a truss like structure which would provide a relatively stiff and efficient means of transferring motion between the basilar membrane and the reticular lamina. It is known that microtubules are relatively stiff structures,[6] and therefore it is predicted that the longitudinal stiffness of the pillar cells may be large.

2 Material and Methods

Guinea pigs were killed by cervical dislocation and their cochleae removed. The organs of Corti were dissected from the cochlear spiral in Liebovitz L-15 (GIBCO) solution and cells were dissociated by rapidly cycling the organ of Corti repeatedly through a pipette tip. Preparations for pillar cells were incubated for 30 minutes in collagenase (SIGMA, type VII) prior to dissociation. Dissociated cells were mounted on glass slides containing a well of about 400μl of L-15 solution and a cocktail of enzyme inhibitors (100μg/ml Phenylmethyl-sulphonylflouride, 1 μg/ml Pepstatin, 1μg/ml Leupeptin, and 2mM Benzamidine). Cells were viewed through a Nikon Diaphot inverted microscope and images were recorded in real time with a super VHS video recorder. Quantitative analysis was performed by replaying the video through image analysis software (Brian Reece Scientific Ltd.).

A three point bending test was used to measure the bending and extensional moduli of both hair cells and pillar cells. Two relatively large rigid glass probes were placed against each end of one side of the cell. A calibrated measurement probe was applied to the opposite side of the cell midway between the stationary points. The calibrated probe was driven by a piezoelectric bender element connected to a Feedback FG601 signal generator at about 1 Hz with 6μm maximum free displacement. The difference in the probe displacement under free conditions and when in contact with the cell gave the force at the probe tip and, therefore, the force on the cell. Maximum axial strains induced in the cell were about 3%.

Measurements of the outer hair cell cytoskeletal lattice were made from cells whose membranes were extracted with 0.1% Triton X-100. Longitudinal stiffness measurements of the cytoskeletal lattice were made from cells held to the slide at their cuticular plates. The measurement probe was attached to the basal end of the lattice and pretensioned by adjusting the micromanipulator. Maximum prestrain was about 10% while the oscillating load induced strains of about 3%.

Cells prepared for circumferential stiffness measurements were dissociated more vigorously in order to remove their cuticular plates. Both rigid and measurement probes were then inserted into the cell and pretensioned.

Displacement of the measurement probe was initiated once the probes were located and the cell membranes were then extracted with 0.1% Triton X-100. Maximum circumferential strains were about 10% with an additional 10% prestrain.

3 Results

3.1 Outer Hair Cells

Three point bending of isolated outer hair cells was used to determine the bending and Young's moduli of the intact cell cortex. The calculations depend on the application of Euler beam theory where the bending modulus is defined as the product of the Young's modulus and the moment of inertia. For a load applied at the midpoint of a simply supported beam the bending modulus is

$$EI = \frac{F L^3}{u\,48} \tag{1}$$

where E is the Young's modulus, F is the normal component of applied force, u is the normal component of displacement, I is the moment of inertia, and L is the length between fixed probes. For 17 cells tested the bending modulus was $EI = 1 \pm 0.7 \times 10^{-18}$ Nm^2 ($\pm$standard deviation). The moment of inertia is a purely geometric term which for a thin cylinder is $I = \pi r^3 t$ where r is the cell radius and t is the cortex thickness. Using a radius of $r = 5$ μm gives the resultant Young's modulus as $Et = 3 \pm 1.5 \times 10^{-3}$ N/m, where the modulus was found to be independent of cell length. The axial compliance of the cylindrical cell is $C = L/2\pi r Et$ and therefore the total compliance for a cell 65 μm in length is 690 m/N. This is within previous experimentally measured values.[3,7,13]

The compliance of the cytoskeletal lattice was measured using a uniaxial tension test where the resultant Young's modulus is

$$Et = \frac{F\,l}{u\,w} \tag{2}$$

where l is the length of the area being tested and w is the width of the area. The resultant Young's modulus for 20 cells was $5 \pm 2 \times 10^{-4}$ N/m. Again, these results were independent of cell length. The corresponding lattice compliance for a cell of 65 μm length was $C = 4100$ m/N. Thus the lattice appears to contribute very little to the axial cortex stiffness in agreement with a previous report.[3] In contrast, the Young's modulus in the circumferential direction from 13 cells was $3 \pm 2 \times 10^3$ N/m. Therefore, the circumferential stiffness of the lattice may contribute significantly to the stiffness of the intact cell cortex.[12]

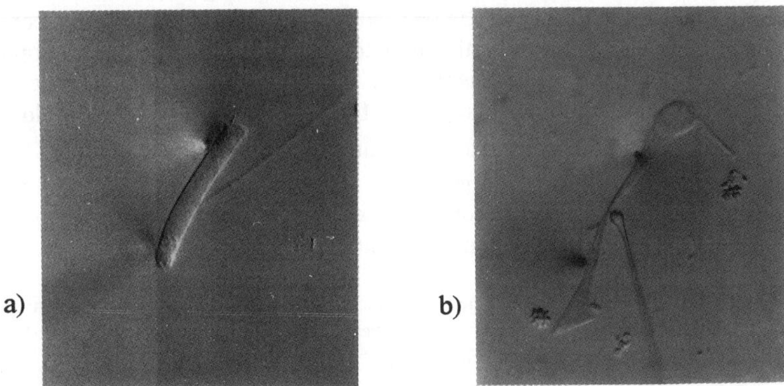

Figure 1 Three point bending of **a)** an outer hair cell (length 65 mm) and **b)** pillar cell (length 95 mm).

3.2 Pillar Cells

The three point bending test was also used to determine the bending and Young's moduli of the cytoskeletal proteins within pillar cells. Equation 1 still holds for the bending modulus where the only difference is in the definition of the moment of inertia as will be described. The bending modulus was measured from 23 cells to be $EI=4\pm3\times10^{-19}\text{Nm}^2$.

The axial Young's modulus can be computed from the bending modulus given an estimate of the moment of inertia. It is assumed that most of the axial stiffness is due to the microtubules. There are about 2500 microtubules within the central rod portion of the cell and each has a diameter of approximately $d=27$ nm.[4] Experimental observations suggested that there was very little effective elasticity linking individual microtubules together. Therefore the total moment of inertia is the sum of the moments of inertia from each individual microtubule, or $I=2500\pi d^4/64$. This gives a Young's modulus for the microtubules of about $E=6.5\pm5\times10^9$ N/m^2 which compares well with previous reported values of $E=1.2\times10^9$ N/m^2 measured from isolated microtubules.[6] Our measured Young's modulus corresponds to an axial compliance for a 100 µm length cell of $C=0.01$m/N. This is about 10^4 times stiffer than a comparable outer hair cell.

The pillar cells were extremely difficult to dissociate intact even after incubation in collagenase. Cells were generally chosen for appearance which included an intact process, well defined outline, and smooth foot plate. However, phalloidin fluorescence studies showed that the membranes had been disrupted in the majority of the dissociated cells.

3.3 Deiters' Cells

The demonstrated correlation between morphology and measured mechanical properties found for the pillar cell can be used to make predictions of the mechanical properties of other elements within the organ of Corti. The Deiters' cells support the outer hair cells above the basilar membrane. The Deiters' cell bodies are known to possess about 500 microtubules that extend from the region of the cup holding the outer hair cell down to the basilar membrane.[4] It is assumed that the Young's modulus for these microtubules is the same as those in the pillar cells. For a Deiters' cell 65μm in length this predicts a total cell axial compliance of $C=0.04$N/m This is still at least 10^3 times stiffer than the outer hair cell.

Table 1 Summary of measured and predicted mechanical properties. The circumferential stiffness of the cortical lattice is similar to the stiffness of the intact cell cortex. The pillar cells and Deiters' cells are relatively rigid compared to the outer hair cells.

Cell Type		
outer hair cell bending modulus	$1\pm0.7 \times 10^{-18}$	Nm^2
outer hair cell compliance (length = 65mm)	690	m/N
outer hair cell cortex axial resultant modulus	$3\pm1.5 \times 10^{-3}$	N/m
outer hair cell lattice axial resultant modulus	$5\pm2 \times 10^{-4}$	N/m
outer hair cell lattice circum. resultant modulus	$3\pm2 \times 10^{-3}$	N/m
pillar cell bending modulus	$4\pm3 \times 10^{-19}$	Nm^2
pillar cell axial compliance (length = 100mm)	0.01	m/N
Deiters' cell axial compliance (length = 65mm)	0.04	m/N

4 Discussion

4.1 Outer Hair Cells

The measurements of outer hair cell stiffness support the hypothesis that the cytoskeletal lattice significantly reinforces the lateral cortex in the circumferential direction, but provides negligible axial stiffness. The clear morphological anisotropy of the lateral cortex is directly reflected in the measured mechanical properties. If the membrane layers are isotropic, then it would be reasonable to expect that the cell cortex, per unit area, is about twice as stiff in the circumferential direction as the axial direction. The direct implication that the membrane layers dominate the axial stiffness of the cell is also consistent with the idea that the plasma membrane is the location of high frequency force generation.

The axial compliance of the cell is the fundamental mechanical property determining how much force the cell can deliver in relation to the stiffness of the surrounding structure. Our compliance measurements were within the range of previous experimental values. In contrast, theoretical compliance estimates based on a single degree of freedom model[8] and the assumption of isotropy[9] tend to overestimate the axial compliance with calculated values of 16 m/N and 82 m/N respectively. Anisotropic material properties are required to describe the deformation response of the outer hair cell for general load conditions[10,11]

4.2 *Pillar Cells*

The pillar cell membranes were frequently broken during mechanical dissociation. The effect of this would be to release soluble intracellular proteins, some of which may be structurally important. This means that our estimates of axial stiffness are likely to be lower than the actual values *in vivo*. However, The microtubules are extremely stable and do not depolymerize even following the addition of the detergent Triton X-100.

The large stiffness of the pillar cells indicates that the arch of Corti may rotate as a nearly rigid body during basilar membrane motion. This would ensure efficient transfer of motion from the basilar membrane into shearing motion of the reticular lamina. The predicted relative stiffness of the Deiters' cell body compared to the outer hair cell indicates that they may transfer force and displacement between the basilar membrane and the outer hair cell in an efficient manner. This is important for current cochlear models which rely on force generation from the outer hair cell as a form of energy input into the basilar membrane. However, a more detailed micromechanical analysis of the organ of Corti structure is needed to account for the effects of geometry. The generation of bending moments may be significant in determining the load paths and effective compliance of each cellular structure.

References

1. Kalinec, F., Holley, M.C., Iwasa, K., Lim, D.J., and Kachar, B. (1992) A membrane-based force generation mechanism in auditory sensory cells, *Proc Natl. Acad. Sci. USA.* **89** 8671-8675.
2. Holley, M.C. and Ashmore, J.F. (1990) Spectrin, actin and the structure of the cortical lattice in mammalian cochlear outer hair cells, *J. Cell. Sci.* **96** 283-291.
3. Holley, M.C. and Ashmore, J.F. (1988) A cytoskeletal spring in cochlear outer hair cells, *Nature* **335** 635-637.
4. Angelberg, C. and Engstrom, H. (1972) Supporting elements in the organ of Corti. I. Fibrillar structures in the supporting cells of the organ of Corti of mammals, *Acta. Otolaryngol. Suppl.* **301** 49-60.
5. Slepecky N. and Chamberlain, S.C. (1983) Distribution and polarity of actin in inner ear supporting cells, Hear. Res. **10** 359-370.
6. Gittes F., Mickey, B., Nettleton, J., and Howard, J. (1993) Flexural rigidity of microtubules and actin filaments measured from thermal fluctuations in shape, *J. Cell Bio.* **120** 923-934.
7. Hallworth, R. (1995) Passive compliance and active force generation in the guinea pig outer hair cell, *J. of Neurophys.* **74** 2319-2328

8. Mountain, D.C. and Hubbard, A.E. (1994) A piezoelectric model of outer hair cell function, *J. Acoust. Soc. Am.* **95** 350-354.

9. Iwasa, K.H. and Chadwick, R.S. (1992) Elasticity and active force generation of cochlear outer hair cells, *J. Acoust. Soc. Am.* **92** 3169-3173.

10. Dallos, P., Hallworth, R., and Evans, B.N. (1993) Theory of electrically-driven shape changes of cochlear outer hair cells, *J. Neurophys.* **70** 299-323.

11. Tolomeo, J.A. and Steele, C.R. (1995) Orthotropic piezoelectric properties of the cochlear outer hair cell wall, *J. Acoust. Soc. Amer.* **97** 3024-3029.

12. Tolomeo, J.A., Steele, C.R., and Holley, M.C. (1996) Mechanical properties of the lateral cortex of the mammalian outer hair cell, *Biophys J.* (accepted for publication).

13. Russel, I.J. and Schauz, C. (1995) Salicylate otoxicity: effects on the stifffness and electromotility of outer hair cells isolated from the guinea pig cochlea, *Aud. Neurosci.* **1** 309-320.

MECHANICAL MODELS OF THE STEREOCILIA BUNDLE OF THE MAMMALIAN COCHLEAR HAIR CELL

D.E. ZETES AND C.R. STEELE

Division of Applied Mechanics, Stanford University
Stanford, CA 94305, USA
dzetes@am-sun2.stanford.edu
chas@am-sun2.stanford.edu

Mechanotransduction in the mammalian cochlea is mediated by deflection of the stereocilia bundle. To investigate the motion of the stereocilia at auditory frequencies, multi-degree of freedom equations of motion for the fluid-structure interaction of the stereocilia bundle have been developed. Solutions have been compared for several measured bundle geometries from the guinea pig cochlea. Results indicate that motion of the stereocilia may exist without substantial attenuation at least up to the frequency corresponding to the location of the outer hair cell along the cochlear duct. In addition, an analytical model of charged flow through ion channels located in the stereocilia walls indicates that flow through the mechanotransduction channel may significantly effect stereocilia motion.

1   Introduction

Current models of mechanotransduction hypothesize that deflection of the stereocilia bundle causes ion flow through stretch-activated channels located along the stereocilia surface.[1] We report on two aspects of the stereocilia bundle that have been investigated by mathematical modeling. First, the fluid-structure interaction of the stereocilia bundle is modeled to consider its frequency response in relation to mechanotransduction. Second, the mechanotransduction channel of the stereocilia bundle is modeled by ionized flow through an elastic orifice to investigate forces caused by the flow of ions through the channel.

2   Frequency Response of the Stereocilia Bundle

Qualitative models of mechanotransduction have in common a reliance on relative motion of the stereocilia for operation of ion channels at auditory frequencies. At present, however, it is not clear how the motion of the fluid and surrounding structures influence displacement of the stereocilia. The viscosity of the endolymphatic fluid will attenuate the magnitude of stereocilia motion for higher excitation frequencies.[2] The dynamic fluid-structure interaction of the stereocilia bundle must therefore be investigated. In this analysis, the viscous contributions of fluid surrounding the stereocilia are addressed and incorporated into linear dynamic equations of motion. Solutions are compared for several measured geometries of guinea-pig stereocilia bundles along the cochlear duct as obtained in transmission electron microscopy (TEM).

2.1 Measured Geometric Variation

Whole guinea-pig cochleas were embedded and cut into hemicoils with a mounted annular diamond blade.[3] Ultra-thin radial sections (80 nm) were cut from each hemicoil, collected onto copper grids, stained with uranyl acetate and lead citrate, and photographed in a JEOL 100CX TEM at X8,300 and X13,000. The magnification was calibrated in each observation session with a grating of 2160 lines/mm (Agar Scientific). Stereociliary lengths were measured from the apical density to the intersection of the center of the rootlet and apical membrane[4]. Multiple measurements (2-11) of all dimensions were made at each location. After sectioning, the location from which the ultra-thin sections had been taken was measured and Greenwood's function[5] used to obtain an estimate of the corresponding characteristic frequency.

2.2 Model Development

The tapered base of a stereocilium is such that when the stereocilium is loaded at its tip, the upper cylindrical portion appears to rotate in a rigid fashion.[6] Each stereocilium has therefore been treated as a rigid body with an apparent rotational spring at its basal attachment. This equivalent system is derived from Euler-Bernoulli beam theory for a beam of cross-section similar to a stereocilium. The tip links connecting the stereocilia have been treated as linear elastic springs.

With these assumptions, multi-degree of freedom equations of motion of a single column of three or more stereocilia have been derived[4]. The frequency response of the stereocilia bundle is considered for the loading case of a harmonic force applied to the tip of the tallest stereocilia. These solutions may be valid until the amplitude of stereocilia motion causes the net force in the tip links to become compressive.

2.3 Viscous Contributions

For small, physiologically reasonable displacements of the stereocilia, hydrodynamic contributions to the dynamic equations of motion are predominately linear and viscous. The stereocilia bundle may therefore be treated within the realm of lubrication theory as having two bearing surfaces, where the first bearing surface is between stereocilia of differing heights in the same column, and the second is between stereocilia of the same height in different columns.

For journal bearings of relatively small width and finite length, the pressure variation in the long direction is negligible in comparison to the pressure variation in the short direction.[7] It is therefore reasonable and consistent to assume that the pressure gradient in the axial direction of the stereocilia is small for both bearing surfaces of the stereocilia bundle, since the diameter of the stereocilia is much smaller than the stereocilium length. Then, between stereocilia of differing height, in the same column, the velocity profiles u and v, in the x and y direction respectively, are approximated by the familiar Poiseuille and Couette flows

$$u \approx \frac{1}{2\mu} \frac{\partial p}{\partial x} \left(z^2 - h(x,y)\, z \right) \qquad\qquad v \approx \frac{V z}{h(x,y)} \tag{1}$$

where x is the rotational axis for deflection of the bundle in the excitatory/inhibitory direction, y is the longitudinal axis of the stereocilia, V is the y component of the velocity of the stereocilia surfaces sliding relative to each other, and $h(x,y)$ is the separation between the stereocilia surfaces. Similar equations can be written for stereocilia in adjacent columns. The stereocilia may also separate with a velocity component in the excitatory/inhibitory direction which does not affect the above equations and is considered when satisfying continuity. Although these relationships (1) are strictly valid only for x and y within the stereocilia radius, the pressure solutions satisfy regularity at infinity.

2.4 Results

Solutions to the equations of motion can be used to consider the hypothesis that tension in the tip links promotes opening of the transduction channels.[1] Using the previously described measured stereocilia dimensions, diameter of 200 nm, rootlet separation of 400 nm, Young's modulus E = 20 MPa, and viscosity of water, the solution for the frequency response of the tension in the tip link is similar to a low pass filter.

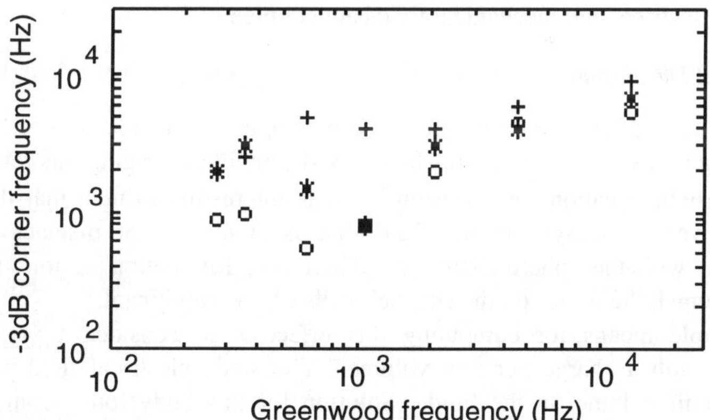

Figure 1: Corner frequency for the tension in the first tip link versus corresponding Greenwood's frequency for seven measured guinea-pig stereocilia bundle geometries along the cochlear duct. All frequencies are in Hz. (+ = OHC1, * = OHC2, o = OHC3)

The corner frequency, defined as 3 dB below the quasi-static solution, is shown in Figure 1 for stereocilia bundles geometries at seven different frequency-locations along the cochlear duct. The resulting range of corner frequencies is not sufficient to encompass the entire auditory range of the guinea pig. However, consideration of variation in stereocilia diameter and rootlet separation may further increase the range of solutions. From this analysis, it appears that the variation in morphology of the stereocilia bundle provides consistent solutions in the frequency domain, with viscous effects dominating at higher frequencies for bundles from higher frequency-locations and at lower frequencies for bundles from lower frequency-locations. This behavior supports the proposition that sufficient relative motion of the stereocilia occurs to operate ion channels at frequencies appropriate to the corresponding outer hair cell location. Further analysis with this model may allow comparison of alternate hypotheses regarding mechanotransduction.

3   Ionized Flow Through a Channel

Previous models for ion pumping,[8] are based on open and closed state configurations. It appears that computations in terms of fundamental mechanical and electrical properties for transition between the two states have not been carried out. It is likely that the forces caused by the flow of ions through the channel have a significant effect on stereocilia motion. A purely mechanical analog model of the hair cell[9] demonstrates that fluid flow through the channel has the effect of a negative spring in the system, as observed experimentally.[1]   A substantial improvement in the model is offered by consideration of an ionized fluid, with which the electrical and mechanical fields are coupled.

3.1   Model Development

The motion of a dilute suspension of ions can be approximated from Stokes' solution for the drag of a sphere in a viscous fluid. With suitable averaging this results in the Stokes-Einstein equation for diffusion.[10] It is interesting to note that the Stokes' solution gives a pressure in the fluid that is significant at distances large in comparison with the sphere diameter. Therefore, for motion of ions through a narrow channel, the forces on the channel walls can be significant.

A simple means for computing this effect is to consider a viscous fluid continuum with a charge per unit volume. The static electrical field produces a force per unit volume on the fluid. Solution for this body force from Laplace's equation is subsequently included in the Navier-Stokes equations which are solved for the fluid motion. For the channel configuration shown in Figure 2, the inlet and exit regions are approximated by spherically symmetric solutions, and the straight and tapered channel regions are approximated by laminar flow solutions

$$
V - V_{ref} = \begin{cases} \beta \left(\frac{1}{a} - \frac{1}{r} \right) & \text{spherical region} \\[2ex] 2\,\beta \int \frac{dz}{r^2(z)} & \text{tapered tube} \end{cases}
$$

$$
P - P_{ref} = \begin{cases} -q\,\beta \left(\frac{1}{a} - \frac{1}{r} \right) - \frac{2\,\mu\,Q}{\pi} \left(\frac{1}{a^3} - \frac{1}{r^3} \right) & \text{spherical region} \\[2ex] -2\,q\,\beta \int \frac{dz}{r^2(z)} - \frac{2\,\mu\,Q}{\pi} \int \frac{dz}{r^4(z)} & \text{tapered tube} \end{cases}
$$

$$
\tag{2}
$$

where V is the voltage, P is the pressure, β is the flow of the electrical field, Q is the flow rate of the fluid, q is the charge per unit volume, μ is the fluid viscosity, r is the radius, a is the inner radius, and z is the axial coordinate.

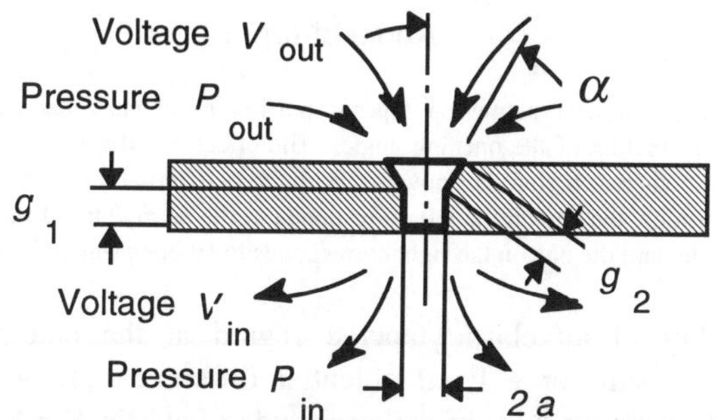

Figure 2: Flow of ionized fluid through a channel. The channel consists of a stiff portion with radius a, length g_1, and a tapered entrance region with taper length g_2 and taper angle a.

For the channel in Figure 2 with straight sides ($\alpha = 0$) and zero pressure on the inside and outside, the result for the conductance and the pressure at the entrance is

$$
Cond = \frac{q^2\,\pi\,a^4}{8\,\mu\,L \left(1 + \frac{a}{2\,L} \right)} \qquad\qquad P_{entrance} = \frac{q\,a \left(V_{out} - V_{in} \right)}{4\,L \left(1 + \frac{a}{2\,L} \right) \left(1 + \frac{a}{L} \right)}
$$

$$
\tag{3}
$$

where the total length is $L = g_1 + g_2$. For $a = 0.85$ nm, $L = 2.5$ nm, the viscosity of water $\mu = 0.0007$ Ns/m^2, and a 155 mM solution, the above result gives a conductivity of 22 pS, which is similar to the estimate for a single channel.[11] The pressure at the entrance for the same geometry and a potential difference of 140 mV is $P_{entrance} = 0.11$ MPa. Thus, according to this calculation, a localized pressure of relatively large positive magnitude exists at the channel entrance while a negative pressure of the same magnitude occurs at the outlet. Such a pressure distribution tends to open the channel at the entrance and close the channel at the outlet.

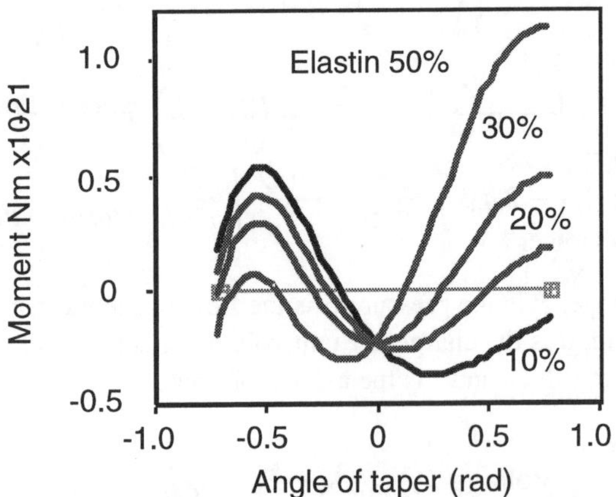

Figure 3: External moment acting on tapered portion of channel necessary to maintain equilibrium as a function of the opening angle. The effect of different values of the elastic modulus of the tapered region is shown. With zero external moment, there are three equilibrium positions, the one on the left corresponds to the nearly closed state, the one in the middle is unstable, and the one on the right corresponds to an open state.

The possibility of an elastic tapered region at the entrance can also be considered. The result for a fixed potential difference of 140 mV and elastic material with a Young's modulus of the magnitude of elastin $E = 4$ MPa, is shown in Figure 3. For zero external moment acting on the tapered region, there is a stable open position and a stable closed position. For fluctuations in the moment, for example, due to the passage of the discrete ions, the channel can pop between open and closed positions. The smaller the local maximum on the left portion of Figure 3, the less time the channel will be in the closed state. Thus mediation of the stiffness of the tapered region by electrical or chemical means can control the percentage of time in the open state.

Results from this model show that there are significant forces acting on the wall of the channel during passage of ions. It is interesting to note that the pressure acting on the entrance region of a channel has a negative spring behavior. For a high stiffness of the protein in the region of the entrance, the fluid effect is negligible. However, for a reasonable protein stiffness value, 10-50% of elastin, the fluid effect is significant and yields both closed and open equilibrium states. This channel model may provide a basis for the computation of the mechano-electrical interaction of the hair cell and stereocilia bundle as a whole.

Acknowledgment

The authors would like to thank Carole Hackney and Dave Furness for their help in preparation and processing of material for TEM.

References

1. Hudspeth, A.J. (1989) How the ear's works work, *Nature* **341** 397-404.
2. Steele, C.R., Baker, G., Tolomeo, J. and Zetes, D. (1993) Electro-mechanical models of the outer hair cell, in Biophysics of Hair Cell Sensory Systems, ed. Duifhuis, H. (World Scientific, Singapore) pp. 207-213.
3. Jiang, D., Furness, D.N., Hackney, C.M. and Lopez, D.E. (1993) Microslicing of the resin-embedded cochlea in comparison with the surface preparation technique for analysis of hair cell number and morphology, *Brit. J. Audiol.* **27**, 195-203.
4. Zetes, D.E., (1995) Mechanical and morphological study of the stereocilia bundle in the mammalian cochlea, Stanford University, Ph.D. Thesis.
5. Greenwood, D.D. (1990) A cochlear frequency-position function for several species - 29 years later, *J. Acoust. Soc. Am.* **87** 2592-2605.
6. Flock, A., Flock, B. and Murray, E. (1977) Studies on the sensory hairs of receptor cells in the inner ear, *Acta oto-laryngologica* **83** 85-91.
7. Ocvirk, F.W. (1952) Short bearing approximation for full journal bearings, *NACA Tech. Note*, 2808.
8. Markin, V.S. and Tsong, T.Y. (1991) Reversible mechanosensitive ion pumping as a part of mechanoelectrical transduction, *Biophys. J.* **59** 1317-1324.
9. Steele, C.R. (1992) Electro-elastic behavior of auditory receptor cells, *J. Biomimetics* **1** 3-22.
10. Hille, B. (1992) Ionic Channels of Excitable Membranes, (Sinauer Associates Inc., Massachusetts).
11. Pickles, J.O. (1988) An Introduction to the Physiology of Hearing, (Academic Press, London).

Part Six

Synthetic models of cellular elements

OUTER HAIR CELL ELECTRO-ANATOMY

W.E. BROWNELL, M. ZHI, J.A. HALTER

Baylor College of Medicine, Houston, TX 77030, USA
brownell@bcm.tmc.edu, mzhi@bcm.tmc.edu, jah@bcm.tmc.edu

The outer hair cell (OHC) possesses an inner subsurface cisterna (SSC) along its lateral wall that is within 30 nm of the outer cytoplasmic membrane. The SSC is a continuous membrane-bound structure extending from the cell's apical end to just below its nucleus and separating the OHC's axial core from the narrow extracisternal space. Measurements of intracellular pH reveal longitudinal proton-gradients in the axial core demonstrating the SSC is a functional as well a structural barrier. We have modeled the transmembrane potential of the OHC lateral-wall cytoplasmic-membrane using a distributed-parameter triaxial cable-model. The model describes the influence of the SSC on the transmembrane potential and indicates that the lateral-wall cytoplasmic-membrane cannot be isopotential.

1 The Outer Hair Cell Subsurface Cisterna

1.1 Structural Features of the Lateral Wall

The OHC has features common to all hair cells including a stereocilia bundle at its apical end and synaptic specializations at its basal end. Its lateral wall is a unique trilaminate structure composed of: 1) the cytoplasmic membrane, 2) the extracisternal space, and 3) the membrane-bound subsurface cisterna. The extracisternal space is a fluid-filled compartment bounded by the cytoplasmic membrane and the SSC. All three layers are located within 100 nm of the cell's outer surface.

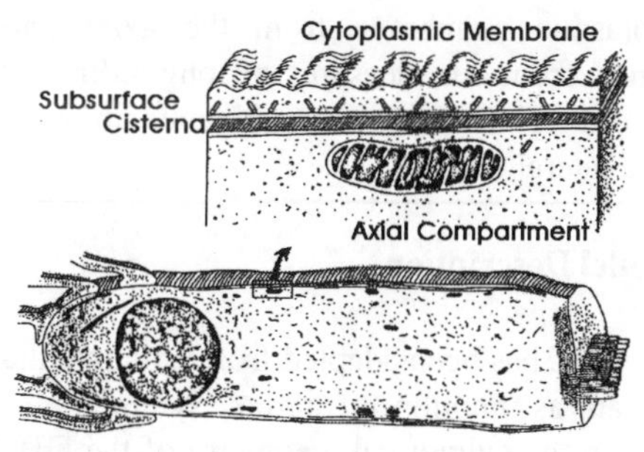

Figure 1. Drawing of an OHC (bottom) with a high magnification rendering of the lateral wall (top). The OHC is an 8 μm diameter cylinder capped at one end by the flattened cuticular plate and at the other by a hemisphere. OHC lengths vary from less than 20 μm in the high frequency region to more then 80 μm in the low frequency regions of the cochlea. The nucleus is displaced basally and occupies most of the hemispheric end. The cell's largest cytoplasmic filled compartment is the axial core located between the cuticular plate and the nucleus and bounded by the lateral wall.

The lateral wall extends from just below the tight junctions at the apical end of the cell to below the nucleus at its base. The extracisternal space contains cytoskeletal fibers known as the cortical lattice. The SSC and the cytoplasmic membrane are concentric cylinders.

574

1.2 pH Gradients in the Axial Core Suggest the SSC is Impermeable to Protons

We have measured the intracellular pH of isolated guinea pig OHCs using quantitative confocal scanning microscopy (see Chu et al.[1] for methods). The cells were loaded *in situ* with the fluorescent dye carboxy-SNARF-1 and placed in a constant flow chamber following isolation. The system was calibrated using the K^+-H^+ antiporter nigericin. Normal - untreated cells had a higher pH in the basal regions of the axial core near the nucleus. Similar pH gradients were found in nigericin treated cells. Longitudinal pH gradients were observed immediately after acidification by salicylate but were not seen after 30 minutes of exposure (see Fig. 2). Ultrastructural studies[2] have demonstrated that the SSC remains intact up to 10 minutes after the beginning of salicylate exposure but undergoes progressive dialation and vesiculation until it is completely disrupted by 30 minutes. Our pH results attest to the functional integrity of the SSC membranes in normal cells. They suggest that the axial core, bounded by the subsurface cisterna and the cuticular plate, is compartmentilized from the rest of the cytoplasm and communicates with it basally either around or through the nucleus.

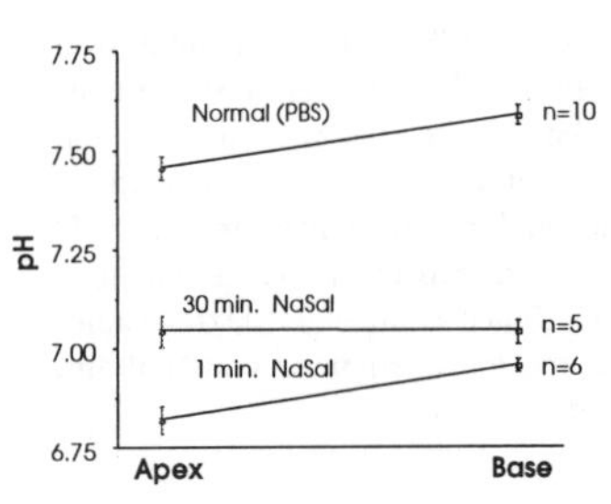

Figure 2. Longitudinal cytoplasmic pH gradients in normal and 10 mM sodium salicylate treated OHCs. The pH values were measured in the apical region (20-40 μm from cuticular plate), and basal portion (near nucleus). Error bars show standard error.

The SSC has at least two membranes for most of the lateral wall and should electrically insulate the adjacent cytoplasmic membrane from the axial core. Evidence for its insulating properties comes from our measures of longitudinal pH gradients. Additional evidence comes from voltage-clamp experiments in which ionic currents were not measured along the lateral wall[3].

2   Triaxial Distributed-parameter Model Description

A distributed-parameter model of the OHC has been adapted from a mammalian myelinated nerve fiber model[4]. Using an assumption of radial symmetry, an electrical equivalent network is derived from the cylindrical geometry of the OHC. This network is presented in Figs. 3&4. It is described by a coupled system of partial differential equations which is numerically integrated with an implicit algorithm similar in form to the Crank-Nicolson method. The system is based on two coupled partial differential equations:

$$C_{ssc}\frac{\partial V^{ax}}{\partial t} = \frac{a}{2\rho^{ax}}\frac{\partial^2 V^{ax}}{\partial x^2} + C_{ax}\frac{\partial V^{ec}}{\partial t} - J_{ssc}$$

and

$$(a\,C_{ssc} + b\,C_m)\frac{\partial V^{ec}}{\partial t} = \frac{a^2 + b^2}{2\rho^{ec}}\frac{\partial^2 V^{ec}}{\partial x^2} + a\,C_{ssc}\frac{\partial V^{ax}}{\partial t} + a\,J_{ssc} - b\,J_m$$

where V^{ax} and V^{ec} are the axial and extracisternal potentials relative to an external common reference potential; a is the radius of the SSC (4 μm) and b - a is the width of the extracisternal space (30 nm); $J_{ssc} = G_{ssc}\,(V^{ax} - V^{ec})$ is the leakage current density across the SSC and $J_m = G_m \cdot V^{ec}$ is the leakage current density across the cytoplasmic membrane. Axial and extracisternal resistivities (ρ^{ax} and ρ^{ec}) are 70 Ωcm, specific conductances for the basal, intermediate, and apical regions of the cytoplasmic membrane (G_m) are 1, 0.001, and 100 mS/cm^2, respectively. A low conductivity for the intermediate region is based on the absence of voltage dependent ion channels in this region[3] and examples of comparable conductivities for the photoreceptor outer-segment membrane[5]. The cytoplasmic membrane in the apical region of the model represents the entire apical region of the cell including the stereocilia. The surface area of the apical end is > 25% of the entire cell surface but in the model it remains fixed regardless of cell length. The resting state membrane potential is -78 mV. Simulations are performed with a Silicon Graphics Indigo R4400 computer. Sealed end conditions are assumed and a temporal step size of 1 μs is used.

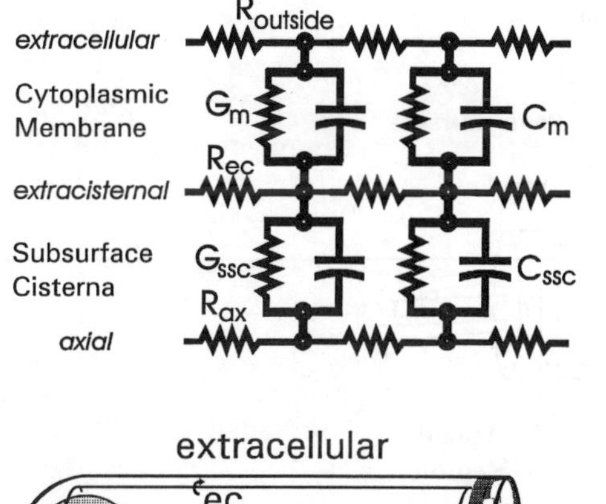

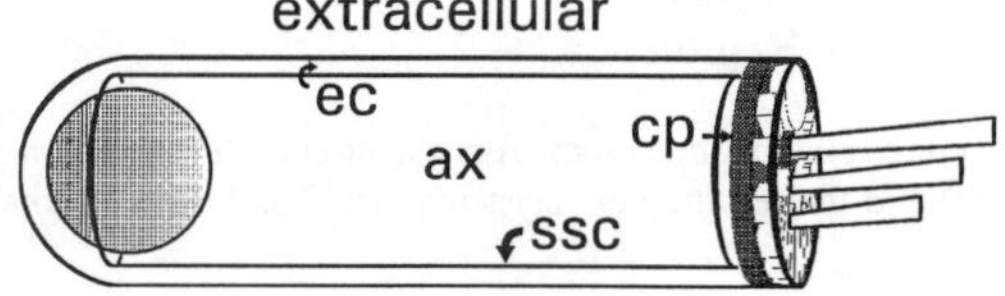

Figure 3. Equivalent electrical circuit of the OHC lateral-wall and cartoon of OHC. The membranes of the subsurface cisterna (ssc) separate the cytoplasm into an extracisternal space (ec) and an axial compartment (ax) which is capped apically by the cuticular plate (cp). The lateral-wall equivalent circuit contains three sets of resistors in series *Routside*, *Rec*, *Rax*. The resistors represent the specific resistivity of the fluid in the extracellular space, ec, and ax, respectively. The electrical properties of the cytoplasmic membrane are represented by *Gm* and *Cm*. Those of the two membranes of the subsurface cisterna are lumped into *Gssc* and *Cssc*. *Rec* varies inversely with the square of the width of the extracisternal space and *Rec>Rax>Routside*.

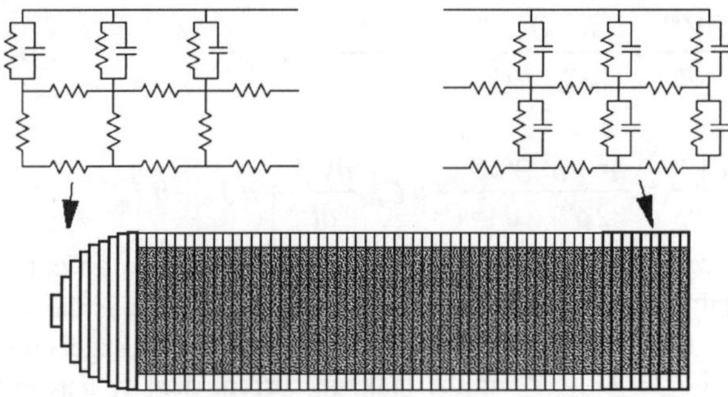

Figure 4. Schematic of model terminations with cartoon showing segmentation of the outer hair cell. Basal and apical regions are on the left and right respectively with the intermediate region in between (see Fig. 5, below). The cell is represented by a total 221 discrete spatial segments. The basal and apical regions are each 4 μm long. The specific conductance of the SSC (G_{ssc}) is 0.1 mS/cm^2 except in the basal region where it is 10^6 mS/cm^2. G_{ssc} represents the conductance of the cuticular plate in the apical region of the model. The specific capacitance for the cytoplasmic membrane and SSC (C_m & C_{ssc}) is 1 μF/cm^2 except in the basal region where the SSC terminates and C_{ssc} is 0 μF/cm^2.

3 Results

3.1 Current-clamp simulation

The model was used to explore the distribution of electrical potentials in the different compartments of the OHC (the OHCs electro-anatomy). Application of a constant-current step to the basal end of the OHC produced spatially-varying extracisternal and transcisternal potentials.

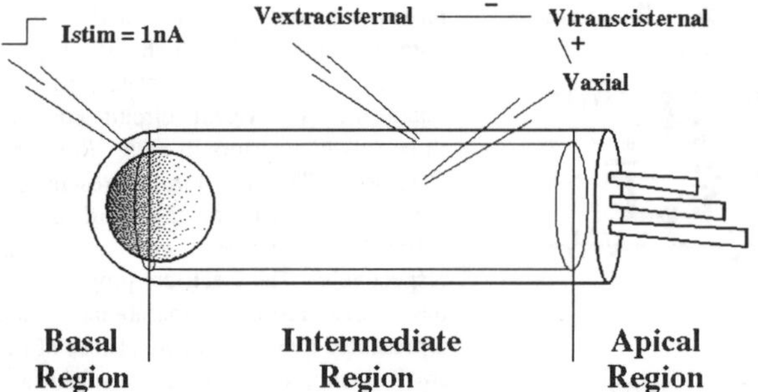

Figure 5. Scheme showing configuration for voltage clamp simulations. A constant-current step of 1 nA was applied to the basal end of the OHC model and the resulting extracisternal, axial and transcisternal potentials predicted.

3.2 Comparison with Experimental Data

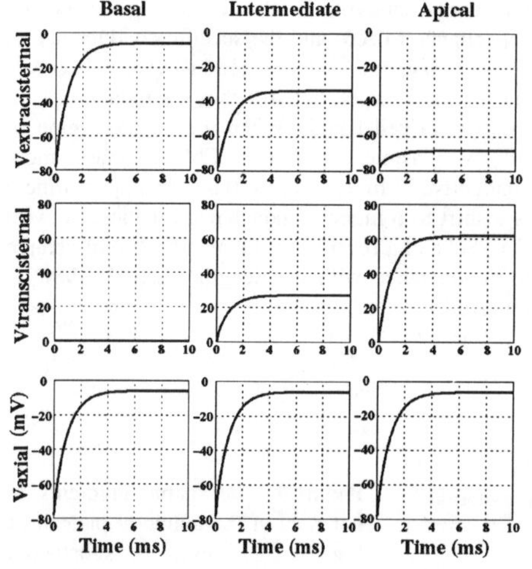

Figure 6. The resulting potentials show spatially-dependent temporal properties, where the extracisternal potentials are largest at the basal end and smallest at the apical end, the transcisternal potentials are complementary to these, being smallest at the basal end and greatest at the apical end and the axial potentials are approximately uniform in amplitude. This simulation is for an 80 µm long OHC.

Experimental data of Housley and Ashmore[6] for a population of OHCs reveals a decrease in the conductance with an increase in cell length. The model was used to compute input conductances for OHCs of different length. A good fit was made to the experimental data. The fit was achieved by assuming a relatively low specific conductivity of the cytoplasmic membrane in the medial regions of the OHC.

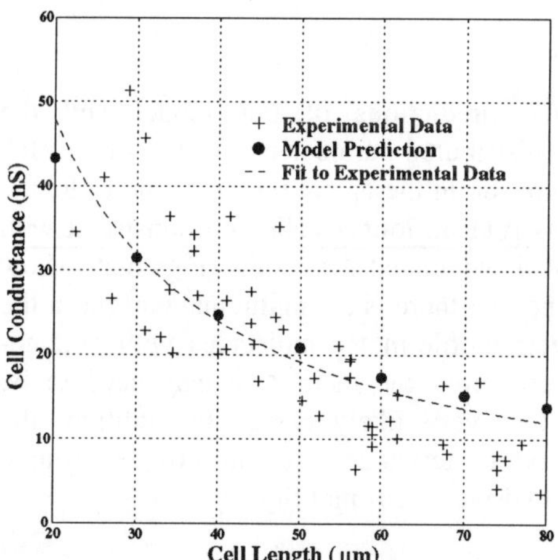

Figure 7. OHC conductance as a function of OHC length. Experimental data was provided by G.D. Housley. The experimental data is fit (dashed line) to the general expression for the conductivity of a conductive cylinder $G = A/\rho L$. The best fit to the data leads to the expression $G = 958$ nS-µm $/L$. The coefficient 958 nS-µm is close to the value of the cross sectional area of the extracisternal annulus divided by the resistivity of the cytoplasm. Our predicted conductance values as simulated by current pulse injection to the basal region of the OHC model are superimposed as solid black dots.

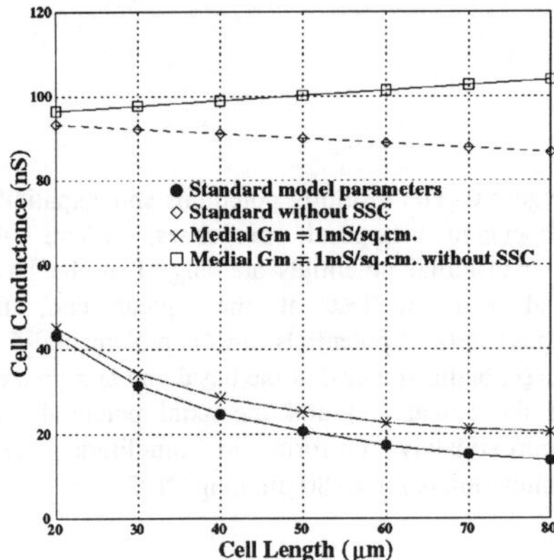

Figure 8. Predicted change in OHC conductance properties with and without the SSC present. Using standard model parameters as in Fig. 6 and effectively removing the SSC by setting the specific capacitance to zero and the specific conductance to 10^6 mS/sq.cm., the conductance becomes substantially larger, but still shows a reduction with increase in cell length. When the medial region of the cytoplasmic membrane (CM) is made more conductive (1 mS/sq.cm. vs. 0.001 mS/sq.cm.) there is a shift to a higher conductance for the case with the SSC and a reversal in the relationship of change in conductance with cell length when the SSC is removed.

3.3 Longitudinal Potential Gradients

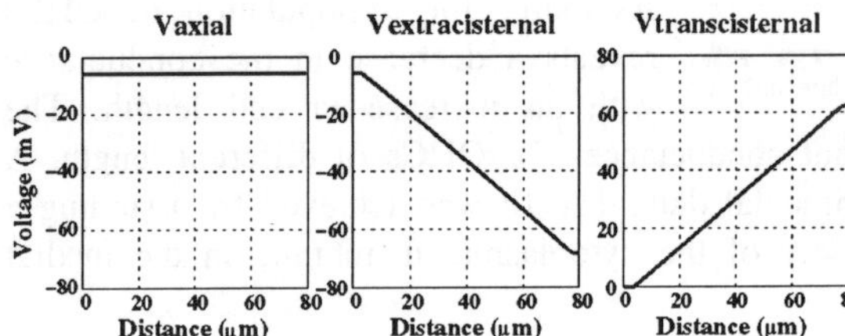

Figure 9. The spatial gradients in potential at the temporal plateau of Fig. 5 reveal substantial longitudinal currents in the extracisternal space as well as the possibility for a non-uniform spatial distribution of potential across the cytoplasmic membrane.

4 Discussion

The qualitative agreement between the predictions of our model and the experimental data are supportive of this distributed-parameter model of the OHC. Since purinergic receptors are thought to reside in the apical region of the OHC the the smaller currents evoked by exogenous ATP in longer cells[7] are consistent with the model. When the influence of the SSC is simulated the results (Figs 6&9) show that the OHC cannot be space-clamped and that there is a longitudinal current in the extracisternal space. Speculation on electromotile-motor molecules with voltage-sensors responsive to potential difference across the membrane may need to be revised to accommodate the gradient that very likely exists. In addition, the longitudinal voltage gradients within the extracisternal space could provide a source of potential energy that might be utilized to drive electromotility.

The model assumes that the axial compartment is capped by the cuticular plate (a dense matrix of cytoskeletal proteins that anchor the stereocilia). Furthermore, the model assumes no impediment for ion movement into the apical end of the extracisternal space. Structural features of the OHC cuticular plate support this possibility. The OHC cuticular plate is different than those of other hair cells. It is concave apically while cuticular plates in all other hair cells are convex[8]. It also extends to the periphery of the lateral wall while other hair cell cuticular plates do not[8,9]. The OHC cuticular plate is structurally anisotropic with cytoskeletal proteins radiating away from stereocilia rootlets towards the lateral wall[9]. The cuticular plates of other hair cells are morphologically isotropic. The fact that the OHC stereocilia rootlets do not penetrate the cuticular plate as they do in other hair cells[10] raises the intriguing possibility that transducer current through the stereocilia is directed radially towards the extracisternal space.

Acknowledgments

We appreciate the efforts of Kareem Zaghoul, John Criscione and Howard Fine for their contributions during the early stages of model development and Brian Phillips for his data analysis of the intracellular pH experiments. Work supported by research grant DC-00354 to WEB as well as funds from the Whitaker Foundation, the Vivian L. Smith Foundation for Restorative Neurology and the W.M. Keck Center for Computational Biology to JAH.

References

1. Chu, S. Brownell, W.E. and Montrose, M.H. (1995) Quantitative confocal imaging along the crypt-to-surface axis of colonic crypts. *Am. J. Physiology* **268** (*Cell Physiology 38*) C1557-1564.
2. Dieler, R., Shehata-Dieler, W.E. and Brownell, W.E. (1991) Concomitant salicylate-induced alterations of outer hair cell subsurface cisternae and electromotility. *J. Neurocytol.* **20** 637-653.
3. Santos-Sacchi, J. and Huang, G.-J. (1996) Electrical dissection of ionic conductances in the outer hair cell. *Abstracts of the Midwinter Research Meeting of the Association for Research in Otolaryngology* **19** 50.
4. Halter, J.A. and Clark, J.W. Jr. (1991) A distributed-parameter model of the myelinated nerve fiber. *J. Theor. Biol.* **148** 345-382.
5. Baylor, D.A. and Nunn, B.J. (1986) Electrical properties of the light-sensitive conductance of rods of the salamander *ambystoma tigrinum*. *J. Physiol.* **371** 115-145.
6. Housley, G.D. and Ashmore, J.F. (1992) Ionic currents of outer hair cells isolated from the guinea pig cochlea. *J. Physiol.* **448** 73-98.
7. Chen, C., Nenov, A. and R.P. Bobbin (1995). Noise exposure alters the OHC response to ATP. *Hear. Res.* **88** 215-21.
8. Liberman, M.C. (1987) Chronic ultrastructural changes in acoustic trauma: Serial-section reconstruction of sterocilia and cuticular plates. *Hear. Res.* **26** 65-88.
9. Raphael, Y., Athey, B.D., Wang, Y., Lee, M.K., and Altschuler, R.A. (1994) F-actin, tubulin and spectrin in the organ of Corti: comparative distribution in different cell types and mammalian species. *Hear. Res.* **76** 173-187.
10. Takasaka, T., Shinkawa, H., Hashimoto, S., Watanuki, K., and Kawamoto, K. (1983) High voltage electron microscopic study of the inner ear. *Ann. Otol. Rhinol. Laryngol. Suppl 92.* **101** 1-12.

MOTOR MECHANISMS OF THE OUTER HAIR CELL
FROM THE COCHLEA

K. H. IWASA

Biophysics Section, NIDCD, NIH
Bethesda, MD 20892-0922
iwasa@nih.gov

The membrane capacitance of the outer hair cell has a bell-shaped dependence on the membrane potential. This singular property is a manifestation of numerous charges mobile across the membrane. If this charge transfer is directly coupled with mechanical changes in the membrane, electrical energy obtained at the plasma membrane is used for cell motility. This mechanism is confirmed by the observation that the membrane capacitance is also dependent on membrane tension. The mechanical changes of the motor so far examined are limited to area changes. The mechanical energy, however, may consist of two terms. One is due to area changes and the other due to stiffness changes. To clarify the characteristics of these two terms and to evaluate their relative significance, two extreme cases are examined. In one extreme, changes in stiffness are ignored, as in previous treatments. In the other extreme, only stiffness changes are considered. Comparison with experimental data indicates that the motility of the outer hair cell is primarily based on area changes.

1 Introduction

It has been shown that the fast motility of the outer hair cell,[1] which is important for tuning of the mammalian ear, is independent of ATP,[2, 3] the energy source of usual cellular motilities. It is also insensitive to Ca ion,[3, 4] a common messenger for these motilities. Such a unique motility can only be based on a membrane motor which directly converts electrical energy into mechanical energy. The direct utilization of electrical energy is possible if a charge movement across the cell membrane is coupled with mechanical changes in the membrane. The existence of such mobile charges is confirmed by measuring the membrane capacitance[5, 6] and transient currents[7] similar to the 'gating current' of ion channels. It has further been shown that electrical energy obtained with this mechanism is sufficient for the mechanical work done by the cell.[8] Direct mechano-electrical coupling is evidenced by the observation that a change in membrane tension, as well as in the the membrane potential, affects the state of the motor.[6, 9, 10] Mechanical work associated with such a membrane motor can be based on a membrane area change of the motor.[6, 11,12] This mechanism can be referred to as 'area motor.' Alternatively, a change in the elastic compliance of the motor associated with the charge movement can also contribute to mechanical work. The latter mechanism can be called 'stiffness motor.' These two effects may also appear in the description of stretch-activated channels.[13]

While it has been shown that models based solely on area changes of the motor (area-change model) are satisfactory in explaining the experimental data so far obtained, models based on stiffness changes of the motor (stiffness motor) have not been examined. This problem is addressed in this report.

2   Motor Mechanisms

and contributes to the total strain of the cell. One mode of the contribution is by changes in the membrane area of this motor. This effect is described by different cross-sectional areas the motor occupies in the membrane in the two states. The other mode is by motor stiffness changes. This effect is described by different elastic moduli in the two states. In the absence of external forces, membrane tension T_z in the axial direction and T_c in the circumferential direction are balanced by the pressure difference P across the membrane,

$$T_z = \tfrac{1}{2} rP, \tag{1a}$$

$$T_c = rP, \tag{1b}$$

where r is the radius of the cell in the standard condition.[8]   If an axial force is applied to the cell, the axial tension is represented by $rP/2 + T_x$, where T_x is tension due to an external axial force.

The values F_0 and F_1 of the free energy of the motor in two conformational state are,

$$F_0 = E_0 + q_0 V + [\tfrac{1}{2}(\varepsilon_a - \varepsilon_{a0})^2 K_0 + \tfrac{1}{2}(\varepsilon_s - \varepsilon_{s0})^2 \mu_0 - \varepsilon_z T_z - \varepsilon_c T_c] s_0, \tag{2a}$$

$$F_1 = E_1 + q_1 V + [\tfrac{1}{2}(\varepsilon_a - \varepsilon_{a1})^2 K_1 + \tfrac{1}{2}(\varepsilon_s - \varepsilon_{s1})^2 \mu_1 - \varepsilon_z T_z - \varepsilon_c T_c] s_0, \tag{2b}$$

Here E_0 and E_1 are constants. The quantities q_0 and q_1 represent charges in the two states and V the membrane potential. The area and shear moduli of the motor are, respectively, K_0 and μ_0 in the standard state (state 0), and K_1 and μ_1 in the other state (state 1). The membrane area occupied by the motor in the standard state is represented by s_0. The area and shear strains in the standard state are ε_{a0} and ε_{s0}, respectively. The strains in state 1 are represented by suffix 1. Area strains and length strains are related by,

$$\varepsilon_a = \varepsilon_z + \varepsilon_c,$$

$$\varepsilon_s = \varepsilon_z - \varepsilon_c,$$

The free energy difference $\Delta F(T_z, T_c)$ between the two states is determined as the difference in the minimum values of these two functions with respect to variables ε_z and ε_c. This leads to

$$\Delta F(T_z, T_c) = \Delta E - qV + \Delta F_{stiff} + \Delta F_{area},$$

with

$$\Delta F_{stiff} = -\frac{s_0}{8}[(K_1^{-1} - K_0^{-1})(T_z + T_c)^2 + (\mu_1^{-1} - \mu_0^{-1})(T_z - T_c)^2] \qquad (3)$$

$$\Delta F_{area} = -s_0[(\varepsilon_z - \varepsilon_{z0})T_z + (\varepsilon_c - \varepsilon_{c0})T_c]. \qquad (4)$$

The first mechanical term (3) is the energy due to elasticity change and the second (4) due to a change in the area in the two states. The ratio P_1 of the motor in state 1 follows the Boltzmann distribution,

$$\frac{P_1}{1 - P_1} = \exp[-\frac{\Delta F(T_z, T_c)}{k_B T}], \qquad (5)$$

where k_B is the Boltzmann constant and T the temperature.

In order to evaluate the relative importance of the two mechanical terms, two extreme cases in which the other term is omitted, are examined in the following.

3 Stiffness motor

If area changes are unimportant, the free energy difference in the two states is represented by,

$$\Delta F(T_z, T_c) = \Delta E - qV + \Delta F_{stiff}.$$

How is the elasticity change in the motor related to the motility of the cell? Because of a turgor pressure, a reduction of stiffness results in an expansion of the motor, bringing about a displacement of the cell as a whole. It would be reasonable to assume that the lateral membrane is represented by a mosaic of passive elements and motor elements, each of which has two states. In a 'homogenization' approximation, in which local stresses at the borders of passive and motor elements are neglected, strains are related to the membrane tensions,

$$T_z = Kp\varepsilon_{ap} + \mu_p\varepsilon_{sp} = K_0\varepsilon_{a0} + \mu_0\varepsilon_{s0} = K_1\varepsilon_{a1} + \mu_1\varepsilon_{s1},$$

$$T_c = Kp\varepsilon_{ap} - \mu_p\varepsilon_{sp} = K_0\varepsilon_{a0} - \mu_0\varepsilon_{s0} = K_1\varepsilon_{a1} - \mu_1\varepsilon_{s1},$$

Here the subscript p indicates the passive component. It is convenient to put $K_p=K_0$ and $\mu_p=\mu_0$ to reduce the number of parameters. With this simplification,

$$\varepsilon_a = \tfrac{3}{4}\, rP[K_0^{-1} + (K_1^{-1} - K_0^{-1})aP_1],$$

$$\varepsilon_s = \tfrac{1}{4}\, rP[\mu_0^{-1} + (\mu_1^{-1} - \mu_0^{-1})aP_1],$$

where the parameter a on the rhs represents the fraction of the membrane occupied by the motors. It is related to the area s_0 of the motor with $aS=ns_0$, where n is the number of the motors in the membrane area S. The magnitude of the motor strain due to elasticity changes between the two states increases with increasing pressure P. A change in the elasticity alters the internal pressure, resulting in a shift in the fraction P_1 of the motors in the state 1 for a given membrane potential. The axial strain ε_z is expressed in the form,

$$\varepsilon_z = \tfrac{1}{8}\, rP(k_{11} + ak_{12}P_1),$$

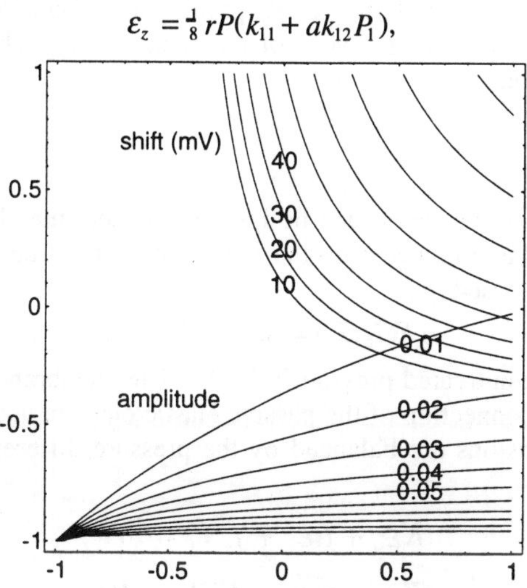

Figure 1: Stiffness motor. Contour plots for amplitude of voltage-dependent strain and for shift of peak capacitance due to a pressure increase. The abscissa is relative change $(\mu_1-\mu_0)/\mu_0$ of the shear modulus and the ordinate is relative change $(K_1-K_0)/K_0$ of the area modulus in the two states of the motor. Values used: motor covers 1/3 of the membrane area. K=0.07 N/m, μ=0.007 N/m, the turgor pressure at the standard state 1 kPa. The voltage shift is for 0.5 kPa increase of the pressure. Experimentally the amplitude is around 0.04 to 0.05 and the shift is around 20 mV. Within the plotted area there is no point which satisfies both conditions.

where k_{11} and k_{12} are constants related to the stiffness. The volume constant condition leads to[8]

$$(k_{21} + ak_{22}P_1)P = (k_{21} + ak_{22}P_1^{(0)})P^{(0)},$$

where $P_1^{(0)}$ and $P^{(0)}$ are, respectively, the probability that the motor in the cell is in state 1 and the internal pressure in the standard condition. Constants k_{21} and k_{22} are related to the stiffness.

By considering the two limits of the membrane potential the amplitude for voltage dependent motility is obtained. Shifts due to pressure are determined by the membrane potential which satisfies $P_1=0.5$ for given values for pressure.

The results on the amplitude and pressure sensitivity are illustrated in Fig. 1. It shows that experimental values for the amplitude and shifts require an extremely large changes in the shear modulus. Other predictions include a significant pressure dependence of the amplitude and shift of the capacitance peak proportional to the square of the pressure.

4   Area motor

If stiffness changes of the motor can be ignored, namely the change in mechanical energy of the motor is dominated by the area change, the free energy difference in the two states is expressed by,

$$\Delta F(T_z, T_c) = \Delta E - qV + \Delta F_{area}.$$

This problem has been treated previously.[11, 14] The membrane equation is derived by assuming series connection of the passive elastic element and the motor element. Since membrane tensions are balanced by the pressure difference, the constitutive equations are

$$K\varepsilon_a + \mu\varepsilon_s + f_z^0 P_1 = \tfrac{1}{2} rP,$$

$$K\varepsilon_a - \mu\varepsilon_s + f_c^0 P_1 = rP,$$

where f_z^0 and f_c^0 are constants determined by $f_z^0 = -ns_0[K(\varepsilon_{a1}-\varepsilon_{a0}) + \mu(\varepsilon_{s1}-\varepsilon_{s0})]$, $f_c^0 = -ns_0[K(\varepsilon_{a1}-\varepsilon_{a0}) - \mu(\varepsilon_{s1}-\varepsilon_{s0})]$. The constant volume condition ($\varepsilon_z + 2\varepsilon_c = $ const.) leads to

$$rPb_1 + b_2 P_1 = c.$$

A constant b_1 is determined by the elasticity of the cell, a constant b_2 reflects area changes of the motor, and a constant c reflects the standard state of the cell. The axial strain is represented by,

$$\varepsilon_z = \tfrac{1}{8}(3K^{-1} - \mu^{-1})rP + ns_0 P_1(\varepsilon_{z1} - \varepsilon_{z0}).$$

It is shown that the amplitude of the voltage-dependent motility is independent of pressure. Relatively small strains in the motor can explain both amplitude of the motility and shifts due to pressure changes experimentally observed (Fig. 2).

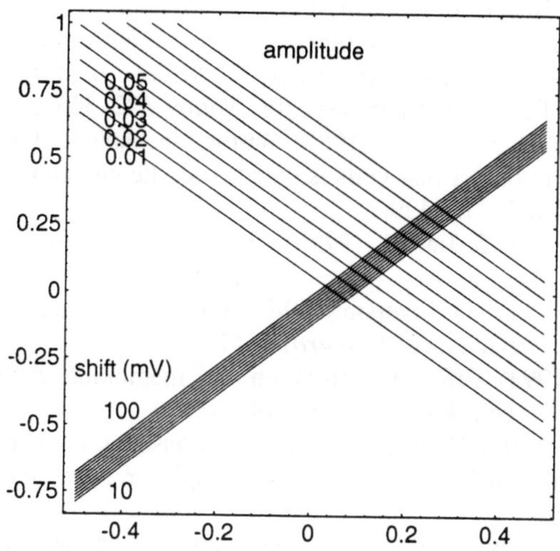

Figure 2: Area motor. Contour plots for amplitude of voltage-dependent strain and for shift of peak capacitance due to pressure increase. The abscissa is relative change $(\varepsilon_{s1}-\varepsilon_{s0})/\varepsilon_{s0}$ of the shear and the ordinate is relative change $(\varepsilon_{a1}-\varepsilon_{a0})/\varepsilon_{a0}$ of the area in the two states of the motor. Values used: motor covers 1/3 of the membrane area. K=0.07 N/m, μ=0.007 N/m. The voltage shift is for 0.5 kPa increase of the pressure. Experimentally the amplitude is around 0.04 to 0.05 and the shift is around 20 mV. The area which satisfies both conditions has relatively small values for both $(\varepsilon_{s1}-\varepsilon_{s0})/\varepsilon_{s0}$ and $(\varepsilon_{a1}-\varepsilon_{a0})/\varepsilon_{a0}$.

5   Conclusion

The experimentally observed amplitude of the membrane-potential dependent length changes and the sensitivity of the membrane capacitance to the intracellular pressure virtually determine the parameters in both mechanisms examined. It was found that the stiffness motor mechanism requires an extremely large difference in the elastic moduli in the two states whereas a relatively small difference in the area is sufficient for the area motor mechanism. For this reason it is unlikely that the stiffness effect is the dominant term in the membrane motor. Indeed, experimentally the axial stiffness of the cell does not have a significant voltage dependence, although it could be somewhat lower when hyperploarized. The amplitude of the membrane-potential dependent length change is also not very sensitive to the intracellular pressure.

References

1. Brownell, W., Bader, C., Bertrand, D. & Ribaupierre, Y. (1985) Evoked mechanical responses of isolated outer hair cells, *Science* **227** 194–196.
2. Kachar, K., Brownell, E.B., Altschuler, R. & Fex, J. (1986) Electrokinetic shape changes of cochlear outer hair cells, *Nature* **322** 365–367.
3. Holley, M.C. & Ashmore, J.F. (1988) On the mechanism of a high-frequency force generator in ouater hair cells isolated from the guinea pig cochlea, *Proc. R. Soc. Lond. B* **232** 413–429.
4. Iwasa, K.H., Li, M. & Jia, M. (1995) Can membrane proteins drive a cell?, *Biophys. J.* **68** 214s.
5. Santos-Sacchi, J. (1991) Reversible inhibition of voltage-dependent outer hair cell motility and capacitance, *J. Neurosci.* **11** 3096–3110.
6. Iwasa, K.H. (1993) Effect of stress on the membrane capacitance of the auditory outer hair cell, *Biophys. J.* **65** 492–498.
7. Ashmore, J.F. (1990) Forward and reverse transduction in guinea-pig outer hair cells: the cellular basis of the cochlear amplifier, *Neurosci. Res. Suppl.* **12** S39–S50.
8. Iwasa, K.H. & Chadwick, R.S. (1992) Elasticity and active force generation of cochlear outer hair cells, *J. Acoust. Soc. Am.* **92** 3169–3173.
9. Gale, J.E. & Ashmore, J.F. (1994) Charge displacement induced by rapid stretch in the basolateral membrane of the guinea-pig outer hair cell, *Proc. R. Soc. Lond. B* **255** 233–249.
10. Kakehata, S. & Santos-Sacchi, J. (1995) Membrane tension directly shifts voltage dependence of outer hair cell motility and associated gating charge, *Biophys. J.* **68** 2190–2197.
11. Iwasa, K.H. (1994) A membrane model for the fast motility of the outer hair cell, *J. Acoust. Soc. Am.* **96** 2216–2224.
12. Dallos, P., Hallworth, R. & Evans, B. (1993) Theory of electrically driven shape changes of cochlear outer hair cells., *J Neurophysiol* **70** 299–323.
13. Sachs, F. & Lecar, H. (1991) Stochastic models for mechanical transduction, *Biophys. J.* **59** 1143–1145.
14. Iwasa, K.H. (1996) Membrane motors in the outer hair cell of the mammalian cochlea, *Comments Theoret. Biol.* (in press).

THE RECEPTOR POTENTIAL NON-LINEARITIES GENERATED BY THE MECHANOELECTRICAL TRANSDUCER TO TWO-TONE STIMULATION

A.N. LUKASHKIN, I.J. RUSSELL

School of Biological Sciences, University of Sussex, Falmer, Brighton, BN1 9QG, UK.

A.Lukashkin@sussex.ac.uk

This paper describes a model of the hair cell receptor potential based on a second-order Boltzmann function. Two levels of discription are presented; one which includes only resistive elements of the hair cell membranes and a second, which also includes the series resistance of the external return path of the transducer current through the tissue of the cochlea and the capacitances of the hair cell membranes. The model provides a qualitative description of signal processing by the hair cell transducer and demonstrates that the non-linearity of the hair cell transducer can give rise to the non-linear phenomena, such as intermodulation distortion products and two-tone suppression which have been recorded from the peripheral auditory system. One interesting outcome of the model is the demonstration that two-tone suppression depends not on the saturation of the receptor potential, but on the behaviour of the hair cell transducer function close to the operating point.

1   Introduction

All stages involved in the processing of auditory signals distort their input to some extent and contribute to the overall non-linearity of the cochlea's response to sound. The mechano-electrical transducer of the hair cell is an early, crucial, stage in auditory sensory processing with strong non-linear characteristics. This non-linear relationship between hair bundle displacement and transducer conductance has been fitted, in turtle hair cells (Crawford et al.[3]) and outer hair cells (OHCs) in organotypic culures of the mouse cochlea (Kros et al.[7]) by a second-order Boltzmann function which describes the probability of transducer channel opening to the displacement of the hair bundle. The basis of this paper is a model based on a second-order Boltzmann function with one open and two closed states and displacement-dependent transitions between them. The parameters used in the model are based on the measurements by Kros et al.[7]. The model provides a qualitative description of signal processing by the hair cell transducer and demonstrates that the non-linearity of the hair cell transducer can give rise to the non-linear phenomena which have been recorded from the peripheral auditory system.

2   Description of the Model

The conductance of the transducer is given by

$$G_{tr}(x(t)) = R_{tr}(x(t))^{-1} = G_{tr\,max}\,[1 + K_2\,[1 + K_1]]^{-1} \tag{1}$$

where $G_{tr\,max}$ is the maximal transducer conductance, R_{tr} is the inverse of the transducer conductance G_{tr}. K_1 is the equilibrium constant between the open state and the first closed state and K_2 is the equilibrium constant between the two closed states. K_1 and K_2 can be described in terms of the position of the hair bundle (Crawford et al.[3])

$$K_1 = \exp[a_1\,[x_1 - x(t)]], \quad K_2 = \exp[a_2\,[x_2 - x(t)]] \tag{2}$$

were a_1, a_2, x_1, x_2 are constants and $x(t)$ is the displacement of the hair bundle from its resting position. An example of $G_{tr}(x)$ as a function of hair bundle displacement for the mammalian OHC is given in figure 1a. The parameters which are used in this figure and throughout the paper are derived from data provided by Kros et al.[7]. The function is a concave-convex asymmetrical function with a point of inflection which lies closer to the lower saturation level. Let us define biasing of the transducer operating point as a steady state displacement x_{set} of the hair bundle. When x_{set} is positive the operating point of the transducer moves in the direction indicated by the arrow in figure 1a.

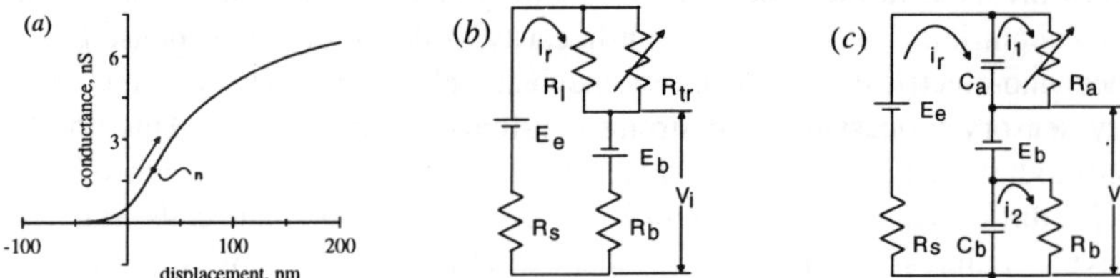

Figure 1:   Electrical circuit representing an OHC *in vivo*. *a*. Transducer conductance of the mammalian OHC as a function of bundle displacement. The curve was described by Kros et al.[7] and was fitted to eq.1 with $G_{tr\,max} = 7$ nS, $a_1 = 0.065$ nm^{-1} $a_2 = 0.016$ nm^{-1}, $x_1 = 24$ nm, $x_2 = 41$ nm. **n** indicates the point of inflection of the transducer function ($x=24.4$ nm). *b*. Resistive circuit. *c*. Circuit with reactive elements of the cell's membranes. R_a is the resistance of the cell's apical pole which consists of the transducer resistance R_{tr} (eq.1 with parameters of figure 1) and the leakage resistance R_l (500 MΩ) connected in parallel. C_a (3 pF) is the capacitance of the cell's apical pole. R_b (50 MΩ) and C_b (30 pF) are resistance and capacitance of the basolateral membrane. These values correspond to a OHC about 0 μm long from guinea pig cochleae (Housley & Ashmore[6]). R_s is the resistance of the cochlear tissue. E_b (90 mV) is an electromotive force of the basolateral membrane determined by the potassium reversal potential . (from Lukashkin and Russell[8])

The non-linearities of the receptor current through conductance $G_{tr}(x(t))$ are manifested in the changes in intracellular potential (the receptor potential). The model of transduction has been examined in conjunction with simple electrical circuits (figure 1b and c). A resistive model (figure 1b) may be useful for describing the distortion products created by the transducer itself because in this circuit the amplitudes of the distortion products are not modified by reactive elements of the cell's membranes. In fact, this circuit approximates the electrical properties of the hair cells *in vivo* in response to low frequency tones. Any models which describe the frequency-dependent behaviour of the voltages through the cell's membranes must take into account the reactive elements of the membranes (figure 1c).

3   Application of the Model for Two-Tone Stimulation.

When two signals of different frequencies f_1 and f_2 are used as input to the transducer, the output signal includes not only these primary frequencies but also intermodulation distortion components (IDCs). The output magnitude of the primaries is also a result of the interference between the input signals. The output signals are also shaped by the hair cell's passive electric characteristics in that the high frequency IDCs are attenuated by the membrane filter. In order to account for the non-linear interaction between two tones in the cochlea, Engebretson and Eldredge[4] developed a model which showed that, when two signals were present at the input of a non-linear system which had an input-output function that could be approximated by a power series, interference between the two signals could be observed. Notably, the output magnitude of one signal was linearised and suppressed when the input magnitude of the other signal was increased. A similar effect might also be expected for the transducer under consideration (figure 1a) because a power series approximation is valid in this case.

In order to examine behaviour of the IDCs and fundamentals when two primary frequencies are used as an input signal to the model, let us expand the transducer function $G_{tr}(x)$ in a Taylor's series about $x=0$:

$$G_{tr}(x) = \sum_{n=0}^{\infty} a_n x^n \qquad \text{where} \qquad a_n = \frac{1}{n!}\left[\frac{d^n G_{tr}(x)}{dx^n}\right]_{x=0} \qquad (3)$$

If two signals, with peak displacement amplitudes A_1 and A_2, are present in the input then

$$x = A_1 \sin\left(2\pi f_1 t\right) + A_2 \sin\left(2\pi f_2 t\right) \qquad (4)$$

590

By substituting this equation into eq.3 one can find the output magnitude of $G_{tr}(x)$ of the frequency f_1 when the peak displacement amplitude A_1 is much smaller than the peak amplitude A_2 of frequency f_2 (see equation 2 from Engebretson and Eldredge[4]):

$$G_{tr}(x)_{f1} \approx A_1\left[a_1 + \frac{3}{2}a_3 A_2^{\,2} + \frac{15}{8}a_5 A_2^{\,4} + \frac{35}{16}a_7 A_2^{\,6} + \cdots \right]_{A_1 \ll A_2} \quad (5)$$

where $G_{tr}(x)_{f1}$ is the magnitude $G_{tr}(x)$ at frequency f_1. Therefore, $G_{tr}(x)_{f1}$ depends linearly on the amplitude A_1 when $A_1{\ll}A_2$. The slope of this dependence is defined by a linear combination of even-order powers of A_2; each power being weighted by a_n, which is defined by the appropriate order derivative of $G_{tr}(x)$ evaluated at the operating point. Some of the first odd-order derivatives of $G_{tr}(x)$ are shown in figure 2.

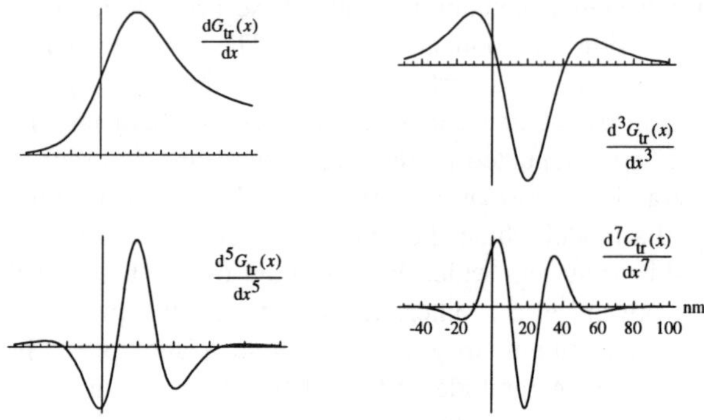

Figure 2: First four even-order derivatives for the function $G_{tr}(x)$ that is shown in figure 1. (from Lukashkin and Russell[8])

It is seen from figure 2 that the sign and value of a_n is heavily dependent on the operating point of the hair cell transducer function (x_{set}). When n>1, a_n may be positive as well as negative, depending on the position of the transducer operating point along the x axis (see figure 2). Therefore, the slope of the level function for the frequency f_1 ($G_{tr}(x)_{f1}$) may be positive as well as negative (figure 3). It worth noting that, with the appropriate x_{set}, interference between f_1 and f_2 leads to facilitation of the $G_{tr}(x)_{f1}$ magnitude rather than to its suppression. In the particular case under consideration this effect occurs when $x_{set}=$ -25nm and 3rd and 5th order derivatives are positive as shown in figure 3c. The interference turns to suppression only when the negative term with 7th order derivative is dominant, which is when the amplitude of A_2 exceeds 30 dB.

From their measurement of the response of the CM to two tones, Geisler et al.[5] proposed that there was a correlation between saturation of the OHC receptor current and two-tone suppression. In the model presented here, suppression depends only on the value of the derivatives of the transducer function $G_{tr}(x)$ at the operating point and does not depend on the behaviour of the function far away from the operating point and into saturation.

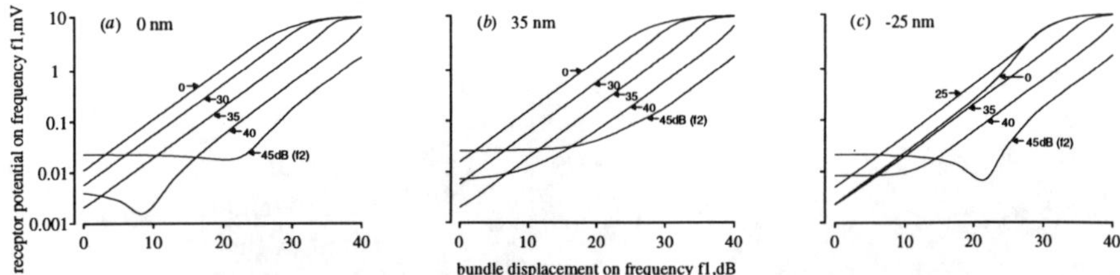

Figure 3: Level functions for the spectral component of the receptor potential on frequency f_1 evaluated at different transducer operating points when the input signal consists of two frequencies f_1 and f_2. Circuit B. Panels a, b and c present responses with x = 0 nm, 35 nm and -25 nm respectively. Parameter indicated near each function is amplitude of f_2 in decibels. 0 dB amplitude for the displacement is equal to 0.1 nm The same model parameters as in figure 1 were used. (from Lukashkin and Russell[8])

By using the same technique one can show that it is possible to obtain non-monotonic level functions for the odd- and even-order IDCs of $G_{tr}(x)$. It is possible to derive the equation for the magnitude of any IDC from eq.3. For example, the $G_{tr}(x)$ magnitude of the distortion product $2f_1\text{-}f_2$ (equation 5 from Engebretson and Eldredge[4]) is given by:

$$G_{tr}(x)_{2f1-f2} = A_1^{\,2}A_2\left[\frac{3}{4}a_3 + \frac{5}{8}a_5\left(2A_1^{\,2} + 3A_2^{\,2}\right) + \right.$$

$$\left. +\frac{105}{64}a_7\left(A_1^{\,4} + 4A_1^{\,2}A_2^{\,2} + 2A_2^{\,4}\right) + \cdots \right] \tag{6}$$

The relative weight of different terms of the linear combination in eq.6 depends on the amplitude of the primaries and on the position of the transducer operating point because a_n depends on the n-th order derivative of $G_{tr}(x)$ evaluated at the operating point. The amplitude of IDCs of the receptor potential as a function of displacement are shown in figure 4 (right) for two primary frequencies of equal amplitude when the set point of the transducer x_{set} is fixed at 26nm. It is possible to see that the even IDCs show local minima together with monotonic growth of the fundamentals and the odd IDCs. These minima are also accompanied by a phase change of 180°. If, instead of keeping a constant operating point of the transducer, we fix the amplitude of the primaries and alter the operating point, we can observe the appearance and disappearance of the notches at the odd and even IDCs (figure 4, left).

592

When the reactive parts of the membrane's impedance are taken into account, (circuit *c*) the behaviour of the IDCs of the receptor potential is not altered qualitatively but the notches become wider. Moreover, the phase changes are not so abrupt as for the circuit B and we can trace the direction of the phase change (lag or lead).

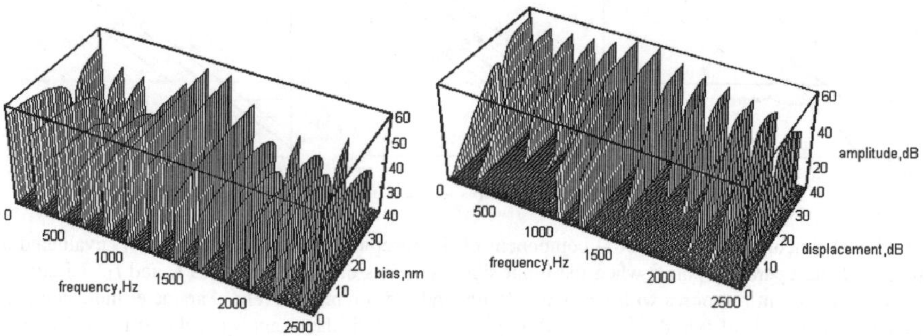

Figure 4: Frequency spectrum of the receptor potential for circuit B. Right. Level function of the frequency spectrum. Primary frequencies of 1000 and 1200 Hz and of equal amplitude were used as an input. x_{set} is equal to 26nm. 0 dB amplitude is equal to 0.1 nm for the displacement and 0.001 mV for the potential. Left. Frequency spectrum with bias of the transducer operating point. Primary frequencies of 1000 and 1200 Hz and of equal amplitude (100 nm peak-to-peak) were used as an input. 0 dB of the receptor potential amplitude is equal to 0.001 mV. The same model parameters as in figure 1 were used. (from Lukashkin and Russell[8])

4   Conclusion

Changes in the operating point of the transducer function could account for the complex, sometimes reciprocal, level dependent changes in the magnitude of odd and even-order IDCs measured at the tympanic membrane (Schmiedt and Adams[11], Brown[2], Whitehead et al.[12], Popelka et al.[9]). The interaction of two-tones with the transducer function can generate two-tone suppression (Arthur et al.[1]) and depending on the set point of the transducer function and the level of the second tone, two-tone facilitation (Russell and Kössl[10]). In the model presented here, suppression depends only on the behaviour of the transducer function close to the operating point and does not depend on saturation of the transducer function (Geisler et al.[5]).

Acknowledgments

We thank Drs. Ann Brown, Cornè Kros, Gunnar Sandberg and Aleksandr Sobolev for valuable discussion. This work was supported by grants from the Medical Research Council and Hearing Research Trust. Andrei Lukashkin is supported by a Wellcome Trust Prize Studentship.

References

1. Arthur, R.M., Pfeiffer, R.R. and Suga, N. (1971) Properties of two-tone inhibition in primary auditory neurons, *J. Physiol. (Lond.)* **212** 593-609.
2. Brown, A.M. (1987) Acoustic distortion from rodent ears: A comparison of responses from rats, guinea pigs and gerbils, *Hear. Res.* **31** 25-38.
3. Crawford, A.C., Evans, M.G. and Fettiplace, R. (1989) Activation and adaptation of transducer currents in turtle hair cells, *J. Physiol. (Lond.)* **419** 405-434.
4. Engebretson, A.M. and Eldredge, D.H. (1968) Model for the nonlinear characteristics of cochlear potentials, *J. Acoust. Soc. Am.* **44** 548-554.
5. Geisler, C.D., Yates, G.K., Patuzzi, R.B. and Johnstone, B.M. (1990) Saturation of outer hair cell receptor currents causes two-tone suppression, *Hear. Res.* **44** 241-256.
6. Housley, G.D. and Ashmore, J.F. (1992) Ionic currents of outer hair cells isolated from the guinea-pig cochlea, *J. Physiol. (Lond.)* **448** 73-98.
7. Kros, C.J., Lennan, G.W.T. and Richardson, G.P. (1995) Transducer currents and bundle movements in outer hair cells of neonatal mice, in *Active hearing*, eds. A. Flock, D. Ottoson, and M. Ulfendahl (Elsevier Science, Amsterdam) pp. 113-125.
8. Lukashkin, A.N. and Russell, I.J. (1996) Model description of the receptor potential non-linearities generated by the hair cell mechanoelectrical transducer, (in preparation).
9. Popelka, G.R., Osterhammel, P.A., Nielsen, L.H. and Rasmussen, A.N. (1993) Growth of distortion product otoacoustic emissions with primary-tone level in humans, *Hear. Res.* **71** 12-22.
10. Russell, I.J. and Kössl, M. (1992) Modulation of hair cell voltage responses to tones by low-frequency biasing of the basilar membrane in the guinea pig cochlea, *J. Neurosci.* **12** 1587-1601.
11. Schmiedt,R.A. and Adams, J.C. (1981) Stimulated acoustic emissions in the ear canal of the gerbil, *Hear. Res.* **5** 295-305.
12. Whitehead, M.L., Lonsbury-Martin, B.L. and Martin, G.K. (1992) Evidence for two discrete sources of $2f_1$-f_2 distortion - product otoacoustic emission in rabbit: I.Differential dependence on stimulus parameters, *J. Acoust. Soc. Am.* **91** 1587-1607.

HARMONIC DISTORTION OF CUPULAR MECHANICS GENERATED BY THE GATING SPRINGS OF LATERAL LINE HAIR CELLS

S.M. VAN NETTEN

Department of Biophysics, University of Groningen, Nijenborgh 4
9747 AG Groningen, The Netherlands
s.van.netten@bcn.rug.nl

1 Introduction

Experiments on saccular hair cells *in vitro* revealed that the opening probability of the mechanosensitive transduction channels is related to the hair bundle's stiffness[1]. The observed reduction in stiffness of a hair bundle when it is deflected can be accounted for by theoretical models in which the transduction channels are opened via elastic elements[2], termed gating springs[1]. The precise mechanism of the mechanical engagement of the transduction channels, however, is still unknown.

The gating spring theory not only describes the mechanical characteristics of individual hair bundles driven by a flexible glass probe, but also explains several features of the nonlinear cupular dynamics of the lateral line organ observed under *in vivo* conditions. The changes in sliding stiffness of the lateral line cupula can be explained by the characteristic reductions in hair bundle stiffness resulting from the opening of the transduction channels[3]. This result is in line with the notion that the sliding stiffness of the cupula can almost completely be attributed to the summed stiffness of the hair bundles protruding into the cupular base[4,5].

The characteristics of the lateral line organ are relatively simple with regard to several other hair cell organs. In a typical supraorbital neuromast some thousands of hair cells receive their identical mechanical stimulus from the cupula, which is driven by the canal fluid flowing past it. The lateral line organ thus allows for the possibility to further investigate the gating spring hypothesis in an intact hair cell organ and may provide estimates of the parameters related to it, such as gating force and gating compliance.

Estimates of these parameters in the lateral line organ, sofar, were obtained by indirect comparison[3] of experimental data with solutions of a nonlinear hydrodynamic model of cupular mechanics[6]. Since the nonlinearity of the gating springs in this model interferes with the frequency dependent mechanics of the cupula, only numerical solutions to the model could be obtained. Estimates of the transduction parameters thus resulted from a trial and error process between the numerical solutions and the measured data.

In the present study, the same hydrodynamic model is considered. However, at low frequencies a simplified equation of motion can be derived, which is solved in analytical terms. These analytical solutions can be used to express the distortion components as a function of the relevant mechanical transduction parameters and thus facilitate the extraction of these parameters from measured data more directly than with the use of numerical solutions. The method applied is also usefull to obtain expressions for the mechanical distortion components produced by the gating mechanism in individual hair bundles in response to hydrodynamic stimuli.

2 Results

2.1 Distortion Components from Numerical Solutions to the Full Model Equation

The equation of motion for the cupula, including the two-state gating springs of the transduction channels, has been described previously[6]. It dictates the displacement of the cupula, X, (normalized with respect to the position at which half of the transduction channels are open, (X_0)), as a function of normalized time, τ $(=\omega_r t)$, in response to a frequency dependent boundary layer around the cupula generated by a spatially uniform fluid displacement far from the cupula, $D(\tau)$, and is given by:

$$\ddot{X} + \tfrac{2}{3}\varepsilon\dot{X} + \tfrac{2}{3}\frac{F_{tot}(X)}{K} = \tfrac{2}{3}\varepsilon\dot{D}(\tfrac{\omega}{\omega_r}\tau) + \ddot{D}(\tfrac{\omega}{\omega_r}\tau). \tag{1}$$

Here, F_{tot}, which is an odd function of X, is the restoring force on the cupula resulting from the hair bundles. The linear component of F_{tot} can be associated with the sum of the pivotal stiffness of the hair bundles (S_{piv}) plus the linear part of the gating springs ($KX = (S_{piv} + N_{g.s.}\gamma K_{g.s.})X$), where γ denotes the lever ratio of cupular displacement to gating spring extension, $K_{g.s.}$ the gating spring constant and $N_{g.s.}$ the total number of gating springs. The nonlinear component of F_{tot} is related to the relief in tension of the gating springs when the channels open ($= -N_{g.s.}Z/[1 + \exp(-Z \cdot (X - X_0)/kT)]$, where $Z = \gamma K_{g.s.} \cdot d$ is the (gating) force needed to extend a gating spring over the swing (d) of the transduction channel[1]. The two terms on the right-hand side of Equation 1 consist of the viscous and inertial fluid force driving the cupula, $(\omega_r)/2\pi$ is the (linear) resonance frequency of the cupula, while ε is given by $6\pi a\mu/\sqrt{(KM)}$, and can be interpreted as the inverse of the quality factor of the system (M is cupular mass, a is cupular radius and μ is canal fluid viscosity). A fourth-order Runge-Kutta algorithm was used to solve Equation 1 with typical parameters of supraorbital lateral line neuromasts[5,6]. Results of the response levels at the fundamental tone $(f = 15$ Hz) and distortion components at $3 \cdot f$ and $5 \cdot f$, are shown in Figure 1 as a function of normalized input level of the fluid force.

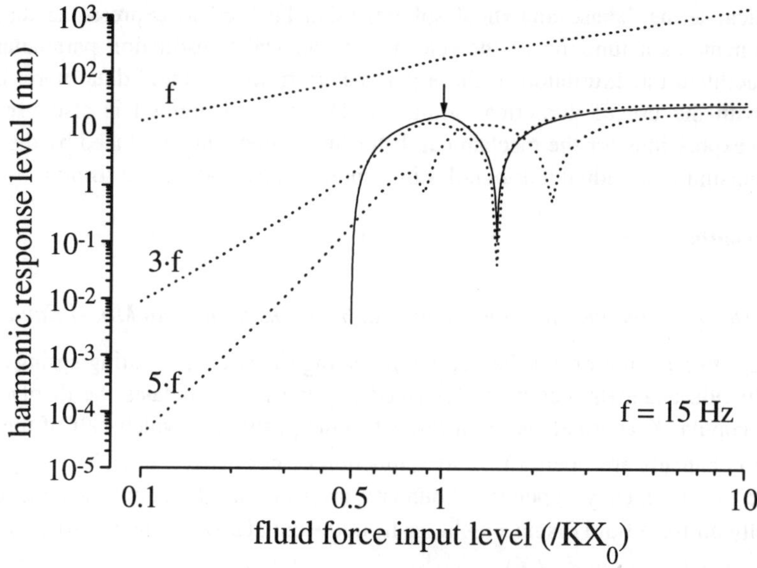

Figure 1: Harmonic distortion components calculated from the full equation of motion of the fish lateral line cupula (dotted lines) in response to fluid flow at 15 Hz, as a function of fluid force input level normalized to $KX_0 = 2 \cdot 10^{-8}$ N. The solid line shows the analytical solution for the third harmonic (see text). The arrow indicates the transition between the two sections of this solution. Parameters used are based on estimates from previous studies[5,6]: $\varepsilon = 0.65$; $\omega_r = 2\pi \cdot 140/s$; $K=0.16$ N/m; $Z=100$ fN; $N_{g.s.} = 10^5$; $X_0 = 125$ nm.

The fundamental component almost linearly increases with input level over the two decades shown, except for an extra increase at input levels close to 1. At low levels the harmonic components typically increase with input level to the power of their harmonic number. When the input level approaches 1.5, the third harmonic steeply declines and becomes zero. Further increase of the input results in a steep increase of the distortion. At high input levels the distortion saturates. At low levels, up to the notch, the third harmonic is out of phase with the driving fluid force, beyond the notch it is in phase. The same behaviour is found for the fifth harmonic but here two notches occur and a lower saturation level is reached. At low levels, the fifth harmonic is in phase with the fluid force and turns 180 degrees at each notch.

2.2 Simplified Equation of Motion of the Cupula

To obtain mathematical expressions in closed form for the distortion levels, we simplified Equation 1, by focusing on those frequencies, at which the cupular response is stiffness controlled $(f<<\omega_r/2\pi)^5$. In that case, the first two terms of the left-hand side of Equation 1 are small and are neglected. Furthermore, we assume that the driving fluid flow far from the cupula, $D(\tau)$, is not affected by the distortions caused by the cupula. This is a reasonable assumption since distortions propagate back into the fluid inversely proportional to the cubed distance from the cupula. In the case of a sinusoidally varying fluid flow, Equation 1 (unnormalized) reduces to:

$$F_{tot}(X) = A\sin(\omega t) \quad \text{and thus:} \quad X = F_{tot}^{-1}(A\sin(\omega t)) \tag{2}$$

where A is the effective amplitude of the combination of viscous and inertial fluid forces. Thus, for the solution of X, only the inverse function of F_{tot} has to be found. Unfortunately, there is no analytical expression for this inverse function known (to the author). Therefore, a linearized three-section approximation to F_{tot} has been constructed, on both sides of the origin. The positive part of this (unnormalized) function is schematically shown in Figure 2a, together with the original F_{tot}. It consists of two linear sections coinciding with the two asymptotes of F_{tot}, together with a third linear section connecting the asymptotes and having a slope equal to the slope of F_{tot} at its inflection point at $X=X_0$. The approximating function, $F_{tot,app.}$, therefore, is completely characterized by the two intersection points X_1, F_1 and X_2, F_2 and thus involves four parameters. The physical meaning of these parameters can most easily be interpreted when the associated stiffness profile, $S(X)=dF/dX$, is considered (Figure 2b). The (unnormalized) stiffness profile that results from $F_{tot,app}$ has two sections with a constant stiffness K, and by virtue of its construction, a square dip (gating compliance) with a depth, Δ, equal to:

$$\Delta = K - \left.\frac{dF_{tot}}{dX}\right|_{X=X_0} = N_{g.s.}\frac{Z^2}{4kT}. \tag{3}$$

Since the area of the dip, $\Lambda\cdot\Delta$, equals per definition the vertical distance, $N_{g.s.}\cdot Z$, of the two asymptotes of $F_{tot}(X)$, the width of the dip, Λ, must equal:

$$\Lambda = \frac{N_{g.s.}Z}{\Delta} = \frac{4kT}{Z}. \tag{4}$$

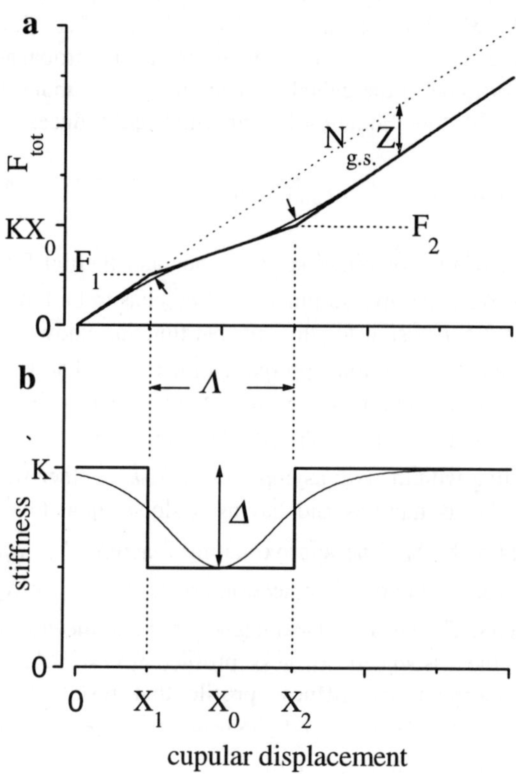

Figure 2: Relationship between (a.) the restoring force function, F_{tot}, (thin smooth lines, indicated by small arrows) and (b.) the related stiffness function. The four characterizing parameters of the mechanical transduction $\Lambda = X_2 - X_1$, X_0, Δ, and K are indicated. The approximating linearized functions are shown as thick lines. F_1 and F_2 are the values of the approximating function at X_1 and X_2 respectively.

Together with K and X_0, the shape parameters Δ and Λ completely characterize both F_{tot} and $F_{tot,app}$. The inverse function of $F_{tot,app}$ is readily found and also consists of three linear sections:

$$\text{I:} \quad X = \frac{F}{K}, \qquad\qquad F < F_1$$

$$\text{II:} \quad X = \frac{F - \Delta(X_0 - \frac{\Lambda}{2})}{K - \Delta}, \qquad\qquad F_1 < F < F_2$$

$$\text{III:} \quad X = \frac{F}{K} + \frac{\Lambda\Delta}{K}, \qquad\qquad F > F_2. \qquad (5)$$

Because of the symmetry in the model, only odd components will be generated of which the third harmonic will be dominant. Therefore, the remaining analysis is restricted to this component. The method used, however, can be applied to higher harmonics as well. To mathematically express the third harmonic, resulting from

Equation 5 with input $F = A \cdot \sin(\omega \cdot t)$, the product of X and $\sin(3\omega \cdot t)$ is integrated over a complete period T resulting in:

$$X_{f3}(A) = \frac{8}{T} \left[\int_{\frac{T}{2\pi}\arcsin\frac{F_1}{A}}^{\frac{T}{2\pi}\arcsin\frac{F_2}{A}} \left[\frac{\Delta\, A \sin(\omega t)}{K(K-\Delta)} - \frac{\Delta(X_0 - \frac{\Lambda}{2})}{K-\Delta} \right] + \int_{\frac{T}{2\pi}\arcsin\frac{F_2}{A}}^{\frac{T}{4}} \frac{\Delta\,\Lambda}{K} \right] \sin(3\omega t)\, dt.$$

(6)

The factor $8/T$ arises from the definition of the Fourier sum in combination with the symmetry of the integral, requiring only evaluation from 0 to $T/4$. The integration limits are related to the different sections of the approximating function (see Figure 2). Performing the integral yields:

$$X_{f3}(A) = -\frac{4}{\pi}\frac{\Delta}{K-\Delta}\left[\sqrt{1-\left(\frac{F_1}{A}\right)^2}\left(X_1\left(\frac{1}{3} - \frac{1}{3}\left(\frac{F_1}{A}\right)^2\right)\right)\right] \qquad F_1 < A < F_2 \quad \text{and}$$

$$X_{f3}(A) = \frac{4}{\pi}\frac{\Delta}{K-\Delta}\left[\sqrt{1-\left(\frac{F_2}{A}\right)^2}\left(\frac{X_1}{3} + \left(\frac{F_2}{A}\right)^2\left(\frac{F_2}{K} - 4\frac{X_1}{3}\right)\right) - \sqrt{1-\left(\frac{F_1}{A}\right)^2}\left(X_1\left(\frac{1}{3} - \frac{1}{3}\left(\frac{F_1}{A}\right)^2\right)\right)\right]$$

$$+ \frac{4}{3\pi}\frac{\Delta\,\Lambda}{K}\left[\sqrt{1-\left(\frac{F_2}{A}\right)^2}\left(1 - 4\left(\frac{F_2}{A}\right)^2\right)\right] \qquad\qquad A > F_2. \qquad (7)$$

This analytic solution has been added to Figure 1, for the same parameters as the results of the full model also depicted in Figure 1. The analytical solution accurately describes the numerical solution, showing the notch and the saturation in the range $A>F_2(=1)$. The saturation level, calculated from Equation 7 for $A \rightarrow \infty$, gives the value $\frac{4}{3\pi}\frac{\Delta\,\Lambda}{K} = \frac{4}{3\pi}\frac{N_{g.s.}Z}{K}$, which equals $8/(3\pi)$ times the distance the cupula would move if all the transduction channels of one hair cell population would suddenly go from one state to the other. Using the estimates for the lateral line, this would amount to about 25 nm. Obviously, there is no solution for $A<F_1(=0.5)$, since in this range the approximating function consists of a linear function through the origin and thus does not produce distortion.

3 Conclusions

Analysis of the harmonic distortion generated by the nonlinear mechanics of the transduction channels of hair cells on the basis of the two state gating spring model, shows that the levels of the generated spectral components exhibit a typical behaviour. Similar behaviour has previously been discussed in hair cell physiology and has been related to hyperbolic tangent like functions describing input-output relations[7]. In fact, the force function used in this study is intimately related to the current-displacement relationship, $I(X)$, of hair cells. This is also reflected in the parameter Λ, which in this study gives a measure of the width of the stiffness dip, but has previously been derived to indicate the range of deflections at which the hair cell is most sensitive, using a linearized approximation to the $I(X)$ curve[8].

The analytical expression derived for the third harmonic of cupular motion can be used to fit measured data. The saturation level gives a direct measure of the total gating force and can be experimentally tested.

The method used to obtain analytic expressions for the harmonic distortion components can also be applied to transduction channels in single hair bundles driven by a sinusoidally varying fluid jet, because hair cells operate under stiffness controlled conditions[9] and are predominantly viscously driven when stimulated at low (< 5 kHz) acoustic frequencies.

References

1. Howard, J. and Hudspeth, A.J. (1988) Compliance of the hair bundle associated with gating of mechanoelectrical transduction channels in the bullfrog's saccular hair cells, *Neuron* **1** 189-199.
2. Corey, D.P. and Hudspeth, A.J. (1983) Kinetics of the receptor current in bullfrog saccular hair cells, *J. Neurosci.* **3** 962-976.
3. van Netten, S.M. and Khanna, S.M. (1994) Stiffness changes of the cupula associated with the mechanics of hair cells in the fish lateral line, *Proc. Natl. Acad. Sci. USA* **91** 1549-1553.
4. van Netten, S.M. and Kroese, A.B.A. (1987) Laser interferometric measurements on the dynamic behaviour of the cupula in the fish lateral line, *Hearing Res.* **29** 55-61.
5. van Netten, S.M. (1991) Hydrodynamics of the excitation of the cupula in the fish canal lateral line, *J. Acoust. Soc. Am.* **89** 310-319.
6. van Netten, S.M. (1993) A nonlinear model of cupular mechanics including the gating springs of the transduction channels of hair cells, in: *Biophysics of hair cell sensory systems,* eds: H. Duifhuis, J.W. Horst, P. van Dijk and S.M. van Netten, pp. 391-397. World Scientific, London.
7. Weiss, T.F. and Leong, R. (1985) A model for signal transmission in an ear having hair cells with free-standing stereocilia, IV Mechanoelectric transduction stage, *Hearing Res.* **20** 175-195.
8. Markin, V.S. and Hudspeth, A.J. (1995) Gating-spring models of mechano-electrical transduction by hair cells of the inner ear, *Ann. Rev. Biophys. Biomol. Struct.* **24**, 59-83.
9. Kros, C.J., Rüsch, A., Lennan, G.W.T. and Richardson, G.P. (1993) Voltage dependence of transducer currents in outer hair cells of neonatal mice, in: *Biophysics of hair cell sensory systems,* eds: H. Duifhuis, J.W. Horst, P. van Dijk and S.M. van Netten, pp. 141-150. World Scientific, London.

IS THE OUTER HAIR CELL WALL VISCOELASTIC?

J.T. RATNANATHER*, A.A. SPECTOR, A.S. POPEL

*Dept. of Biomedical Engineering, The Johns Hopkins University School of Medicine
720 Rutland Avenue, Baltimore, MD 21205, USA
email: tratnana@bme.jhu.edu

W.E. BROWNELL

*Bobby R. Alford Department of Otorhinolaryngology and Communicative Sciences
Baylor College of Medicine, One Baylor Plaza, Houston, TX 77030, USA*

1 Introduction

A growing body of evidence suggests that the cochlear outer hair cell (OHC) contributes to the active feedback process in the mammalian cochlea. The OHC is a hydrostat [1]: its lateral wall is both elastic and mechanically reinforced and its shape is maintained by a pressurized fluid core. Mechanical properties of the OHC wall have been both modeled and measured [2-5]. In particular, Brundin and Russell [6] subjected isolated OHCs to mechanical stimuli and found that OHC deformations could be described in terms of a damped mechanical oscillator. Our goal is to determine whether the damping results from either (i) the viscosity of the cytoplasm and the surrounding fluid as suggested by Tolomeo [7] or (ii) the cell wall which may possess the characteristics of a viscoelastic material or (iii) both.

2 Theory

The Brundin and Russell [6] experiment is difficult to model because the mechanical stimuli is an oscillating water jet aimed at the lateral wall. We, thus, consider an isolated OHC as cylindrical viscoelastic membrane of length, l_0, and radius, r_0, with one fixed closed end and an applied sinusoidal force at the other closed end. This model can be adapted to analyse the experiments described in this book by Hemmert *et al.* [8] The viscoelastic OHC wall incorporates the effects of membrane viscosity [9] together with a model of a cylindrical elastic membrane [2]. The longitudinal membrane tension is balanced by the fluid stresses from inside and outside the OHC. Our analysis differs from the approach taken by Jen and Steele [10]. A slender body perturbation approximation [11] based on the OHC aspect ratio, $\epsilon = r_0/l_0$, is used to determine equations for the longitudinal tension and pressure difference across the membrane.

2.1 *Fluid analysis*

The fluid inside and outside the OHC is modeled by the normalized unsteady axisymmetric Stokes equations:

$$St\frac{\partial u_z}{\partial t} = -\epsilon\frac{\partial p}{\partial z} + \frac{1}{r}\frac{\partial}{\partial r}\left(r\frac{\partial u_z}{\partial r}\right) + \epsilon^2\frac{\partial^2 u_z}{\partial z^2}$$

$$St\frac{\partial u_r}{\partial t} = -\frac{1}{\epsilon}\frac{\partial p}{\partial r} + \frac{\partial}{\partial r}\left(\frac{1}{r}\frac{\partial(ru_r)}{\partial r}\right) + \epsilon^2\frac{\partial^2 u_r}{\partial z^2}$$

$$\frac{1}{r}\frac{\partial(ru_r)}{\partial r} + \frac{\partial u_z}{\partial z} = 0$$

where $St = \omega r_0^2/\nu$ is the Stokes number; ω is the frequency of the disturbance; $\nu = \tilde{\mu}/\rho$ is the kinematic viscosity of the fluid. The fluid boundary conditions are related to the displacement of the membrane:

$$u_z = 0 \text{ at } z = 0; u_z = \frac{\partial \delta_z}{\partial t} \text{ at } z = 1; u_r = \frac{\partial \delta_r}{\partial t} \text{ at } r = 1; u_z = \frac{\partial \delta_z}{\partial t} \text{ at } r = 1$$

where δ_z and δ_r are the normalized longitudinal and radial displacement of the elastic cylinder respectively. The symmetry boundary condition is applied at $r = 0$ inside the cell and at $r = a$ outside the cell. At $r = 1$, the normalized fluid stress is:

$$\tau = \pm\left(\frac{\partial u_z}{\partial r} + \epsilon^2\frac{\partial u_r}{\partial z}\right)$$

where the sign indicates whether the fluid is inside or outside the cell.

Since we are modelling the response of the OHC to a sinusoidal force applied at $z = 1$, we consider harmonic oscillations:

$$u_r = U_r e^{it}; u_z = U_z e^{it}; p = P e^{it}; \delta_z = \Delta_z e^{it}; \delta_r = \Delta_r e^{it}$$

The OHC aspect ratio, ϵ, is chosen as the perturbation parameter so that variables, U_r, U_z and P can be expanded in a power series in ϵ: $Y = Y_0 + \epsilon Y_1 + \epsilon^2 Y_2 + ...$ The superscripts I and E pertain to variables inside and outside the OHC respectively. Then in the limit as $a \to \infty$, the leading order expressions up to and including $O(\epsilon)$ for the fluid pressure and stress at $r = 1$ inside and outside the cell are:

$$\frac{d^2 P_0{}^I}{dz^2} = \frac{\imath \beta^{I\,2}}{\epsilon} \frac{\left(Q^I \dfrac{d\Delta_z}{dz} + \Delta_r \right)}{\left(\frac{1}{2} - Q^I \right)}; \qquad \tau^I = -Q^I \left[\epsilon \frac{dP_0{}^I}{dz} + \imath \beta^{I\,2} \Delta_z \right]$$

$$\frac{d^2 P_0{}^E}{dz^2} = \frac{\imath \beta^{E\,2}}{\epsilon} \frac{\left(Q^E \dfrac{d\Delta_z}{dz} - \Delta_r \right)}{\left(\dfrac{a^2 - 1}{2} - Q^E \right)}; \qquad \tau^E = -\frac{\tilde{\mu}^E}{\tilde{\mu}} Q^E \left[\epsilon \frac{dP_0{}^E}{dz} + \imath \beta^{E\,2} \Delta_z \right]$$

$$(1)$$

where

$$Q^I = \frac{I_1(\beta^I)}{\beta^I I_0(\beta^I)}; \qquad Q^E = \frac{K_1(\beta^E)}{\beta^E K_0(\beta^E)}; \qquad \beta^I = e^{\imath \pi/4}\sqrt{St^I}; \qquad \beta^E = e^{\imath \pi/4}\sqrt{St^E}$$

where I_n and K_n are the modified Bessel functions of the nth kind.

2.2 Membrane analysis

The normalized tensions, T_θ and T_z, are related to the fluid pressure and wall shear stress from inside and outside the OHC:

$$T_\theta = (P_0{}^I - P_0{}^E); \qquad \frac{dT_z}{dz} = -\frac{1}{\epsilon}\left(\tau^I + \tau^E \right) \tag{2}$$

The membrane undergoes strains given by $e_\theta = \delta_r$ and $e_z = d\delta_z/dz$ which are related to the membrane tensions by a viscoelastic model[9]:

$$\begin{bmatrix} \Delta_r \\ \dfrac{d\Delta_z}{dz} \end{bmatrix} = \frac{\mathcal{T}}{\mathcal{D}} \begin{bmatrix} \mathcal{A} & -\mathcal{B} \\ -\mathcal{B} & \mathcal{A} \end{bmatrix} \begin{bmatrix} T_\theta \\ T_z \end{bmatrix} \tag{3}$$

where $\mathcal{A} = K + \mu + \imath\omega(\kappa + \eta)$; $\mathcal{B} = K - \mu + \imath\omega(\kappa - \eta)$; $\mathcal{D} = 4(K + \imath\omega\kappa)(\mu + \imath\omega\eta)$; $\mathcal{T} = \tilde{\mu}\omega l_0$; K and μ are the elastic area and shear moduli respectively; κ and η are the wall area and shear viscosities respectively.

2.3 Solution

If $P_0 = P_0{}^I - P_0{}^E$ then eqs. (1) through (3) are combined to describe the fluid-membrane interaction problem:

$$\frac{d^2}{dz^2} \begin{bmatrix} T_z \\ P_0 \end{bmatrix} = M \begin{bmatrix} T_z \\ P_0 \end{bmatrix} \tag{4}$$

604

The boundary conditions at $z = 0$ and $z = 1$ are:

$$\left.\frac{dP_0}{dz}\right|_{z=0} = \left.\frac{dT_z}{dz}\right|_{z=0} = 0; \quad \left.\frac{dP_0}{dz}\right|_{z=1} = -\frac{i\gamma\beta^{I^2}\,\Delta_z|_{z=1}}{\epsilon}; \quad P_0|_{z=1} - 2\,T_z|_{z=1} = F \tag{5}$$

where $\gamma = 1 + \dfrac{\beta^{E^2}}{\beta^{I^2}}\dfrac{(2Q^E+1)}{(a^2-1-2Q^E)}$; $\Delta_z|_{z=1}$ is obtained from eq. (3); F is the normalized sinusoidal force applied at $z = 1$. If $\lambda_1{}^2$ and $\lambda_2{}^2$ are the eigenvalues of M and

$$R_{11} = \sinh\lambda_1 \left[\frac{\mathcal{T}i\beta^{I^2}\gamma(\mathcal{A}(M_{22}-\lambda_1{}^2)+\mathcal{B}M_{21})/\mathcal{D} - \epsilon M_{21}\lambda_1{}^2}{\lambda_1}\right]$$

$$R_{12} = \sinh\lambda_2 \left[\frac{\mathcal{T}i\beta^{I^2}\gamma(\mathcal{A}(M_{22}-\lambda_2{}^2)+\mathcal{B}M_{21})/\mathcal{D} - \epsilon M_{21}\lambda_2{}^2}{\lambda_2}\right]$$

$$R_{21} = 2\cosh\lambda_1\left(2(M_{22}-\lambda_1{}^2)+M_{21}\right)$$

$$R_{22} = 2\cosh\lambda_2\left(2(M_{22}-\lambda_2{}^2)+M_{21}\right)$$

then, with a pressure of n Nm^{-2} at $z = 1$, we obtain the dimensional OHC displacement, $\delta_z{}^* = l_0\delta_z$:

$$\left.\delta_z{}^*\right|_{z^*=l_0} = \frac{2nr_0{}^2 M_{21}\sinh\lambda_1\sinh\lambda_2(\lambda_1{}^2-\lambda_2{}^2)(\mathcal{A}M_{22}+\mathcal{B}M_{21})}{\mathcal{D}\lambda_1\lambda_2\det(R)} \tag{6}$$

3   Results

In our simulations, $r_0 = 5\mu$m which is a typical OHC radius; $\mu = 0.007$ Nm^{-1} and $K = 0.07$ Nm^{-1} are the OHC elastic moduli[2]; $\tilde{\mu}^E = 10^{-3}$ kgm^{-1}s^{-1} and $\rho^E = 10^3$ kgm^{-3} by assuming that the external fluid is similar to water; $\tilde{\mu} = 3\tilde{\mu}^E$ and $\rho^I = 1.06\rho^E$ by assuming that the cytoplasm is more viscous and denser than the surrounding fluid. Figure 1 shows the displacement of the OHC for lengths in the range $20-80\mu$m for a purely elastic wall; the OHC response is similar to the simulations of Tolomeo[7] in which the mechanical stimulus was applied uniformly on the lateral wall. The flat low frequency asymptote is numerically equal to the static displacement value of $2nr_0l_0/(9\mu+K)$. Figure 2a shows the effect of wall shear viscosity on the displacement of a 60μm long OHC for values of $\eta = 0, 10^{-8}, 10^{-7}$ and 10^{-6} Nsm^{-1}. Evidently as η increases, the OHC peak displacement becomes diminished leading to a band pass filter behavior. Figure 2b shows the effect of η on the mechanical impedance, $Z = n\pi r_0{}^2/(i\omega\delta_z{}^*|_{z^*=l_0})$, for a 60μm long OHC. The high frequency asymptote for $\eta = 0$ behaves like $\omega^{-1/4}$.

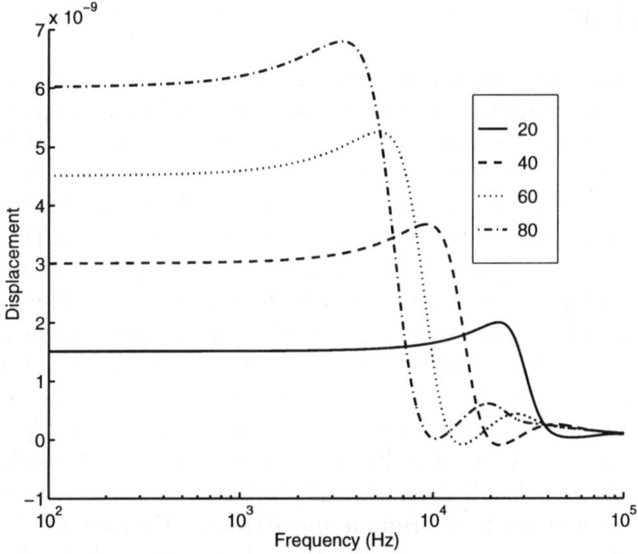

Figure 1: Displacement against frequency of applied pressure of magnitude 1 Nm^{-2} for purely elastic OHCs of length between 20μm (bottom) and 100μm (top).

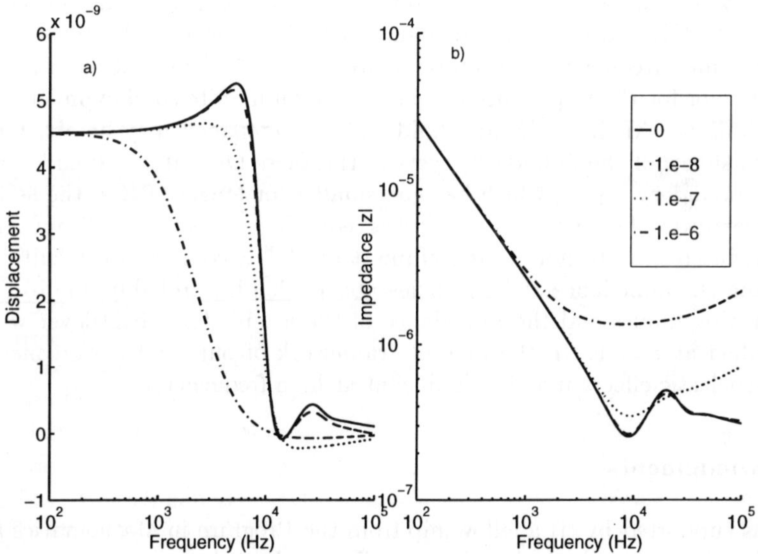

Figure 2: Effect of wall viscosity with $\eta = 0, 10^{-8}, 10^{-7}, 10^{-6}$ Nsm^{-1} on a) displacement and b) mechanical impedance for OHC of length 60μm.

4 Discussion

A model of the OHC viscoelastic wall has been developed to determine the nature of viscous damping in OHC motility. Results for a purely elastic wall suggest that when a mechanical stimulus is applied at one end of the OHC, a peak displacement is attained at a length-dependent frequency location. This location can be influenced by the choice of the membrane model. For example, a reduction in K and μ leads to a corresponding reduction in the break frequency location, which may explain why the break frequency data is an order of magnitude larger than that reported by Hemmert at $al.$ [8] The highly organized structure of the OHC wall[5] suggests that the analysis may be improved if the isotropic model in eq. (3) is replaced by an orthotropic model. Results for a viscoelastic wall indicate that the peak displacement at the break frequency decreases with increasing wall shear viscosity resulting in a band pass filter for $\eta = 10^{-7}$ Nsm^{-1} which incidentally is an order of magnitude smaller than the value of red blood cell wall shear viscosity[9]. But if the OHC is to be mechanically tuned as suggested by Brundin and Russell[6], then the OHC wall shear viscosity has to be significantly smaller than that for the red blood cell (RBC). This suggests that the characteristic time, $t_c = \eta/\mu$, for the OHC is less than 10^{-4}s in contrast with 0.1s for the RBC[9]. Such a low value of t_c would allow the OHC wall to deform rapidly at acoustic frequencies. Also, η affects the behavior of the OHC mechanical impedance at high frequencies. However, when $\eta = 0$ the high frequency asymptote behaves like $\omega^{-1/4}$ in contrast with the $\omega^{1/2}$ behavior for the impedance on the wall of an infinite solid cylinder oscillating along its axis in an infinite fluid. This discrepancy may be attributed to the existence of the boundary layers of thickness $O(\epsilon)$ at $z = 0$ and $z = 1$; in these boundary layers, which become smaller for longer OHCs, the second order streamwise derivatives in the Stokes' equations become significant. It is, however, interesting to note that Hemmert at $al.$ [8] encountered difficulties in measuring the impedance at frequencies above 5000 Hz probably due to both the vibration modes and the impedance of the atomic force cantilever which was applied at $z = 1$. In the present framework of our model, we conclude that viscoelastic effects may be significant at high frequencies.

Acknowledgments

JTR was supported by (i) a fellowship from the Program in Mathematics and Molecular Biology at the University of California Berkeley, which is supported by the NSF under Grant No. DMS-9406348 (ii) DRF. NIDCD DC-00354 and DC-02775 research grants are also acknowledged.

References

1. W. E. Brownell. (1990) Outer hair cell electromotility and otoacoustic emissions. *Ear and Hearing* **11** 82–92.
2. K. H. Iwasa and R. S. Chadwick. (1993) Elasticity and active force generation of cochlear outer hair cells. *J. Acoust. Soc. Am.* **92** 3169–3173.
3. J. T Ratnanather, M. Zhi, W. E. Brownell, and A. S. Popel. (1996) The ratio of elastic moduli of cochlear outer hair cells derived from osmotic experiments. *J. Acoust. Soc. Am.* **99** 1025–1028.
4. A. A. Spector, W. E. Brownell, and A. S. Popel. (1996) A model for cochlear outer hair cell deformations in micropipette aspiration experiments: an analytical solution. *Annals Biomed. Engng.* **24** 241–249.
5. J. A. Tolomeo and C. R. Steele. (1995) Orthotropic piezoelectric properties of the cochlear outer hair cell wall. *J. Acoust. Soc. Am.* **97** 3006–3011.
6. L. Brundin and I. J. Russell. (1994) Tuned phasic and tonic motile responses of isolated outer hair cells to direct mechanical stimulation of the cell body. *Hearing Research* **73** 35–45.
7. J. A. Tolomeo. (1996) *Models of the structure and motility of the auditory outer hair cell.* PhD thesis, Stanford University.
8. W. Hemmert, C. Schauz, H-P. Zenner, and A. W Gummer. (1996) Force generation and mechanical impedance of outer hair cells. In *Diversity in Auditory Mechanics*, ed. E. R. Lewis (World Scientific, Singapore).
9. E. A. Evans and R. Skalak. (1980) *Mechanics and Thermodynamics of Biomembranes.* CRC Press, Boca Raton, FL.
10. D. H. Jen and C. R. Steele. (1987) Electrokinetic model of cochlear outer hair cell motility. *J. Acoust. Soc. Am.* **82** 1667–1678.
11. J. Kevorkian and J. D. Cole. (1981) *Perturbation Methods in Applied Mathematics.* Springer-Verlag, NY.

AN ELASTIC COMPOSITE MODEL OF THE OUTER HAIR CELL WALL

A.A. SPECTOR

*Department of Biomedical Engineering, The Johns Hopkins University School
of Medicine, 720 Rutland Avenue, Baltimore, MD 21205, USA
aspector@bme.jhu.edu*

W.E. BROWNELL

*Department of Otorhinolaryngology and Communicative Sciences,
Baylor College of Medicine, One Baylor Plaza, Houston, TX 77030, USA
brownell@bcm.tmc.edu*

A.S. POPEL

*Department of Biomedical Engineering, The Johns Hopkins University School
of Medicine, 720 Rutland Avenue, Baltimore, MD 21205, USA
apopel@bme.jhu.edu*

A model of elastic behavior of the outer hair cell (OHC) located in the inner ear is
proposed. The cell lateral wall is treated as a cylindrical composite shell consisting
of two layers connected by elastic liaisons. Such a model reflects the OHC wall
microstructure. The outer layer is isotropic; the inner layer is a composite made
of two sublayers, isotropic and orthotropic, bonded to each other. The general
Flügge-type equations for the OHC wall are derived. The model is applied to the
analysis of two experiments with axial and torsion modes of OHC loading.

1 Introduction

We consider the elastic properties of the wall (composite membrane) of the
OHC. The unique ability of the OHC to change its length in response to
changes of the transmembrane potential[1] provides additional energy for vibration of the surrounding elements of the inner ear. These properties of the
OHC are believed to be crucial for the sharp frequency selectivity of the ear.
The magnitude of the forces exerted by OHC on the surrounding elements
directly depends on the elastic properties of the cell wall. The OHC is an
elongated cylinder with a pressurized liquid inside. The OHC wall consists
of three distinct approximately cylindrical elements: the innermost subsurface
cisternae, the outermost plasma membrane, and the intermediate cortical lattice adjacent to the subsurface cisternae. The composite layer consisting of the
two adjacent elements is attached to the plasma membrane by radial elastic
pillars. The elastic pillars are located within the extracisternal space which
is filled with the same liquid that is in the core bounded by the subsurface

cisternae. The outermost and innermost layers can be considered isotropic. The cortical lattice is comprised of two networks (actin filaments and spectrin crosslinks) with different elastic properties. The angles between the filaments and the circumferential direction are distributed along the wall surface with the mean value about $10^o - 15^o$.[2,3] Iwasa and Chadwick[4], Ratnanather *et al.*[5] treated the OHC wall as a single isotropic elastic membrane and determined its characteristics. Steele[6] suggested a model of the wall as a composite membrane. Steele *et al.*[7] and Tolomeo and Steele[8] also proposed a single piezoelectric membrane model with separate mechanical and electrical terms. They treated the mechanical properties of the membrane as elastic orthotropic and estimated the corresponding Young's moduli and Poisson's ratios. Spector *et al.*[9] proposed a single-layer shell model for the OHC wall, demonstrated the relatively high value of bending modulus and the importance of bending effects. In the present paper, we develop a composite shell model for the cell wall that includes its basic microstructural components.

2 General equations

We derive Flügge-type equations[10] for the composite wall of OHC. We choose a cylindrical coordinate system $x\theta r$ where the surface $r = 0$ is located in the middle between the external and internal surfaces of the wall (Fig. 1). We treat the plasma membrane as an isotropic shell layer 1 and characterize it by deformations $\bar{\epsilon}^1(\epsilon_x^1, \epsilon_\theta^1, \epsilon_{x\theta}^1)$, curvatures/twist $\bar{k}^1(k_x^1, k_\theta^1, k_{x\theta}^1)$, and displacements (u^1, v^1, w^1). We consider the subsurface cisternae as another isotropic layer and treat the cortical lattice

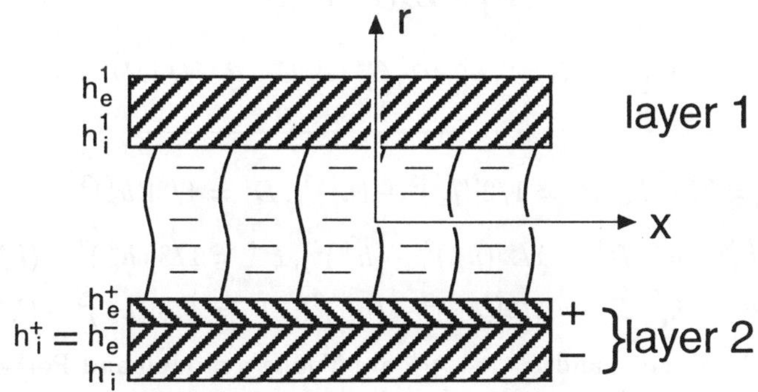

Figure 1: Illustration of the proposed model

as a homogeneous orthotropic layer with the local axes of orthotropy inclined at angle κ with respect to the natural axes of the cell. This angle can be interpreted as an average angle of the fiber directions. We treat the combination of the two adjacent components as a composite shell layer 2 with characteristics $\bar{\epsilon}^2(\epsilon_x^2, \epsilon_\theta^2, \epsilon_{x\theta}^2)$, $\bar{k}^2(k_x^2, k_\theta^2, k_{x\theta}^2)$, and (u^2, v^2, w^2) of the neutral surface. We use indices $+$ and $-$ to specify the elastic and geometrical characteristics of the cortical lattice and the subsurface cisternae, respectively. We assume that the liaisons connecting the layers 1 and 2 behave like linear elastic springs with respect to the radial direction $(u^1 = u^2, v^1 = v^2)$. By using Flügge's approximations[10], we can express the vector of the membrane forces $\overline{N}^1(N_x^1, N_\theta^1, N_{x\theta}^1, N_{\theta x}^1)$, $\overline{N}^2(N_x^2, N_\theta^2, \dot{N}_{x\theta}^2, N_{\theta x}^2)$ and bending/twisting moments $\overline{M}^1(M_x^1, M_\theta^1, M_{x\theta}^1, M_{\theta x}^1)$, $\overline{M}^2(M_x^2, M_\theta^2, M_{x\theta}^2, M_{\theta x}^2)$ in the following form

$$\overline{N}^1 = [\mathbf{E_1^1}]\bar{\epsilon}^1 + [\mathbf{E_2^1}]\bar{k}^1, \overline{M}^1 = -[\mathbf{E_3^1}]\bar{\epsilon}^1 - [\mathbf{E_4^1}]\bar{k}^1 \tag{1}$$

$$\overline{N}^2 = [\mathbf{E_1^2}]\bar{\epsilon}^2 + [\mathbf{E_2^2}]\bar{k}^2, \overline{M}^2 = -[\mathbf{E_3^2}]\bar{\epsilon}^2 - [\mathbf{E_4^2}]\bar{k}^2 \tag{2}$$

The strains $\bar{\epsilon}^1$, $\bar{\epsilon}^2$ and curvatures $\bar{k}^1, \bar{k}^2$ are determined by the displacements and their derivatives[10,11], and $[\mathbf{E_j^i}]$ $i = 1, 2; j = 1, .., 4$ are 4×3 matrices which have the following form for $j = 1, 2, 3$[12]

$$\mathbf{E_j^1} = \mathbf{E_j^1}(E^1, \nu^1, A^1, B^1, D^1) \tag{3}$$

$$\mathbf{E_j^2} = \mathbf{E_j^2}(E^+, e^+, \nu^+, G^+, \kappa, E^-, \nu^-, A^+, B^+, D^+, A^-, B^-, D^-) \tag{4}$$

For $j = 4$, the matrices are expressed by the equations[12]

$$\mathbf{E_4^1} = \mathbf{E_4^1}(E^1, \nu^1, D^1) \tag{5}$$

$$\mathbf{E_4^2} = \mathbf{E_4^2}(E^+, e^+, \nu^+, G^+, \kappa, E^-, \nu^-, D^+, D^-) \tag{6}$$

where

$$A^1 = h_e^1 - h_i^1, B^1 = 1/2[(h_e^1)^2 - (h_i^1)^2], D^1 = 1/3[(h_e^1)^3 - (h_i^1)^3] \tag{7}$$

$$A^+ = h_e^+ - h_i^-, B^+ = 1/2[(h_e^+)^2 - (h_i^+)^2], D^+ = 1/3[(h_e^+)^3 - (h_i^+)^3] \tag{8}$$

$$A^- = h_e^- - h_i^-, B^- = 1/2[(h_e^-)^2 - (h_i^-)^2], D^- = 1/3[(h_e^-)^3 - (h_i^-)^3] \tag{9}$$

Here E^1, ν^1; E^-, ν^-, and E^+, e^+, ν^+ are Young's moduli and Poisson's ratios of the plasma membrane, the subsurface cisternae, and the cortical lattice, respectively, G^+ is independent shear modulus of the cortical lattice (layer $+$).

We assume that the fluids located outside and inside the cell and within the extracisternal space create pressures p^e, p^i, and p and tangential stresses

$\bar{\tau}^e$, $\bar{\tau}^i$, $\bar{\tau}$, respectively, which act on the corresponding elements of the wall. The components of the displacements u^1, v^1, w^1 and w^2 satisfy the following equations

$$\frac{\partial(N_x^1 + N_x^2)}{\partial x} + \frac{\partial(N_{\theta x}^1 + N_{\theta x}^2)}{a\partial\theta} + \tau_x^e + \tau_x^i + 2\tau_x = 0 \qquad (10)$$

$$\frac{\partial(N_\theta^1 + N_\theta^2)}{a\partial\theta} + \frac{\partial(N_{x\theta}^1 + N_{x\theta}^2)}{\partial x} - \frac{\partial(M_\theta^1 + M_\theta^2)}{a^2\partial\theta} - \frac{\partial(M_{x\theta}^1 + M_{x\theta}^2)}{a\partial x} + \tau = 0 \qquad (11)$$

$$\frac{\partial^2 M_\theta^1}{a^2\partial\theta^2} + \frac{\partial^2(M_{x\theta}^1 + M_{\theta x}^1)}{a\partial x\partial\theta} + \frac{\partial^2 M_x^1}{\partial x^2} + \frac{N_\theta^1}{a} - k\frac{(w^1 - w^2)}{a} + p - p^e = 0 \qquad (12)$$

$$\frac{\partial^2 M_\theta^2}{a^2\partial\theta^2} + \frac{\partial^2(M_{x\theta}^2 + M_{\theta x}^2)}{a\partial x\partial\theta} + \frac{\partial^2 M_x^2}{\partial x^2} + \frac{N_\theta^2}{a} + k\frac{(w^1 - w^2)}{a} + p^i - p = 0 \qquad (13)$$

Here a is the radius of the middle surface of the wall, k is a characteristic of the stiffness of the liaisons (pillars), and $\tau = \tau_\theta^e + \tau_\theta^i + 2\tau_\theta$. Note that to find two different radial components of the displacements of layers 1 and 2, we use two separate equations (12) and (13).

3   Application to the Interpretation of the Experiments

3.1   Axial loading[2,13]

We apply our model to the analysis of the measurement of the axial stiffness of OHC. In this experiment, one end of the cell is fixed, the other end is under the action of an axial force , and the axial displacement u_o is measured (Fig. 2).

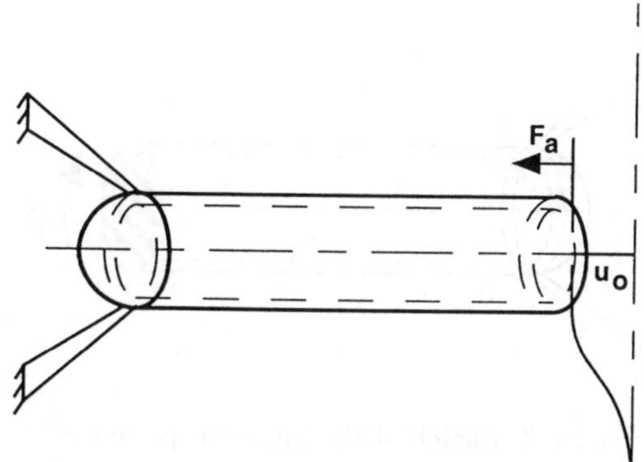

Figure 2: Sketch of the axial stiffness measurement

We assume that the stress-strain state of the wall is axisymmetric, and the fluid inside is incompressible. We also neglect any inertial effects in the fluids and in the wall. Under such approximation, pressures p_i and p inside the intracellular space and the extracisternal space are equal and constant throughout the whole volume. A purely membrane homogeneous stress-strain state satisfies all the conditions except the fixed end conditions. It can be shown[12] that a boundary layer solution which is valid in a narrow zone adjacent to the fixed end can be considered as a correction of the homogeneous solution, and this correction has a small effect on the homogeneous solution. Solving the problem and determining the components of the displacements and the pressure change caused by the application of the axial force, we finally obtain an expression for the axial stiffness of the cell

$$K_a = \frac{\pi a}{L}\left\{\frac{4(E_{11}^1 + E_{11}^2) - 4E_{12}^1 + E_{11}^1 + ka}{4} - \right.$$

$$\frac{(E_{33}^1 + E_{33}^2)(2E_{12}^2 + ka)^2 + 4ka E_{13}^2(E_{13}^2 - E_{23}^2)}{4[(E_{33}^1 + E_{33}^2)(E_{22}^2 + ka) - (E_{23}^2)^2]} -$$

$$\left. \frac{E_{13}^2(E_{13}^2 E_{22}^2 - E_{23}^2 E_{12}^2)}{(E_{33}^1 + E_{33}^2)(E_{22}^2 + ka) - (E_{23}^2)^2}\right\} \tag{14}$$

where $2L$ is the length of the cell.

3.2 Torsion

We consider also a conceivable experiment with torsion of OHC when one end is fixed and the other is rotated by an applied torque (Fig. 3). The unfixed end is prevented from any radial and axial displacement.

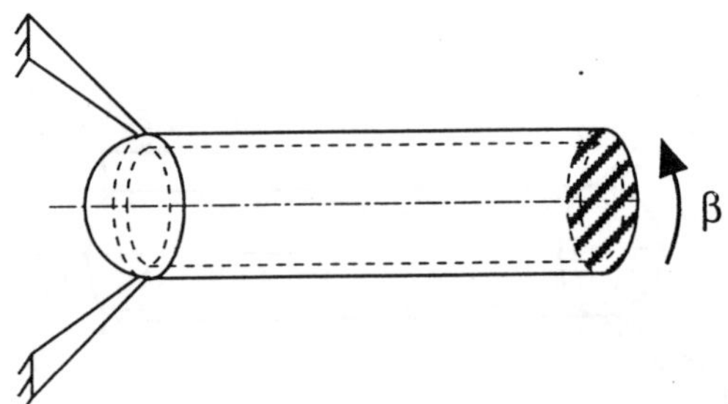

Figure 3: Sketch of the torsion experiment

In this case, the corresponding stress-strain state is purely homogeneous. Because of this, there are no radial and axial components of the displacement, and stresses and strains are determined by the angular component. The relationship between the applied torque M, the axial reaction F and the angle of torsion β is expressed by the following equations

$$M = \frac{\pi\beta a^3}{L}(E^1_{33} + E^2_{33}) \tag{15}$$

$$F = \frac{\pi\beta a^2}{L}E^2_{13} \tag{16}$$

Assuming angle κ small and keeping the leading terms in the asymptotic expansions of M and F, we obtain the expressions for the torque and the axial reaction in terms of Young's moduli, Poisson's ratios, and shear modulus of the wall components

$$M = \frac{\pi\beta a^3}{L}[\frac{E^1 A^1}{2(1+\nu^+)} + \frac{E^- A^-}{2(1+\nu^-)} + G^+ A^+] \tag{17}$$

$$F = \frac{2\pi\beta a^2 A^+}{L}[\frac{(1-\nu^+)e^+}{1-\alpha^+(\nu^+)^2} - 2G^+]\kappa \tag{18}$$

where $\alpha^+ = e^+/E^+$.

4 Discussion

The composite anisotropic wall model exhibits some qualitative effects of the wall behavior. One of them is torsion of the cell under the action of the axial force. The angle ψ of torsion can be expressed by the following formula

$$\psi = \frac{2L}{a}\frac{\partial v^1}{\partial x} = \frac{F_a}{aK_a}\frac{2E^2_{13}E^2_{22} - 2E^2_{23}E^2_{13} + ka(2E^2_{13} - E^2_{23})}{2(E^1_{33} + E^2_{33})(E^2_{22} + ka) - 2(E^2_{23})^2} \tag{19}$$

The angle of torsion is approximately proportional to the angle of the orthotropy axes inclination. Another effect is related to the different radial displacements of the wall components (w^1 and w^2). The direct measurement of these effects can provide additional information on the elastic properties of cell elements. The axial stiffness is important for characterization of the OHC behavior *in vivo*. The first two terms in (14) are determined by the longitudinal and circumferential rigidities of the wall and also by the stiffness of the pillars. The last term is determined by the inclination of the directions of the filaments. If we neglect this inclination and the compliance of the pillars, we obtain the axial stiffness corresponding to the Tolomeo and Steele model. The experiment with torsion of the OHC has an advantage of the straightforward interpretation because only the angular component of the displacements is involved. As a result, this experiment can provide two additional equations for the determination of the elastic constants of the OHC elements.

References

1. W.E. Brownell, C.R. Bader, D. Bertrand, and Y. de Ribaupierre. (1985) Evoked Mechanical Responses of Isolated Cochlear Outer Hair Cells, *Science* **227** 194-196.
2. M.C. Holley and J.F. Ashmore. (1988) A Cytoskeletal Spring in Cochlear Outer Hair Cell, *Nature* **335** 635-637.
3. M.C. Holley, F. Kalinec, and B. Kachar. (1992) Structure of the Cortical Cytoskeleton in Mammalian Outer Hair Cells, *J. Cell Science* **102** 569-580.
4. K.H. Iwasa and R.S. Chadwick. (1992) Elasticity and Active Force Generation of Cochlear Outer Hair Cells, *J. Acoust. Soc. Am.* **92** 3169-3173.
5. J.T. Ratnanather, M. Zhi, W.E. Brownell, and A.S. Popel. (1995) The Ratio of Elastic Moduli of Cochlear Outer Hair Cells Derived from Osmotic Experiments *J. Acoust. Soc. Am.* **99** 1025-1028.
6. C.R. Steele. (1990) Elastic Behavior of the Outer Hair Cell Wall. In: *The Mechanics and Biophysics of Hearing*, eds. P. Dallos, C.D. Geisler, J.W. Matthews, M.A. Ruggero, C.R. Steele (Springer-Verlag, Berlin) 121-130.
7. C.R. Steele, G. Baker, J. Tolomeo, and D. Zetes. (1993) Electro-Mechanical Models of the Outer Hair Cell Sensory Systems. In: *Biophysics of Hair Cell Sensory Systems*, eds. H. Duifhuis, J.H. Horst, P. van Dijk, S.M. van Netten (World Scientific) 207-214.
8. J.A. Tolomeo and C.R. Steele, Orthotropic Piezoelectric Properties of the Cochlear Hair Cell Wall. (1995) *J. Acoust Soc. Am.* **97** 3006-3011.
9. A.A. Spector, W.E. Brownell, and A.S. Popel. (1996) A Model for Cochlear Outer Hair Cell Deformations in Micropipette Aspiration Experiment: An Analytical Solution, *Ann. Biomed. Engin.* **24** 241-249.
10. W. Flügge. (1960) *Stresses in Shells*, Springer-Verlag, Berlin.
11. V.V. Novozhilov. (1959) *The Theory of Thin Shells*, Noordhoff, Groningen.
12. A.A. Spector, W.E. Brownell, and A.S. Popel. (1996) A Model of Elastic Properties of Cell Membrane. In: *The Eriksen Symposium on Recent Developments in Elasticity*, eds. R.C. Batra and M.F. Beatty, International Center for Numerical Methods in Engineering, Barcelona, Spain (in press).
13. R. Hallworth. (1995) Passive Compliance and Active Force Generation in the Guinea Pig Outer Hair Cell, *J. Neurophysiology* **74** 2319-2328.

AUTHOR INDEX